The Anterior Cruciate Ligament
Current and Future Concepts

The Anterior Cruciate Ligament
Current and Future Concepts

Editor

Douglas W. Jackson, MD
Director
Southern California Center for Sports Medicine
Long Beach, California

Associate Editors

Steven P. Arnoczky, DVM
Wade O. Brinker Endowed Professor of Surgery
Director
Laboratory of Comparative Orthopaedic Research
College of Veterinary Medicine
Michigan State University
East Lansing, Michigan

Savio L-Y. Woo, PhD
Professor
Orthopaedic Surgery and Mechanical Engineering
Vice Chairman for Research
University of Pittsburgh School of Medicine
Pittsburgh, Pennsylvania

Cyril B. Frank, MD
Professor
McCaig Centre for Joint Injury and Arthritis Research
Department of Surgery
The University of Calgary
Calgary, Alberta
Canada

Timothy M. Simon, MS
Director of Research
Southern California Center for Sports Medicine
Long Beach, California

Raven Press ✆ *New York*

Raven Press, Ltd., 1185 Avenue of the Americas, New York, New York 10036

Made in the United States of America

Library of Congress Cataloging-in-Publication Data

The Anterior cruciate ligament: current and future concepts/editor-in-chief,
    Douglas W. Jackson; section leaders, Steven P. Arnoczky . . . [et al.].
       p. cm.
     Includes bibliographical references and index.
     ISBN 0-7817-0039-6
      1. Anterior cruciate ligament—Surgery. 2. Anterior cruciate ligament.
      [DNLM: 1. Anterior Cruciate Ligament. 2. Jackson, Douglas W.
    3. Arnoczky, Steven P.   We 870 A6273 1993]
    RD561.A59   1993
    617.5'82—dc20
    DNLM/DLC
    for Library of Congress   93-18586
                                                          CIP

9 8 7 6 5 4 3 2 1

Contents

SECTION III: INJURY, HEALING, REPAIR, AND RECONSTRUCTION
Section Editor: *Cyril B. Frank*

SECTION IV: ACL RECONSTRUCTION AND SUBSTITUTES (BIOLOGIC)
Section Editor: *Douglas W. Jackson*

Contributing Authors

Wayne H. Akeson, MD
Professor/Chairman
Department of Orthopaedics
School of Medicine
University of California, San Diego
9500 Gilman Drive, 0630
La Jolla, California 92093

David Amiel, PhD
Director, Connective Tissue Biochemistry
Professor of Orthopaedic Surgery
School of Medicine
University of California, San Diego
9500 Gilman Drive 0630
La Jolla, California 92093

Thomas P. Andriacchi, PhD
Professor
Department of Orthopaedic Surgery
Rush Presbyterian/St. Lukes Medical Center
1653 W. Congress Parkway
Chicago, Illinois 60612

Steven P. Arnoczky, DVM
Wade O. Brinker Endowed Professor of
* Surgery*
Director, Laboratory for Comparative
* Orthopaedic Research*
College of Veterinary Medicine
Michigan State University
East Lansing, Michigan 48824

Geethani Bandara, PhD
Research Associate
Ferguson Laboratory
Department of Orthopaedic Surgery
University of Pittsburgh School of Medicine
986 Scaife Hall
Pittsburgh, Pennsylvania 15261

Bruce D. Beynnon, PhD
Research Assistant Professor
McClure Musculoskeletal Research Center
Department of Orthopaedics
University of Vermont Medical School
C-444 Given Building
Burlington, Vermont 05402

Gail Blomstrom, PhD
Research Associate
Musculoskeletal Research Center
Department of Orthopaedic Surgery
University of Pittsburgh
Pittsburgh, Pennsylvania 15261

Richard A. Brand, MD
Professor
Department of Orthopaedic Surgery
University of Iowa Hospital
Iowa City, Iowa 52242

Joseph A. Buckwalter, MD
Professor
Department of Orthopaedic Surgery
University of Iowa Hospital and Clinics
Iowa City, Iowa 52242

Arnold I. Caplan, PhD
Professor
Department of Biology
Case Western Reserve
Cleveland, Ohio 44106

Pascal S. Christel, MD, PhD
Orthopaedic Research Laboratory and
* Orthopaedic Surgery Department*
Lariboisiere Saint-Louis Medical School
University of Paris
9 Square Clignan Court
75018 Paris, France

Kelly J. Cole, PhD
Assistant Professor
Department of Exercise Physiology
University of Iowa
Iowa City, Iowa 52242

Dale M. Daniel, MD
Staff Orthopaedic Surgeon
Kaiser Permanente, San Diego
Clinical Associate Professor
Department of Orthopaedic Surgery
University of California, San Diego
4647 Zion Avenue
La Jolla, California 92020

Lars Engbretsen, MD, PhD
Department of Orthopaedic Surgery
Trondheim University Hospital
Rosenborg Sportsklinik, A.S.
Postboks 4150
7002 Trondheim, Norway

Christopher H. Evans, PhD
Associate Professor
Ferguson Laboratory
Department of Orthopaedic Surgery
Department of Molecular Genetics and
*   Biochemistry*
University of Pittsburgh School of Medicine
986 Scaife Hall
Pittsburgh, Pennsylvania 15261

David J. Fink, PhD
President
Bio-Integration, Inc.
1445 Summit Street
Columbus, Ohio 43201

Braden C. Fleming, MS
McClure Musculoskeletal Research Center
Department of Orthopaedics
University of Vermont Medical School
C-444 Given Building
Burlington, Vermont 05402

Scott K. Forman, MD
Sports Medicine Fellow
Southern California Center for Sports
*   Medicine*
Long Beach Memorial Medical Center
2760 Atlantic Avenue
Long Beach, California 90806

Peter J. Fowler, MD, FRCS(C)
Professor
Orthopaedic Surgery
Head, Section of Sport Medicine
University of Western Ontario
Department of Orthopaedics
University Hospital
339 Windmere Road
London, Ontario N6A 5A5
Canada

Cyril B. Frank, MD
Professor
McCaig Centre for Joint Injury and Arthritis
*   Research*
The University of Calgary
Department of Surgery
3330 Hospital Drive NW
Calgary, AB T2N 4N1
Canada

Marc J. Friedman, MD
Southern California Orthopaedic Institute
15211 Vanowen Street, #300
Van Nuys, California 91405
and
Assistant Clinical Professor
University of California, Los Angeles
Los Angeles, California 90024

Anthony D. Frogameni, MD
Sports Medicine Fellow
Southern California Center for Sports
*   Medicine*
Long Beach Memorial Medical Center
2760 Atlantic Avenue
Long Beach, California 90806

Freddie H. Fu, MD
Professor
Department of Orthopaedics
University of Pittsburgh School of Medicine
3471 Fifth Avenue, Suite 1010
Pittsburgh, Pennsylvania 15213

Helga I. Georgescu, BS
Research Specialist
Ferguson Laboratory
Department of Orthopaedic Surgery
University of Pittsburgh School of Medicine
3471 Fifth Avenue
Pittsburgh, Pennsylvania 15213

Donald F. Gibbons, DSc, PhD
3M Biosciences Lab
3M Center
Building 270-2A-08
St. Paul, Minnesota 55144

Joseph C. Glorioso, PhD
Department of Molecular Genetics and
*   Biochemistry*
University of Pittsburgh School of Medicine
3471 Fifth Avenue
Pittsburgh, Pennsylvania 15213

Victor M. Goldberg, MD
Professor
Department of Orthopaedic Surgery
Case Western Reserve
University School of Medicine
Cleveland, Ohio 44106

Mark A. Gomez, PhD
Assistant Professor
University of Colorado Health Sciences
*   Center*
Department of Orthop B202
4200 E. 9th Avenue
Denver, Colorado 80262

Tatsuhiko Goto, MD
Department of Orthopaedic Surgery
National Defense Medical College
3-2 Namiki, Tokorozawa 354
Japan

Ben K. Graf, MD
Assistant Professor
Division of Orthopaedic Surgery
University of Wisconsin
600 Higland Avenue
Madison, Wisconsin 53792

Edward S. Grood, PhD
Professor and Director
University of Cincinnati
Noyes-Giannestras Biomechanics Lab
2900 Reading Road CSB
Cincinnati, Ohio 45221

Christopher D. Harner, MD
Assistant Professor
Department of Orthopaedics
University of Pittsburgh School of Medicine
3471 Fifth Avenue, Suite 1010
Pittsburgh, Pennsylvania 15213

David A. Hart, PhD
Professor
University of Calgary Health Science Center
McCaig Center for Joint Injury and Arthritis
  Research
Department of Microbiology and Infectious
  Diseases
3330 Hospital Drive NW
Calgary, AB T2N 4N1, Alberta
Canada

Roger C. Haut, PhD
Professor
Department of Biomechanics
Michigan State University
East Lansing, Michigan 48824

Stephen E. Haynesworth, PhD
Professor
Skeletal Research Center
Department of Biology
Case Western Reserve University
Cleveland, Ohio 44106

Mohamed Samir Hefzy, PhD, PE
Professor and Co-Director
Biomechanics Laboratories
Department of Mechanical Engineering
University of Toledo, Toledo, Ohio 43606
and
Adjunct Associate Professor
Department of Orthopaedic Surgery
Medical College of Ohio
Toledo, Ohio 43699-0008

J. Marcus Hollis, PhD
Assistant Professor
Department of Orthopaedic Surgery
University of Arkansas for Medical Sciences
4301 W. Markham, MS 531
Little Rock, Arkansas 72205

James J. Irrgang, MS
Sports Medicine Institute
University of Pittsburgh Medical Center
Pittsburgh, Pennsylvania 15213

Douglas W. Jackson, MD
Director
Southern California Center for Sports
  Medicine
2760 Atlantic Avenue
Long Beach, California 90806

James Jamison, MD
Department of Orthopaedics
University of Pittsburgh School of Medicine
3471 Fifth Avenue, Suite 1010
Pittsburgh, Pennsylvania 15213

Robert J. Johnson, MD
Professor and Head of Sports Medicine
  Section
McClure Musculoskeletal Research Center
Department of Orthopaedics
University of Vermont Medical School
C-444 Given Building
Burlington, Vermont 05402

Kenton R. Kaufman, PhD
Director of Orthopedic Research
Motion Analysis Laboratory
Children's Hospital, San Diego
and
Assistant Adjunct Professor
University of California, San Diego
4647 Zion Avenue
San Diego, California 92020

Mark J. Lemos, MD
Sports Medicine Fellow
Southern California Center for Sports
* Medicine*
Long Beach Memorial Medical Center
Long Beach, California 90806

William D. Lew, MS
Research Fellow
Department of Orthopaedic Surgery
University of Minnesota
Minneapolis, Minnesota 55455

Jack L. Lewis, PhD
Professor
Department of Orthopaedic Surgery
University of Minnesota
Minneapolis, Minnesota 55455

Anne E. Linton, MD
Department of Emergency Medicine
MetroHealth Medical Center
2500 MetroHealth Drive
Cleveland, Ohio 44109–1998

Steven M. Madey, MD
Department of Orthopaedic Surgery
University of Iowa
Iowa City, Iowa 52242

Jose Marcelino, BS
Graduate Student
Cleveland State University, and Cleveland
* Clinic Foundation*
Section of Musculoskeletal Biology
Department of Biomedical Engineering
The Cleveland Clinic Foundation Research
* Institute*
Cleveland, Ohio 44106

Keith L. Markolf, PhD
Adjunct Professor
Division of Orthopaedic Surgery
University of California, Los Angeles
21-67 UCLA Rehab Center
1000 Veterans Avenue
Los Angeles, California 90024

John Robert Matyas, PhD
Post-Doctoral Fellow
University of Calgary
Department of Medicine
3330 Hospital Drive, NW
Calgary, Alberta T2N OW6
Canada

Donal M. McCarthy, MD
Musculoskeletal Research Laboratories
Department of Orthopaedic Surgery
University of Pittsburgh
3471 Fifth Avenue, Suit 1010
Pittsburgh, Pennsylvania 15213

Cahir A. McDevitt, PhD
Staff Scientist
Section of Musculoskeletal Biology
Department Biomedical Engineering
Cleveland Clinic Foundation Research
* Institute*
9500 Euclid Avenue
Cleveland, Ohio 44106

Robert Meislin, MD
The Orthopaedic Specialty Hospital
5848 S 300 East
Salt Lake City, Utah 84107

Nicholas G. H. Mohtadi, MD, MSc,
* FRCS(C)*
Clinical Assistant Professor
University of Calgary
Sports Medicine Center
2500 University Drive, NW
Calgary, Alberta 22N 1N4
Canada

Gunhild M. Mueller, PhD
Department of Molecular Genetics and
* Biochemistry*
University of Pittsburgh School of Medicine
3471 Fifth Avenue
Pittsburgh, Pennsylvania 15213

Patricia G. Murphy, PhD
Post-Doctoral Fellow
Joint Injury and Arthritis Research Group
University of Calgary
Calgary, Alberta
Canada

Marcel Nimni, PhD
Professor
University of Southern California
Orthopaedic Hospital
D&T, Fifth Floor
2400 South Flower Street
Los Angeles, California 90007

Barry W. Oakes, MD
Department of Anatomy
Monash University
Two Reeve Center, Cheltenham
Melbourne, 3192
Australia

John J. O'Connor, BE, MA, PhD
Research Director
Oxford Orthopaedic Research Centre
University Lecturer in Engineering Science
Fellow of St. Peter's College
University of Oxford
Parks Road
Oxford OX1 3PJ
England

Lonnie E. Paulos, MD
The Orthopaedic Specialty Hospital
5848 S. 300 East
Salt Lake City, Utah 84107

Malcolm H. Pope, MD
Professor and Director
McClure Musculoskeletal Research Center
University of Vermont Medical School
C-444 Given Building
Burlington, Vermont 05402

Paul D. Robbins, PhD
Department of Molecular Genetics and
*   Biochemistry*
University of Pittsburgh School of Medicine
3471 Fifth Avenue
Pittsburgh, Pennsylvania 15213

Paul J. Schreck, MD
Department of Orthopaedics
University of California, San Diego
9500 Gilman Drive
La Jolla, California 92093

Les Schwendeman, MD
Musculoskeletal Research Laboratories
Department of Orthopaedic Surgery
University of Pittsburgh School of Medicine
3471 Fifth Avenue, Suite 1010
Pittsburgh, Pennsylvania 15213

Timothy M. Simon, MS
Director of Research
Southern California Center for Sports
*   Medicine*
2760 Atlantic Avenue
Long Beach, California 90806

Jeremy Stern, MD
The Orthopaedic Specialty Hospital
5848 S. 300 East
Salt Lake City, Utah 84107

Brad S. Tolin, MD
Southern California Orthopaedic Institute
15211 Vanowen Street, #300
Van Nuys, California 91405

Ray Vanderby, Jr., PhD
Division of Orthopaedic Surgery
University of Wisconsin
Madison, Wisconsin

Shigeyuki Wakitani, MD
Department of Environmental Medicine
Osaka University Hospital Medical School
2-2 Yamadaoke, Suita
Osaka 565 Japan

Monica Wiig, MD
Post-Doctoral Fellow
School of Medicine
University of California, San Diego
9500 Gilman Drive
La Jolla, California 92093

Savio L-Y. Woo, PhD
Professor
Department of Orthopaedic Surgery
Vice Chairman for Research
Musculoskeletal Research Center
University of Pittsburgh School of Medicine
3471 Fifth Avenue, Suite 1010
Pittsburgh, Pennsylvania 15213

Virgil L. Woods, Jr., MD
School of Medicine
University of California, San Diego
9500 Gilman Drive
La Jolla, California 92093

Randell G. Young, DVM
Skeletal Research Center
Department of Biology
Case Western Reserve University
Cleveland, Ohio 44106

Amy Zavatsky, BSE
Research Student
Department of Engineering Science
University of Oxford
Parks Road
Oxford OX1 3PJ
England

Preface

The anterior cruciate ligament is the most commonly ruptured ligament in the human knee. It has been estimated that annually one half million individuals in the United States sustain a clinically significant ACL injury. ACL injuries are seen in active and athletic individuals and are commonly described by the lay press and on the sports pages. Surgeons are inundated with information on the subject of the ACL, with a large number of sometimes contradictory and confusing surgical, clinical, and basic science articles, symposia, scientific reviews, and text books. In spite of all the data and literature to date, our understanding of the structure, function, and biology of the ACL is not to the point where this complicated ligament can be repaired or reconstructed to its pre-injury state.

This text is devoted to summarizing what is presently known about the anterior cruciate ligament. It reviews pertinent orthopaedic research and clinical observations from different disciplines. The scope of this review is related to the structure, function, and biology of injury and healing, reconstruction, and rehabilitation of the ACL. The authors include authorities from the fields of cellular biology, biochemistry, anatomy, veterinary surgery, biomechanics, bioengineering, and orthopaedic surgery. Each section is presented and referenced by investigators who are active in the field.

A planning group, consisting of Douglas Jackson, Steven Arnoczky, Savio Woo, Cyril Frank, and Tim Simon reviewed current ideas and data on the ACL in interdisciplinary discussions. The additional contributing authors were selected by the group on the basis of their current and past research excellence. The collective efforts and support of these authors made the organization, the editorial workshop, and final text possible in a timely manner.

Our specific aim was to:
1. Review and interpret the most current basic science and clinical understanding of the ACL.
2. Stimulate and promote clinicians and basic scientists to collaborate on specific areas dealing with repairing and reconstructing the ACL.
3. Identify and suggest directions for future work on the ACL.

The book is organized into six sections. The first section examines the structure of the ACL from gross to ultrastructural appearance and characteristics. The second section deals with the function of the normal ACL. This section includes discussions of the tensile, mechanical, and viscoelastic properties of the ACL; the loads that affect both the normal ACL and the grafts, methods of evaluating strain and ACL forces during activity, the ACL's interaction with muscle function, and the gait variations in the ACL deficient knee.

Sections three and four review our understanding of the cell and molecular biology of the anterior cruciate ligament, its potential for healing, and the collagen remodeling that occurs following a reconstruction. This basic science information is presented in Section III, then expanded in Section IV to the clinical setting. The clinical discussions include the status of the current knee laxity testers, considerations for patient selection, factors in selecting a graft, present surgical techniques, complications associated with surgery, and the rehabilitation techniques following ACL reconstruction.

New directions are presented in Section V to expand our present understanding and suggest future treatments and research, including the application of growth factors and bioactive molecules, the introduction of unique cell populations, mesenchymal stem cells, gene therapy, integrin receptors, and new biologic substitutes. Finally, methods for the future assessment of ACL treatment are discussed in Section VI.

The authors contributing to this text and the workshop participants agreed the next decade will see many advancements in our understanding and replacement of the anterior cruciate ligament. We hope this text will serve as a stepping stone to the understanding of how to regenerate, duplicate, or at least optimize the replacement of this amazing structure.

Douglas W. Jackson

Acknowledgments

This volume, *The Anterior Cruciate Ligament:Current and Future Concepts*, has been made possible through the work and support of many individuals. We would like to thank all of the contributing authors for their time in meeting the manuscript deadlines and bringing their expertise to this project. The participation in the author's workshop by the clinicians and scientists resulted in an exchange of multidisciplinary ideas. The insightful discussions that followed contributed positive input to the final book organization and content.

Funding of the authors' workshop was made possible through the donation of two equal grants. This financial support was provided by the 3M Corporation and the Douglas W. Jackson Orthopaedic Research Trust.

In addition, we thank Valerie Stoker, 3M Corporation, for participation in organizing and coordinating the workshop logistics. Becky Yannatone, Southern California Center for Sports Medicine, showed diligence in contacting authors, assisting at the workshop, and in her expert wordprocessing skills. As well, Dennis Kunishima provided assistance with computerizing the chapters and coordinating the computer editing room at the workshop. The text emerged from all of these individuals' contributions.

SECTION I

Structure

The anterior cruciate ligament (ACL) is, perhaps, the most intriguing component of the knee joint. Initially referred to as a crucial ligament because of the cruciate or crossed arrangement of the anterior and posterior ligaments within the knee, the irony of the anterior cruciate ligament being crucial to the well-being of the joint has only recently been appreciated. The axiom of "form reflects function" is especially relevant to the anterior cruciate ligament as its construction and design are directly related to its function as a constraint of knee motion. From the microanatomy of its insertion into bone to the interactions of its matrix components, the complex structure of the anterior cruciate ligament reflects its important contribution to knee joint function.

In addition to its role as a static stabilizer of the knee, there is evidence that the anterior cruciate ligament is an integral component of a proprioceptive feedback mechanism of the joint. Although the exact contribution of the ACL to this neurosensory loop is still unclear, new studies continue to explore this relationship.

In this section, Chapter 1 provides a detailed examination of the gross, microscopic, and vascular anatomy of the anterior cruciate ligament. In addition, the biochemical makeup of the ligament is discussed. Chapter 2 is a comprehensive discussion of the neuroanatomy of the anterior cruciate ligament with special emphasis on the neurosensory role of the ligament. These chapters are intended to provide a prologue for the remaining sections on function, injury, healing, and repair.

Steven P. Arnoczky

The Anterior Cruciate Ligament: Current and Future Concepts, edited by D.W. Jackson, et al. Raven Press, Ltd., New York © 1993.

CHAPTER 1

Anatomy of the Anterior Cruciate Ligament

Steven P. Arnoczky, John R. Matyas, Joseph A. Buckwalter, and David Amiel

Understanding the anatomy of the knee is crucial to understanding its function; this is especially true of the cruciate ligaments. The anatomy of the anterior cruciate ligament is closely related to its function as a constraint of knee joint motion (5,9,11,26,27,29,38,40,41,53–55,67). Its spatial orientation within the knee along with its composition and microstructure provide the anterior cruciate ligament with unique properties that allow it to help "guide" the knee through the range of motion.

In addition to its functional role as a static stabilizer of the knee, the anterior cruciate ligament has a unique neurovascular system (7,8,14,45,62,68). The vascular anatomy of the ACL plays a crucial role in the repair and reconstruction of the ligament, and the neuroreceptors found in its substance suggest a possible proprioceptive role for the ligament (10,32,39,44,63,64,71,72).

The anterior cruciate ligament is a complex structure, and knowledge of its anatomy is a prerequisite for any basic science or clinical discussions. This chapter examines the design and construct of the anterior cruciate ligament to provide a prologue for the ensuing chapters on function, injury, and repair.

DEVELOPMENTAL ANATOMY

The development of the knee joint and its component structures has been the topic of many elegant and detailed embryonic investigations in both humans and animals (6,22,28,30,47). Studies have shown that the human knee joint develops as a cleft between the mesenchymal rudiments of the femur and tibia in about the 8th week of development (28,30,47). As the mesenchyme in the region of the future knee joint condenses to form the precartilage of the joint and the joint capsule, some vascular mesenchyme becomes isolated within the joint (28). This tissue is the precursor to the intraarticular structures of the knee (cruciate ligaments and menisci) (28).

Early investigators considered the intraarticular structures of the knee to be derived from extraarticular muscles and ligaments, which they thought were "drawn" onto the joint during its embryonic evolution (66). Subsequent studies, however, have demonstrated that the cruciate ligaments develop *in situ,* presumably in response to some genetic factor, and are not merely derived secondarily from capsule or muscle (28,30).

The cruciate ligaments of the human knee joint first appear as condensations of vascular synovial mesenchyme at about 7 to 8 weeks of development (28,30). By 9 weeks the cruciate ligaments are composed of numerous immature fibroblasts having scanty cytoplasm and fusiform nuclei, the long axes of which are parallel to the course of the ligaments (28,30).

At 10 weeks the ACL and the posterior cruciate ligament (PCL) are separate from each other and are easily distinguished from one another by the direction of their parallel fibers (Fig. 1). Although no blood vessels are seen in the cruciate ligaments at this time, capillaries are noted in the blastema adjacent to the ligaments (Fig. 2) (28,30).

Over the next 4 weeks the cruciate ligaments continue to differentiate from the adjacent tissues and the insertion sites seem to become more specialized. Blood vessels are also seen in the loose tissue surrounding the cruciate ligaments at this time (9,28,30).

By 18 weeks the cruciate ligaments stand almost alone, and a few vascular elements are to be found within their substance. During the following weeks the

S. P. Arnoczky: Laboratory for Comparative Orthopaedic Research, College of Veterinary Medicine, Michigan State University, East Lansing, Michigan 48824.

J. R. Matyas: Department of Medicine, University of Calgary, Calgary, Alberta, Canada T2N 0W6.

J. A. Buckwalter: Department of Orthopaedic Surgery, University of Iowa Hospital and Clinics, Iowa City, Iowa 52242.

D. Amiel: Department of Orthopaedic Surgery, University of California San Diego School of Medicine, La Jolla, California 92093.

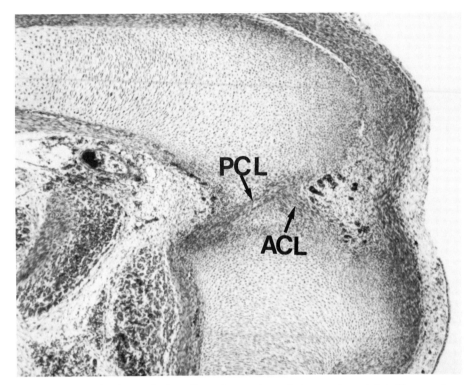

FIG. 1. Photomicrograph of a sagittal section of an embryonic human knee joint. The condensation of mesenchymal tissue forming the anterior (*ACL*) and posterior (*PCL*) cruciate ligaments is clearly visible. (H&E, ×10). (From Arnoczky and Warren, ref. 9, with permission.)

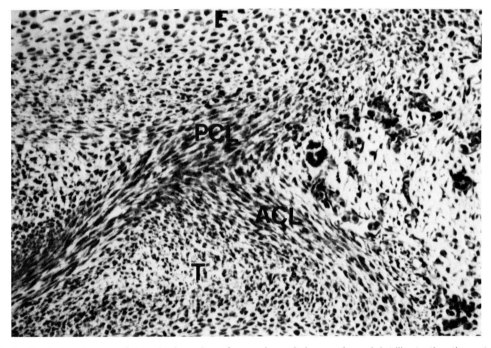

FIG. 2. Photomicrograph of a sagittal section of an embryonic human knee joint illustrating the anterior (*ACL*) and posterior (*PCL*) cruciate ligaments and the adjacent vascular tissue. *F,* femur; *T,* tibia. (H&E, ×100). (From Arnoczky and Warren, ref. 9, with permission.)

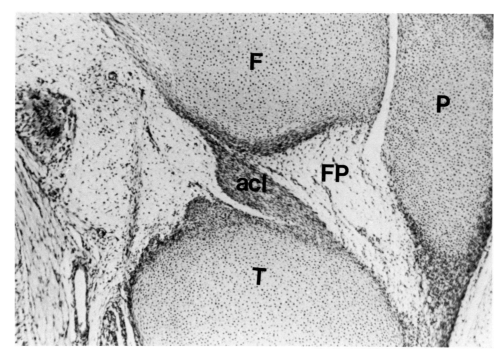

FIG. 3. Photomicrograph of a sagittal section of a human knee joint in approximately the 20th week of development. The anterior cruciate ligament (*ACL*), infrapatellar fat pad (*FP*), and patella (*P*) are clearly visible. *F*, femur; *T*, tibia. (H&E, ×40). (From Arnoczky and Warren, ref. 9, with permission.)

major changes, in addition to growth, are the increase in vascularity and the appearance of definite fat cells in the mass of connective tissue anterior to the cruciate ligaments and inferior to the patella; thus, the infrapatellar fat pad forms at this time (Fig. 3) (9,28,30).

By 20 weeks of development the cruciate ligaments resemble those of the adult. Their remaining develop-

ment consists of marked growth with little change in form (Fig. 4) (9,28,30).

THE GROSS ANATOMY OF THE ANTERIOR CRUCIATE LIGAMENT

The anterior cruciate ligament is a band of regularly oriented, dense connective tissue that connects the femur and tibia. It is surrounded by a mesentery-like fold of synovium that originates from the posterior intercondylar area of the knee and completely envelopes both the anterior and the posterior cruciate ligaments. Thus, although the cruciate ligaments are intraarticular they are also extrasynovial (7,11,29,31).

Bony Attachments

The normal anatomy of the ACL attachments has received considerable attention because of the emphasis of reestablishing a so-called "anatomical" position of the insertion to attain as close to an "isometric" position as possible when reconstructing or replacing the ACL (5,7,11,13,19,26,27,29,35,37,40,41,49,52,53,61,65). The attachments of the human ACL to the femur and tibia have been carefully mapped with respect to bony landmarks by several authors (7,11,26,29,35,40,49,53,55, 61,65). The anterior cruciate ligament is attached to a fossa on the posterior aspect of the medial surface of the

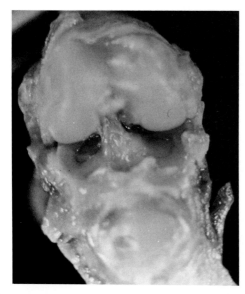

FIG. 4. A human knee joint in approximately the 20th week of development. The cruciate ligaments and menisci are fully formed at this time. (From Arnoczky and Warren, ref. 9, with permission.)

lateral femoral condyle. The femoral attachment is in the form of a segment of a circle, with the anterior border straight and the posterior border convex. The long axis of the femoral attachment is tilted slightly forward from the vertical, and the posterior convexity is parallel to the posterior articular margin of the lateral femoral condyle (Fig. 5).

The anterior cruciate ligament is attached to a fossa in front of and lateral to the anterior tibial spine (Fig. 6). At this attachment the ACL passes beneath the transverse meniscal ligament, and a few fascicles of the ACL may blend with the anterior attachment of the lateral meniscus. In some instances fascicles from the posterior aspect of the tibial attachment of the ACL may extend to, and blend with, the posterior attachment of the lateral meniscus. The tibial attachment of the ACL is somewhat broader than the femoral attachment.

The ACL begins to "fan out" in the proximal one-third of the ligament such that it terminates in a larger tibial attachment compared to the femoral attachment (29). Schutte et al. reported that the characteristic "twist" of the ACL begins approximately 5 mm distal to the femoral insertion, corresponding to the beginning of the "fanning out" (64). Recent magnetic resonance imaging (MRI) studies of human knees have shown that the tibial attachment "flares" to nearly twice the bulk width of the ACL in the sagittal plane, with a distinct anterior "toe" right at the tibial attachment that lies against and "adapts to the contour of the intercondylar roof when the joint is in full extension" (37).

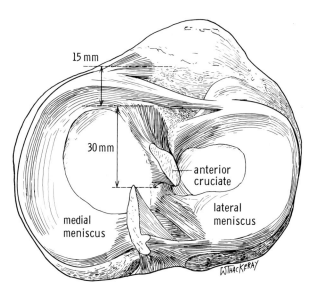

FIG. 6. The tibial plateau showing the average measurements and relations of the tibial attachments of the anterior cruciate ligaments. (From Arnoczky, ref. 7, with permission.)

Spatial Orientation

The cruciate ligaments, as their names signify, cross each other as they pass from the femur to the tibia. This spatial orientation is critical to the function of the cruciate ligaments as constraints of joint motion.

The ACL courses anteriorly, medially, and distally across the joint as it passes from the femur to the tibia (Fig. 7). It also seems to turn on itself in a slight outward

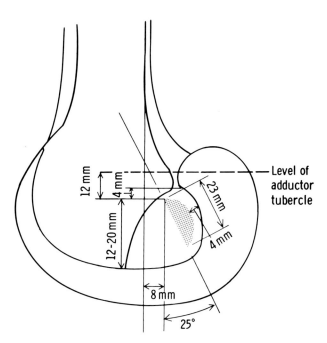

FIG. 5. The medial surface of the right lateral femoral condyle showing the average measurements and body relations of the femoral attachment of the anterior cruciate ligament. (From Arnoczky, ref. 7, with permission.)

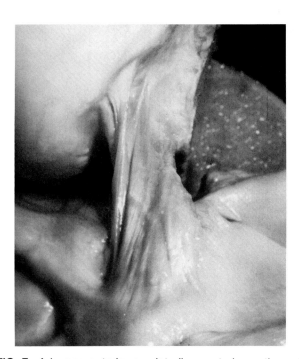

FIG. 7. A human anterior cruciate ligament shows the outward (lateral) spiral of the ligament as it passes from the femur to the tibia.

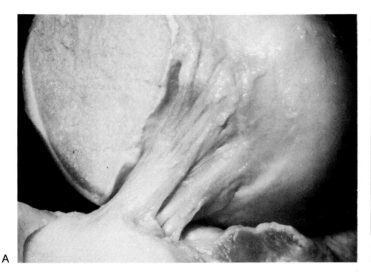
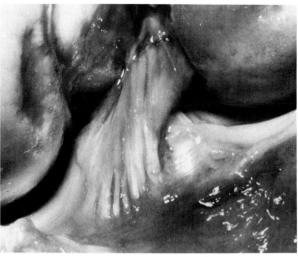

FIG. 8. The femoral (**A**) and tibial (**B**) attachments of the anterior cruciate ligament, demonstrating its broad attachment area and its multifascicular structure. (From Arnoczky, ref. 7, with permission.)

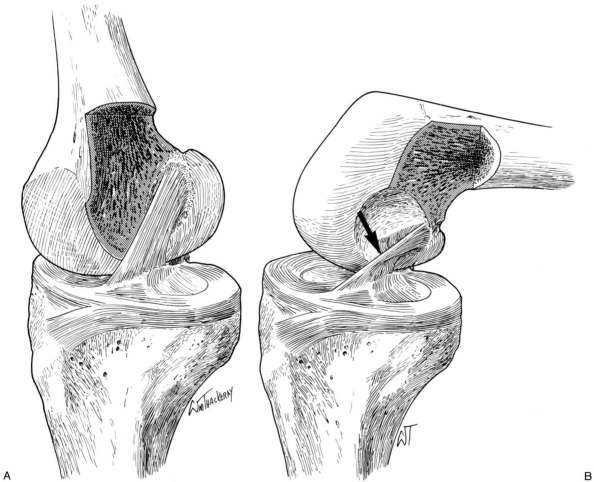

FIG. 9. The anterior cruciate ligament with the knee in extension (**A**) and flexion (**B**). Note the presence of an anteromedial band (*arrow*). (From Arnoczky, ref. 7, with permission.)

(lateral) spiral. This twist is most likely a result of the orientation of its bony attachments (29).

The orientation of the femoral attachment of the anterior cruciate ligament in flexion and extension is also responsible for the relative tension of the ligament throughout the range of motion. The anterior cruciate ligament is attached to the femur and tibia not as a singular cord but as a collection of individual fascicles that fan out over a broad, flattened area (Fig. 8). In the anterior cruciate ligament these fascicles have been summarily divided into two groups: the anteromedial band (AMB)—those fascicles originating at the proximal aspect of the femoral attachment and inserting at the anteromedial aspect of the tibial attachment—and the posterolateral bulk (PLB)—the remaining bulk of fascicles that are inserted at the posterolateral aspect of the tibial attachment. When the knee is extended, the PLB is tight and the AMB is moderately lax. However, as the knee is flexed, the femoral attachment of the ACL assumes a more horizontal orientation, causing the AMB to tighten and the PLB to loosen (Fig. 9).

Although this two-part designation provides a general idea of the dynamics of the anterior cruciate ligament through the range of motion, it is an oversimplification. Indeed, these macroscopic bundles lack a corresponding microstructure in the substance of the ACL (19,54). The functional significance attributed to the ACL by its fascicular structure is that different groups of fascicles may function together throughout the range of joint motion.

THE MICROANATOMY OF THE ANTERIOR CRUCIATE LIGAMENT

The microarchitecture of the cruciate ligaments has often been likened to the hierarchical arrangement described for tendon in which collagen fibrils are grouped into fibers that, in turn, make up subfascicular units that are bound together to form a fasciculus (21,25). However, a recent anatomical study has demonstrated only two distinct orders of separation (19). This study found that the anterior cruciate ligament is composed of multiple 20-μm-wide collagen fiber bundles separated by columns of cells in fibrous capsules (19). These bundles were, in turn, grouped into fascicles that varied in size from 20 to 400 μm in diameter. As noted previously, this study did not demonstrate an anatomical delineation of bands within the ligament, further supporting the concept that this description is functional rather than anatomical (19).

INSERTIONS

The anterior cruciate ligament attaches to the femur and tibia by way of an incorporation of collagen fibers of the ligament within the mineralized bone (20,46,69).

The abrupt change from flexible ligamentous tissue to rigid bone is mediated through a transition zone of fibrocartilage and mineralized fibrocartilage (20,46,69). This alteration in microstructure from ligament to bone presumably allows a graduated change in stiffness and prevents stress concentration at the attachment sites (69). Classically, this "transition zone" has been divided into four morphologically distinct zones (Fig. 10) (20,46,69).

Zone 1 is essentially ligamentous tissue consisting of Type I collagen in an extracellular matrix. The collagen fibers vary in diameter from 25 to 300 nm and are interspersed with a few elastin fibers. The major cell type is the fibroblast, and small vessels (capillaries, arterioles, and venules) are located in the endoligamentous tissues (see below) and run parallel to the collagen fibers (20,36,69).

Zone 2 is composed of fibrocartilage. The collagen fibers extend into this zone without any noticeable change in orientation or size. The cells of Zone 2 are somewhat larger than those of Zone 1 and are characterized by a rounded, ovoid shape, frequently visible lacunae, and relatively abundant pericellular proteoglycan matrix (Fig. 11). Although these characteristics define the morphology of "chondroid" cells, the distinctly fibrous matrix in which these cells are embedded characterizes them as fibrochondrocytes. The transition between the ovoid fibrocytes of the midsubstance (see below) and the fibrochondrocytes of the insertion is gradual, and a demarcation between these two zones is indistinct. In general, these fibrochondrocytes are typically arranged in columns that vary in cell number, although the fibrochondrocytes are said to be more numerous on this side of the line of mineralization. Although this zone seems to be microscopically similar to other fibrocartilaginous tissues, the narrow extent (150 to 400 μm in dogs) of this region has made biochemical characterization difficult (46,69).

As collagen fiber bundles traverse the fibrocartilaginous zone, they gradually bend to meet the mineralization front of the insertion. The radius of bend varies within the insertion, and it has been hypothesized that the abundant pericellular matrix of this zone is responsible for supporting a smooth bending of the fibers. This bending aligns the collagen fiber bundles so that they penetrate into the mineralized fibrocartilage zone at angles nearly perpendicular to the mineralization front (Fig. 12). This arrangement (bending through a matrix rich in pericellular proteoglycans) may aid in reducing the mechanical stress of the collagen fibers as they pass from nonmineralized to mineralized tissue. No vascular or neural elements have been observed in this zone (46,69).

Zone 3 is characterized by mineralized fibrocartilage and is highlighted by a basophilic line (staining blue with hematoxylin) or "tidemark," which sharply demarcates the outer limit of mineralization (calcification) (Fig. 13).

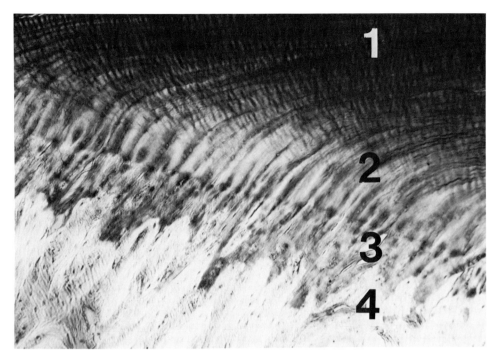

FIG. 10. Low-magnification light photomicrograph of the tibial insertion of the anterior cruciate ligament of an adult dog. Periodic collagen crimp is visible in Zone 1. Collagen fibers enter Zone 2 obliquely but curve to meet Zone 3 at nearly right angles. Pericellular proteoglycans are shown to advantage in Zones 2 and 3 in this section, as is the demarcation between Zones 3 and 4. (Safranin O, partially polarized light and Nomarski optics.)

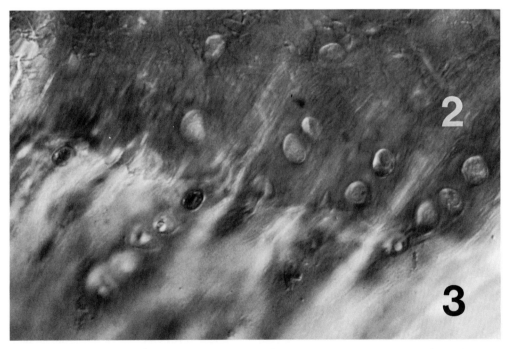

FIG. 11. High-magnification photomicrograph of Fig. 10 at the border between Zones 2 and 3. Note the rounded fibrochondrocytes with abundant safranin O-staining pericellular matrix, indicating the presence of acidic proteoglycans. (Partially polarized light and Nomarski optics.)

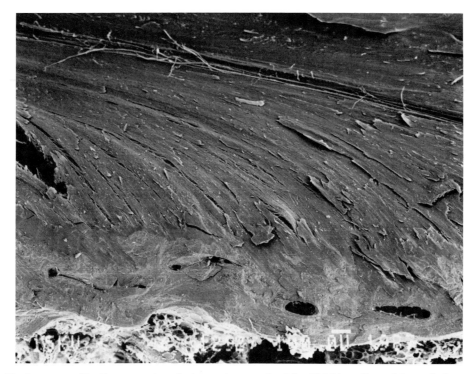

FIG. 12. Low-magnification scanning electron micrograph of the tibial insertion of the anterior cruciate ligament in an adult human being. This preparation technique highlights the curvature of the collagen fibers. The orientation of the curving fibers is opposite to the orientation of the fibers in Fig. 10. (From Clark and Sidles, ref. 19, with permission.)

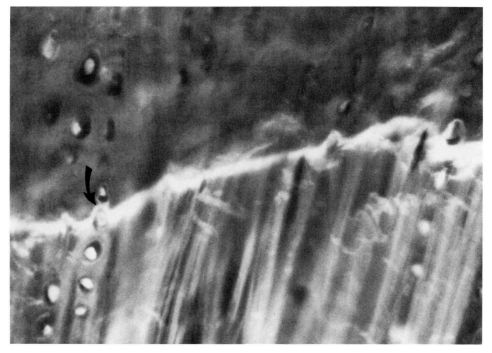

FIG. 13. Ultraviolet light photomicrograph of the femoral insertion of the anterior cruciate ligament of an adult rat. A parenteral dose of oxytetracycline localizes along the tidemark, indicating that the insertion continually advances and cements the ligament fibers to the surface of the bone. Note the contour of the tidemark, particularly as it "cups" the base of a fibrochondrocyte in Zone 2.

The tidemark is usually smooth in contour but can be irregular. In addition, multiple basophilic staining lines lying parallel and deep to the mineralization front have been observed. However, the significance of these "duplicated tidemarks" has not been determined (69).

As noted above, the transition from nonmineralized to mineralized tissue is sudden. Although individual mineral crystals are seen within collagen fibrils near the tidemark, the crystals soon (approximately 12 μm into the zone) markedly increase in number. These crystals aggregate into masses, and individual crystals become less obvious. Although the mineralization also encloses the fibrocartilaginous cell lacunae, the cells seem to remain active within this mineralized matrix. The total width of the mineralized zone is approximately 100 to 300 μm (69).

Zone 4 is composed of bone. Here, the mineralized matrix of the inserting tissues interdigitates with the mineralized matrix of the bone (46,69).

THE COMPOSITION OF THE ANTERIOR CRUCIATE LIGAMENT

The anterior cruciate ligament consists of fibroblasts surrounded by an extracellular matrix formed by two components: a solid, highly ordered arrangement of macromolecules (primarily Type I collagen) and water, which fills the macromolecular framework (1,18,25). The specialized mechanical properties of the ligament depend on the composition of the matrix, the organization of the matrix macromolecules, and the interaction between the matrix macromolecules and the tissue water (1,25).

Although the exact composition of ligaments has not been determined, the available evidence shows that different ligaments and different regions of the same ligament may vary slightly in matrix composition and in cell shape and density and that ligament composition may change slightly with age (1,3,24,25). Presumably, these small differences in the composition reflect subtle but potentially important differences in mechanical function. Furthermore, dense fibrous tissues can respond to changes in their mechanical environment by changing their matrix composition. For example, patellar tendon grafts used to replace the anterior cruciate ligament change their matrix composition so that the tendon graft matrix becomes nearly the same as the matrix of an anterior cruciate ligament (4).

Cells

The anterior cruciate ligament comprises several distinct tissue regions, and each is populated with different types of intrinsic cells. Different types of intrinsic cells are distinguished principally by the tissue region in which they are located. However, they also possess a range of characteristic shapes and sizes.

The Epiligament

Beneath the extrinsic investing layers of the synovium, the outermost intrinsic layer of the ACL is known variously as the epiligament, peritenon, or periligament (7,25). A clearly distinguishable plane of transition between the synovial subintima and the epiligament is not visible by scanning electron or transmission electron microscopy. Similarly, a strict distinction between the cell types of the synovial subintima and the epiligament is not possible. Like the subintima, the intrinsic cells of the epiligament include small fibrocytes and adipocytes (Fig. 14). Fibrocytes are distributed rather evenly throughout the epiligament, whereas the adipocytes typically occur in clusters (25).

The Endoligament

At certain locations, the epiligament continues into the substance of the ACL as the endoligament (also referred to as the endotenon) (Fig. 15). The endoligament

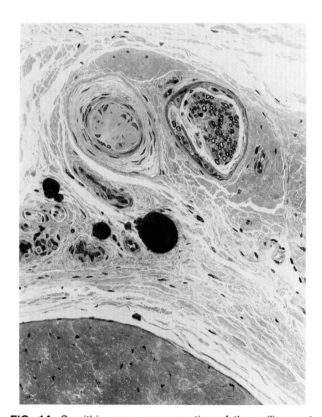

FIG. 14. Semithin epoxy cross-section of the epiligament-ligament junction of a human anterior cruciate ligament. At the bottom, densely packed collagen fibers and ligament fibrocytes are characteristic of ligament substance. (In cross-section, ligament fibrocytes appear stellate.) In the overlying epiligament, the collagen fibers are less densely packed and the small fibroblasts are elongate. Darkly stained fat cells are located just below a large neurovascular bundle that contains a lamellar corpuscle mechanoreceptor (*left*) and a nerve fascicle with both unmyelinated and myelinated fibers (*right*). (×210.) (From Halata and Haus, ref. 32, with permission.)

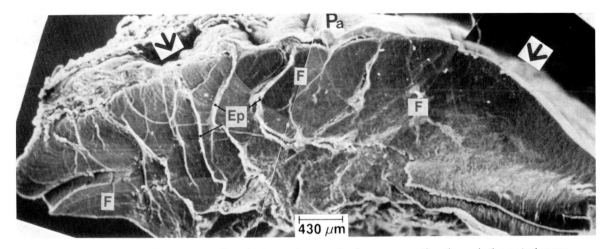

FIG. 15. Low-magnification scanning electron micrograph of a cross-section through the anterior cruciate ligament of a young adult dog. The epiligament (here labeled peritenon—*Pa*) covers the surface of the ACL and is continuous at various locations around the circumference of the ACL with the endoligament (epitenon—*Ep*). The endoligament subdivides the ACL into discrete fascicles. (From Yahia and Drouin, ref. 70, with permission.)

not only serves to support the entering neurovascular structures but also subdivides the ligament through a "network of membranous septae" that separate collagen fibers into "bundles" and "fascicles" (19). Reportedly, the amount of endoligament is greater in the human ACL than in the rabbit ACL (19). Endoligament cells are basically fibrocytes that appear similar in size and shape to cells in the epiligament. Adipocytes have not been described as a component of the endoligament of the ACL.

Immunohistochemical studies at the light microscopic level indicate that endoligamentous septae are enriched with fibronectin and Type III collagen (43). Whether these products are produced endogenously by the endoligament cells, by extrinsic cells of the ACL (e.g., vascular pericytes), or by some source of cells outside the ACL is unknown.

The Ligament Substance Cells

Cell shape (more often nuclear shape) and the presence of a lacunar space are the chief morphological characteristics used to distinguish between cells of the ACL substance. The limits of the cytoplasm usually cannot be discerned without special optics (e.g., Normarski differential interference contrast) or electron microscopy.

Cells between the longitudinal collagen fibers of the ACL have a variety of shapes ranging from ovoid to fusiform, with many intermediate shapes (Fig. 16) (3). Because cell shapes vary widely, it is unclear whether the cells that populate the ACL substance form a single population or whether two or more populations of cells have shapes that overlap. As different descriptions of cells in the substance of the ACL are based on observations from different animals, it is unclear what factors (e.g., area of

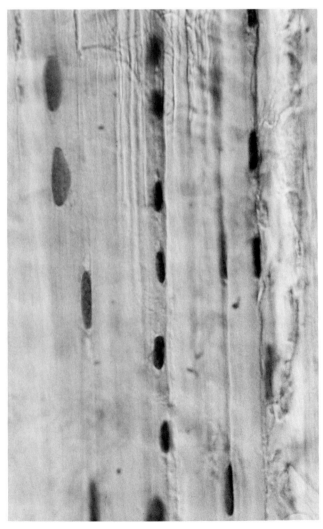

FIG. 16. Light photomicrograph of cells from the midsubstance of the anterior cruciate ligament of an adult dog. Note the variety in cell shapes. (Nomarski optics.)

sampling, stage of skeletal maturation, mechanical state), if any, influence cell shape.

Ovoid cells are typically arranged in columns that are sandwiched between collagen fibers (3,42,70). Scanning electron microscopy of the rabbit ACL reveals that these cells are more "cuboid" than ovoid (Fig. 17) (19). These ovoid cells sometimes appear to be located within chondrocytic lacunae and are surrounded by a fibrous capsule that is made up of fine fibrils and amorphous ground substance (19,42,70). This fine-fibered capsule is said to resemble the pattern of territorial networks of articular cartilage lacunae (19). Unlike the more elongated fibroblasts in the ACL and other ligaments, ovoid cells lack extensive cytoplasmic processes (42).

Positive periodic acid-Schiff staining in the pericellular regions has been observed in ovoid cell columns throughout the human ACL, suggesting an accumulation of glycosaminoglycans in this region (19). In addition, immunohistochemical localization of fibronectin has been reported to be associated with ovoid cells in the skeletally immature rabbit ACL (42). The functional significance of these findings is unclear.

Fusiform fibrocytes, as well as cells with intermediate shapes, are less well described than are the ovoid cells of the ACL. More elongated than the ovoid cells and usually found closely approximating the dense collagen bundles, these cells, either singularly or in groups, are distributed throughout the midsubstance of the ACL (2,4,13,32,43). A clear pattern of the distribution of ovoid, fusiform, and intermediately shaped cells in the ACL has not been described in any species.

In addition to the intrinsic cells described above, there are also vascular and neural cells found within the ligament. In longitudinal sections, vascular endothelial cells seem to be flanked by cells described as pericytes, although these may also be cells of the endoligament (31,40). There is also evidence for at least a diminutive lymphatic supply within the ACL, but as yet the anatomy of the lymphatic vasculature of the ACL has not been investigated systematically (32).

Nerve fibers and sensory receptors have been described throughout the ACL, including the insertions (see Chapter 2). Various investigations have reported a preponderance of mechanoreceptors at the femoral and tibial insertions of the human and feline ACL (35,39,44,63,64,71,72). Schutte et al. reported that nociceptive free nerve endings were found predominantly at the femoral insertion proximal to the "twist"(64). At the insertions, sensory receptors were located mainly in the synovial subintima and the epiligament layers, but they have also been described deep in the substance of the insertions.

The Extracellular Matrix

Water

Water contributes 60% or more of the wet weight of most ligaments (1,3,23,25). A significant part of this water is associated with the ground substance (the ground substance is the term used to refer to the portion

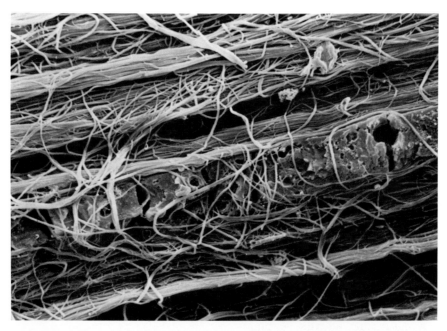

FIG. 17. Scanning electron photomicrograph of cells within the substance of the anterior cruciate ligament of an adult human. Note the cuboidal shape of the cells and their arrangement into a column between the collagen fibrils of the midsubstance, giving them the appearance of "boxcars." Also note that most of the collagen fibers are aligned along the axis of the ACL, although some other fibers crisscross through the matrix. (From Clark and Sidles, ref. 19, with permission.)

of the matrix consisting of proteoglycans). Water, in association with the ground substance, provides the lubrication and spacing that are crucial to the gliding function at the intercept points where fibers cross in the tissue matrices (1,3,25). Gliding is an essential physical property of ligaments. Water and ground substance also confer viscoelastic properties to ligamentous tissue (1,3,25). The movement of water in this system is inhibited by its entrapment between the large, highly charged molecules of proteoglycans. In addition, because many ligaments lie at some distance from vessels, these cells must depend on diffusion of nutrients and metabolites through tissue fluid.

The Matrix Macromolecules

Four classes of molecules [collagens, proteoglycans, elastin, and noncollagenous proteins (glycoproteins)] form the molecular framework of the ligament matrix and contribute approximately 40% of the wet weight of most ligaments (1,3,16,18,23,25). Although the macromolecules will be discussed individually, it is the interactions among these molecules that creates the three-dimensional structure of the matrix and gives the tissue its cohesiveness and unique mechanical properties.

The Collagens

Collagen is the single most abundant animal protein in mammals, accounting for up to 30% of all proteins (50,51). It is the major constituent of the anterior cruciate ligament and makes up approximately 75% of the dry weight of the ligament (1,3,25). The collagen molecules, after being secreted by the cells, assemble into characteristic fibers responsible for the functional integrity of the tissue (50,51).

Although 16 different collagen types have been found in human tissues, the ligaments contain predominantly Types I and III (1,3,25). Type I collagen is composed of three chains, two identical alpha 1 chains and one alpha 2 chain. It comprises approximately 90% of the collagen in ligaments. Type III collagen accounts for approximately 10% of the collagen in ligaments and is composed of three identical chains (1,3,50,51). Because the ratio of Type I to Type III collagen changes with age, Type III being predominant in the fetus, this collagen is sometimes referred to as fetal or embryonic collagen (50,51).

The Collagen Molecule and Biosynthesis. The arrangement of amino acids in fibrillar collagen molecules is shown schematically in Fig. 18. Every third amino acid is glycine. Proline and hydroxyproline follow each other relatively frequently, and the (Gly,Pro,Hyp) sequence makes up about 10% of the molecule. This triple helical structure generates a symmetrical pattern of three left-handed helical chains that are, in turn, slightly displaced to the right, superimposing an additional "supercoil" with a pitch of approximately 8.6 nm. The exact number of hydrogen bonds that stabilize the triple helical structure has not been determined. One model describes two hydrogen bonds for every three amino acids, whereas another assumes one. In addition to these intramolecular conformational patterns, there seems to exist a supramolecular coiling. Microfibrils, possibly representing intermediate stages of packing, have also been described.

For an organism to develop an extracellular network of collagen fibers, the cells involved in the biosynthetic process must first synthesize a precursor known as procollagen. This molecule is later enzymatically trimmed of its nonhelical ends, giving rise to a collagen molecule that spontaneously assembles into fibers in the extracellular space.

The tendency of collagen molecules to form macromolecular aggregates is well known. However, the exact mode by which the collagen molecules pack into microfibrils (precursors of the larger fibrils) still remains a subject for speculation.

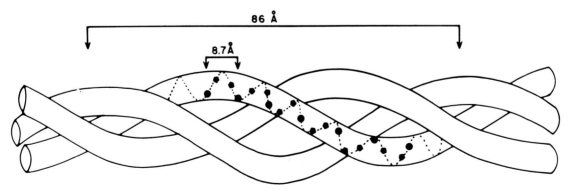

86 Å

8.7 Å

● GLYCINE

● PREDOMINANTLY AMINO ACIDS

FIG. 18. The amino acid arrangement in a collagen molecule.

Cross-linking. Cross-linking renders the collagen fibers stable and provides them with a degree of tensile strength and viscoelasticity adequate to perform their structural role. The degree of cross-linking, the number and density of the fibers in a particular tissue, and their orientation and diameter combine to provide this function. Cross-linking begins with the oxidative deamination of the e-carbon of lysine or hydroxylysine to yield the corresponding semialdehydes and is mediated by the enzyme lysyloxidase (Fig. 19). In general, lysine-derived cross-links seem to predominate in soft connective tissues such as skin and tendon, whereas hydroxylysine-derived cross-links are prevalent in the harder connective tissues such as bone, cartilage, and dentin.

Collagen Fibril Diameter. Recently, a great deal of attention has been paid to the diameter of collagen fibrils and their distribution within the ligament. Several studies have shown that the anterior cruciate ligament of humans has a bimodal profile of collagen fibrils, the majority of which are 30 to 100 nm in diameter, with a small number of fibrils greater than 100 nm in diameter (25,56,57). Animal and human data suggest that this profile changes with age (see Chapter 19) (57). These studies demonstrated a unimodal profile of small-diameter collagen fibers at birth (57). The fibril size increased in diameter until maturity, when the profile became bimodal, with the majority being small-diameter fibrils (57). As the individuals became elderly, the diameter of the fibrils seemed to decrease (57).

The importance of this fibril size is not understood. Although it is intriguing to link fibril diameter with some measure of functional strength, there is currently no scientific basis for these theories (56).

Elastin

The anterior cruciate ligament contains only a small amount of elastin (less than 5%), but this molecule probably makes important contributions to the organization and function of the ligament matrix (16,18). Elastin forms networks interdigitated among ligament collagen fibril fascicles, an arrangement similar to that seen in dermis (16,18). It lacks the cross-banding pattern of fibrillar collagens and differs in amino acid composition, including two amino acids not found in collagen, desmosine and isodesmosine (16,18). Elastic fibers consist of two components: elastin and fibrillin, a glycoprotein that forms beaded tubules. Cells synthesize elastin and the fibrillin and then assemble the elastic fibers in grooves on the cell surface (Fig. 20) (16,18).

When unstretched, the elastin molecule takes on a complex coiled arrangement. When stretched, this coiled arrangement is stretched into a more ordered configuration. Upon removal of the tension, the molecule returns to its random coil conformation. This organiza-

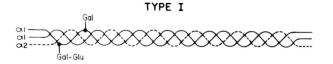

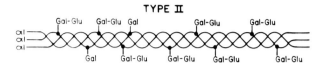

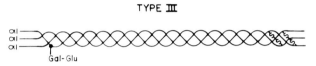

FIG. 19. The intramolecular and intermolecular cross-links.

tion of the amino acid chains in the elastin molecule makes it possible for elastin to undergo some deformation without rupturing or tearing and then, when unloaded, return to its original size and shape (16,18). This behavior probably supplies at least a small part of the tensile resistance in ligament tissue and some of its elastic recoverability. In particular, it may help restore the crimp pattern of the collagen fibrils after deformation (16,18).

The Proteoglycans

Proteoglycans consist of small amounts of protein bound to negatively charged polysaccharide chains referred to as glycosaminoglycans. In articular cartilage, proteoglycans form a large portion of the macromolecular framework (commonly about 30% to 35% of the tissue dry weight), but in ligaments they form only a small portion of this framework, usually less than 1% of the dry weight (1,3,25). Nonetheless, proteoglycans may have an important role in organizing the extracellular matrix and in interacting with the tissue fluid (12,15–18,33,34,48).

Like tendon, meniscus, and articular cartilage, ligaments contain two known classes of proteoglycans: large, articular cartilage type proteoglycans containing long, negatively charged chains of chondroitin and keratan sulfate (syndecan) and smaller proteoglycans that contain dermatan sulfate (16–18). Because of their long chains of negative charges, the articular cartilage type proteoglycans tend to expand to their maximum domain until restrained by the collagen fibril network. As a result, they maintain water within the tissue, alter fluid flow within the tissue during loading, and exert a swelling pressure, thereby contributing to the mechanical properties of the tissue and filling the regions between collagen fibrils.

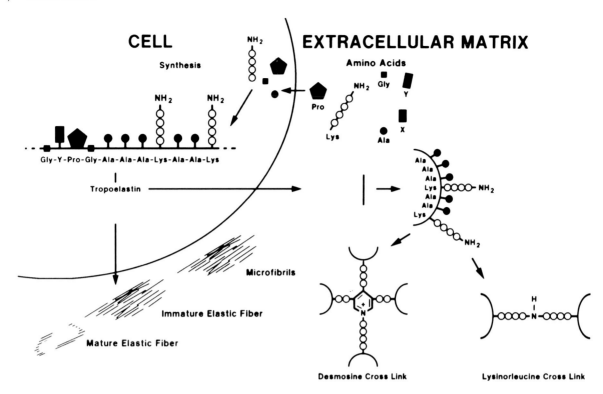

FIG. 20. Elastin synthesis and the assembly of elastin fibers. (From Buckwalter and Cooper, ref. 16, with permission.)

Small dermatan sulfate proteoglycans (decorin and biglycan) usually lie on the surface of collagen fibrils and seem to affect the formation, organization, and stability of the extracellular matrix, including collagen fibril formation and diameter (58,59). These molecules may also affect the ability of mesenchymal cells to repair ligament injuries. They can inhibit fibroblast adhesion to other matrix macromolecules (especially the noncollagenous protein fibronectin) and thereby may limit the ability of the cells to bind to the matrix and form new tissue (60).

The concentration of glycosaminoglycans (GAGs) present in rabbit knee ligaments differs significantly from that present in tendinous tissue (1,3). The ACL has the highest proportion of GAGs, two to four times the amount observed in tendons (1,3). Although the functional importance of these differences is unknown, it is clear that the higher the GAG content, the more water that is associated with the complex. This naturally alters the viscoelastic properties of these tissues and may represent an additional "shock-absorbing" feature in ligaments (optimized in the cruciate ligaments) that is less important in tendon.

The Noncollagenous Proteins (Glycoproteins)

These molecules consist primarily of protein, but many of them also contain a few monosaccharides and oligosaccharides (16,18,25). Although noncollagenous proteins such as fibronectin contribute only a few percentage points to the dry weight of ligaments, they have an important role in the complex interaction of ligament cells and their environment during growth, healing, and remodeling. However, this role is poorly understood.

Fibronectins are important in an array of cellular functions, particularly those involving a cell's interaction with its surrounding extracellular matrix. They are high-molecular-weight extracellular glycoproteins whose functions include (modulating?) intra- and extracellular matrix morphology, cellular adhesion (both cell to cell and cell to substratum), and cell migration. Examined by electron microscopy, fibronectins appear as fine filaments or granules coating the surface of fibrillar collagens or associated with cell membranes. Fibronectins have an adhesive domain specific to fibrin, actin, hyaluronic acid, cell surface factors, and collagen. They function to attract and couple key elements in normal healing and in growing tissue.

Quantitative studies of fibronectin concentrations in rabbit ligaments demonstrate significantly (two to three times) higher amounts of fibronectin in the cruciate ligaments as compared to the collateral ligaments (3). This difference may reflect the fact that the cruciate ligaments are surrounded by a synovial sheath and therefore have a higher degree of cellularity as compared to the extraarticular ligaments.

Cell-Matrix Interactions

The maintenance of ligament tissue and its ability to respond to changes in loading depend on interactions between the cells and the matrix. Normally, the matrix macromolecules are slowly but continually degraded and replaced. The cells must synthesize new macromolecules to balance the losses due to normal degradation or microtrauma. The matrix provides to the cells protection from mechanical injury during normal loading and transmits signals generated by loading to the cells.

Cells bind to the matrix primarily through a family of cell surface proteins called integrins. These molecules mechanically link the matrix macromolecules, including fibronectin, to the internal cell cytoskeleton. They participate in cell adhesion, migration, and proliferation and in regulation of cell synthesis of new matrix macromolecules.

The Vascular Supply to the Anterior Cruciate Ligament

The blood supply to the knee is derived from branches of the following major arteries: the descending genicular artery, the medial and lateral superior genicular arteries, the medial and lateral inferior genicular arteries, the middle genicular artery, and the anterior and posterior tibial recurrent arteries (Fig. 21) (7,8,45,62,68). The major blood supply to the anterior cruciate ligament arises from the ligamentous branches of the middle genicular artery as well as some terminal branches of the medial and lateral inferior genicular arteries (7,8,62).

The anterior cruciate ligament is covered by a synovial fold that originates at the posterior inlet of the intercondylar notch and extends to the anterior tibial insertion of the ligament, where it joins with the synovial tissue of the joint capsule distal to the infrapatellar fat pad. This synovial membrane, which forms an envelope about the ligament, is richly endowed with vessels that originate predominantly from the ligamentous branches of the middle genicular artery (Fig. 22). A few smaller terminal branches of the lateral and medial inferior genicular arteries also contribute some vessels to this synovial plexus through its connection with the infrapatellar fat pad. The synovial vessels arborize to form a web-like network of periligamentous vessels that ensheathe the entire ligament. These periligamentous vessels then give rise to smaller connecting branches that penetrate the ligament transversely and anastomose with a network of endoligamentous vessels (Fig. 23). These vessels, along with their supporting connective tissues, are oriented in a longitudinal direction and lie parallel to the collagen bundles within the ligament (7,8,62).

The anterior cruciate ligament is supplied with blood predominantly from soft tissue origins (fat pad and synovium). Although the middle genicular artery gives off additional branches to the distal femoral epiphysis and proximal tibial epiphysis, the ligamentous-osseous junctions of the anterior cruciate ligament do not contribute

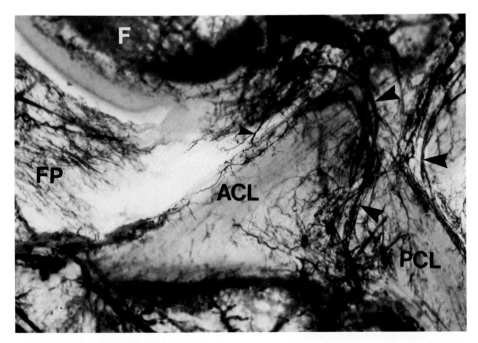

FIG. 21. Five-millimeter-thick sagittal section of a human knee (Spalteholz technique) showing the branches of the middle genicular artery that supply the cruciate ligaments (*arrowheads*). *F,* femur; *T,* tibia; *FP,* fat pad; *P,* popliteal artery; *ACL,* anterior cruciate ligament; *PCL,* posterior cruciate ligament. (From Arnoczky, ref. 8, with permission.)

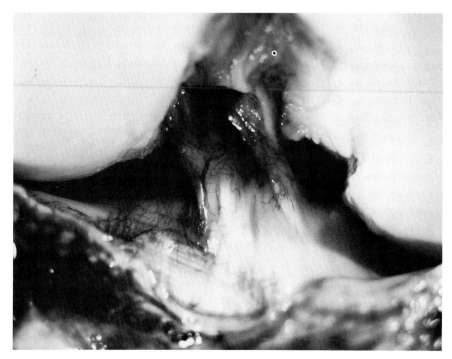

FIG. 22. A human knee specimen injected with India ink demonstrating the synovial (periligamentous) vasculature on the surface of the anterior cruciate ligament. (The infrapatellar fat pad has been removed for better visualization.) (From Arnoczky, ref. 8, with permission.)

significantly to the vascular scheme of the ligament itself (7,8).

The role of the vascular soft tissues in anterior cruciate ligament injury, repair, and reconstruction has been documented in both the experimental and the clinical situation. A study in dogs showed that the synovium and fat pad provide the origin for the vascular response of the cruciate ligaments after injury (10).

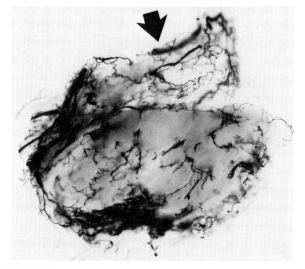

FIG. 23. Cross-section of a human anterior cruciate ligament (Spalteholz technique) demonstrating the periligamentous as well as endoligamentous vasculature. The fold of synovial membrane (*arrow*) can be seen supplying vessels to the synovial covering of the ligament. (From Arnoczky, ref. 7, with permission.)

The Neural Anatomy

Nerve fibers and sensory receptors have been described throughout the ACL, often accompanying vessels in the form of neurovascular bundles (32,39,63, 71,72). It is via these neurovascular bundles that nerve fibers enter the ligament from the synovial subintima and epiligament. Some nerve fibers and a variety of sensory end organs are also located in the ligament apart from the vasculature (39,44). The nerve fibers that lead to these endings may be either unmyelinated or myelinated (32). In addition, four morphologically distinct types of sensory endings have been described in the human ACL, including two types of Ruffini end organs, Pacinian corpuscles, and free nerve endings (44,64). It has been estimated that 1% of the volume of the ACL is occupied by specialized nerve receptors and free nerve endings (64). The sensory nerve endings are located along the entire length of the ACL, including both insertions, and are found primarily in the subintimal later of the synovium and the epiligament (44) (see Chapter 2).

SUMMARY

The human anterior cruciate ligament is a complex structure at every level ranging from its gross structure to its molecular organization. The ligament is designed to act as a stabilizer of the knee joint while allowing normal joint movement throughout the functional range of motion. This is accomplished through the precise orientation and composition of the ligament, but the exact relationship of form to function remains unknown. The ACL is also a vital biological structure possessing a unique blood supply that plays a crucial role in the repair process of the ligament. The ligament also possesses neural elements that may serve a proprioceptive function.

NEW DIRECTIONS

In this chapter we have attempted to assemble a comprehensive review of the structure of the normal human anterior cruciate ligament. However, many aspects of this review are limited by the amount and quality of information that is currently available about the human anterior cruciate ligament. The direct extrapolation of animal data (both morphological and biochemical) on the ACL still awaits conformation from similar studies on "normal" human tissue.

Another area warranting further study is the relationship between the structure (including composition) and functions of the ACL. Although intriguing speculations about the relationships of form to function have been made, the exact relationship between the mechanical properties of the ACL and collagen fiber diameter, collagen cross-linking, or matrix interactions remains unknown.

The limitations of this chapter and of the scientific literature both warrant caution and offer opportunity. Clinicians and basic scientists are encouraged to evaluate the original literature critically and make firsthand observations before making conclusions about the anatomy of the ACL, particularly if they plan on repairing or reconstructing it. There are still many opportunities to carry out original studies of ACL anatomy that would further our understanding of this clinically important structure. We hope that this chapter will serve as a foundation for those who desire a reference on ACL structure and as a catalyst for others who are searching for a springboard for new ideas and directions of study.

REFERENCES

1. Amiel D, Billings E, Akeson WH. (1990): Ligament structure, chemistry, and physiology. In: Daniel D, Akeson W, O'Connor J, eds. *Knee ligaments: structure, function, injury and repair.* New York: Raven Press, pp 77–91.
2. Alm A, Ekstrom H, Gillquist J, Stromberg B. (1974): The anterior cruciate ligament: a clinical and experimental study on tensile strength, morphology, and replacement by patellar ligament. *Acta Chir Scand,* 445[Suppl]:1–49.
3. Amiel D, Frank C, Harwood F, Fronek J, Akeson W. (1984): Tendons and ligaments (1984): a morphological and biochemical comparison. *J Orthop Res,* 1:257–265.
4. Amiel D, Kleiner JB, Roux RD, Harwood FL, Akeson WH. (1986): The phenomenon of "ligamentization": anterior cruciate ligament reconstruction with autogenous patellar tendon. *J Orthop Res,* 4:162–172.
5. Amis AA, Dawkins GPC. (1991): Functional anatomy of the anterior cruciate ligament: fibre bundle actions related to ligament replacements and injuries. *J Bone Joint Surg [Br],* 73B:260–267.
6. Anderson H. (1961): Histochemical studies on the histogenesis of the knee joint and superior tibio-fibular joint in human foetuses. *Acta Anat (Basel),* 46:279–303.
7. Arnoczky SP. (1983): Anatomy of the anterior cruciate ligament. *Clin Orthop,* 172:19–25.
8. Arnoczky SP. (1985): Blood supply to the anterior cruciate ligament and supporting structures. *Orthop Clin North Am,* 16:15–28.
9. Arnoczky SP, Warren RF. (1988): Anatomy of the cruciate ligaments. In: Feagin JA Jr, ed. *The cruciate ligaments.* New York: Churchill Livingstone, pp 179–195.
10. Arnoczky SP, Rubin RM, Marshall JL. (1979): Microvasculature of the cruciate ligaments and its response to injury. *J Bone Joint Surg [Am],* 61A:1221–1229.
11. Brantigan OC, Voshell AF. (1941): The mechanics of the ligaments and menisci of the knee joint. *J Bone Joint Surg [Am],* 23A:44–66.
12. Bray DF, Frank CB, Bray RC. (1990): Cytochemical evidence for a proteoglycan-associated filamentous network in ligament extracellular matrix. *J Orthop Res,* 8:1–12.
13. Bray R, Frank C, Miniaci A. (1991): Structure and function of diathrodial joints. In: McGinty JB et al., eds. *Operative arthroscopy.* New York: Raven Press, pp 79–123.
14. Bray RC, Fisher AWF, Frank CB. (1990): Fine vascular anatomy of adult rabbit knee ligaments. *J Anat,* 172:69–79.
15. Buckwalter JA. (1991): Cartilage. In: Dulbecco, ed. *Encyclopedia of human biology.* San Diego: Academic Press, vol 2, pp 201–215.
16. Buckwalter JA, Cooper RR. (1987): The cells and matrices of skeletal connective tissues. In: Albright, Brand, eds. *The scientific basis of orthopaedics.* Norwalk, CT: Appleton and Lange, pp 1–29.
17. Buckwalter JA, Cruess R. (1991): Healing of musculoskeletal tissues. In: Rockwood, Greene, eds. *Fractures.* Philadelphia: Lippincott, pp 181–222.
18. Buckwalter JA, Maynard JA, Vailas AC. (1987): Skeletal fibrous tissues: tendon, joint capsule and ligament. In: Albright, Brand, eds. *The scientific basis of orthopaedics.* Appleton and Lange.
19. Clark JM, Sidles JA. (1990): The interrelation of fiber bundles in the anterior cruciate ligament. *J Orthop Res,* 8:180–188.
20. Cooper RR, Misol S. (1970): Tendon and ligament insertion: a light and electron microscopic study. *J Bone Joint Surg [Am],* 52A:1–20.
21. Danylchuk KD, Finlay JB, Krcek JP. (1978): Microstructural organization of human and bovine cruciate ligaments. *Clin Orthop,* 131:294–298.
22. Ellison AE, Berg EE. (1985): Embryology, anatomy, and function of the anterior cruciate ligament. *Orthop Clin North Am,* 16:3–14.
23. Frank CB, Hart DA. (1990): The biology of tendons and ligaments. In: Mow, Radcliffe, Woo, eds. *Biomechanics of diarthrodial joints.* Berlin: Springer-Verlag.
24. Frank CB, McDonald D, Leiber RL, et al. Biochemical heterogeneity within maturing rabbit medial collateral ligament. *Clin Orthop,* 236:279–285.
25. Frank CB, Woo SL-Y, Andriacchi T, Brand R, Oakes B, Dahners L, DeHaven K, Leis J, Sabiston P. (1988): Normal ligament: structure, function, and composition. In: Woo, Buckwalter, eds. *Injury and repair of the musculoskeletal soft tissues.* Park Ridge, Ill: American Academy of Orthopaedic Surgeons.
26. Furman W, Marshall JL, Girgis FG. (1976): The anterior cruciate ligament: a functional analysis based on post-mortem studies. *J Bone Joint Surg [Am],* 58A:179–185.
27. Fuss FK. (1989): Anatomy of the cruciate ligaments and their function in extension and flexion of the human knee joint. *Am J Anat,* 184:165–176.
28. Gardner E, O'Rahilly R. (1968): The early development of the knee joint in staged human embryos. *J Anat,* 102:289–299.
29. Girgis FG, Marshall JL, Monajem ARS. (1975): The cruciate ligaments of the knee joint. *Clin Orthop,* 106:216–231.
30. Gray DJ, Gardner E. (1950): Prenatal development of the human knee and superio-tibiofibular joints. *Am J Anat,* 86:235–288.
31. Gray H, Gross CM, ed. (1975): *Anatomy of the human body.* 29th ed. Philadelphia: Lea & Febiger.
32. Halata Z, Haus J. (1989): The ultrastructure of sensory nerve endings in human anterior cruciate ligament. *Anat Embryol (Berl),* 179:415–421.

33. Hardingham TE. (1981): Proteoglycans: Their structure, interactions, and molecular organization in cartilage. *Biochem Soc Trans,* 9:489–497.

34. Hascall VC. (1977): Interactions of cartilage proteoglycans with hyaluronic acid. *J Supramol Structure,* 7:101–120.

35. Hefzy MS, Grood ES. (1986): Sensitivity of insertion locations on length patterns of anterior cruciate ligament fibers. *J Biomech Eng,* 108:73–82.

36. Heinegaard D, Paulsson M. (1984): Structure and metabolism of proteoglycans. In: Piez KA, Reddi AH, eds. *Extracellular matrix biochemistry.* New York: Elsevier, pp 278–328.

37. Howell SM, Clark JA, Farley TE. (1991): A rationale for predicting anterior cruciate graft impingement by the intercondylar roof: A magnetic resonance imaging study. *Am J Sports Med,* 19:276–282.

38. Kaplan EB. (1962): Some aspects of functional anatomy of the human knee joint. *Clin Orthop,* 23:18–29.

39. Kennedy JC, Alexander IJ, Hayes KC. (1982): Nerve supply of the human knee and its functional importance. *Am J Sports Med,* 10:329–335.

40. Kennedy JC, Weinberg HW, Wilson AS. (1974): The anatomy and function of the anterior cruciate ligament as determined by clinical and morphological studies. *J Bone Joint Surg [Am],* 56A:223–235.

41. Last RJ. (1948): Some anatomical details of the knee joint. *J Bone Joint Surg [Br],* 30B:683–688.

42. Lyon RM, Akeson WH, Amiel D, Kitabayashi LR, Woo SL-Y. (1991): Ultrastructural differences between the cells of the medial collateral and anterior cruciate ligaments. *Clin Orthop,* 272:279–286.

43. Makisalo SE, Paavolainen PP, Lehto M, Skutnabb K, Slatis P. (1989): Collagen Types I and III and fibronectin in healing anterior cruciate ligament after reconstruction with carbon fiber. *Injury,* 20:72–76.

44. Marinozzi G, Ferrante F, Gaudio E, Ricci A, Amenta F. (1991): Intrinsic innervation of the rat knee joint articular capsule and ligaments. *Acta Anat (Basel),* 141:8–14.

45. Marshall JL, Arnoczky SP, Rubin TL, Wickiewicz TL. (1979): Microvasculature of the cruciate ligaments. *Phys Sports Med,* 7:87–91.

46. Matyas JR. (1985): *The structure and function of tendon and ligament insertions to bone* [Thesis]. New York: Cornell University Medical College.

47. McDermott LJ. (1943): Development of the human knee joint. *Arch Surg,* 46:705–719.

48. Muir H. (1983): Proteoglycans as organizers of the extracellular matrix. *Biochem Soc Trans,* 11:613–622.

49. Muller W. (1983): *The knee: form, function and ligamentous reconstruction.* New York: Springer-Verlag.

50. Nimni ME, Harkness RD. (1988): Molecular structures and functions of collagen. In: Nimni ME, ed. *Collagen: biochemistry.* Cleveland, OH: CRC Press, vol 1, p 77.

51. Nimni ME. (1983): Collagen: structure, function, and metabolism in normal and fibrotic tissues. *Semin Arthritis Rheum,* 13:1–86.

52. Norwood LA, Cross MJ. (1977): The intercondylar shelf and the anterior cruciate ligament. *Am J Sports Med,* 5:171–176.

53. Norwood LA, Cross MJ. (1979): Anterior cruciate ligament: functional anatomy of its bundles in rotary instability. *Am J Sports Med,* 7:23–26.

54. Odensten M, Gillquist J. (1985): Functional anatomy of the anterior cruciate ligament and a rationale for reconstruction. *J Bone Joint Surg [Am],* 67A:257–262.

55. Palmer I. (1938): On the injuries to the ligaments of the knee joint: a clinical study. *Acta Chir Scand,* 81[Suppl 53]:2–282.

56. Parry DAD, Barnes GRG, Craig AS. (1978): A comparison of the size distribution of collagen fibrils in connective tissues as a function of age and a possible relationship between fibril size distribution and mechanical properties. *Proc R Soc Lond [Biol],* 203:305–321.

57. Parry DAD, Craig AS. (1988): Collagen fibrils during development and maturation and their contribution to the mechanical attributes of connective tissue. In: Nimni M, ed. *Collagen.* Cleveland, OH: CRC Press, vol 2.

58. Poole AR, Webbed C, Pidoux I, Choi H, Rosenberg LC. (1986): Localization of a dermatan sulfate proteoglycan (DSPGII) in cartilage and the presence of an immunologically related species in other tissues. *J Histochem Cytochem,* 34:619–625.

59. Rosenberg LH, Choi HU, Neame PJ, Sasse J, Roughley PJ, Poole AR. (1990): Proteoglycans of soft connective tissues. In: Leadbetter, Buckwalter, Gordon, eds. *Sports induced inflammation—basic science and clinical concepts.* Park Ridge, Ill: American Academy of Orthopaedic Surgeons.

60. Rosenberg LC, Choi HU, Poole AR, Lewandowska K, Culp LA. (1986): Biological roles of dermatan sulfate proteoglycans. *Ciba Found Symp,* 124:47–61.

61. Sapega AA, Moyer RA, Schneck C, Komalahiranya N. (1990): Testing for isometry during reconstruction of the anterior cruciate ligament: anatomical and biomechanical considerations. *J Bone Joint Surg [Am],* 72A:259–267.

62. Scapinelli R. (1968): Studies on the vasculature of the human knee joint. *Acta Anat (Basel),* 70:305–331.

63. Schultz RA, Miller DC, Kerr CS, Micheli L. (1984): Mechanoreceptors in human cruciate ligaments. *J Bone Joint Surg [Am],* 66A:1072–1076.

64. Schutte MJ, Dabezies EJ, Zimny ML, Happel LT. (1987): Neural anatomy of the human anterior cruciate ligament. *J Bone Joint Surg [Am],* 69A:243–247.

65. Sidles JA, Larson RV, Garbibi JL, Downey DJ, Matsen FA. (1988): Ligament length relationships in the moving knee. *J Orthop Res,* 6:593–610.

66. Sutton JB. (1887): *Ligaments: their nature and morphology.* Philadelphia, Blakiston and Son.

67. Welsh RP. (1980): Knee joint structure and function. *Clin Orthop,* 147:7–14.

68. Wladmirow B. (1968): Arterial sources of blood supply of the knee joint in man. *Acta Med,* 47:1–10.

69. Woo SL-Y, Maynard J, Butler D, Lyon R, Torzilli PA, Akeson WH, Cooper RR, Oakes B. (1987): Ligament, tendon, and joint capsule insertions to bone. In: Woo SL-Y, Buckwalter JA, eds. *Injury and repair of the musculoskeletal soft tissues.* Park Ridge, Ill: American Academy of Orthopaedic Surgeons, pp 133–166.

70. Yahia LH, Drouin G. (1989): Microscopical investigation of canine anterior cruciate ligament and patellar tendon: Collagen fascicle morphology and architecture. *J Orthop Res,* 7:243–251.

71. Zimny ML. (1988): Mechanoreceptors in articular tissues. *Am J Anat,* 182:16–32.

72. Zimny ML, Schutte M, Dabezies E. (1986): Mechanoreceptors in the human anterior cruciate ligament. *Anat Rec,* 214:204–209.

The Anterior Cruciate Ligament: Current and Future Concepts, edited by D.W. Jackson, et al. Raven Press, Ltd., New York © 1993.

CHAPTER 2

The Sensory Role of the Anterior Cruciate Ligament

Steven M. Madey, Kelly J. Cole, and Richard A. Brand

Numerous studies demonstrate neural elements within the anterior cruciate ligament of a diverse group of species, most notably the cat and human being (15,36,47, 50,51,61,62,66,84,85,89,90,93,95,96). Furthermore, mechanical stimulation of the ACL produces discharge of peripheral afferent fibers supplying the knee joint of experimental animals (63,78). Based on these findings and the continuing controversy that surrounds treatment and long-term outcome of the ACL-injured patient (1,6,24,58,59,74,77,94), some authors have suggested a sensory role for ligaments (3,17,18,31,61,94) and specifically the ACL (17,18,53,56,57,62,63,89,96). However, the functional significance of input to the central nervous system (CNS) from these neural elements remains unclear.

THE INNERVATION OF THE ANTERIOR CRUCIATE LIGAMENT

The human knee joint has a rich afferent and efferent neural supply. Although several authors have noted variability of nerve branches that innervate the joint (38,52), Kennedy et al. (61) described two distinct patterns and categorized the joint sensory branches into anterior and posterior groups. These general patterns of knee joint innervation are similar in the cat (36,39,90).

The anterior group consists of articular branches from the femoral, common peroneal, and saphenous nerves. The femoral nerve gives rise to small articular branches after it pierces the three vastus muscles. The common peroneal nerve gives rise to the lateral articular nerve (LAN) and the recurrent peroneal nerve. The saphenous nerve (itself a branch of the femoral nerve) gives rise to the medial articular nerve (MAN).

The posterior group consists of articular branches from the tibial and obturator nerves. The tibial nerve gives rise to the posterior articular nerve (PAN). The obturator forms articular branches at its terminus (61).

The innervation of the ACL has most often been attributed to the PAN in the human being (38,52,61) and the cat (5,33,36,78). The PAN is generally the largest and most consistent articular branch supplying the joint in both cat and human, although its origin is variable in both species (38,75). However, most authors acknowledge that other articular branches may make some contribution to the ACL. By injecting the neuronal tracer wheat germ agglutinin-horseradish peroxidase (WGA-HRP) into distinct regions of cat ACL and allowing retrograde axonal transport to label cell bodies in the lumbar dorsal root ganglion, Gomez Barrena et al. (40) documented that the MAN and LAN innervate a significant portion of the ACL along with the PAN.

THE NERVE FIBERS WITHIN THE ACL

Several authors (61,84,85) identified various nerve fibers within the human ACL. Specifically, Haus and Halata (50) differentiated four types of fibers: those composed of only unmyelinated axons; mixed (composed of both myelinated and unmyelinated axons); mixed, associated with one to three blood vessels at their margins; and mixed, associated with vessels at their margins and possessing an additional perineural sheath. These fibers are characteristically found in the loose and fibrous subsynovial connective tissue as it encompasses the entire ACL and invests between collagen fascicles (50,51,84).

S. M. Madey and R. A. Brand: Department of Orthopaedic Surgery, University of Iowa Hospital, Iowa City, Iowa 52242.

K. J. Cole: Department of Exercise Science, University of Iowa, Iowa City, Iowa 52242.

THE NERVE ENDINGS OF JOINTS AND THE ACL

Various investigators have described four types of neural receptors in both the cat (89) and human ACL (85,95). Their function remains speculative because no studies of the ACL correlate histology and physiologic response, but functions (inferred from discharge properties similar to those of morphologically well-defined receptors in skin, tendon, and periarticular tissues) are both mechanoreceptive and nociceptive (14,16,47,50, 61,84,85,89,96). Freeman and Wyke (36), by examining receptor size and shape as well as morphologic characteristics of capsule, parent axon, feeding axon, and terminal axon, described four types of endings in the cat knee joint at the light microscope level. Their nomenclature continues to be used today and is applicable to the endings of the ACL at the light microscope level.

Type I endings are bean-shaped, globular corpuscles with average dimensions of 40 × 100 μm; they are surrounded by a thin capsule consisting of one to two layers of connective tissue cells. Each corpuscle is fed at its hilum by a myelinated branch of a parent axon measuring 5 to 8 μm in diameter. The branch axon loses its myelination upon entering the corpuscle and arborizes into multiple terminal axons.

Type II endings are elongated, conical corpuscles (average dimensions of 120 × 280 μm) surrounded by a thick multilayered capsule composed of connective tissue and fibroblasts. The corpuscle is fed at its base by a myelinated branch of a parent axon averaging 8 to 12 μm in diameter. The branch axon loses its myelination upon entering the corpuscle but becomes "ensheathed" by columnar cells (Fig. 1).

Type III endings are fusiform with average dimensions of 100 × 600 μm and are surrounded by a thin capsule composed of one to three layers of connective tissue and cells. Freeman and Wyke (36) reported that Type III endings were confined to ligaments. The long axis of the ending parallels the long axis of the ligament, and the receptor capsule is intimately associated with ligamentous collagen fascicles. These endings are fed directly by a myelinated parent axon that enters from the side, losing its myelin sheath to form a dense arborization of axons with numerous globular expansions along their length.

Type IV endings are noncorpuscular, unmyelinated nerve filaments with an average diameter of 0.5 to 1.5 μm. They have no capsule, and they are fed by both myelinated and unmyelinated parent axons, whose average diameter is 1 to 5 μm.

Joint receptors (as well as those of nonarticular tissue) show a certain degree of variability. Freeman and Wyke specifically chose a numerical classification system so as not to "homologize" joint receptors with those of nonarticular tissue (36). However, each joint receptor has a nonarticular analog with well-characterized physiological properties. Based on morphological criteria, Type I endings resemble slowly adapting, low-threshold Ruffini endings of subcutaneous tissue and are also referred to as "spray" type endings (15); Type II endings resemble rapidly adapting, low-threshold Pacinian corpuscles of subcutaneous tissue and are also referred to as "lamellar" type endings (15); Type III endings resemble slowly adapting, low-threshold Golgi tendon organs; and Type IV endings resemble free nerve endings (16,47,50,62, 84,89,93). Furthermore, by linking receptor histology in the joint capsule to discharge patterns of its feeding axon, Boyd (15) characterized "spray" type endings as slowly adapting and "lamellar" type endings as rapidly adapting receptors, whereas Grigg and Hoffman (45) concluded that "Ruffini" afferents respond to tension and shear stress directed along the long axis of the joint capsule but not to pressure.

In the human ACL all four types of endings that fit the morphological criteria put forth by Freeman and Wyke have been described at the light (36) and at the electron microscopic (47) level. Most authors, however, refer to Ruffini, Pacinian, Golgi tendon organs, and free nerve endings, respectively, rather than using Freeman and Wyke's nomenclature (14,16,47,50,62,84,85,89,93,95, 96). Golgi tendon organs have been described in the cat (15,36,89,90) and human ACL (84,85) at the light microscope level, but descriptions and published photomicrographs do not always clearly distinguish them from Ruffini endings. Realizing that at times it is difficult to classify a given receptor based upon light microscopy and that functional homology to nonarticular receptors remains to be fully established, we will use eponyms throughout this section.

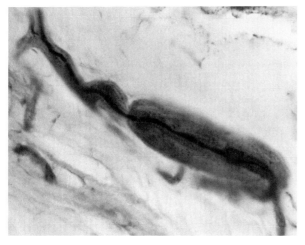

FIG. 1. Pacinian receptor of the posterior capsule in the cat. Note the single parent axon, thick inner core, and large capsule. (Gold chloride stain, ×400) (Courtesy of Robert McClain.)

At the ultrastructural level in the human ACL, Halata and Haus (47) distinguished Ruffini corpuscles, Pacinian corpuscles, and free nerve endings based on terminal axon association with Schwann cells, endoneurium, and perineurium. The terminal axons of Ruffini corpuscles are incompletely covered by Schwann cells, which allows the axolemma to come into direct contact with the collagen of the endoneurium. In addition, the capsules of Ruffini corpuscles have gaps at their distal ends, which allows the endoneurium to blend with collagen matrix outside the ending. The terminal axons of Pacinian corpuscles, on the other hand, are completely covered by Schwann cells and do not contact the endoneurium. The Schwann cells often form layers, the composite of which is referred to as the "inner core." These "inner cores" are completely surrounded by a perineural capsule up to 35 layers thick. This gives a characteristic "lamellar" appearance.

No study to date definitively reports the number or location of receptors within the cat or human ACL, although Schutte (85) reported that 1% of the "area" of the human ACL is composed of neural elements and that Pacinian corpuscles outnumbered Ruffini endings. Haus and Halata (50) examined 26 human ACLs and found 21 total Ruffini corpuscles and 5 Pacinian corpuscles, whereas Schultz et al. (84) reported 1 to 3 endings, morphologically similar to Golgi tendon organs, per ligament. After viewing the ACL in sagittal section, Zimny et al. (96) reported that most receptors were found at the tibial attachment, whereas Schultz et al. (84) and Haus and Halata (50) reported more at the femoral attachment.

Most investigators agree that, in cross-section, receptors are more frequently found in the subsynovial connective tissue that both surrounds the entire ligament and is interspersed between adjacent collagen fascicles (47,61,84). Although endings are not reported in the thin synovial lining, they are occasionally found within collagen fascicles (89) (Fig. 2).

Ambiguities among reports on joint and ACL receptors stem in part from limitations in histological processing techniques and interpretation and/or classification of stained structures. Gold, silver, and methylene blue are the most frequently used stains for investigation in both cats (16,36,89,90) and humans (50,61,84,85,95–97) but lack specificity for neural elements in joint tissue (9). Because of this significant problem, De Avila et al. (30) questioned the validity of certain joint receptor descriptions and suggested more rigid criteria when discerning between neural and nonneural tissue, such as identification of nodes of Ranvier in axons and the "lattice work" pattern of endothelial junctions in blood vessels. The use of thicker serial sections for preservation of axon and receptor continuity allows confirmation that a putative axon in fact ends within a receptor, and modifications in staining technique (97) decrease background artifact. Ultrastructural histological techniques afford increased specificity and resolution of joint receptors (7) but do so at the expense of viewing range (9).

The neuronal tracer horseradish peroxidase (conjugated with wheat germ agglutinin) may solve the problem of specificity. Madey et al. (66) pressure-injected WGA-HRP into the dorsal root ganglia, which house the cell bodies of joint afferents (28,40), and obtained excellent definition of receptors in the cat knee, including the ACL, with little background artifact (Figs. 3–6). Presumably only nerve structures can be labeled, avoiding confusion with other structures. However, this technique does not seem to allow for the detailed appearances required for novel classification schemes.

Also, the small sample sizes used for all studies on human ACL to date most likely do not represent a true population cross-section and can introduce age and pathological bias. Indeed, Salo and Tatton (82) showed a 37% decrease in labeling of mouse joint afferents between the ages of 3 to 4 months and 16 to 18 months, implying a significant reduction in receptor number with age. Such changes imply at least the possibility that

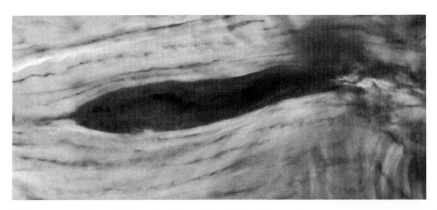

FIG. 2. ACL receptor within collagen fascicles of cat ACL. The receptor is parallel to collagen bundles. (Gold chloride stain, ×400) (Courtesy of Robert McClain.)

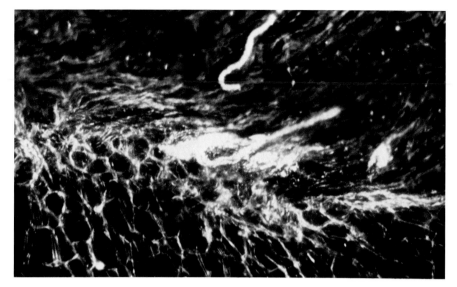

FIG. 3. Ruffini ending of the posterior capsule in the cat. Note two axons feeding two corpuscles. The background is adipose and fibrous connective tissue. (WGA-HRP stain, ×100)

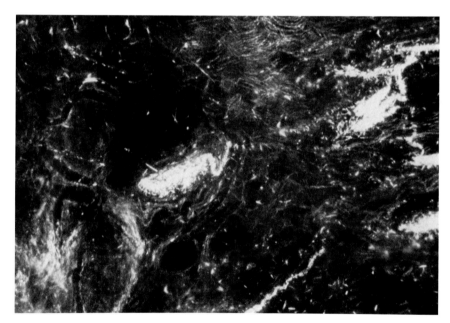

FIG. 4. Pacinian ending of the posterior capsule in the cat. Note the single parent axon, thick inner core, and thickened capsule. The background is fibrous connective tissue, and other neural elements are visible. (WGA-HRP stain, ×100)

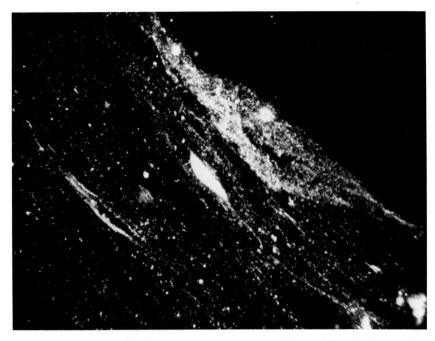

FIG. 5. Ellipsoid receptor of cat ACL. Note the homogeneous staining and the single parent axon parallel to collagen bundles. (WGA-HRP stain, ×40)

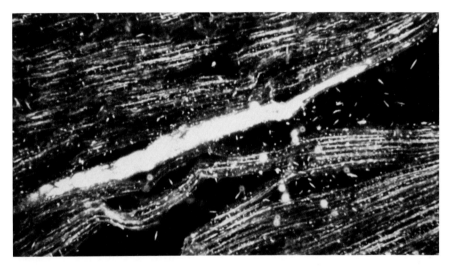

FIG. 6. Golgi tendon organ of cat ACL. Note segmentation within the receptor and the thin capsule parallel to collagen bundles. Demonstrated in 14 consecutive 30-μm-thick sections. (WGA-HRP stain, ×40)

ligament mechanoreceptors play a more important role in the development of central motor patterns in the young but become less important with age once the central patterns become established. On the other hand, the reduction in mechanoreceptors may represent a more simple attrition process with aging that is consistent with loss of receptors in other regions, such as the glabrous skin (23). Indeed, knee joint position sense declines with age (11).

THE PHYSIOLOGICAL CHARACTERISTICS OF ACL MECHANORECEPTORS

Recent studies have correlated mechanical stimulation of the cat ACL and axonal discharge properties of peripheral afferents. Pope et al. (78) recorded from single PAN afferents during increased tension or punctate pressure stimulation of the ACL and described afferents sensitive to tension or pressure, or both. The threshold sensitivities to tension or direct pressure ranged from a few to 10 g. In addition, these afferents were low threshold, slowly adapting; low threshold, rapidly adapting; or high threshold, slowly adapting. The investigators did not establish which receptors were innervated by these axons nor the conduction velocities of the axons. In all, 36 afferents were identified in 39 knees, but the largest number of afferents in a single knee was 3 (Figs. 7 and 8).

In a subsequent study, by Krauspe et al. (63), 26 afferents were identified in 13 cat knees. Based on conduction velocities, 24 of these axons comprised 79% Group II (thick myelinated), 13% Group III (thin myelinated), and 8% Group IV (unmyelinated). Mechanical thresholds, tested with von Frey hairs, ranged from 0.7 to 15 g (similar to those reported by Pope et al.), with the largest receptive field, of high sensitivity, less than 0.5 mm. No units were reported active in the resting knee at 30° of flexion, but all units responded to movement (rotation of the extended knee, flexion, and extension). Increased firing was noted as the knee loads were increased over physiological ranges. Finally, Ferrell (33) reported that 26 slowly adapting cruciate afferents (not specified further) were active throughout the midrange of joint movement.

KNEES	TOTAL AFFERENTS	TENSION	PRESSURE	TENSION/ PRESSURE
39	36[1]	15	4	3

The maximum number of discriminable units from a single knee was three.

FIG. 7. Recording from 39 afferents in PAN during mechanical stimulation of cat ACL with the tibial insertion freed from the tibia with bone block. (Courtesy of Pope et al.)

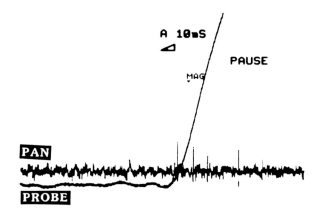

CH1 50mV CH2 10mV

FIG. 8. Recording of a rapidly adapting, pressure-sensitive afferent during mechanical stimulation of cat ACL with a blunt probe. Spike average potentials were utilized for isolation of the single afferent. (Courtesy of Pope et al.)

THE CONTRIBUTIONS OF ACL AND JOINT SENSORY ELEMENTS TO MOTOR CONTROL

Attempts to define a specific role for the sensory elements of the ACL by direct effects on skeletal motoneurons in the cat have led to equivocal results. Solomonow et al. (91) showed hamstring EMG activity of chloralose-anesthetized cats by loading the ACL. Responses were elicited at supraphysiological loads (four to five times body weight), supporting the existence of a ligamento-muscular reflex. However, Pope et al. (79) were unable to show any hamstring or quadriceps EMG activity using a similar experimental protocol. Possible explanations for this discrepancy, given by the latter authors, include the unpredictable effect of chloralose on reflex hyperexcitability at varying time and dosages (8) and the variable effect of joint angle on reflex activity (29,42).

Apparent contradictions may be explained in part by a lack of clear understanding about peripheral afferent contributions to the motor control system in general, as well as the fact that joint receptors have a weak direct influence on alpha motoneurons. Although electrical stimulation of knee joint afferents facilitates Ib interneurons (48,65), thus indicating that synaptic connections exist for reflex modulation by joint afferents, the specific role of joint afferents in lower limb control is difficult to interpret because of the indiscriminate, nonphysiological activation of afferents by electricity (44).

Furthermore, experimental designs that have utilized more physiological loading conditions have led to contradictory results. Focal loads applied to discrete areas of the joint have shown both facilitation (2,13) and inhibition (31) of quadriceps (the latter study also showing hamstring facilitation); mechanical stimulation of joint receptors by knee flexion has produced both facilitation

(2,26) and inhibition of muscles that contribute to knee movement (90). Possible explanations for the ambiguity in the results of these studies include the variable effect of knee joint angle on joint afferent input to the CNS (29,42); unpredictable effects on segmental reflexes of removing supraspinal and cortical influences on the spinal cord by spinalization and decortication (68); and bias of experimental design that yields anticipated results as opposed to systematic or random experimental conditions (42). However, even though the specific results seem contradictory, most studies document some effect of joint afferents on skeletal motoneurons. Indeed, Freeman and Wyke (35) severed the MAN and PAN in the cat and produced significant alterations in posture and movement, whereas Marshall and Tatton (68) demonstrated unbalancing of EMG output to muscles acting at the knee when the joint was anesthetized with lidocaine in the awake cat and changes in the latency, amplitude, and duration of EMG responses to joint load perturbations.

Perhaps the most compelling evidence supporting a functional role of sensory input from the ACL in motor control comes from a series of investigations by Johansson and colleagues (53–57,89). They have shown that mechanical stimulation of the sensory elements of the ACL (and PCL) has a significant effect on Ia afferent discharge from muscle spindles, presumably through gamma motor neurons. Tensile loads of 500 to 2,000 g (5 to 20 N) applied to the intact ACL produced a significant change in response patterns in many of the muscle spindles in sinusoidally stretched knee flexors (73% of triceps surae and 55% of posterior biceps and semitendinosus). In light of muscle spindle afferent influence on muscle stiffness (73,80), the findings by Johansson et al. provide indirect evidence for a sensorimotor role of the ACL by influences on the gamma motor neuron system.

THE ROLE OF ACL SENSORY ELEMENTS IN PROPRIOCEPTION

The term *proprioception* is often used to describe the ability of the CNS to determine relative position and movement of body segments to one another, whether manipulated actively or passively at both the conscious and the unconscious levels (92). When considering this definition one must keep several points in mind. First, this description varies from that originally intended by Sherrington in 1906 (86), who clearly distinguished the proprioceptive system from the exteroceptive system as one that could respond to stimuli "traceable to the organism's own actions." However, exteroceptive cutaneous ("nonproprioceptive") receptors probably contribute to position sense (37). Second, active and passive movement of limb segments produces different patterns of mechanoreceptor discharge (32). This is important in the interpretation of experimental data, when most limb

movements are passive. Third, peripheral sensory information diverges (60) throughout the CNS and contributes to unconscious motor control at many levels (86). It enters into subjective awareness and is *sensed,* per se, only upon reaching the primary somatic sensory cortex (60,71). Furthermore, evidence supports the ability of individuals to distinguish between position sense and movement sense and detect the latter at smaller increments of displacement (92). It seems likely, but is unproven, that this distinction is also made at the unconscious level.

The importance of joint receptors to conscious sensation of joint motion or position remains unclear. Investigations by Boyd (15), Andrew and Dodt (4), Freeman and Wyke (36), and Skoglund (90) indicated that joint receptors could be activated throughout the full range of joint movement and thus supported joint receptors as major contributors to proprioceptive input. Later evidence refuted these initial findings and thrust muscle spindles into this role (20,25,41,69). However, a role for joint receptors is suggested by studies of Gandevia and McCloskey (37), who took advantage of the anatomical characteristics of the human hand that permit functional disengagement of flexors and extensors of the distal phalanx of the long finger. Their results showed that muscle, joint, and cutaneous receptors were all important in position sense. In addition, Ferrell (33) confirmed that some knee joint receptors and cruciate ligament receptors were capable of signaling position through the entire range of physiological movement. Also, Krauspe et al. (63) showed that receptors of the ACL were capable of firing afferents from full extension through 60° of flexion (but not at 30° flexion). Tensile loads on the joint capsule enhance the activation of joint afferents; thus, the range of knee angles over which joint receptors are active is dependent on the state of contraction of muscles crossing the knee (42,43). Also, joint afferents may preferentially signal movement over position (81).

There is a question as to whether injury of the ACL leads to abnormal subjective awareness of joint position and motion. Harter et al. (49) observed no difference in ability to reproduce knee position in ACL-reconstructed versus normal contralateral knee with an average follow-up of 48 months. Barrack et al. (10), on the other hand, noted a significant difference between ACL-deficient and normal knees in detecting slow movements. This study was conducted on average 3 months after injury treated conservatively. However, comparison of these studies is somewhat limited. The longer follow-up time of Harter et al. could have allowed CNS adaptation for loss of certain receptor groups. The study of Barrack et al. focused on detection of movement, whereas Harter et al. focused on matching static positions of experimental and control knees, a maneuver that can be affected by memory (19). However, a recent study of joint position sense in ACL-deficient knees examined both detection of movement and the ability to reproduce static position and found both deficient in cruciate-injured patients 2 to 14 years postinjury (27).

THE IMPLICATIONS OF THE SENSORY ROLE OF THE ACL

The existence of free nerve endings connected to fine, unmyelinated afferents within the ACL provides the potential for nociception (46). Many of these fine, myelinated and unmyelinated afferents also are activated preferentially by normal movements in the presence of inflammatory mediators (83). Ruffini endings, Pacinian corpuscles, and Golgi tendon organs provide for potential mechanoreception. Ruffini endings and Golgi tendon organs most likely respond to tension and Pacinian endings to pressure. And, indeed, these two modalities of ACL mechanical stimulation elicit axonal responses in the cat (63,78). Close association of receptors with collagen bundles of the ACL provide a mechanism of signal transduction of loads that create tension within the ligament, such as anterior translation of the tibia on the femur, varus-valgus stress, and rotation at the knee joint. However, this is not the only potential mechanism for ACL receptor stimulation. Several areas of the ACL are juxtaposed with other knee structures. The femoral insertion is associated with the posterior capsule, the midportion with the posterior cruciate ligament, and the tibial insertion with the anterior insertion sites of both the medial and the lateral menisci. In addition, the synovial and subsynovial tissue of the ACL is continuous with that of these other structures. This places the receptors of the ACL in a position to respond to both pressure and tension created by the interaction of ACL and juxtaposed structures.

Both tension and pressure ACL receptors in the cat are responsive to a wide range of loads, from as little as a few grams (63,78) to much higher loads generated by forced hyperextension or internal and external rotation (63). Furthermore, the response pattern seems to be graded with increasing signals corresponding to increased loads. Thus, ACL receptors may contribute information on both the position of the knee in physiological ranges as well as during the limits of joint motion, which could be integrated into the CNS in a manner similar to that of joint receptors, namely at the level of spinal reflexes (2,12,13,15,26,31,44,65,90), the cerebellum (64) dorsal column nuclei, the thalamus, and areas of primary somatic sensory cortex (70).

If sensory information provided by ACL receptors is important, its loss could lead to the unbalancing of muscle forces acting about the knee, with consequent subtle instability and long-term progression to osteoarthritis (76). Indeed, muscles that cross the knee joint contribute not only to posture and movement of the lower limb, but also to joint stability (34). Markolf et al. (67) demonstrated that contraction of the muscles acting at the knee substantially increases knee joint stiffness. Normal subjects tested during voluntary contraction of knee flexors and extensors showed a decrease in anterior/posterior displacement of the tibia on the femur as well as a 2.2 to 4.2 increase in joint stiffness during varus-valgus loads. Furthermore, Nichols and Houk (73) reported decreased stiffness of muscles crossing the knee with loss of sensory input, with rapid yielding of muscles subjected to constant displacement. However, with the afferent input intact, the muscles did not yield and exhibited a substantial increase in stiffness.

Some EMG studies seem consistent with the notion of unbalancing of muscles after ligament injury. In comparing ACL-deficient and normal individuals, Sinkjaer et al. (88) showed changes in muscle recruitment, while Shiavi et al. (87) showed subtle (but in our opinion functionally questionable) changes in EMG patterns during walking. Carlsoo and Nordstrand (21), on the other hand, reported no difference in muscle coordination. Whether or not there are abnormal patterns of muscle firing after ACL injury, one must keep in mind that even minimal subluxation of the tibia on the femur (i.e., resulting from loss of passive joint stability) will most likely activate a wide array of joint, tendon, and muscle receptors, the input of which to the CNS could explain altered muscle firing patterns (79). Thus, it would be difficult to know whether any functionally significant changes were in fact primary (i.e., due to loss of sensory input from the torn ACL) or secondary (i.e., due to increased sensory input from non-ACL periarticular receptors during subluxation).

Current information about mechanoreceptors raises certain questions about the treatment of ACL injuries: (a) What degree of disability after injury relates to structural loss, and what degree relates to neurosensory loss? (b) Does neurosensory loss ever constitute the major degree of disability? (c) Can we distinguish structural from neurosensory disability? (d) If neurosensory loss is functionally important, to what degree can the neuromuscular system adapt? (e) Can we enhance adaptation? (f) Can we restore neurosensory loss?

These more general questions imply more immediate considerations: (a) Are the receptors remaining (particularly near the femoral and tibial attachments) sufficiently important to retain? (b) Can mechanoreceptors regrow into repaired or reconstructed ligaments? With our present knowledge, it seems questionable that retention or repair of a stump would lead to mechanically competent mechanoreceptors. To restore normal function, one would need to mimic the normal mechanical environment for the receptors. Given that they are sensitive to a few grams of load and that our ability to restore functional tension is probably no better than many Newtons of load (at least 3 orders of magnitude greater), any restoration would not likely be sufficiently sensitive, even assuming an enormous capacity of receptors to adapt to a new mechanical environment. Further, although peripheral nerves have the potential to regenerate into ligament, denervated receptors atrophy with time (22) and in skin even reinnervated receptors may be significantly altered histologically and functionally (72).

CONCLUSIONS

A number of pieces of evidence strongly point to a functionally important role for ligament mechanoreceptors: (a) Both cat and human ACLs contain nerve fibers and endings resembling mechanoreceptors. (b) Mechanical stimulation of the ACL in experimental animals reveals slowly and rapidly adapting, low-threshold neural elements within the ligament. (c) Afferent impulses generated by mechanical stimulation of these neural elements affect the central nervous system at virtually all levels, although the most compelling available evidence suggests that ligament mechanoreceptors affect muscle spindle output through influences on gamma motoneurons. (d) Some patients with ACL tears exhibit abnormal proprioception and altered EMG patterns. Taken together, these findings imply that the ACL has a sensory role and can make contributions to segmental reflexes, supraspinal levels of the motor system, and conscious awareness of joint movement and position through projections to primary somatic sensory cortex and other higher cortical centers. However, it remains unclear whether or not known and potential connections are functionally significant and whether their loss after injury contributes to disability.

ACKNOWLEDGMENTS

The authors acknowledge the help of Drs. Brian J. Daley and David F. Pope in the design and conduct of some of the experiments reported in the text. This work was supported in part by NIH Grants AR40199 and AR07075 and by a Bristol-Myers/Squibb/Zimmer Award for Excellence in Research administered through the Orthopaedic Research and Education Foundation.

REFERENCES

1. Andersson C, Odensten M, Good L, Gillquist J. (1989): Surgical or non surgical treatment of acute rupture of the anterior cruciate ligament. *J Bone Joint Surg [Am]*, 71A:965–974.
2. Andersson C, Stener B. (1959): Experimental evaluation of the hypothesis of ligamentomuscular protective reflexes: II. A study in cat using the mediocollateral ligament of the knee joint. *Acta Physiol Scand*, 48[Suppl 166]:27.
3. Andrew BL. (1954): The sensory innervation of the medial ligament of the knee joint. *J Physiol (Lond)*, 123:241–250.
4. Andrew BL, Dodt E. (1952): The deployment of sensory nerve endings at the knee joint of the cat. *Acta Physiol Scand*, 28:287–296.
5. Arnoczky SP. (1983): Anatomy of the anterior cruciate ligament. *Clin Orthop*, 172:19.
6. Arnold, JA, Coker TP, Heaton LM, Park JP, Harris W. (1979): Natural history of anterior cruciate tears. *J Sports Med*, 7:305–313.
7. Badalamente MA, Dee R, Propper M. (1984): Ultrastructural study of joint innervation. *Orthop Rev*, 8:212–216.
8. Balis G, Monroe R. (1964): The pharmacology of chloralose: A review. *Psychopharmacology*, 6:1–30.
9. Bancroft JD, Stevens A. (1990): *Theory and practice of histological techniques*. 3rd ed. London: Churchill Livingstone.
10. Barrack RL, Skinner HB, Buckley SL. (1989): Proprioception in the anterior cruciate deficient knee. *Am J Sports Med*, 17:1–6.
11. Barrett DS, Cobb AG, Bentley G. (1991): Joint proprioception in normal, osteoarthritic, and replaced knees. *J Bone Joint Surg [Br]*, 73B:53–56.
12. Baxendale RH, Ferrell WR. (1980): Modulation of transmission in flexion reflex pathways by knee joint afferent discharge in the decerebrate cat. *Brain Res*, 202:497–500.
13. Baxendale RH, Ferrell WR, Wood L. (1987): The effect of mechanical stimulation of knee joint afferents on quadriceps motor unit activity in the decerebrate cat. *Brain Res*, 415:353–356.
14. Bessette GC, Hunter RE. (1990): Anterior cruciate ligament. *Orthopedics*, 13:551–562.
15. Boyd IA. (1953): The histological structure of the receptors in the knee joint of the cat correlated with their physiological response. *J Physiol (Lond)*, 124:476–488.
16. Boyd IA, Roberts TDM. (1954): Proprioceptive discharges from stretch receptors in the knee-joint of the cat. *J Physiol (Lond)*, 122:38–58.
17. Brand RA. Knee ligaments: a new view. *J Biomech Eng*, 108:106–109.
18. Brand RA. (1989): A neurosensory hypothesis of ligament function. *Med Hypotheses*, 29:245–250.
19. Brooks VB. (1986): *The neural basis of motor control*. New York: Oxford University Press.
20. Burgess PR, Clark FJ. (1969): Characteristics of knee joint receptors in the cat. *J Physiol (Lond)*, 203:317–335.
21. Carlsoo S, Nordstrand A. (1968): The coordination of the knee-muscles in some voluntary movements and in the gait in cases with and without knee joint injuries. *Acta Chir Scand*, 134:423–426.
22. Carlstedt T, Lugnegard H, Andersson M. (1986): Pacinian corpuscles after nerve repair in humans. *Periph Nerve Rep Reagen*, 1:37–40.
23. Cavna N. (1965): The effects of aging on the receptor organs of the human dermis. In: Montagna W, ed. *Advances in biology of the skin*. New York: Pergamon Press, pp 63–96.
24. Clancy WG, Ray JM, Zoltan DJ. (1988): Acute tears of the ACL. *J Bone Joint Surg [Am]*, 70A:1483–1488.
25. Clark FJ, Burgess PR. (1975): Slowly adapting receptors in the cat knee joint: can they signal joint angle? *J Neurophysiol*, 38:1448–1463.
26. Cohen LA, Cohen ML. (1956): Arthrokinetic reflex of the knee. *Am J Physiol*, 184:433–437.
27. Corrigan JP, Cashman WE, Brady MP. (1992): Proprioception in the cruciate deficient knee. *J Bone Joint Surg [Br]*, 74B:247–250.
28. Craig AD, Heppelmann B, Schaible HG. (1988): The projection of the medial and posterior articular nerves of the cat's knee to the spinal cord. *J Comp Neurol*, 276:279–288.
29. Davis T, Lader M. (1983): Effects of ankle joint angle on reflexes and motor threshold intensities of soleus in man. *J Physiol (Lond)*, 339:228.
30. De Avila GA, O'Connor BL, Visco DM, Sisk TD. (1989): The mechanoreceptor innervation of the human fibular collateral ligament. *J Anat*, 162:1–7.
31. Ekholm J, Eklund G, Skoglund S. (1960): On the reflex effects from the knee joint of the cat. *Acta Physiol Scand*, 50:167–174.
32. Evarts EV. (1985): Sherrington's concept of proprioception. In: Evarts EV, Wise SP, Bousfield D, eds. *The motor system in neurobiology*. Amsterdam: Elsevier, pp 183–186.
33. Ferrell WR. (1980): The adequacy of stretch receptors in the cat

knee joint for signalling joint angle throughout a full range of movement. *J Physiol (Lond)*, 299:85–99.

34. Fischer LP, Guyot J, Gonon GP, Carret JP, Courcelles P, Dahhan P. (1978): The role of the muscles and ligaments in stabilization of the knee joint. *Anat Clin*, 1:43–54.

35. Freeman MAR, Wyke B. (1966): Articular contributions to limb muscle reflexes. *Br J Surg*, 53:61–69.

36. Freeman MAR, Wyke B. (1967): The innervation of the knee joint: an anatomical and histological study in the cat. *J Anat*, 101:505–532.

37. Gandevia SC, McCloskey DL. (1976): Joint sense, muscle sense, and then combination as position sense, measured at the distal interphalangeal joint of the middle finger. *J Physiol (Lond)*, 260:387.

38. Gardner E. (1948): The innervation of the knee joint. *Anat Rec*, 101:109–130.

39. Gardner E. (1944): The distribution and termination of nerves in the knee joint of the cat. *J Comp Neurol*, 80:11–32.

40. Gomez-Barrena E, Munurea L, Martinez-Moreno E. (1992): Neural pathways of anterior cruciate ligament traced to the spinal ganglia. Presented at the 38th meeting of the Orthopaedic Research Society, Washington, DC, February 17–20.

41. Goodwin GM, McCloskey DL, Matthews PBC. (1972): Proprioceptive illusions induced by muscle vibration: contribution by muscle spindles to perception. *Science*, 175:1382.

42. Grigg P. (1975): Mechanical factors influencing response of joint afferent neurons from cat knee. *J Neurophysiol*, 38:1473–1484.

43. Grigg P, Greenspan BJ. (1977). Response of primate joint afferent neurons to mechanical stimulation of knee joint. *J Neurophysiol*, 40:1–8.

44. Grigg P, Harrigan EP, Fogarty KE. (1978): Segmental reflexes mediated by joint afferent neurons in cat knee. *J Neurophysiol*, 41:9–14.

45. Grigg P, Hoffman AH. (1982): Properties of Ruffini afferents revealed by stress analysis of isolated sections of cat knee capsule. *J Neurophysiol*, 47:41–54.

46. Grigg, P, Schaible HG, Schmidt RF. (1986): Mechanical sensitivity of Group III and IV afferents from posterior articular nerve in normal and inflamed cat knee. *J Neurophysiol*, 55:635.

47. Halata Z, Haus J. (1989): The ultrastructure of sensory nerve endings in human ACL. *Anat Embryol*, 179:415–421.

48. Harrison PJ, Jankowska E. (1985): Sources of input to interneurones mediating Group I non-reciprocal inhibition of motoneurones in the cat. *J Physiol (Lond)*, 361:379–401.

49. Harter RA, Ostering LR, Singer KM, James SL, Larson RL, Jones DC. (1988): Long-term evaluation of knee stability and function following surgical reconstruction for anterior ligament insufficiency. *Am J Sports Med*, 16:434–443.

50. Haus J, Halata Z. (1990): Innervation of the anterior cruciate ligament. *Int Orthop*, 14:293–296.

51. Haus J, Refior HJ. (1987): A study of the synovial and ligamentous structure of the ACL. *Int Orthop*, 11:117–124.

52. Jeletsky AG. (1931): On the innervation of the capsule and epiphysis of the knee joint. *Vestn Khir*, 22:74–112.

53. Johansson H, Lorentzon R, Sjolander P, Sojka P. (1990): The anterior cruciate ligament. *Neuro-orthopedics*, 9:1–23.

54. Johansson H, Sjolander P, Sojka P. (1986): Actions on gamma-motoneurones elicited by electrical stimulation of joint afferent fibers in the hind limb of the cat. *J Physiol (Lond)*, 375:137–152.

55. Johansson H, Sjolander P, Sojka P. (1988): Fusimotor reflexes in triceps surae muscle elicited by natural and electrical stimulation of joint afferents. *Neuro-orthopedics*, 6:67–90.

56. Johansson H, Sjolander P, Sojka P. (1991): A sensory role for the cruciate ligaments. *Clin Orthop*, 268:161–178.

57. Johansson H, Sjolander P, Sojka P. (1991): Receptors in the knee joint ligaments and their role in the biomechanics of the joint. *Crit Rev Biomed Eng*, 18(5):341–367.

58. Johnson RJ, Eriksson E, Haggmark T, Pope MH. (1984): Five to ten year follow-up evaluation after reconstruction of the anterior cruciate ligament. *Clin Orthop*, 183:122–140.

59. Jokl P, Kaplan N, Stovell P, Keggi K. (1984): Non-operative treatment of severe injuries to the medial and anterior cruciate ligaments of the knee. *J Bone Joint Surg [Am]*, 66A:741–744.

60. Kandel ER, Schwartz JH, Jessell TM. (1991): *Principles of neuroscience*. 3rd ed. New York: Elsevier.

61. Kennedy JC, Alexander IJ, Hayes KC. (1982): Nerve supply of the human knee and its functional importance. *Am J Sports Med*, 10:329–335.

62. Kennedy JC, Weinberg HW, Wilson AS. (1974): The anatomy and function of the anterior cruciate ligament. *J Bone Joint Surg [Am]*, 56A:223–235.

63. Krauspe R, Schmidt M, Schaible HG. (1992): Sensory innervation of the anterior cruciate ligament. *J Bone Joint Surg [Am]*, 74A:390–397.

64. Lindstrom S, Takata M. (1972): Monosynaptic excitation of dorsal spinocerebellar tract neurons from low threshold joint afferents. *Acta Physiol Scand*, 84:430–432.

65. Lundberg A, Malmgren K, Schomburg ED. (1978): Role of joint afferents in motor control exemplified by effects on reflex pathways from Ib afferents. *J Physiol (Lond)*, 284:327–343.

66. Madey SM, Wolff AJ, Brand RA, Cole KJ. (1993): Joint receptors anterogradely labelled with WGA-HRP. *ORS*.

67. Markolf KL, Graff-Radford A, Amstutz HC. (1978): *In vivo* knee stability: A quantitative assessment using an instrumented clinical testing apparatus. *J Bone Joint Surg [Am]*, 60A:570.

68. Marshall KW, Tatton WG. (1990): Joint receptors modulate short and long latency muscle responses in the awake cat. *Exp Brain Res*, 83:137–150.

69. Matthews PBC. (1982): Where does Sherrington's "muscle sense" originate? Muscles, joints, corollary discharges? *Ann Rev Neurosci*, 5:189–218.

70. Mountcastle VB. (1957): Modality and topographic properties of single neurons of cat's somatic sensory cortex. *J Neurophysiol*, 20:408–434.

71. Mountcastle VB. (1975): The view from within: Pathways to the study of perception. *Johns Hopkins Med J*, 136:109.

72. Munger BL. (1988): The reinnervation of denervated skin. *Prog Brain Res*, 74:259–262.

73. Nichols TR, Houk JC. (1973): Reflex compensation for variations in the mechanical properties of a muscle. *Science*, 181:182–184.

74. Noyes FR, McGinniss GH, Mooar LA. (1984): Functional disability in the anterior cruciate insufficient knee syndrome. *Sports Med*, 1:278–302.

75. O'Connor BL, Seipel J. (1983): Anatomical variations of the posterior articular nerve to the cat knee joint. *J Anat*, 136:27–34.

76. O'Connor BL, Visco DM, Brandt KD, Myers SL, Kalasinski LA. (1992): Neurogenic acceleration of osteoarthrosis. *J Bone Joint Surg [Am]*, 74A:367–376.

77. Odensten M, Hamberg P, Nordin M, Lysholm J, Gillquist J. (1985): Surgical or conservative treatment of the acutely torn anterior cruciate ligament. *Clin Orthop*, 198:87–93.

78. Pope DF, Cole KJ, Brand RA. (1990): Discharge properties of mechanoreceptive afferents in the cat anterior cruciate ligament. In: *Transactions of the 36th Annual Meeting of the Orthopaedic Research Society*, New Orleans, vol 15, p 31.

79. Pope DF, Cole KJ, Brand RA. (1990): Physiologic loading of the ACL does not activate quadriceps or hamstrings in the anesthetized cat. *Am J Sports Med*, 18:595–599.

80. Prochazka A, Hulliger M, Zangger P, Appenteng K. (1985): Fusimotor set: New evidence for alpha-independent control of gamma-motoneurons during movement in the awake cat. *Brain Res*, 339:136–140.

81. Proske U, Schaible HG, Schmidt RF. (1988): Joint receptors and kinesthesia. *Exp Brain Res*, 72:219–224.

82. Salo PT, Tatton WG. (1991): Age-related loss of joint innervation. Presented at the Combined Meeting of the Orthopedic Research Society of the United States, Japan, and Canada, Banff, Alberta, October 21–23.

83. Schaible HG, Schmidt RF, Willis WD. (1987): New aspects of the role of articular receptors in motor control. In: Struppler A, Weindl A, eds. *Clinical aspects of sensory motor integration*. Berlin: Springer-Verlag, pp 34–45.

84. Schultz RA, Miller DC, Kerr CS, Micheli L. (1984): Mechanoreceptors in human cruciate ligaments. *J Bone Joint Surg [Am]*, 66A:1072–1076.

85. Schutte MJ, Dabezies EJ, Zimny ML, Happel LT. (1987): Neural

anatomy of the human anterior cruciate ligament. *J Bone Joint Surg [Am]*, 69A:243–249.

86. Sherrington CS. (1906): On the proprioceptive system, especially in its reflex aspects. *Brain, 29:*467.

87. Shiavi R, Limbird T, Borra H, Edmondstone M. (1991): Electromyography profiles of knee joint musculature during pivoting: Changes induced by anterior cruciate ligament deficiency. *J Electromyogr Kinesiol, 1:*49–57.

88. Sinkjaer T, Arendt-Nielsen L, Le Fevre S, Petersen ML, Kaalund S, Lass P. (1989): EMG measurements of muscle coordination in ACL injured subjects. Presented at the meeting of the European Society of Biomechanics, Denmark, July 8–11.

89. Sjolander P, Johansson H, Sojka P, Rehnholm A. (1989): Sensory nerve endings in the cat cruciate ligaments: a morphological investigation. *Neurosci Lett, 102:*33–38.

90. Skoglund S. (1956): Anatomical and physiological studies of knee joint innervation in the cat. *Acta Physiol Scand, 36:*1–100.

91. Solomonow M, Baratta R, Zhou BH, et al. (1987): The synergistic action of the anterior cruciate ligament and thigh muscles in maintaining joint stability. *Am J Sports Med, 15:*207–213.

92. Williams WJ. (1981): A systems-oriented evaluation of the role of joint receptors and other afferents in position and motion sense. *Crit Rev Biomed Eng, 8:*23–77.

93. Wink CS, Elsey RM, St. Onge M, Zimny ML. (1989): Neural elements in the cruciate ligaments and menisci of the knee joint of the American alligator, *Alligator mississippiens. J Morphol,* 202: 165–172.

94. Wroble RR, Brand RA. (1990): Paradoxes in the history of the anterior cruciate ligament. *Clin Orthop, 259:*183–191.

95. Zimny ML. (1988): Mechanoreceptors in articular tissues. *Am J Anat, 182:*16–32.

96. Zimny ML, Schutte M, Dabezies E. (1986): Mechanoreceptors in the human anterior cruciate ligament. *Anat Rec, 214:*204–209.

97. Zimny ML, St. Onge M, Schutte M. (1985): A modified gold chloride method for the demonstration of nerve endings in frozen sections. *Stain Tech, 60:*305–306.

SECTION II

Function

Continued advances in the treatment of ACL injuries will require better understanding of the structural properties of the femur-ACL-tibia complex, the mechanical properties of the ACL substance, the *in situ* forces and strains of the ACL, and the role of this ligament in knee function. The 11 chapters in this section describe the current knowledge about ACL properties, the roles played by the ACL in knee function, and up-to-date techniques for studying the ACL.

As an introduction, the geometry of the knee joint is described along with changes in the geometry that occur with knee motion. A four-bar linkage model of the knee ligaments is used to describe and predict knee motion. Next, methods for measuring both structural and mechanical properties of the ACL are detailed, with emphasis on the importance of ligament orientation with respect to the tensile load and knee flexion angle. The effects of age and exercise on the tensile properties of the ACL also are discussed. Additionally, the properties of the ACL are compared to those of other knee ligaments. This material is followed by a description of the nonlinear and viscoelastic properties of the ACL, as well as models used to explain these properties.

Next, the changes in knee motion resulting from ACL deficiency are noted, together with the contributions of the other soft tissues to knee joint stability. Three chapters deal with methods to measure forces and strains in the ACL. The advantages and disadvantages of indirect and direct methods of force measurement are detailed. Methods for measuring strains in the ACL are described, with special emphasis placed on techniques that can be used *in vivo,* where muscle forces also affect the strains in the ACL.

To evaluate the ACL and the kinematics and kinetics of the knee thoroughly, we consider the contributions of the muscles that cross the knee joint. A chapter describes *in vitro* studies that simulate quadriceps and hamstrings stabilization of cadaveric knees. Engineering models used to predict ACL forces during various activities are also discussed. These models are potentially useful for the evaluation of various rehabilitation protocols used after ACL reconstruction. Methods for describing complex knee motion are presented, and *in vitro* studies employing these methods are used to define the contributions of the ACL. The final chapter details gait analysis studies that evaluate functional changes occurring as a consequence of ACL deficiency.

Overall, the series of chapters in this section present diverse methods that are used to study ACL function, particularly its contributions to knee joint stability. With this background information, we will be able to characterize further the normal and reconstructed ACL, and to provide appropriate data on a rational basis for improving reconstruction and rehabilitation techniques.

Savio L-Y. Woo

The Anterior Cruciate Ligament: Current and Future Concepts, edited by D.W. Jackson, et al. Raven Press, Ltd., New York © 1993.

CHAPTER 3

Anterior Cruciate Ligament Function in the Normal Knee

John J. O'Connor and Amy Zavatsky

The ligaments of the knee have several distinct mechanical functions. They define the motion limits of the bones with respect to each other. They stretch and transmit tensile forces to resist movement outside those limits, pulling the articular surfaces together into compression. Within the motion limits, they control and guide the relative movements of the bones. They also work in partnership with the muscles and articular surfaces to transmit the loads of activity across the joint.

All knee structures interact geometrically and mechanically; to explain the function of one, its interactions with the others must be considered. Although this chapter concerns the functional role of both cruciate ligaments, the anterior cruciate ligament is emphasized. The roles of the ligaments in limiting joint movements are summarized, and then a simple geometrical and mechanical model of the knee is presented and used to explain other important, yet more subtle functions of the cruciate ligaments. The model is based on ligament functional architecture and represents a series of hypotheses about the way the natural joint works; comparing model predictions with the results of experimental observations on human specimens tests the validity of these hypotheses. The simplest model treats the ligaments as inextensible straight lines. This model is sufficient to explain how the ligaments control the rolling movements of the bones relative to each other during flexion and extension. It illustrates the relationship between the geometry of the cruciate ligaments and the geometry of the articular surfaces of the tibiofemoral joint. An elaboration of this model treats the ligaments as ordered arrays of fibers and is used to explain the changing shapes of the ligaments and the patterns of strain induced in them

during passive flexion/extension. It elucidates the concept of ligament isometry and its limitations. Finally, the model is used to show how ligament fibers are progressively recruited to bear load and how the effective ligament cross-sectional area increases to resist increasing anterior-posterior (A-P) movements of the bones.

These models will be further developed in Chapter 9 to investigate interactions between ligaments and muscles during activity. The possible proprioceptive functions of the ligaments will not be discussed.

THE RESTRAINTS TO JOINT MOTION

The ligaments limit the movement of the bones relative to each other and define the range of passive movement (5). In the simplest terms, the ACL resists anterior subluxation of the tibia; the posterior cruciate ligament resists posterior subluxation; the medial collateral ligament (MCL) resists abduction; the lateral collateral ligament (LCL) resists adduction; and the posterior capsule resists hyperextension. This description is, however, oversimplified. The ligaments act together in groups to limit these motions. For instance, all of the ligaments limit distraction of the joint. Shoemaker and Daniel (41) summarized the large body of experimental evidence defining the primary and secondary ligamentous restraints to various movements, and Hefzy and Grood present a similar review in Chapter 6. Thus, the following is only a brief review of these restraining functions.

The Anterior Cruciate Ligament

The major function of the ACL is to resist anterior displacement of the tibia with respect to the femur at all

J. J. O'Connor and A. Zavatsky: Department of Engineering Science, University of Oxford, Oxford OX1 3PJ, England.

flexion positions (8,11,12,15,19,30,39). The anteromedial part of the ACL reportedly is most important in flexion, whereas the posterolateral part contributes most to stability in extension (3,16). The ACL also helps to resist hyperextension (16,19). It contributes to the rotational stability of the fully extended knee for both internal and external tibial rotation (12,16,19). In flexion, it resists internal rotation only (38) or both directions of rotation, depending on the part of the ligament considered (16). The ACL resists medial displacement of the tibia (38), but it is believed to play only a small role in maintaining the varus-valgus stability of the knee (20).

The Posterior Cruciate Ligament

The major function of the PCL is to resist posterior displacement of the tibia (8,11,12,15,16,19,30,38). It also resists lateral tibial movement, but contributes only minimally to rotational stability (12,19,20) and to varus-valgus stability (12,20,38).

THE GUIDES TO JOINT MOTION

The cruciate ligaments contain fibers that rotate about their points of origin and insertion on the bones to allow and control movement within the motion limits of the knee. These actions can be described by reference to a theoretical model of the joint. The model is based on the four-bar cruciate linkage first described by Strasser in 1917 (43), further developed by Menschik (31) and Huson (24) and rediscovered by Goodfellow and O'Connor (21) to explain the movements of the meniscal bearings in a knee prosthesis. This four-bar linkage model not only highlights the role of the cruciate ligaments in guiding flexion of the knee, but also relates ligament anatomy to some important aspects of knee function.

The Four-Bar Cruciate Linkage

The cruciate ligaments and the bones form a mechanical linkage that guides the movements of the bones relative to each other during flexion and extension. A simplified version of this mechanism is the four-bar cruciate linkage ABCD (Fig. 1) (35,37). Two links, AB and CD, represent the ACL and PCL, respectively, and two links, BC and AD, join their points of attachment on the femur and on the tibia, respectively. Changes in the flexion angle of the joint result in equal changes in the angle between the femoral link BC and the tibial link AD. Figure 2 shows the linkage at extension and at 70° and 140° of flexion with the tibial link fixed. The shape of the linkage changes as the ligament links rotate about their attachment points. The three diagrams of Fig. 2 are shown superimposed in Fig. 3. With the femur flexing and extending on a fixed tibia (Fig. 3A), the femoral attach-

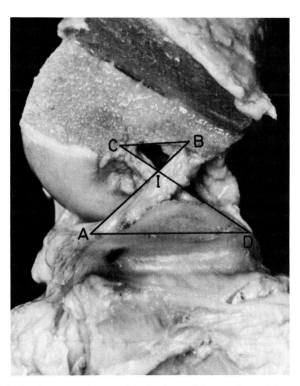

FIG. 1. A human knee with the lateral femoral condyle removed, exposing the cruciate ligaments. Superimposed is a diagram of a four-bar linkage comprising the anterior cruciate ligament AB, the posterior cruciate ligament CD, the femoral link CB joining the ligament attachment points on the femur, and the tibial link AD joining their attachments on the tibia. (From ref. 33a, with permission.)

ments B and C of the cruciate ligaments rotate on circular arcs about their tibial attachments A and D, respectively, while the ligament links AB and CD remain isometric. Similarly, in Fig. 3B, with the tibia flexing and extending on a fixed femur, the tibial attachments A and D of the ligament links rotate isometrically about their femoral attachments B and C, respectively.

The Instantaneous Center of the Linkage

The instantaneous center of the linkage lies at point I (Figs. 1 and 3), where the ligament links cross. The flexion axis of the joint, about which the bones flex and extend, passes through I. Because the geometry of the linkage changes during flexion and extension, the instantaneous center moves backward and forward relative to the two bones. It moves relative to the tibia along the curve marked "tibial centrode" (Fig. 3A) and relative to the femur along the curve marked "femoral centrode" (Fig. 3B).

The Relation Between Ligament Geometry and Articular Surface Shape

The shapes of the articular surfaces of the bones must be compatible with the changing geometry of the cru-

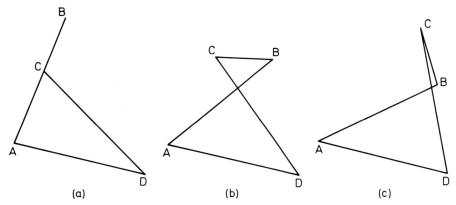

FIG. 2. The cruciate linkage *ABCD* drawn by the computer at full extension (**A**) and at 70° (**B**) and 140° (**C**) of flexion. Between A and C, the femoral link *CB* rotates through 140° relative to the tibial link *AD*, and the cruciate ligaments *AB* and *CD* rotate through 40° about their tibial attachments *A* and *D* and through 100° about their femoral attachments *B* and *C*. (From ref. 37, with permission.)

ciate linkage. They must allow passive flexion and extension while maintaining the isometricity of the cruciate links. If the shape of one of the articular surfaces is chosen arbitrarily, what should be the compatible shape of the other surface? An alternative statement of the problem is to ask where a compatible femoral surface should touch a specified tibial surface.

The theoretical solution is illustrated in Fig. 4, wherein the shape of the tibial surface is chosen to be flat and the shape of the femoral surface is sought. If the position of the contact point on the tibia can be found, its position relative to the femoral link *BC* can be calculated. When this is done over the flexion range, the shape of the compatible femoral condyle is obtained. In Fig. 4, contact must occur at the point *F* where the line perpen-

dicular to the tibial plateau passes through the instantaneous center *I*. Because, with the tibia stationary, all points on the femur rotate in circles centered at *I*, only point *F* on the femur can move tangentially to the tibial plateau while maintaining the isometry of the ligament links. Contact at F_1 would cause interpenetration of the bones or tightening of the cruciate links. In contrast, contact at F_2 would cause separation of the bones or slackening of the cruciate links. The shape of the femoral surface shown in Fig. 5 was calculated on this basis.

Similar methods have been used to calculate the shapes of femoral surfaces compatible with concave and convex tibial plateaus (35,37). The calculated shapes have proven to be very similar to the medial and lateral femoral condyles of the human knee. Upon detailed ex-

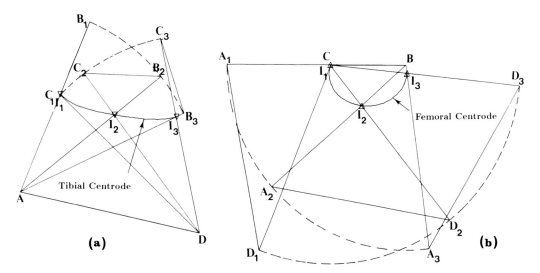

FIG. 3. The cruciate linkage drawn by computer with the tibial link fixed (**A**) and the femoral link fixed (**B**). The *relative* positions of the links are the same in both diagrams for each of the corresponding three configurations. In A, the femoral attachments of the ligaments move on circular arcs about their tibial attachments; in B, the tibial attachments move on circular arcs about the femoral attachments. The curves marked *Tibial Centrode* and *Femoral Centrode* are the tracks of the flexion axis of the joint on the tibia and femur, respectively, and are drawn through successive intersections of the ligaments. (From ref. 37, with permission.)

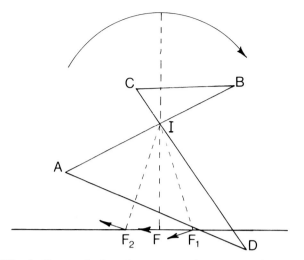

FIG. 4. Demonstration that contact between a flat tibial plateau occurs at point F, where the normal to the articular surfaces at their point of contact pass through the flexion axis at I. With the surface of the tibia fixed, all points on the femur move on circular arcs centered on the flexion axis. Contact between the bones at F_1 would lead to interpenetration and at F_2 to separation of the bones. Contact at F allows the bones to slide upon each other without interpenetration or separation.

amination, the curvature of the calculated surface shapes appears nearly circular in the sagittal plane, consistent with the conclusion of Kurosawa et al. (26) that the posterior femoral condyles of the human knee are spherical.

The Movements of the Bones

The rolling and sliding of the femoral condyles on the tibial plateaus was first described by Weber and Weber in 1836 (46). An elaboration of the computer-generated model shown in Fig. 5 demonstrates this movement. The contact point between the bones in the model follows the movement of the instantaneous center, shown in Fig. 3, and moves backward during flexion and forward during extension. Because the articulation lies distal to the instantaneous center, the femur not only rolls backward but also slides forward on the tibia during flexion and vice versa during extension (35). The movements of the model femur on the tibia during flexion/extension agree well with *in vitro* measurements on human cadaveric specimens (35,37).

Conclusions

The four-bar linkage model suggests that each human cruciate ligament has one point within its tibial attachment area that remains a constant distance from a corresponding point within its femoral attachment area during passive flexion and extension of the knee. If these points are joined by an actual ligament fiber [the "neutral fiber" (7) or "guiding bundle" (17)], then that fiber remains isometric during passive knee movements. This idea is used as the basis for the following further development of the four-bar linkage model in which the ligaments are treated as ordered arrays of fibers.

MODELING OF THE LIGAMENTS

The simple model just described cannot explain the functional subtleties of the ligaments, for example, the patterns of strain that develop within the ligaments dur-

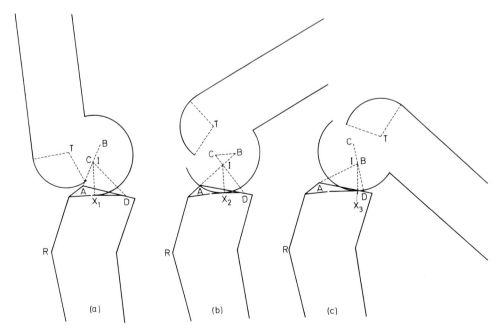

FIG. 5. Model bones and cruciate linkage shown in three flexion positions. *ABCD*, four-bar cruciate linkage; I, instantaneous center; *T*, center of trochlear facet of the femur; *R*, tibial tubercle; X_1, X_2, X_3, tibiofemoral contact points. (From ref. 33a, with permission.)

ing passive movements and load transmission. To do this, it is necessary to consider the ligaments as arrays of fibers and to calculate the geometric and mechanical relationships between the fibers.

When the knee is unloaded, ligament fibers are assumed to be transmitting little, if any, force. Passive movement of the joint, in the absence of loads, can thus be considered as an unresisted movement from one state of neutral equilibrium to another.

Geometric representation of ligament-fiber architecture involves a description of the bony attachment areas of the ligaments and of the relationships between the femoral and tibial attachment positions of each fiber, that is, the fiber mapping. The position of the neutral fiber within each cruciate ligament, corresponding to the ligament link of the previously described four-bar linkage, also must be specified, as well as the zero-tension reference position at which all other fibers within each ligament are just tight. Although the cruciate and collateral ligaments have been modeled using this method (3,49), this section describes only its development for the ACL.

Attachment Lines

A sagittal view of the femoral and tibial attachment areas of the ACL is shown in Fig. 6. The attachments are modeled as straight line segments (*heavy black lines*).

Fiber Mapping

The fibers between the tibial and femoral attachment lines must be mapped. The human ACL has been described as having a flat band-like appearance in the sagittal plane at full extension of the knee (19,40), with consistently matched origins and insertions (17,33). Therefore, a map was used that had individual model fibers originating and inserting at the same proportional distance along each bony attachment line. In extension, the model ACL thus consists of a sheet of fibers, all more or less parallel. The model fibers are defined as straight lines connecting points on the tibia and femur. In reality, slack fibers tend to buckle into curved shapes, whereas tight fibers remain straight.

The Neutral Fiber and the Zero-Tension Reference Position

In developing four-bar linkage theory to analyze ligaments of finite size, the positions of the neutral fibers within the cruciate ligaments must be chosen. Based on a radiographic study of cruciate ligament fiber lengths, Fuss (17) concluded that in extension the neutral fiber in the human ACL originates anteriorly within the femoral attachment area, and inserts anteriorly within the tibial

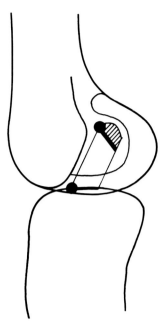

FIG. 6. The tibial and femoral attachment areas of the ACL. *Heavy lines* represent the model ligament attachment lines; *light lines* connect the attachment areas and the model anterior and posterior fibers. (From ref. 37, with permission.)

attachment area. During passive flexion, ligament fibers that pass anterior to the flexion axis tighten and those that pass posterior to the axis slacken (2,7). The model ACL in extension should therefore lie posterior to the instantaneous center of the joint and, hence, posterior to the neutral fiber. All but the anterior fiber will then slacken with initial flexion. For this reason, the anterior fiber of the model ACL was chosen as the ACL neutral fiber in the four-bar linkage model, and the position of extension was used as the zero-tension reference point for calculating model ACL fiber strain.

Model Parameters

The outcome of the model calculations depends on the choice of model parameters: the locations of the bony attachment lines of the ligament, the zero-tension reference position, and the lengths of the links in the four-bar cruciate ligament mechanism. The results for only one choice of parameters are reported here. They are based primarily on anatomical measurements reported by van Dijk and colleagues (13,44,45). A detailed description of the parameters and arguments leading to their choice is given elsewhere (49).

CHANGES IN ACL SHAPE DURING PASSIVE FLEXION

Several investigators have described separate and distinct fiber bundles within the body of each cruciate liga-

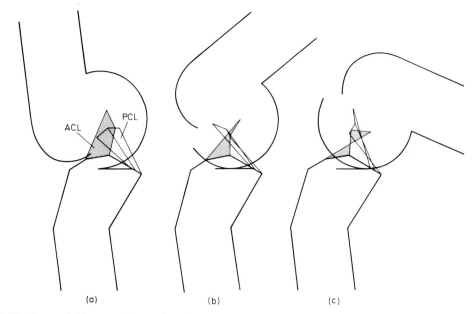

FIG. 7. The model femur, tibia, and cruciate ligaments drawn in 0° (**A**), 60° (**B**), and 120° (**C**) of flexion. The ACL is shaped. Both the anterior and posterior parts of the PCL are shown. As flexion progresses and corresponding tibial and femoral attachment sites rotate relative to each other, the fiber orientations and the overall shapes of the ligaments change. By 120° flexion, some fibers are crossed. (From ref. 37, with permission.)

ment (4,23,25,32). The present work suggests that such bundles are manifest because of the relative movements of the ligament attachment areas during flexion and extension. For instance, the ACL in extension is modeled by a sheet of fibers all more or less parallel (Fig. 7A). At 120° flexion (Fig. 7C), relative rotation of the attachment areas has caused the same fibers to cross. Fibers attached at the front or back of the tibial attachment area are now pointing in very different directions.

The changing shapes of the model ligaments in this figure resemble those of the human ligaments in the sagittal plane as described by Brantigan and Voshell (8), Girgis et al. (19), van Dijk and colleagues (13,44,45), and O'Brien et al. (33). Although the anterior and posterior halves of the human ACL resemble distinct bands in the flexed knee, the same fibers are more or less parallel in the sagittal plane in the extended knee.

The two-dimensional theory can describe only those changes in shape that result from bending-like rotations of the attachment areas relative to each other, leading to crossing of the fibers (Fig. 7). In effect, the model is based on the assumption that the axis of flexion lies parallel to both attachment areas and that the attachment areas lie perpendicular to the sagittal plane. In the human knee, the femoral attachment area of the ACL is not perpendicular to the sagittal plane; thus, a rotation about the flexion axis both twists and bends the ligament. During flexion, the fibers of the ACL, therefore, would be expected both to twist and to cross over each other.

CHANGES IN ACL FIBER LENGTH DURING PASSIVE FLEXION

Figure 8 shows the calculated relative length changes of selected fibers of the model ACL in Fig. 7 plotted against flexion angle. Relative fiber length is defined as calculated fiber length divided by length at the zero-tension reference position. The distance between a pair of points representing the origin and insertion of a fiber

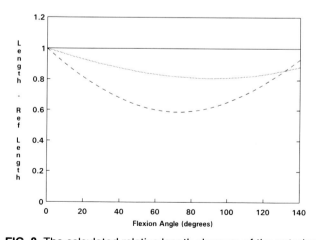

FIG. 8. The calculated relative length changes of the anterior (*solid line*), central (*dotted line*), and posterior (*dashed line*) fibers of the ACL. During passive flexion, relative length equals unity at full extension, the zero-tension reference position. (From ref. 37, with permission.)

on the femur and tibia is calculated and assumed to represent fiber length.

Near extension, the central and posterior fibers of the ACL pass behind the flexion axis. As the attachment areas rotate relative to each other during flexion, the femoral origins of those fibers move forward, and the fibers eventually pass in front of the flexion axis. The slackening and subsequent tightening of the central and posterior model ACL fibers with increasing flexion, as illustrated in Fig. 8, result from their movement from the back to the front of the flexion axis as the knee flexes. Minimum length is reached when the fibers pass through the flexion axis.

Our calculated fiber length changes compare with those measured on human specimens by Sapega et al. (40). They found that fibers attached anteromedially on the femur in extension had the least deviation from isometry during flexion, although their measurements showed an initial slackening as flexion began. They also observed slackening followed by lengthening of the central and posterior fibers with flexion. Amis and Dawkins (4) found similar patterns in central and posterior fibers. The most anterior fiber slackened initially and then tightened beyond its length at full extension.

Fibers that pass through the flexion axis of the joint remain instantaneously isometric. Because it is unlikely that an entire bundle of fibers occupying a finite area could pass through a single point, the concept of fiber isometricity must apply only to individual fibers. Consequently, the clinical objective of implanting a graft or prosthesis so that all of its fibers remain isometric during passive movements cannot be met.

LIGAMENT FIBER RECRUITMENT UNDER LOAD

Geometry

To design grafts or prosthetic replacements for injured ligaments, one must know the forces that knee ligaments withstand under load. However, quantification of such ligament forces *in vitro* is difficult, with only a few attempts reported (1,27–29,34). The problems of calculating the distributions of strain and stress within individual ligaments and the sharing of load between different ligaments are statically indeterminate; force equilibrium conditions alone do not provide sufficient information. Geometric analysis of the deformed configurations of the ligaments can supply the additional compatibility conditions necessary to solve the statically indeterminate ligament-force problem, at least in the absence of muscle action.

In this and the next section, geometric compatibility is used to determine strain distributions and forces in the model ligaments produced by A-P tibial translation. Ligament fiber recruitment occurs when ligament fibers, made slack by passive flexion of the knee, stretch and change their spatial orientations to resist applied loads. The concepts of fiber recruitment and functional architecture as alluded to here were developed mainly by physiologists studying skeletal muscle (18). The chief application of these concepts to the study of ligaments has been in modeling the nonlinear mechanical behavior of ligaments, specifically, in the relationship between fiber crimp and tissue stiffness (48). The ideas of minimal fiber-bundle recruitment length and recruitment probability were recently proposed by Blankevoort et al. (6). They applied these ideas to the results of an experimental study of cruciate ligament fiber bundle lengths. The present work is based on an analysis by FitzPatrick and O'Connor (14). They considered each ligament as consisting of a single extensible line, and they calculated ligament strains and forces compatible with specified flexion angles and anterior tibial translations.

Geometric Development

Figure 9A shows a single fiber connecting the femur and tibia. A forward movement x of the tibia relative to the femur displaces the fiber from its unloaded position, decreases its inclination with the tibial plateau, and increases its length. From the geometry of the triangle in Fig. 9A, the stretched length of the fiber *compatible with* a tibial displacement x can be calculated readily. Figure 9C shows the anterior and posterior fibers of the model ACL (of Fig. 9B) and MCL moved to new positions by successive anterior displacements of the tibia. The distribution of fiber elongation or shortening in these model ligaments compatible with any specified tibial displacement can be calculated (50).

Figure 10 shows the model ACL at 25° and 90° of flexion and at 2-mm intervals of anterior tibial displacement. Because of the relative movements of the ligament attachment areas on the bones, the shape of the ligament in the two positions of flexion differ, as do the directions of its fibers. In the unloaded state in both positions, the fiber inserting into the anterior point on the tibial attachment is the isometric fiber of the ligament that coincides with the ACL link in the four-bar linkage of Fig. 1. During flexion from 25° to 90°, this fiber rotates toward the tibial plateau under the control of the four-bar linkage of Fig. 2. The attachment line of the ligament on the femur at 90° flexion has rotated through 65° relative to its orientation at 25° flexion.

When the tibia is moved forward, all ACL fibers stretch, and their inclinations to the tibial plateau decrease. Fibers rendered slack by passive movement, are *progressively recruited* to offer increasing resistance to tibial translation as shown in Fig. 10. The effective cross-sectional area of the ligament increases as fibers are suc-

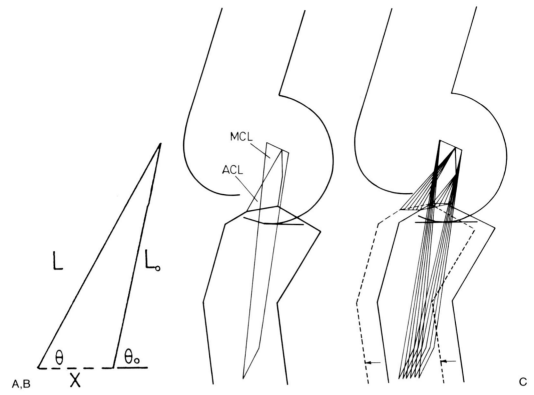

FIG. 9. A: A single fiber connecting femur and tibia. In the unloaded state, the fiber has a length L and is inclined to the tibia at an angle θ_o. When the tibia moves forward a distance x, the fiber stretches to a length L and to an inclination θ compatible with the displacement x. The model bones are shown with the ACL and MCL (anterior and posterior fibers only) drawn in 25° flexion (B) and with tibia translated anteriorly 10 mm in steps of 2 mm (C). (From ref. 37, with permission.)

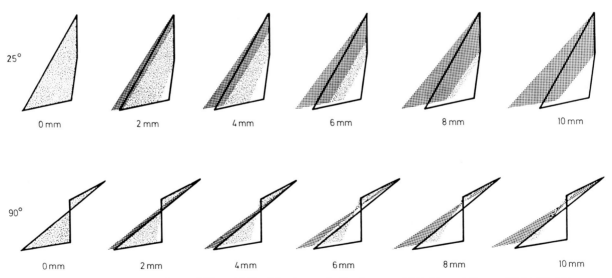

FIG. 10. The model ACL at 25° and 90° of flexion and after imposed tibial translations of 2 to 10 mm. *Heavy lines,* the shape of the ACL as a result of passive flexion; *dark shading,* the taut part of the ACL (stretched beyond its zero-tension reference length); *lighter shading,* the part of the ligament that remains slack. (From ref. 37, with permission.)

cessively recruited, and the mechanical stiffness of the ligament increases. An anterior translation of 8 mm is required to tighten all model ACL fibers at 25°, and an even greater translation is needed at 90°.

Fiber Strain Distributions

To illustrate fiber recruitment further, Fig. 11 shows the calculated fiber lengths for successive increases in anterior tibial translation for anterior, central, and posterior fibers in the model ACL plotted against flexion angle. The model anterior fiber, which remains isometric during passive flexion, stretches as soon as tibial translation begins. The central and posterior fibers tighten with initial translation only when their lengths are near their zero-tension reference lengths in the position of extension. Larger displacements are required to tighten the central and posterior fibers at all other flexion angles. From 35° to 125° flexion, even *10 mm* of anterior translation cannot tighten the model posterior fibers made slack by passive flexion. Similar fiber recruitment occurs in the model PCL, MCL, and LCL.

Many experimental studies of knee ligament fiber isometry have been conducted. Some investigators have reported cruciate ligament isometry regions located outside the anatomical attachment areas of the ligaments (4). Because it is difficult to find truly isometric ligament

fibers experimentally, some have concluded that the concepts of isometricity and the four-bar linkage model, which assumes isometricity, are not valid (4,6). We challenge these assertions. As defined here, the concept of isometricity applies only during passive, unloaded movement of the joint, a condition difficult to achieve experimentally. Figures 10 and 11 show that even small anterior tibial translations result in stretching of the anterior fiber of the model ACL, which is the neutral fiber in the four-bar linkage. Thus, even small loads can stretch or slacken fibers, hampering the interpretation of fiber isometry studies, especially when the conditions for holding and loading the knee specimens are not fully defined (42).

Mechanics

Fiber Stress Distributions

Fiber strain can be calculated for a specified tibial translation. Because fiber elongation can be substantial (up to 20%), a nonlinear elongation/strain relationship was used for these calculations (14,36,50). As a first approximation, a linear stress-strain relationship, with Young's modulus $E = 80$ MPa, was used to deduce approximate fiber stress. Calculations were also performed with a nonlinear stress-strain relationship.

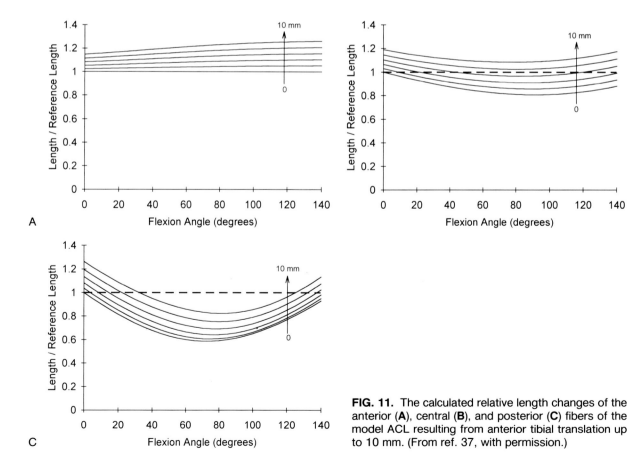

FIG. 11. The calculated relative length changes of the anterior (**A**), central (**B**), and posterior (**C**) fibers of the model ACL resulting from anterior tibial translation up to 10 mm. (From ref. 37, with permission.)

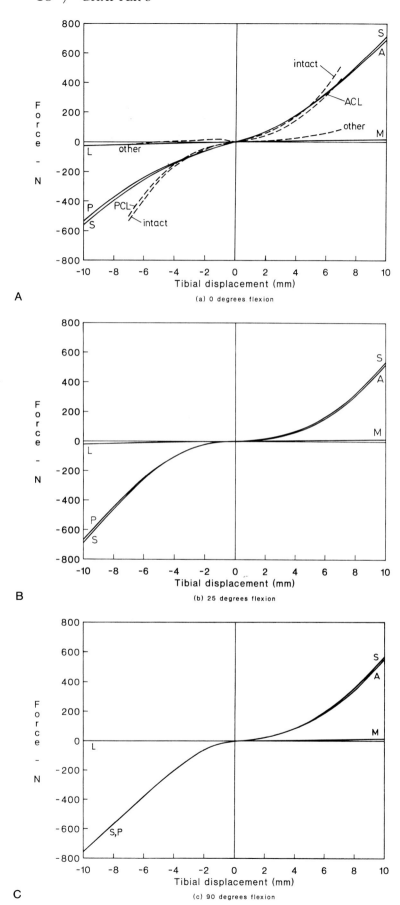

FIG. 12. Applied anteroposterior force versus tibial displacement for extension (**A**), 25° of flexion (**B**), and 90° of flexion (**C**). *A,* ACL; *P,* PCL; *M,* MCL; *L,* LCL; *S,* sum of A, P, M, and L. In (A), *dashed lines* are derived from the experimental results of Piziali et al. (38) for the intact knee, the ACL only, the PCL only, and all structures other than the cruciate ligaments.

Ligament Force Magnitude

The total force in a ligament is the sum of the force contributions from individual fibers in tension. For any chosen tibial displacement, the fiber force acting on a small element of tibial attachment area was calculated by multiplying the fiber stress by the area element, taking account of the fiber direction. The components of ligament force parallel and perpendicular to the tibial plateau were found by summing the contributions from all of those fibers that were stretched beyond their zero-tension reference lengths. Because the direction of a fiber can change considerably as it stretches, particularly when it lies nearly perpendicular to the tibial plateau, the components of fiber force must be calculated in the deformed state. In this study, the mediolateral thickness of each model ligament was taken to be a constant.

Calculated Results

The sum of the horizontal components of the ligament forces must equal the magnitude of the horizontal force that has to be applied to the tibia to achieve the specified A-P displacement. Figure 12 shows applied A-P forces versus tibial displacement for flexion angles of 0°, 25° (the position in which the Lachman test is usually performed), and 90° (the position for the drawer test). The curves illustrate load sharing between the ligaments. For anterior tibial displacement, the model ACL and MCL share the load. For posterior tibial displacement, the model PCL and LCL share the load at 0° and 25° of flexion, whereas the PCL resists all of the load at 90° of flexion. Thus, the ACL and PCL are the primary restraints to anterior and posterior tibial displacement, respectively. The MCL and LCL are secondary restraints.

Piziali et al. (38,39) measured all applied forces and moments necessary to achieve pure A-P tibial translation in cadaveric knee specimens at full extension. Except for the A-P force, they found that almost all of the coupled loads during A-P displacement were small and were directed mainly mediolaterally. The load sharing among the model ligaments is consistent with Piziali's load/displacement data (39); however, the stiffnesses are not the same. Compared to the experimental knees, the model intact knee is slightly stiffer for anterior displacement but is less stiff for posterior translation. When the cruciate ligaments are omitted from the calculation, thus simulating cruciate deficiency, the stiffness of the residual collateral structures is less than that of the experimental knees in anterior translation and is very similar to the experimental knees for posterior translation.

If the posterior oblique ligament, whose fibers are oriented to resist posterior tibial translation, were included in the model or if a higher value were used for the Young's modulus, the results would more closely match Piziali's data for the posterior translations. Use of the nonlinear stress-strain relationship (Fig. 13A) leads to a somewhat better fit with the experimental data, at least in this isolated case (Fig. 13B). The calculated results, however, are not fundamentally changed. The nonlinear relationship between A-P force and A-P displacement in Fig. 13 occurs for several reasons, one being the nonlinear stress-strain relationship of collagen fiber. Other nonlinear effects include the relationship between tibial displacement and fiber length (Fig. 9A), the relation between fiber extension and fiber strain when the strains are large (14,50), the increasing effective area of the ligaments as fibers are recruited under load and the ligament stiffens (Fig. 10), and these combined effects, which produce the nonlinear relationships between force and displacement in Fig. 12.

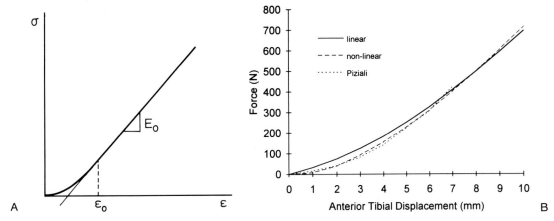

FIG. 13. A: Nonlinear stress-strain relationship used to calculate fiber stress. The *curved region* at the toe of the graph is a parabola, tangential at a strain of $\varepsilon_o = 0.03$ (10) to a straight region where the slope is $E_o = 90$ mPa. **B:** Applied anterior force versus tibial displacement at 0° of flexion for the model ACL. Comparison of calculations using linear and nonlinear stress-strain relationships with the experimental results of Piziali et al. (38). (From ref. 37, with permission.)

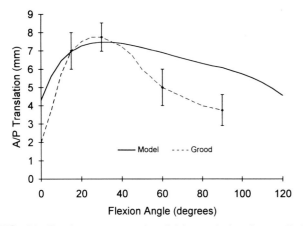

FIG. 14. Total anteroposterior tibial translation for applied anteroposterior forces of 67 N plotted against flexion angle for the model knee with both cruciate and collateral ligaments intact. The *dotted line* is derived from the experiments of Grood and Noyes (22), Fig. 9-9. (From ref. 37, with permission.)

The calculated total A-P tibial translation resulting from forces of 67 N, applied first anteriorly and then posteriorly, were plotted against flexion angle for the model knee with both the cruciate and collateral ligaments intact (Fig. 14). Translation was greatest at 35° flexion, where the ACL was both slack and poorly oriented to resist loads and the PCL was slack. Translation was least when one of the ligaments, although poorly oriented, was completely taut (ACL at extension, PCL at full flexion). The model adequately represents the general trends in A-P knee laxity obtained by Grood and Noyes (22), but it overestimates their experimental translations at extension and from 45° to 120° of flexion. A better fit near extension would be obtained if the posterior capsule and posterior oblique MCL fibers were

included in the model. The discrepancies at higher flexion angles are the result of a greater slackness in the model ACL fibers than in the human ACL fibers.

Model ACL force, expressed as a proportion of the applied anterior force, is plotted against flexion angle in Fig. 15. Included is a curve representing ligament force per unit of anterior load based on the orientation of the inextensible neutral fiber of the four-bar linkage (rigid model). The force ratio decreases with flexion as the ACL becomes more horizontal and thus better oriented to resist the applied load. At any flexion angle, this effect is further accentuated when ligament fibers stretch, as indicated by the reduction in ligament force per unit load as tibial translation increases.

DISCUSSION

We have described the mechanisms whereby the ACL guides the movements of the femur on the tibia during flexion extension and resists movement away from the positions dictated by those mechanisms. Our models show that the apparently separate functions of the ligament, limiting movements of the bones and guiding movements within those limits, are interrelated. These models simplify the description of those relationships but contain the essential elements.

Treating the ligaments as inextensible straight lines explains the rolling and sliding movements of the femur on the tibia during passive flexion and extension and the geometric relationships between the ligaments and the articular surfaces. Elastic ligament theory illustrates the strain patterns within ligaments during passive movements and the progressive fiber recruitment under load. The simple two-dimensional model shows how geometric compatibility can be used to calculate the distributions of strain in all the ligaments of the knee at any position after the following are specified: the sites of the neutral fibers within each cruciate ligament, the attachment lines of ligament fibers on the bones together with the mapping of fibers between these attachment lines, and the zero-tension reference position of all but the neutral fibers. The detailed results depend on the choices of all of these parameters, and a complete parametric analysis represents a formidable task, even with the two-dimensional model. The alternative is direct measurement of strain distributions within the human ligaments, itself a difficult task, even *in vitro*.

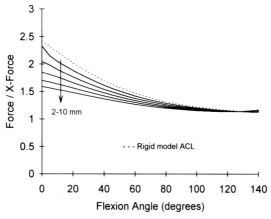

FIG. 15. Model ACL force expressed as a proportion of applied anterior force (the horizontal component of total ligament force) versus flexion angle for 2- to 10-mm anterior tibial translation. For the *dotted line,* the ACL force direction is given by the ACL neutral fiber, calculated from four-bar linkage theory (50). (From ref. 37, with permission.)

Limitations of the Model

Although the theoretical models described here can be further refined and elaborated, they contain most of the important elements. Quantifying their geometric aspects requires a knowledge of only basic trigonometry. A three-dimensional model currently being developed requires more complex mapping functions for the fibers but will enable calculation of fiber strains compatible with mediolateral translation, abduction, adduction, and long-axis tibial rotation, as well as A-P translation. In addition, the present analysis must be further developed to account for possible intra- and interligament variations in material properties (9,10,47). It does not account for the effects of cross-linking and other interactions between ligament fibers. In applying the calculated data to a particular knee, it would be ideal to use measurements of parameters obtained on that same knee.

Clinical Significance

The choice of model parameters necessary to achieve reasonable agreement between theory and observation defines the quantities that control the changing strain patterns within ligaments during passive flexion. These parameters include identification of ligament bony attachment areas, choice of fiber mappings between corresponding areas on the two bones, localization of the neutral fibers of the cruciate linkage within the finite cruciate ligaments, and specification of the zero-tension reference positions for all other fibers. To design and implant a ligament graft or prosthesis that reproduces the natural strain patterns, not only must the implant pass through the natural attachment areas, but also the natural mapping of the ligament fibers must be reproduced and maintained. Then, all fibers would have to be rendered just tight at the appropriate zero-tension reference position. New prostheses designs that adequately emulate these aspects of ligament structure may improve the success rate for ligament replacement surgery.

ACKNOWLEDGMENTS

The work described in this chapter was supported by a grant from the Arthritis and Rheumatism Council. Amy Zavatsky was supported by a Thouron Award and a Wellcome Trust Prize Studentship.

REFERENCES

1. Ahmed AM, Hyder A, Burke DL, Chan KH. (1987): *In-vitro* ligament tension pattern in the flexed knee in passive loading. *J Orthop Res,* 5:217–230.
2. Amis AA. (1985): Biomechanics of ligaments. In: Jenkins DHR, ed. *Ligament injuries and their treatment.* London: Chapman and Hall, pp. 3–28.
3. Amis AA, Dawkins GPC. (1990): Anatomy and function of the anterior cruciate ligament. In: *Proceedings of the Fourth Congress of the European Society for Knee Surgery and Arthroscopy,* Stockholm: pp 95–96.
4. Amis AA, Dawkins GPC. (1991): Functional anatomy of the anterior cruciate ligament: fiber bundle actions related to ligament replacements and injuries. *J Bone Joint Surg [Br],* 73B:260–267.
5. Blankevoort L, Huiskes R, de Lange A. (1988): The envelope of passive knee joint motion. *J Biomech,* 21:705–720.
6. Blankevoort L, Huiskes R, de Lange A (1991): Recruitment of knee joint ligaments. *Trans ASME J Biomech Eng,* 113:94–103.
7. Bradley J, FitzPatrick D, Daniel D, Shercliff T, O'Connor J. (1988): Orientation of the cruciate ligaments in the sagittal plane. *J Bone Joint Surg [Br],* 70B:94–99.
8. Brantigan OC, Voshell AF. (1941): The mechanics of the ligaments and menisci of the knee joint. *J Bone Joint Surg [Am],* 23A:44–66.
9. Butler DL, Guan Y, Kay MD, Cummings JF, Feder SM, Levy MS. (1992): Location-dependent variations in the material properties of the anterior cruciate ligament. *J Biomech,* 25:511–518.
10. Butler DL, Kay MD, Stouffer DC. (1986): Comparison of material properties in fascicle-bone units from human patellar tendon and knee ligaments. *J Biomech,* 19:415–432.
11. Butler DL, Noyes FR, Grood ES. (1980): Ligamentous restraints to anterior-posterior drawer in the human knee. *J Bone Joint Surg [Am],* 62A:259–270.
12. Crowninshield R, Pope MH, Johnson RJ. (1976): An analytical model of the knee. *J Biomech,* 9:397–405.
13. de Lange A, van Dijk R, Huiskes R, Selvik G, van Rens TJG. (1982): The application of roentgen stereophotogrammetry for evaluation of knee-joint kinematics *in vitro.* In: *Biomechanics: principles and applications.* The Hague: Martinus Nijhoff, pp 177–184.
14. FitzPatrick DP, O'Connor JJ. (1989): Theoretical modelling of the knee applied to the anterior drawer test. In: *Proceedings of the Institute of Mechanical Engineers - changing role of engineering in orthopaedics.* London: Institute of Mechanical Engineers, pp 79–83.
15. Fukubayashi T, Torzilli PA, Sherman MF, Warren RF. (1982): An *in-vitro* biomechanical evaluation of anterior-posterior motion of the knee: tibial displacement, rotation and torque. *J Bone Joint Surg [Am],* 64A:258–264.
16. Furman W, Marshall JL, Girgis FG. (1976): The anterior cruciate ligament—a functional analysis based on postmortem studies. *J Bone Joint Surg [Am],* 58A:179–185.
17. Fuss FK. (1989): Anatomy of the cruciate ligaments and their function in extension and flexion of the human knee joint. *Am J Anat,* 184:165–176.
18. Gans C, Bock WJ. (1965): The functional significance of muscle architecture—a theoretical analysis. *Ergeb Anat Entwgesch,* 38:115–141.
19. Girgis FG, Marshall JL, Al Monajem ARS. (1975): The cruciate ligaments of the knee joint—anatomical, functional and experimental analysis. *Clin Orthop,* 106:216–231.
20. Gollehon DL, Torzilli PA, Warren RF. (1987): The role of the posterolateral and cruciate ligaments in the stability of the human knee. *J Bone Joint Surg [Am],* 69A:233–241.
21. Goodfellow J, O'Connor J. (1978): The mechanics of the knee and prosthesis design. *J Bone Joint Surg [Br],* 58B:358–369.
22. Grood ES, Noyes FR. (1988): Diagnosis of knee ligament injuries: biomechanical precepts. In: Feagin JA, ed. *The crucial ligaments: diagnosis and treatment of ligamentous injuries about the knee.* New York: Churchill Livingstone, pp 245–285.
23. Hughston JC, Bowden JA, Andrews JA, Norwood LA. (1980): Acute tears of the posterior cruciate ligament: results of operative treatment. *J Bone Joint Surg [Am],* 62A:28–450.
24. Huson A. (1974): Biomechanische probleme des kniegelenks. *Orthopade,* 3:119–126.
25. Kapandji IA. (1987): Volume 2: the lower limb. In: *The physiology of the joints.* 5th ed. London: Churchill Livingstone. Honore LH, translator.
26. Kurosawa H, Walker PS, Abe S, Garg A, Hunter T. (1985): Geometry and motion of the knee for implant and orthotic design. *J Biomech,* 18:477–499.
27. Lewis JL, Lew WD, Engebretson L, Hunter RE, Kowalczyk C. (1990): Factors affecting graft force in surgical reconstruction of the anterior cruciate ligament. *J Orthop Res,* 8:514–521.
28. Malcolm L, Daniel D. (1980): A mechanical substitution technique for cruciate ligament force determination. *Trans Orthop Res Soc,* 26:303.
29. Markolf KL, Gorek JF, Kabo M, Shapiro MS. (1990): Direct measurement of resultant forces in the anterior cruciate ligament. *J Bone Joint Surg [Am],* 72A:557–567.

30. Markolf KL, Mensch JS, Amstutz HC. (1976): Stiffness and laxity of the knee—the contributions of the supporting structures: a quantitative *in-vitro* study. *J Bone Joint Surg [Am]*, 58A:583–593.

31. Menschik A. (1974): Mechanik des knielgelenks. *Z Orthop,* 113:225–230.

32. Norwood LA, Cross MJ. (1977): The intercondylar shelf and the anterior cruciate ligament. *Am J Sports Med,* 5:171–176.

33. O'Brien WR, Friederich NF, Muller W, Henning CE. (1989): Functional anatomy of the cruciate ligaments. Unpublished, Kantonsspital, Bruderholz, Switzerland.

33a.O'Connor J. (1993): Can muscle co-contraction protect knee ligaments following injury or repair? *J Bone Joint Surg* [Br] 75-B (*in press*)

34. O'Connor J, Biden E, Bradley J, FitzPatrick DP, Young S, Kershaw C, Daniel DM, Goodfellow J. (1990): The muscle-stabilised knee. In: Daniel DM, Akeson WH, O'Connor JJ, eds. *Knee ligaments: structure, function, injury, and repair.* New York: Raven Press, pp 239–277.

35. O'Connor J, Shercliff T, FitzPatrick D, Bradley J, Daniel D, Biden E, Goodfellow J. (1990): Geometry of the knee. In: Daniel DM, Akeson WH, O'Connor JJ, eds. *Knee ligaments: structure, function, injury, and repair.* New York: Raven Press, pp 163–200.

36. O'Connor J, Zavatsky A. (1990): Kinematics and mechanics of the cruciate ligaments of the knee. In: Mow VC, Ratcliffe A, Woo SL-Y, eds. *Biomechanics of diarthrodial joints.* New York: Springer-Verlag, vol 2, pp 197–241.

37. O'Connor JJ, Shercliff TL, Biden E, Goodfellow JW. (1989): The geometry of the knee in the sagittal plane. *Proc Inst Mech Eng [H],* 203:223–233.

38. Piziali RL, Rastegar J, Nagel DA, Schurman DJ. (1980): The contribution of the cruciate ligaments to the load-displacement characteristics of the human knee joint. *Trans ASME J Biomech Eng,* 102:277–283.

39. Piziali RL, Seering WP, Nagel DA, Schurman DJ. (1980): The function of the primary ligaments of the knee in anterior-posterior and medial-lateral motions. *J Biomech,* 13:777–784.

40. Sapega AA, Moyer RA, Schneck C, Komalahiranya N. (1990): Testing for isometry during reconstruction of the anterior cruciate ligament. *J Bone Joint Surg [Am],* 72A:259–267.

41. Shoemaker SC, Daniel DM. (1990): The limits of knee motion: *in vitro* studies. In: Daniel DM, Akeson WH, O'Connor JJ, eds. *Knee ligaments: structure, function, injury, and repair.* New York: Raven Press, pp 153–162.

42. Sidles JA, Larson RV, Garbini JL, Downey DJ, Matsen FA. (1988): Ligament length relationships in the moving knee. *J Orthop Res,* 6:593–610.

43. Strasser H. (1917): *Lehrbuch der muskel und gelenkmechanik, III.* Berlin: Springer-Verlag.

44. van Dijk R. (1983): *The behaviour of the cruciate ligaments of the knee* [Thesis]. Nijmegen, The Netherlands: Catholic University.

45. van Dijk R, Huiskes R, Selvik G. (1979): Roentgen stereophotogrammetric methods for the evaluation of the three dimensional kinematic behavior and cruciate ligament length patterns of the human knee joint. *J Biomech,* 12:727–731.

46. Weber WE, Weber EFW. (1836): *Mechanik der menschlichen Gehwerkzeuge in der Dietrichschen Buchhandlung.* Gottingen.

47. Woo SL-Y, Newton PO, MacKenna DA, Lyon RM. (1992): A comparative evaluation of the mechanical properties of the rabbit medial collateral and anterior cruciate ligaments. *J Biomech,* 25:377–386.

48. Woo SL-Y, Young P, Kwan MK. (1990): Fundamental studies in knee ligament mechanics. In: Daniel DM, Akeson WH, O'Connor JJ, eds. *Knee ligaments: structure, function, injury and repair.* New York: Raven Press, pp 115–134.

49. Zavatsky AB, O'Connor JJ. A model of human knee ligaments in the sagittal plane: Part I. Response to passive flexion. *Proc Inst Mech Eng [H]* [*in press*].

50. Zavatsky AB, O'Connor JJ. A model of human knee ligaments in the sagittal plane: Part II. Fibre recruitment under load. *Proc Inst Mech Eng [H]* [*in press*].

The Anterior Cruciate Ligament: Current and Future Concepts, edited by D.W. Jackson, et al.
Raven Press, Ltd., New York © 1993.

CHAPTER 4

The Tensile Properties of the Anterior Cruciate Ligament as a Function of Age

Savio L-Y. Woo and Gail L. Blomstrom

As one of the major knee stabilizers, the ACL restrains excessive anterior translation of the tibia and also limits varus-valgus and axial tibial rotations of the knee. The ACL is one of the most frequently injured ligaments in the body, and surgical replacement is often required to restore knee stability after a midsubstance rupture. Ideally, a replacement graft should possess the same properties as the natural ACL; therefore, knowledge about the tensile load-elongation relationship for the human ACL is necessary for the selection, design, and evaluation of ACL substitutes. Additionally, these data are useful in kinematic analyses of the human knee.

STRUCTURAL PROPERTIES VERSUS MECHANICAL PROPERTIES

In discussing the tensile properties of ligaments, it is important to distinguish between the structural properties of the bone-ligament-bone complex and the mechanical properties of the ligament substance. The structural properties describe the tensile behavior of the bone-ligament-bone complex as a functional composite. Values for these properties (e.g., ultimate load, ultimate elongation, linear stiffness, and energy absorbed to failure) can be obtained from the load-elongation curve. A typical load-elongation curve for a bone-ligament-bone complex is shown in Fig. 1. The curve can be divided into two regions: an initial, low-stiffness region (sometimes called the "toe" region) in which small loads are required for elongation and a subsequent high-stiffness region where larger loads are required for further elongation. In this latter region, the load-elongation curve becomes linear and the term *linear stiffness* is used to refer to its slope. The existence of these two distinct regions has been attributed to the microscopically observed undulating or "crimp" pattern of the collagen fibrils along the length of a ligament. If the fibrils are placed in tension, small initial loads are required to straighten the crimp. Once straight, the fibrils begin to elongate, and larger loads are needed for further elongation. Because of the varying degrees of crimping within groups of fibrils in a particular specimen, each group can uncrimp and, thus, begin to bear load at different elongations of the ligament. During a process termed *recruitment*, increasing numbers of the fibrils become load bearing and tissue stiffness gradually increases, resulting in a nonlinear load-elongation curve.

The mechanical properties are measurements of the material characteristics of the ligament substance. Values for these properties (e.g., tangent modulus, tensile strength, and ultimate strain) can be obtained from the stress-strain curve (Fig. 2). Determining the mechanical properties of ligaments presents several technical hurdles, including accurately measuring specimen dimensions and isolating the properties of the tissue substance. The simplest case, tensile testing of an isolated segment of ligament, is complicated by difficulties in effectively securing the cut ends of the specimen. Ligament specimens are typically too short to enable convenient clamping of the isolated substance to be tested. Furthermore, clamping of the free ends can weaken and damage the underlying tissue and induce premature failure. The use of bone-ligament-bone preparations allows more secure clamping and may provide a better approximation of *in situ* loading conditions; however, it is difficult to isolate the tensile properties of the ligament substance from

S. L-Y. Woo and G. L. Blomstrom: Musculoskeletal Research Center, Department of Orthopaedic Surgery, University of Pittsburgh School of Medicine, Pittsburgh, Pennsylvania 15261.

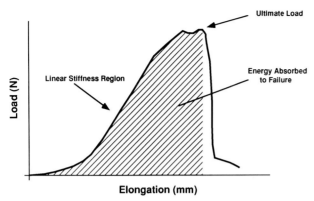

FIG. 1. Load-elongation curve resulting from a tensile test of a FATC. (From ref. 65, with permission.)

those of the insertion sites (61). In this chapter we review the recent progress in this area of study and specifically discuss techniques used in our laboratory to overcome some of these difficulties.

THE DETERMINATION OF CROSS-SECTIONAL AREA

If the load on the ligament and its cross-sectional area are known, a value for stress can be calculated (assuming uniform stress across the ligament). However, determining the cross-sectional area of soft tissue has proven to be challenging. Early attempts to determine soft tissue cross-sectional areas include those by Gratz (20), Cronkite (12), Nunley (45), and Rigby et al. (49). In the 1960s, several investigators used the gravimetric method, which calculated cross-sectional area by dividing the specimen's volume (calculated from its weight) by its length

(1,12,15,37,53). The area has also been calculated on the assumption of a rectangular cross-section using a conventional mechanical method, vernier caliper, which measures both width and thickness. Using this method to measure the ACL can produce large errors because the ligament's shape is irregular and geometrically complex.

In recent years, a number of other methods have been used. Haut and Little (24) assumed the cross-sectional shape of the canine ACL to be elliptical and calculated the cross-sectional area by measuring the major and minor axes with a micrometer. The area micrometer system determines cross-sectional areas by compressing the specimen in a rectangular slot of known width and then measuring the specimen height with a micrometer (9,17). However, measurements made using the area micrometer method are dependent upon the pressure applied to the specimen (2). In our laboratory (59,61) we have used a micrometer system that applied a minimal compressive force to the specimen to measure the thickness of the canine and swine medial collateral ligament. The widths of these specimens were measured with a cathetometer and the areas were calculated assuming a rectangular cross-section. Shrive et al. (50) designed a device consisting of a thickness caliper and a displacement transducer for measuring the area of the rabbit MCL by determining the thickness profile along the width of the tissue. However, the areas measured with this device were reported to be 43% smaller than those obtained by using vernier calipers. This large discrepancy may have been due to distortion of the ligament cross-section as the thickness caliper was dragged across the width of tissue.

A number of noncontact image reconstruction techniques have also been described (16,21,27,42). Ellis (16) used a "shadow amplitude method" to determine the

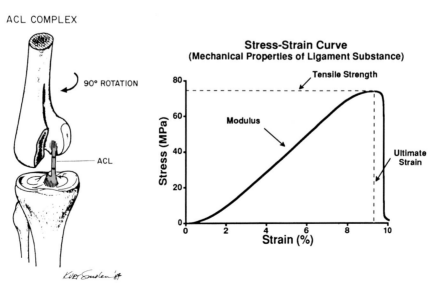

FIG. 2. Stress-strain curve representing the mechanical properties of the ACL. (From ref. 5, with permission.)

radius of specimen profiles and to reconstruct their cross-section. Gupta et al. (21) used a rotating microscope to determine the profile of the canine ACL, from which the cross-sectional area was calculated, and Njus and Njus (42) used a video dimensional analyzer (VDA) system to measure profile widths.

Recently, a laser micrometer method has been developed in our laboratory (33). This is a noncontact, automated system designed to determine the cross-sectional area and shape of ligaments using a collimated laser beam (33). The specimen is placed perpendicular to the collimated beam and is rotated through 180° by a computer-controlled drive system while profile widths for each increment of rotation are recorded via a microprocessor. The center of rotation and upper and lower boundaries of the object are then determined for each incremental rotation, and an iterative procedure is used to reconstruct the cross-sectional shape digitally and calculate the area. For both cross-sectional shape and area determination, the laser micrometer method gives a highly accurate and reproducible reconstruction of the ACL's complex geometry (60). In addition, this technique has been used to measure the variation in shape and cross-sectional area along the length of a ligament (22).

Laser micrometer, digital caliper, and area micrometer methods were used to measure the cross-sectional areas at identical locations along the midsubstance of the rabbit MCL and ACL, and the results were compared (60). For the MCL, the digital calipers and the laser micrometer yielded very similar results, but the constant pressure area micrometer yielded values 20% lower. For the ACL, the values obtained by the digital calipers and the constant pressure area micrometer were 16% and 20% lower, respectively. The digital calipers could not accurately measure the cross-sectional area of the ACL because of its irregular shape. The constant pressure area micrometer yielded lower values for the cross-sectional area of both the MCL and ACL because of the applied pressure, which changed both the cross-sectional shape and the area. These results are consistent with the differences Lee and Woo (33) obtained comparing methods measuring the ACL.

THE DETERMINATION OF STRAIN

Historically, changes in ligament length have been determined based on the testing machine cross-head displacement or clamp-to-clamp displacement. For a bone-ligament-bone complex, these values reflect the elongation of the whole complex, and methods do not isolate the strains of the ligament substance from those of the insertion sites and other interposed soft tissues. Therefore, ligament strain as a mechanical property should be obtained from the ligament substance and expressed as the change in length of the ligament substance normalized to a defined initial length.

Ligament strain has been estimated by a wide variety of methods (6,9,14,34,38,40,51,57). Kennedy et al. (29) performed one of the first important studies of knee ligament strain using a liquid mercury strain gauge sutured to the ligament. Others have also used liquid metal strain gauges to measure strains in the tissue substance (25,38,40). Dorlot et al. (14) implemented a new method that measured the change in insertion-site separation during knee flexion as an indication of ligament strain. The Hall effect strain transducer, developed by Arms et al. (6), uses changes in an electromagnetic field to determine length changes in the ligament.

The video dimensional analyzer is an excellent tool for measuring tissue strain. This technique requires no direct contact with the ligament, relying instead on a recorded video image of the specimen. Before tensile testing, two or more reference lines (markers for gauge length) are stained on the ligament, perpendicular to the loading axis with Verhoff's elastin stain (64). As the ligament is lengthened, the test data are recorded by a video camera and stored on a videocassette for permanent record. The taped image is then played back through the VDA system, which superposes two electronic "windows" over the reference lines. These windows automatically track the movement of the reference lines throughout the test and convert the horizontal scan time between lines into an output voltage. The change in voltage, expressed as a function of the initial voltage, can then be calibrated to correspond to the percentage of strain of the tissue. The frequency response of the VDA system is as high as 120 Hz, and errors in linearity and accuracy are less than 0.5% (58).

For measuring ligament strain, noncontact methods such as the VDA system have several advantages over methods involving mechanical or electronic gauges. With the VDA system, there is no physical contact with the specimen during testing and strains can be measured in the midsubstance, independent of the insertion sites. Strain values can be obtained from different regions of the same specimen simply by selective placement of the reference lines (gauge lengths). High-speed video recorders allow videotaping of high-strain-rate testing with slower playback for subsequent strain analysis (47). Also, video recording of testing enables convenient data analysis after the test and provides a permanent record.

THE STRUCTURAL PROPERTIES OF THE ACL

Data from the Literature

Over the several decades that the ACL has been studied, only a few published works have characterized the human ACL's tensile stiffness and strength properties.

The lack of data is due, in part, to obstacles hindering specimen procurement as well as difficulties in testing this geometrically complex ligament. Proper alignment of the femur-ACL-tibia complex (FATC) for tensile loading is particularly difficult. Although many authors have evaluated the tensile properties of the FATC, most have used animal models, including the rabbit (7,19,54,64), swine (36), dog (3,10,14,18,46,67), goat (28), and monkey (11,44). Some studies have examined the tensile properties of various autografts, including the patellar tendon (7,10), iliotibial tract (10,26,46,52), and semitendinosus tendon (31). Surprisingly little research has been done on the tensile properties of the human ACL. Kennedy et al. (30) measured the strength of the isolated human ACL and found the ultimate loads to be in the range of 480 ± 30 N to 640 ± 20 N. Trent et al. (51) examined the human ACL from donors 29 to 55 years old. The investigators removed the ACL with its bone blocks from the knee and maintained the ligament in a "physiological" position for tensile testing. They reported a linear stiffness of 141 N/mm and an average ultimate load of 633 N. Failures frequently occurred at the ligament insertion site. These two reports provided limited biomechanical data and lower-than-expected ultimate load values for the human FATC. In 1976, Noyes and Grood (44) studied the tensile properties of the human ACL as a function of age. Using an initial strain rate of 100%/sec, the load-deformation relationship was obtained for ACLs from two donor age groups, younger (16 to 26 years) and older (48 to 86 years). Values were 182 ± 33 N/mm (mean ± SE) and 1,725 ± 269 N for linear stiffness and ultimate load, respectively, for the six younger donors. The corresponding values were 129 ± 39 N/mm and 734 ± 266 N, respectively, for 20 older specimens.

Rauch et al. (48) tested the human FATC at 30° flexion from donors ranging in age from 17 to 84 years.

There was a significant correlation between specimen age and ultimate load. The linear stiffness and ultimate load mean values for the five specimens from the younger group (17 to 28 years) were 203 ± 34 N/mm and 1,716 ± 538 N, respectively. For the 44 older specimens (34 to 84 years), the corresponding values were lower (124 ± 39 N/mm and 814 ± 356 N, respectively). The highest individual values obtained for these structural properties were approximately 255 N/mm and 2,500 N.

Data from our Laboratory

The Effects of Knee Flexion Angle, Ligament Orientation, and Age

In our laboratory, testing devices were designed to accommodate the anatomical complexity of the ACL such that the FATC could be tested with the direction of load applied along (a) the long axis of the ligament (anatomical orientation) or (b) along the tibial axis (tibial orientation) at a wide range of knee flexion angles. The effects of both knee flexion angle and the direction of applied tensile load on the structural properties of the FATC were evaluated in both rabbit and human cadaver models.

Rabbit Specimens

We conducted a study to determine the effects of ligament orientation and flexion angle on the structural properties of the rabbit FATC. The rabbit knees were tested at 0°, 30°, 45°, or 90° of flexion while the applied tensile forces were directed along the tibia (tibial orientation) in the sagittal plane or along the longitudinal axis of the ACL (anatomical orientation) in the sagittal plane.

Two series of specimens were tested. The first series of FATCs from 57 rabbits were tensile tested in the anatom-

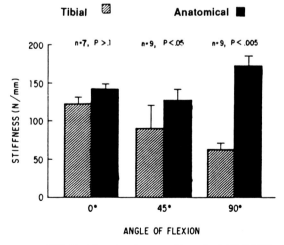
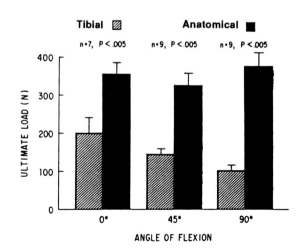

FIG. 3. Structural properties of rabbit FATC obtained at three angles of flexion. Tangent stiffness and ultimate load at failure for paired specimens. (From ref. 64, with permission.)

ical orientation at 0°, 45°, or 90° of knee flexion. In the second group, the FATC from the left leg was tested in the tibial orientation and the FATC from the right leg was tested in the anatomical orientation. The test protocol included preconditioning the specimen and applying a preload of 0.5 N to the FATC. Subsequently, the specimen was stretched to failure at a rate of 200 mm/min (approximately 33%/sec strain rate). The ultimate load, energy absorbed, and elongation at maximum load were obtained. Stiffness was calculated from the linear region of the load-elongation curve (10). The mode of failure of the FATC was also noted.

The ultimate load values for the FATC decreased with increasing knee flexion for those specimens loaded along the tibial axis, whereas no such change was detected for FATCs tested along the ligament axis (Fig. 3). Linear stiffness and energy absorbed at failure followed similar trends. Figgie et al. (18) also systematically studied the strength of the FATC with respect to knee flexion angle. We concluded that the structural properties of the rabbit FATC change minimally with knee flexion (from 0° to 90°) when loaded along the ligament axis but decrease significantly with knee flexion when loaded along the axis of the tibia. When the tensile load was applied along the tibia, the ultimate load decreased as the angle of knee flexion increased. Therefore, data obtained on the structural properties of the ACL can be compared only if the direction of loading with respect to the ACL is the same.

Human Specimens

An experimental device was developed in our laboratory to test the human FATC at any desired angle of knee flexion and in different vertical orientations with respect to the applied tensile load (36,63). Using this device, we tested 27 pairs of cadaveric human knees, equally distributed into three age groups: 22 to 35 (mean of 29) years, 40 to 50 (mean of 45) years, and 60 to 97 (mean of 75) years. One knee from each pair was tested in an orientation in which the long axis of the ligament was aligned with the tensile load while its normal angles of insertion to the bones were maintained (anatomical orientation) (Fig. 4). The contralateral knee was tested with the tensile load aligned vertically with the tibia and the femur translated medially and anteriorly to align the ACL with the tensile load (tibial orientation). This latter alignment did not maintain the normal angles of ACL insertion to the femur and tibia. The effects of specimen orientation as well as specimen age on the structural properties of the paired human FATC were evaluated. The femur and tibia were secured in stiff "universal" clamps with the knee angle fixed at 30°. The FATC was loaded to failure at a rate of 200 mm/min, and the load-elongation curve was recorded. The structural properties of the FATC, as represented by the linear stiffness, ultimate load, and energy absorbed to failure, were then determined.

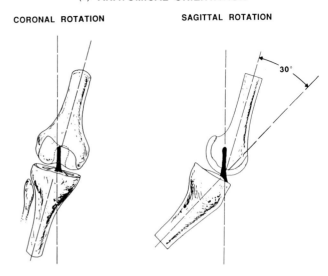

(a) **ANATOMICAL ORIENTATION**

CORONAL ROTATION   SAGITTAL ROTATION

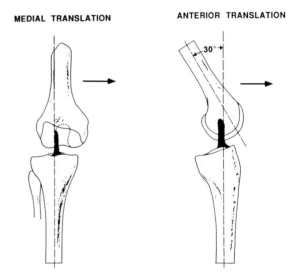

(b) **TIBIAL ORIENTATION**

MEDIAL TRANSLATION   ANTERIOR TRANSLATION

FIG. 4. Schematic of specimen orientation for tensile testing. **A:** For the anatomical orientation, the tensile load is applied along the axis of the ACL. **B:** For the tibial orientation, the tensile load is applied in line with the femoral and tibial insertion sites. (From ref. 63, with permission.)

Figure 5 shows typical load-elongation curves for a paired set of knees from the youngest age group. These two curves typify the differences in the structural properties of the complex due to specimen orientation. Those tested in the anatomical orientation demonstrated higher linear stiffness, ultimate load, and energy absorbed to failure than did those tested in the tibial orientation. These results confirmed our hypothesis that the anatomical orientation allows a greater proportion of the fibers of the ACL to be loaded simultaneously, resulting in higher linear stiffness and higher ultimate load to failure than for those tested in the tibial orientation.

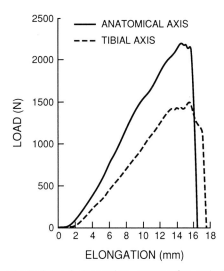

FIG. 5. Typical load-elongation curves for paired FATCs from a donor in the youngest age group, which demonstrates the differences between the anatomical and tibial orientations. (From ref. 63, with permission.)

Age also had a profound effect on the structural properties of the FATC. For specimens tested in the anatomical orientation, the ultimate load to failure of the youngest group was approximately 50% higher than that of the middle-aged group and over three times higher than that of the oldest group. This rapid decline in the ultimate load to failure with increasing age is illustrated in Fig. 6. The linear stiffness and energy absorbed at failure followed similar trends (63). The reasons for the extreme decreases in the structural properties with increasing age are unknown, but changes in the types as well as the levels of strenuous physical activity with age are thought to be partly responsible. It is also possible that changes in joint geometry (and therefore knee kinematics) with aging may play a role. Changes in the structure and integrity of the collagen fibers in the ligament with age may also be a factor. Additional investigations are needed to verify or refute these hypotheses.

THE MECHANICAL PROPERTIES OF THE ACL

In an effort to determine the mechanical properties of the ACL, several investigators have divided the ligament into bundles and tested the bundles individually. Thus, the tensile stress across the ligament can be more evenly distributed. Butler et al. (9) tested bone-fascicle-bone units from human cadaveric specimens. In preparation for tensile testing, they dissected the ACLs into bundles and measured the cross-sectional area and length of each bundle. The average elastic modulus and ultimate tensile strength were measured to be 278 MPa and 40 MPa, respectively. In this study, the ligaments reached their maximum stress at approximately 12% strain, which is a much lower level than that reported for the maximum percentage of elongation (sometimes erroneously referred to as ACL strain) in FATC tests. In a later study, the same group reported the nonuniform properties of the ACL. They showed that the anteromedial and the anterolateral bundles exhibited much higher material properties than did the posterior bundle of the ACL (8). The average modulus of the posterior bundle was approximately 50% lower than that of the anterior bundles, although this was not a statistically significant difference.

In our laboratory, we evaluated and compared the mechanical properties of the ACL and the MCL in rabbits (66). In an effort to control variables such as age, sex, and activity levels, animals were age and sex matched. Additionally, because the ACL is anatomically complex, with portions of the ACL having different lengths, it is impossible to apply a simultaneous and uniform load to all portions of the ACL during a simple tensile test of the FATC. Therefore, the ACL was divided into two portions before testing. The cross-sectional shape and area of both portions were determined using the laser micrometer system (Fig. 7). The cross-sectional shape of the MCL was found to be generally oblong, with a width:thickness ratio of approximately 3:1. The individual portions of the ACL were more ovoid in cross-

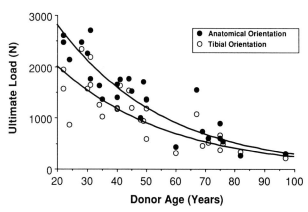

FIG. 6. The effect of age on the ultimate load of the FATC. (From ref. 63, with permission.)

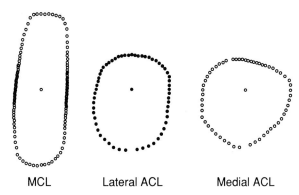

MCL   Lateral ACL   Medial ACL

FIG. 7. Typical cross-sectional shape of the MCL and two portions of the ACL. The reconstructed area and shape were obtained using a laser micrometer system. (From ref. 66, with permission.)

section, and the cross-sectional areas of the ACL portions were similar to each other.

Strain in the ligaments was measured using a VDA. The mechanical properties of the MCL differed from those of the medial and lateral portions of the ACL (Fig. 8). The modulus (slope of the stress-strain curve measured between 4% and 7% strain) was significantly greater for the MCL (1,120 ± 153 MPa) than for either the medial (516 ± 64 MPa) or lateral (516 ± 69 MPa) portions of the ACL. Comparison of the moduli demonstrates large differences between the MCL and the medial and lateral portions of the ACL, as the MCL substance withstands approximately twice the stress at a given strain compared to the medial and lateral portions of the ACL. There was no significant difference in moduli between the medial and lateral portions of the ACL.

The mode of failure for the three different structures also varied. Ninety percent of the lateral FATCs failed due to avulsion, in contrast to the medial FATC and the femur-MCL-tibia complex, in which only 10% and 0%, respectively, failed in this manner. Tensile strength and ultimate strain of the bundles could not be compared because of the differences in failure mode.

When examined under scanning electron microscopy (SEM), differences can be seen between the ACL and MCL. The ACL shows a distinct fascicular structure with large amounts of interfascicular space and loose connective tissue, which is not seen in the MCL. Also, the collagen fibrils in the MCL are more densely packed and more uniformly distributed than are those in the ACL. The cross-sectional area of longitudinally oriented collagen fibers per unit of ligament cross-sectional area appears less in the ACL than in the MCL. It has been shown that the amount of longitudinally oriented collagen in the ligament is higher in the rabbit MCL than in the ACL by approximately 15%. Hart et al. (23) demonstrated that the distribution of the fibril diameters is different for the two ligaments. These observations provide possible explanations for the differences seen in the

lower modulus and the lower stress at failure for the ACL compared to that of the MCL (41).

Biochemical differences between the MCL and ACL have also been noted. The rabbit cruciate ligaments have a higher percentage of Type III collagen (12%) compared to the MCL (9%). The cruciate ligaments also have twice the amount of glycosaminoglycans and larger amounts of reducible collagen cross-links compared to the MCL (4).

Using both light and transmission electron microscopy, we (35) have found that the cells populating the MCL had characteristics typical of fibroblasts, with long cytoplasmic processes. The cells of the ACL were more rounded and devoid of these processes. Additionally, the ACL cells did not seem to be in contact with the collagen matrix; instead they were separated by a region of amorphous ground substance. Interestingly, these differences between the cells in the ACL and MCL diminished after immobilization (41)

Recently, we have also studied the ultrastructural morphometry of the ACL and MCL in the rabbit (23). The collagen subfascicle area fraction and collagen fibril diameter distributions between the two ligaments were compared. The ACL had significantly less subfascicular area fractions than the MCL (.89 ± .02 vs .97 ± .01, respectively). The mean fibril diameter was also less for the ACL than for the MCL (0.059 ± 0.005 μm vs 0.085 ± 0.001 μm, respectively). However, fibril eccentricity (a measure of parallel alignment of collagen fibrils within the ligaments, defined as the ratio of minor to major axes of elliptical fibril outlines) was not significantly different for the two ligaments. These differences may help to explain the differences in mechanical properties between the ACL and MCL.

IMMOBILIZATION

The effect of immobilization on the structural properties of ligaments has been the topic of several studies. In 1974, Noyes et al. (43) studied the effects of immobilization on FATCs of wild primates. They found that, after 8 weeks of immobilization, both the ultimate load to failure and the energy absorbed decreased by 39% and 32%, respectively. After 26 weeks of remobilization, the FATC only partially recovered to its original load to failure. In our laboratory, the effect of immobilization of the knee on the structural properties of the collateral ligaments was studied in the rabbit (58). After an 8-week immobilization period, linear stiffness, ultimate load, and energy absorption to failure were approximately one-third that of the contralateral control. Later, a biomechanical and histological study was performed to investigate further the consequences of immobilization and remobilization in the rabbit (62). Nine weeks of immobilization resulted in reductions in stiffness, ultimate

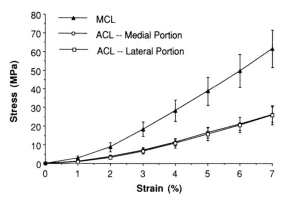

FIG. 8. Stress-strain curve representing the mechanical properties of the midsubstance of the MCL and ACL. (From ref. 66, with permission.)

load, and energy absorption at failure of bone-MCL-bone complexes, as well as increased incidences of failure due to tibial avulsion. Histologically, the tibial insertion site showed increased osteoclastic activity, bone resorption, and disruption of the normal ligament insertion. After 1 year of remobilization, the ultimate load and energy absorption, although improved, had not returned to normal.

EXERCISE

Viidik (54) demonstrated that training throughout life increased both the energy absorbed to failure and the ultimate load. In his study, rabbits were exercised on a running machine during a 40-week period. Both elasticity and tensile tests were performed on the FATCs. Because the specimen failures were not midsubstance, it could be argued that exercise may only affect the bone; however, the load-relaxation phenomenon was larger in the trained group, which indicated that changes were occurring in the ligamentous tissue. In our laboratory, a dog model was used to evaluate the effects of age and life-long exercise on the structural and mechanical properties of the MCL (56). Tensile strength and strain to failure both decreased as a function of age, 30% and 20%, respectively, regardless of the exercise. However, exercise did increase the tangent modulus by 20%.

SUMMARY AND FUTURE DIRECTIONS

Through many recent investigations, we are beginning to comprehend the complex roles in normal joint function played by the ligaments of the knee. Experimental testing has provided the tensile characteristics of the ACL, and kinematic studies have begun to define the role of the ACL in maintaining normal joint motion. Various external factors such as immobilization and exercise have profound effects on the biomechanical properties of the bone-ligament-bone complexes. More information is necessary regarding ACL replacement grafts and reparative techniques; however, standardized test protocols should be developed so that results from different studies can be compared. Further, the collagen-collagen (13,32,55) and the proteoglycan-collagen (39) interactions and their effect on the mechanical properties of the ACL deserve additional investigation.

ACKNOWLEDGMENTS

Some of the work presented in this chapter was done in collaboration with the colleagues of the senior author while he was at the University of California, San Diego. The authors gratefully acknowledge the financial assistance of NIH Grant AR-39683.

REFERENCES

1. Abrahams M. (1967): Mechanical behavior of tendon *in vivo*. *Med Biol Eng*, 5:433–443.
2. Allard P, Thirty PS, Bourgault A, Drouin G. (1979): Pressure-dependence of the "area micrometer" method in evaluation of cruciate ligament in cross-section. *J Biomech Eng*, 1:265–267.
3. Alm A, Ekstrom H, Stromberg B. (1974): Tensile strength of the anterior cruciate ligament in the dog. *Acta Chir Scand [Suppl]*, 445:15–23.
4. Amiel D, Frank C, Harwood F, Fronek J, Akeson W. (1984): Tendons and ligaments: morphological and biochemical comparison. *J Orthop Res*, 1:257–265.
5. Anderson DR, Weiss JA, Takai S, Ohland KJ, Woo SL-Y. (1992): Healing of the medial collateral ligament following a triad injury: a biomechanical and histological study of the knee in rabbits. *J Orthop Res*, 10:485–495.
6. Arms SW, Pope MH, Boyle JB, Davignon PJ, Johnson RJ. (1982): Knee medial collateral ligament strain. *Trans Orthop Res Soc*, 7:47.
7. Ballock RT, Woo SL-Y, Lyon RM, Hollis M, Akeson WH. (1989): Use of patellar tendon autograft for anterior cruciate ligament reconstruction in the rabbit: a long-term histologic and biomechanical study. *J Orthop Res*, 7:474–485.
8. Butler DL, Guan Y, Kay MD, Cummings JF, Feder SM, Levy MS. (1992): Location-dependent variations in the material properties of anterior cruciate ligament subunits. *J Biomech*, 25:511–518.
9. Butler DL, Kay MD, Stouffer DC. (1986): Comparison of material properties in fascicle-bone units from human patellar tendon and knee ligaments. *J Biomech*, 19:425–432.
10. Butler DL, Stouffer DC. (1983): Tension-torsion characteristics of the canine anterior cruciate ligament—Part II: experimental observations. *J Biomech Eng*, 105:160–165.
11. Clancy WG, Narechania RG, Rosenberg TD, Gmeiner JG, Wisnefske DD, Lange TA. (1981): Anterior and posterior cruciate ligament reconstruction in rhesus monkeys: a histological, microangiographic, and biomechanical analysis. *J Bone Joint Surg [Am]*, 63A:1270–1284.
12. Cronkite AE. (1936): The tensile strength of human tendons. *Anat Rec*, 64:173–186.
13. Danielsen CC. (1981): Mechanical properties of reconstituted collagen fibrils. *Connect Tissue Res*, 9:52–57.
14. Dorlot JM, Ait ba Sidi M, Gremblay GM, Drouin G. (1980): Load-elongation behavior of the canine anterior cruciate ligament. *J Biomech Eng*, 102:190–193.
15. Elden HR. (1964): Aging of rat tail tendon. *J Gerontol*, 19:173–178.
16. Ellis DG. (1968): A shadow amplitude method for measuring cross-sectional areas of biological specimens. *21st Ann Conf Eng Med Biol*, 51:6.
17. Ellis DG. (1969): Cross-sectional area measurements for tendon specimens—a comparison of several methods. *J Biomech*, 2:175–186.
18. Figgie HE III, Bahniuk EH, Heiple KG, Davy DT. (1986): The effects of tibial-femoral angle on the failure mechanics of the canine anterior cruciate ligament. *J Biomech*, 19:89–91.
19. Goldberg VM, Burstein A, Dawson M. (1982): The influence of an experimental immune synovitis on the failure mode and strength of the rabbit anterior cruciate ligament. *J Bone Joint Surg*, 64:900–906.
20. Gratz CM. (1931): Tensile strength and elasticity tests on human fascia lata. *J Bone Joint Surg*, 13:334–340.
21. Gupta BN, Subramanian KN, Brinker WO, Gupta AN. (1971): Tensile strength of canine cranial cruciate ligaments. *Am J Vet Res*, 32:183–190.
22. Harner CD, Livesay GA, Choi NY, Fujie H, Fu FH, and Woo SL-Y. (1992): Evaluation of the sizes and shapes of the human anterior and posterior cruciate ligaments: a comparative study. *Trans Orthop Res Soc*, 17:123.
23. Hart RA, Newton PO, Woo SL-Y. (1991): Quantitative morphology of the anterior cruciate and medial collateral ligaments. *Trans Orthop Res Soc*, 16:181.
24. Haut RC, Little RW. (1969): Rheological properties of canine anterior cruciate ligaments. *J Biomech*, 2:289–298.

25. Henning CE, Lynch MA, Glick KR Jr. (1985): An *in vivo* strain gage study of elongation of the anterior cruciate ligament. *Am J Sports Med*, 13:22–26.

26. Holden JP, Grood ES, Butler DL, Noyes FR, Mendenhall VH, Van Kampen CL, Neidich RL. (1988): Biomechanics of fascia lata ligament replacements: early postoperative changes in the goat. *J Orthop Res*, 6:639–647.

27. Iaconis F, Steindler R, Marinozzi G. (1987): Measurements of cross-sectional area of collagen structures (knee ligaments) by means of an optical method. *J Biomech*, 20:1003–1010.

28. Jackson DW, Grood ES, Arnoczky SP, Butler DL, Simon TM. (1987): Cruciate reconstruction using freeze dried anterior cruciate ligament allograft and a ligament augmentation device (LAD): an experimental study in a goat model. *Am J Sports Med*, 15:528–538.

29. Kennedy JC, Hawkins RJ, Willis RB. (1977): Strain gauge analysis of knee ligaments. *Clin Orthop*, 129:225–229.

30. Kennedy JC, Hawkins RJ, Willis RB, Danylchuk KD. (1976): Tension studies of human knee ligaments: yield point, ultimate failure, and disruption of the cruciate and tibial collateral ligaments. *J Bone Joint Surg*, 58:350–355.

31. Kennedy JC, Roth JH, Mendenhall HV, Sanford JB. (1980): Presidential address: intraarticular replacement in the anterior cruciate ligament-deficient knee. *Am J Sports Med*, 8:1–8.

32. Lapiere CM, Nusgens B, Pierard GE. (1977): Interactions between collagen Type I and Type III in conditioning bundles organization. *Connect Tissue Res*, 5:21–29.

33. Lee TQ, Woo SL-Y. (1988): A new method for determining cross-sectional shape and area of soft tissues. *J Biomech Eng*, 110:110–114.

34. Lewis JL, Bhybut GT. (198A): *In vivo* forces in the collateral ligaments of canine knees. *Trans Orthop Res Soc*, 6:4.

35. Lyon RM, Akeson WH, Amiel D, Kitabayashi LR, Woo SL-Y. (1991): Ultrastructural differences between the cells of the medial collateral and anterior cruciate ligaments. *Clin Orthop*, 272:279–286.

36. Lyon RM, Woo SL-Y, Hollis JM, Marcin JP, Lee EB. (1989): A new device to measure the structural properties of the femur-anterior cruciate ligament-tibia complex. *J Biomech Eng*, 111: 350–354.

37. Matthews LS, Ellis D. (1968): Viscoelastic properties of cat tendon—effects of time after death and preservation by freezing. *J Biomech*, 1:65–71.

38. Meglan D, Zuelzer W, Buck W, Berme N. (1986): The effects of quadriceps force upon the strain in the anterior cruciate ligament. *Trans Orthop Res Soc*, 11:55.

39. Minns RJ, Soden PD, Jackson DS. (1973): The role of the fibrous components and ground substance in the mechanical properties of biological tissues: a preliminary investigation. *J Biomech*, 6:153–165.

40. Monahan JJ, Grigg P, Pappas AM, Leclair WL, Marks T, Fowler DP, Sullivan TJ. (1984): *In vivo* strain patterns in the four major canine knee ligaments. *J Orthop Res*, 2:408–418.

41. Newton PO, Woo SL-Y, Kitabayashi LR, Lyon RM, Anderson DR, Akeson WH. (1990): Ultrastructural changes in knee ligaments following immobilization. *Matrix*, 10:314–319.

42. Njus GO, Njus NM. (1986): A non-contact method for determining cross-sectional area of soft tissues. *Trans Orthop Res Soc*, 32:126.

43. Noyes FR, DeLucas JL, Torvik PJ. (1974): Biomechanics of anterior cruciate ligament failure: an analysis of strain-rate sensitivity and mechanisms of failure in primates. *J Bone Joint Surg [Am]*, 56A:236–253.

44. Noyes FR, Grood ES. (1976): The strength of the anterior cruciate ligament in humans and rhesus monkeys: age-related and species-related changes. *J Bone Joint Surg [Am]*, 58A:1074–1082.

45. Nunley RL. (1958): The ligamenta flava of the dog: a study of tensile and physical properties. *Am J Phys Med*, 37:256–268.

46. O'Donoghue DH, Frank GR, Jeter GL, Johnson W, Zeiders JW, Kenyon R. (1971): Repair and reconstruction of the anterior cruciate ligament in dogs—factors influencing long term results. *J Bone Joint Surg [Am]*, 53A:710–718.

47. Peterson RH, Woo SL-Y. (1986): A new methodology to determine the mechanical properties of ligaments at high strain rates. *J Biomech Eng*, 108:365–367.

48. Rauch G, Allzeit B, Gotzen L. (1987): Tensile strength of the anterior cruciate ligament in dependence on age. In: *Proceedings of the meeting on the Biomechanics of Human Knee Ligaments*, University of Ulm, Ulm, Germany p 24.

49. Rigby BF, Hirai N, Spikes JD, Eyring H. (1959): The mechanical properties of rat tail tendon. *J Gen Physiol*, 43:265–283.

50. Shrive NG, Lam TC, Damson E, Frank CB. (1988): A new method of measuring the cross-sectional area of connective tissue structures. *J Biomech Eng*, 110:104–109.

51. Trent PS, Walker PS, Wolf B. (1976): Ligament length patterns, strength, and rotational axes of the knee joint. *Clin Orthop*, 117:263–270.

52. van Rens TJG, van den Berg AF, Huiskes R, Kuypers W. (1986): Substitution of the anterior cruciate ligament—a long term histologic and biomechanical study with autogenous pedicled grafts of the iliotibial band in dogs. *Arthroscopy*, 2:139–154.

53. VanBrocklin JD, Ellis DG. (1965): A study of the mechanical behavior of toe extensor tendons under applied stress. *Arch Phys Med*, 46:369–373.

54. Viidik A. (1968): Elasticity and tensile strength of the anterior cruciate ligament in rabbits as influenced by training. *Acta Physiol Scand*, 74:372–380.

55. Vogel HG. (1974): Correlation between tensile strength and collagen content in rat skin: effect of age and cortisol treatment. *Connect Tissue Res*, 2:177–182.

56. Wang CW, Weiss J, Albright JA, Buckwalter RM, Woo SL-Y. (1990): Life-long exercise and aging effects on the canine medial collateral ligament. *Trans Orthop Res Soc*, 518.

57. Warren RF, Marshall JL, Girgis F. (1974): The prime static stabilizers on the medial side of the knee. *J Bone Joint Surg*, 56:665–674.

58. Woo SL-Y. (1982): Mechanical properties of tendons and ligaments: quasi-static and nonlinear viscoelastic properties. *Biorheology*, 19:385–396.

59. Woo SL-Y, Akeson WJ, Jemmott GF. (1976): The measurements of nonhomogeneous, directional mechanical properties of articular cartilage in tension. *J Biomech*, 9:785–791.

60. Woo SL-Y, Danto MI, Ohland KJ, Lee TQ, Newton PO. (1990): The use of a laser micrometer system to determine the cross-sectional shape and area of ligaments: a comparative study with two existing methods. *J Biomech Eng*, 112:425–430.

61. Woo SL-Y, Gomez MA, Seguchi Y, Endo CM, Akeson WH. (1983): Measurement of mechanical properties of ligament substance from a bone-ligament-bone preparation. *J Orthop Res*, 1:22–29.

62. Woo SL-Y, Gomez MA, Sites TJ, Newton PO, Orlando CA, Akeson WH. (1987): The biomechanical and morphological changes in medial collateral ligament of the rabbit after immobilization and remobilization. *J Bone Joint Surg [Am]*, 69A:1200–1211.

63. Woo SL-Y, Hollis JM, Adams DJ, Lyon RM, Takai S. (1991): Tensile properties of the human femur-anterior cruciate ligament-tibia complex: the effects of specimen age and orientation. *Am J Sports Med*, 19:217–225.

64. Woo SL-Y, Hollis JM, Roux RD, Gomez MA, Inoue M, Kleiner JB, Akeson WH. (1987): Effects of knee flexion on the structural properties of the rabbit femur-anterior cruciate ligament-tibia complex (FATC). *J Biomech*, 20:557–563.

65. Woo SL-Y, Livesay GA, Engle C. (1992): Biomechanics of the human anterior cruciate ligament: ACL structure and role in knee motion. *Orthop Rev*, Jul 21(7):835–842.

66. Woo SL-Y, Newton PO, MacKenna DA, Lyon RM. (1992): A comparative evaluation of the mechanical properties of the rabbit medial collateral and anterior cruciate ligaments. *J Biomech*, 25:377–386.

67. Yoshiya S, Andrish JT, Manley MT, Bauer TW. (1987): Graft tension in anterior cruciate ligament reconstruction: an *in vivo* study in dogs. *Am J Sports Med*, 15:464–470.

The Anterior Cruciate Ligament: Current and Future Concepts, edited by D.W. Jackson, et al. Raven Press, Ltd., New York © 1993.

CHAPTER 5

The Mechanical and Viscoelastic Properties of the Anterior Cruciate Ligament and of ACL Fascicles

Roger C. Haut

The knee is one of the most frequently injured joints in the human body. Epidemiological studies estimate that 1.6 to 1.9 million patients, most between the ages of 15 and 44 years, see a physician for a knee sprain each year (10). Among those who sustain an acute traumatic hemoarthrosis to the knee, the anterior cruciate ligament is partially or completely torn more than 70% of the time (20,58). Many studies conducted over the years discussed the mechanisms of injury to the ACL. Butler et al. (9) introduced the concepts of primary and secondary restraints in the knee. The ACL functions as the primary restraint to limit anterior tibial displacements (9,25). The ACL is the primary ligamentous restraint to anterior tibial displacement up to 5 mm at both 30° and 90° of knee flexion. It provides 85% to 87% of the total ligamentous restraining force. The ACL functions as a secondary restraint to tibial rotation (1,50).

The ACL attaches to the depression in the front of the intercondyloid eminence of the tibia, being blended with the anterior extremity of the lateral meniscus; it passes upward, backward, and laterally and is fixed into the medial and back part of the lateral condyle of the femur. There is a twist of the ACL fibers in the coronal plane with external rotation of the fibers by approximately 90° as they approach the tibial surface (8). This complex anatomy results in significant difficulty in the documentation of mechanical properties for the human ACL.

Recent review articles described the current state of knowledge of the mechanical function and properties of the ACL and of changes due to pathological conditions,

surgical intervention, and the subsequent healing response of this structure (10,11). Although the tensile behavior of the human ACL has been studied for many decades, there are really only a few publications that characterize its stiffness and strength. In these studies the properties vary dramatically with age of the subject (56) and flexion of the joint (71). Another difficulty in the literature is that many biomechanical studies have used animal models. In these cases the anatomy is different than the human (2), so loads in the ACL may not compare to those in the human ligament. The differences may result in an altered morphology (18,26) that could, in turn, cause this structure to respond differently than the human to physiological forces, deformations, surgical interventions, etc. The complex anatomy of the ACL also suggests that individual portions of the structure experience different loading histories. This could be reflected in variable morphology and material properties for the individual fascicles (29). In this chapter I attempt to establish a basis for the characterization of structural and material properties of the ACL, as well as other ligaments and tendons. Some of the recent literature on this subject has been integrated into the following discussion.

MICROSTRUCTURAL-MECHANICAL RESPONSES

The nonlinear, stiffening tensile response of a human ACL has been characterized as consisting of four specific regions. At the levels of strain imposed on the ACL during a typical clinical diagnostic test, the ligament is rarely thought to be extended beyond the nonlinear "toe" response (10) (Fig. 1). The estimated range for the normal

R. C. Haut: Department of Biomechanics, College of Osteopathic Medicine, Michigan State University, East Lansing, Michigan 48824.

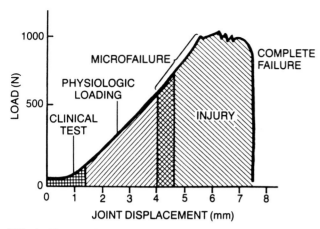

FIG. 1. The tensile response of an anterior cruciate ligament during a simulated anterior drawer. The curve has been divided into four regions: (*1*) clinical response; (*2*) linear range and physiological limits; (*3*) failure region; and (*4*) a region of sequential failure of collagen bundles and ultimate structural collapse of the structure. (From ref. 11a, with permission.)

physiological loading probably encompasses both the nonlinear "toe" and a portion of the linear response (59) (Fig. 2). The actual loads existing in the ACL during normal physiological response are controversial. Morrison (51) estimated *in vivo* forces in the human ACL from force plate analysis in a number of typical daily functions. In level walking the maximum estimated force in the ACL is 169 N; in ascending stairs 27 N; in descending stairs 93 N; in ascending a ramp 67 N; and in descending a ramp approximately 445 N. Because frictional forces were not considered, Morrison estimated that these forces may be approximately 40 N low. Noyes and Grood (56) calculated values of 200 to 400 N for younger humans and 80 to 160 N for older humans. Chen and Black (12) estimated the tensile forces in the ACL during normal function to range from 67 N for ascending stairs to 630 N for jogging. It is clear from these estimates of

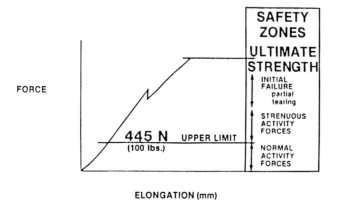

FIG. 2. Schematic load-elongation curve for an anterior cruciate ligament-bone preparation showing zones of safe loading and the estimated limits on normal activity loading. (Adapted from ref. 59, with permission.)

the *in vivo* loads and from recent tensile data from the human ACL that the ligament is normally tensioned over the nonlinear "toe" and the early linear ranges during normal functioning, yet only a few studies have concentrated on the characterization of tensile response at these low levels of elongation. It is generally accepted that the primary structural event during the "toe" part of the tensile response for ligaments and tendons is straightening of initially crimped bundles of collagen (64,65). The human ACL is composed of a complex arrangement of collagen fibrils in bundles called fibers, subfascicles, and fascicles (73) (Fig. 3). The collagen fibrils in the human ACL range from 150 to 250 nm in diameter. The collagen fibrils are grouped into bundles averaging 5 to 10 nm in diameter. Subfascicles averaging 100 to 250 nm are enclosed in a sheath known as the endotenon (18). Fascicles (250 nm to 1 μm in diameter) seem to be composed of subfascicles of different sizes and enclosed together by a connective tissue sheath called the epitenon. Fine fibrils (180 to 650 μm) of unknown origin and function seem to exist between the longitudinally oriented collagenous units.

One of the most significant morphological properties of the human ACL is a waviness or crimping at the level between fiber and fascicle (units ranging from 20 to 640 nm). The waviness period of approximately 20.6 ± 6.7 nm for the human ACL is significantly less, say, than that of the patellar tendon, which is often used as a substitute graft (7,59). The waviness of collagen fascicles in the human ACL is quite complex in nature. Two patterns can be observed, depending on the anatomical site. The posterior band is composed of small fascicles embedded in a loose alveolar tissue, whereas the anterior band is formed of dense and thick collagenous fascicles (73). In addition, there seems to be a possible difference between the periphery and interior of the ACL; the peripheral fascicles often follow a helical pattern, whereas the internal fascicles appear straight and parallel to the longitudinal axis (Fig. 4). Studies with isolated subunits of the human ACL and patellar tendon (PT) show that the crimp period decreases near the bone insertions (63). Although the origin of the variation in crimping of collagen down the length of ligaments is unknown, the feature may serve to protect the insertion sites from damaging loads.

The complex nature of the above-described crimping in collagen of the human ACL currently precludes an accurate microstructurally based model, but a number of structural models have been developed over the years to describe the process of uncrimping in the collagen from other ligaments, tendons, and connective tissues. Viidik (66) was one of the first investigators to develop a mathematical formulation describing the uncrimping of collagen in the rabbit ACL. The nonlinear elasticity model was based on a progressive recruitment of individual linearly elastic components (24). Constitutive equa-

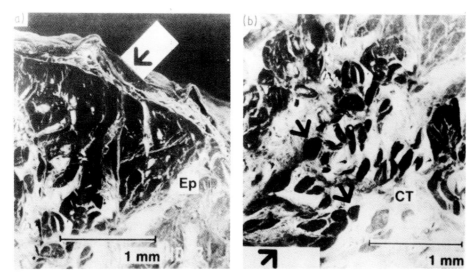

FIG. 3. Transverse sections of a human anterior cruciate ligament showing the delineation of large fascicles of collagen by the epitenon (**A,** *Ep*) and single fibers and subfascicles (**B,** *arrows*). Section A was taken from the anteromedial band, and Section B from the posterolateral band. (Contributed by H. Yahia and reproduced from ref. 73, with permission.)

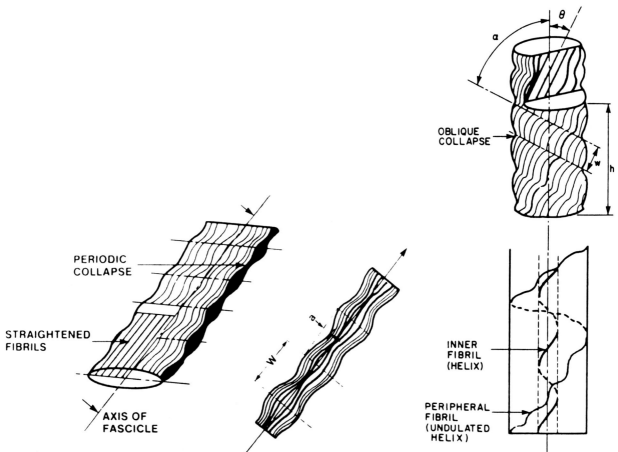

FIG. 4. Schematic diagrams showing the collagen fibril crimp patterns evident in the human anterior cruciate ligament. **A:** The centrally located fascicles are either straight or undulated in a planar wave pattern. **B:** Those at the periphery are arranged in a more helical wave pattern. (Contributed by H. Yahia and reproduced from ref. 74, with permission.)

tions have been proposed based on the crimp unfolding and refolding of collagen during loading and unloading of soft connective tissues. Various crimp shapes have been proposed, including sinusoidal (16,46). Kastelic et al. (42) described a model for the uncrimping of collagen fibrils within a single fascicle from tail tendon of rat (RTT). The "toe" response of the RTT was assumed to be due to a progressive straightening (recruitment) of collagen fibrils, which had planar crimp periods that decreased linearly from the center of the fascicle. The crimp structure was based on earlier studies using x-ray diffraction (28) and electron microscopy (41). The mathematical model of Lanir (46) has recently been adapted to model the tensile response of human patellar tendons (4). This model assumes a naturally occurring waviness (crimp) of collagen in the stress-free state (Fig. 5). As the tendon is deformed, the crimp gradually disappears as collagen becomes straightened. Once straight, the collagen is able to resist deformation and generate load. It is assumed that the collagen is not straightened all at once but sequentially, such that the distribution of slack-lengths is described by a normal Gaussian distribution function. The model analysis is based on a curve-fitting routine and fits well to tensile data on control and irradiated patellar tendons. Qualitatively, the model supports histological impressions that show that gamma irradiation induces crimp into collagen and alters its tensile modulus (19). Although one can introduce sophisticated geometry for the crimp pattern into these types of structure-based models, more research is needed to docu-

ment the microarchitecture of the load-bearing collagenous structures in the ACL and other ligaments and tendons.

The second range of tensile response, in which the ligament exhibits a linear response, is generally thought to represent the tensile response of straightened bundles of collagen. The slope of this region is termed the structural stiffness. It is often used as the parameter on which substitute grafts are selected (35,59). The slope of the corresponding stress-strain response in this region is a measure of the tensile modulus of the ligament. Recently, Haut et al. (37) found that the tensile modulus of the canine PT correlated with the content of mature (cross-linked) collagen. In studies on irradiated patellar tendon, Haut et al. (36) found that a decline in the tangent modulus paralleled with an increase in the solubility of tendon collagen in a weak enzyme (pepsin) solution. Other studies have correlated the tangent modulus of tissue with the content of mature collagen (3). A complete and detailed description of the covalent cross-linkages in collagen responsible for this tensile stiffness is currently lacking (19).

VISCOELASTIC RESPONSES

In one of the earlier reports on the ACL, Haut and Little (30) performed subfailure tests on the canine femur-ACL-tibia preparation. The authors documented that the slope of the stress-strain curve in the "toe" region increased with increased strain rate. These strain rates were low, however, compared to those expected when the ACL sustains an injury. Noyes and coworkers (55) studied how larger variations in the strain rate influenced the stiffness of rhesus monkey ACL-bone units. They found that the stiffness was relatively unaffected by 100-fold increases in strain rate (0.66%/sec to 66%/sec). The authors did document, however, that the ligament preparation failed at higher maximum load and strain and absorbed more energy before failure in the high-strain-rate experiments. Strain rates that occur during ligamentous injury may be much higher (i.e., from 50%/sec to as high as 150,000%/sec) (17). In the engineering literature the notion of a time-dependent tensile response is commonly handled with the concept of viscoelasticity. If it is appropriate to attribute the discovery of viscoelasticity to any one person, the honor may go to Wilhelm Weber (68). He fabricated a name to describe the phenomenon he observed while conducting tensile tests on silk. Weber observed that silk threads obeyed the law of proportionality between stretching load and the resulting elongation (Hooke's Law) but only for a short time after applying the load. If the load was applied for a long time, then elongation would continually increase with time. Roy (62) conducted tensile experiments on a wide variety of animal tissues and found the time-

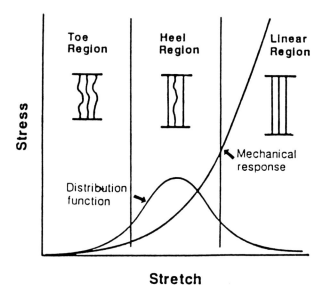

FIG. 5. A typical stress-strain plot representing the tensile response of a ligament or tendon and the proposed distribution of crimps in the collagen according to Lanir (46). During initial stretch the crimped fibrils of collagen straighten. As more and more fibrils are straightened, the response stiffens due to tension being developed in the high-modulus collagen fibers. (Contributed by S. Belkoff and reproduced from ref. 4, with permission.)

dependent elongation (or creep) to be universal. Before Boltzmann (5,6) no unified theory had been developed to describe creep and the associated phenomenon known as load (stress) relaxation. Today the superposition principle of Boltzmann has helped establish a sound basis for the theory of linear viscoelasticity. In the first of two assumptions set forth by Boltzmann, he stated that for linear viscoelasticity the ratio of strain to stress in two separate creep experiments would have to be a constant dependent only on time (called the *creep function*). A plot of this ratio for various levels of load (stress) yields the so-called "isochronal" curve. For linear viscoelastic materials the slope of this curve is a constant.

Assuming superposition of separate creep experiments performed concurrently on a material, this leads to the following hereditary integral formulation

$$\epsilon(t) = \int_0^t \Psi(t - t') \frac{d\sigma(t')dt'}{dt'}$$

or conversely in terms of stress

$$\sigma(t) = \int_0^t \Phi(t - t') \frac{d\epsilon(t')}{dt'} dt'$$

where $\Phi(t)$ is termed the stress relaxation function.

Studies indicate that for tendons and ligaments the isochronal curve is highly nonlinear (Fig. 6). Fung (27) proposed a theoretical formulation to handle the nonlinear viscoelastic response of biological tissues within the

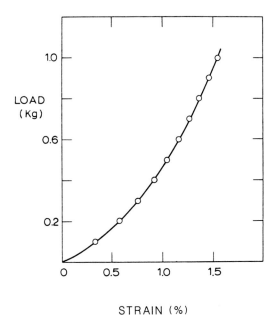

FIG. 6. Representative "isochronal" curve from a human flexor tendon at $t = 20$ sec. The curve is constructed from the ratio of strain to applied load in separate creep experiments. The slope of the line represents the creep function. For most biological tissues the creep and corresponding relaxation functions are nonlinear. This is handled by the quasi-linear viscoelastic formulation according to Fung (27). (From ref. 15, with permission.)

framework of a linear theory. The empirically based formulation assumes that the relaxation (or creep) function is dependent on both strain (stress) and time and can be written as

$$K(\epsilon, t) = \Phi(t)\sigma^e(\epsilon)$$

where σ^e is the "elastic" response (a function of only strain) and $\Phi(t)$ is a reduced relaxation function (function of only time) with $\Phi(0) = 1$. The stress at any time is then given by the convolution integral between the "reduced" relaxation function and the rate of elastic stress, or

$$\sigma(t) = \int_0^t \Phi(t - t') \frac{d\sigma^e(\epsilon)}{d\epsilon} \frac{d\epsilon}{dt'} dt'$$

Given $\Phi(t)$, $\sigma^e(\epsilon)$, and strain history $\epsilon(t)$, the stress $\sigma(t)$ is completely described by a "quasi-linear" viscoelastic law.

The above formulation has been used to characterize the viscoelastic response of tendons (31) and ligaments (40,49,70). Historically, a continuous set of parallel Maxwell elements, with time constants τ_i, modulus E_i, described by the function $H(\tau)/\tau$ and an isolated spring to confer solid properties, have been used to describe stress relaxation for engineering materials (53). Letting $H(\tau)$ be given a box distribution, such that $H(\tau) = 0$ outside the internal $\tau_1 < \tau < \tau_2$ and $H(\tau) = C/\tau$ inside, yields the reduced relaxation function

$$\Phi(t) = \frac{1 + C[E_1(\tau/\tau_2) - E_2(\tau/\tau_2)]}{1 + C \ln (\tau_2/\tau_1)} + O[C]$$

where $E_i(t)$ is the exponential integral and $O[C]$ can be neglected (70). The above equation indicates that the reduced relaxation function is linear in the logarithm of time. This fact has been borne out in the literature (31,40,49,70) (Fig. 7). The formulation has recently been used to describe the time-dependent tensile response of anteromedial bundles of the porcine ACL relaxation experiments, yielding $\Phi(t) = 0.858 - 0.0491\, n(t)$ with an elastic function given by $\sigma^e = 210(e^{0.63\epsilon} - 1)$. The expressions have been used in the quasi-linear viscoelastic formulation to predict the tensile responses in cyclic experiments between 1% and 5% strain (49) (Fig. 8).

The slope of the "reduced" relaxation function determines the relative degree of viscoelastic (time) effect in the tissue. Quasi-linear modeling constants are typically derived from relaxation testing (21). Perhaps the greatest limitation is the inability to perform an infinite rate ramp and hold relaxation test. As a result the initial portion of the measured relaxation function is lost, and the measured elastic function contains a component of relaxation. Dortmans et al. (21) noted the importance of these limitations using a numerical technique to reduce theoretical data. Lin et al. (49) used a normalization process to determine quasi-linear model parameters from finite rate ramp-relaxation experiments. Nigul and Nigul (54) described an interactive technique for the removal of

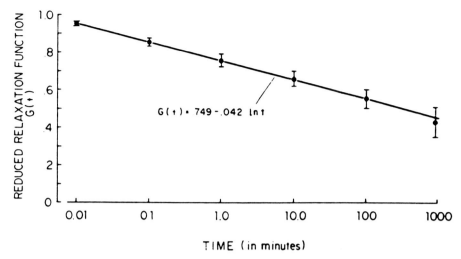

FIG. 7. Reduced relaxation function for canine MCL (n=8). Representative long-term "relaxation" response of a ligament showing a linear curve in the logarithm of time. The slope of this line corresponds to the rate of relaxation and the relative degree of viscoelasticity in the tissue. The rate of relaxation for ligaments and tendons is typically much less than that of articular cartilage. (From ref. 70, with permission.)

these effects from τ_1. Myers et al. (53) corrected for this effect in their studies on the cervical spine by extrapolation of the relaxation data to time zero with a linear least squares fit over the first 200 ms of relaxation. Dramatic effects can be seen in the prediction of the viscoelastic properties of these tissue structures for short time experiments, when the above deficiencies in the experimental methods are corrected (Fig. 9). These factors are important in the characterization of ACL responses during high-speed injury-producing situations.

The basis for a viscoelastic effect in the tensile responses of the ACL is largely unknown, but we can draw some qualitative information from experiments on other tissues. Age-dependent changes in the viscoelastic properties of the rabbit MCL to 3% strain may be a reflection of alterations in the viscoelastic properties of collagen itself, the matrix of proteoglycans, or interactions between these two components (45). In tensile experiments on bovine articular cartilage, Woo et al. (69) found a response with much shorter relaxation time constants compared to the ACL data. A high content of hydrated matrix proteoglycans may serve as a basis for the viscoelastic effect, as viscous shearing stresses may develop

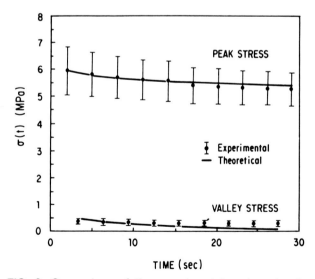

FIG. 8. Comparison of the experimental peak and valley stress relaxation for the cyclic stretching of the anteromedial bundle of the porcine anterior cruciate ligament between 1% and 5% strain at Hz. Note the excellent theoretical fit using the quasi-linear theory of viscoelasticity according to Fung (27). The degree of fit was improved significantly using a new normalization scheme. (From ref. 49, with permission.)

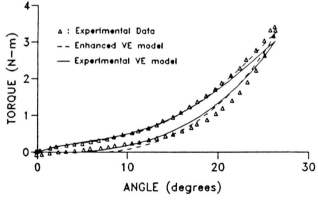

FIG. 9. Comparison of the torsional responses of the human cervical spine using the quasi-linear theory of viscoelasticity and the improved extrapolation deconvolution technique. The method uses a linear extrapolation of the short-time relaxation response to remove the effects of stress relaxation from finite-time ramp functions for determination of the "elastic" response function in the theory according to Fung (27). (From ref. 53, with permission.)

during the uncrimping of collagen (48). The early data of Cohen et al. (14) would support this notion. Lanir (46) used the notion that the matrix acted to support the fibrous elements in tendon and ligament by acting like an elastic foundation in low-speed experiments. In an interesting series of experiments using bovine ligamentum nuchae, Jenkins and Little (40) found that stress relaxation was nearly eliminated after removal of collagenous elements in the ligament. They concluded that the elastin component does not influence the viscoelastic effects. The studies suggest that the source of viscoelastic response in ligaments and tendons is due to the collagen fibers themselves or interactions with the hydrated matrix of proteoglycans and glycoproteins. Studies on rat tissue showed a correlation between age-related changes in the content of glycosaminoglycans and the viscoelastic response of the tissue (32,67). Recent studies with the rabbit MCL indicated that the rate of cyclic stress relaxation is decreased with a decrease in the content of water in the tissue (13). Others have shown an increase in stress relaxation with an increase in water content of the tissue (60). These data suggest that, in part, the viscoelastic effect in ligaments and tendons may depend on the movement of fluids in and out of the tissue, similar to that proposed for cartilage (52). Lanir et al. (47) recently measured the movement of fluids and proteoglycans during cyclic extensions of RTT. Cyclic stress relaxation of the human patellar tendon, for example, can be altered by the testing environment, being more pronounced in a warm, saline bath versus a drip moistening environment (35).

FAILURE RESPONSES

Over the years considerable attention has focused on the tensile failure properties of the human ACL, as well as other ligaments and tendons. It is clinically important to understand the mechanisms of tensile failure for a complete diagnosis of musculoskeletal injuries (23). With increasing participation in a more active life-style by the general population and with more demanding and intensive training regimens by sports people, injuries to the musculoskeletal system occur more frequently and receive more publicity (43). Kennedy et al. (44) conducted tensile failure studies on the isolated, human ACL, PCL, and LCL. In a hallmark paper, Noyes and Grood (56) established the current basis for strength characteristics of the human ACL and its replacements. The nonlinear response curve is typically observed until abrupt unloadings occur near the maximum load (Fig. 1). Their studies suggested that these abrupt unloadings were associated with failure of individual collagen fibrils and bundles, or fascicles. High-speed movies of the ACL under tensile failure experiments indicate that the ligament appears grossly intact well beyond the point of maximum load (57). Photomicrographs of failed ligaments indicate that collagen fibers fail in different portions of the ligament, giving an uneven cleavage line corresponding to the common "mop-end" appearance (Fig. 10).

More recently, SEM has been utilized in detailed studies of ligaments under tensile strain (75). The rabbit MCL was stretched at a low speed to 20% strain and then biologically fixed. The stress-strain response showed a characteristic nonlinear stiffening and a subsequent linear response to approximately 10.5% strain. Above this level a series of abrupt unloadings were observed to strain levels of 20% (Fig. 11). When the ligament was elongated to 10% strain, almost all fibers were able to return to the crimped configuration after unloading. Some straightened fibers, however, were observed. Higher magnifications showed that fine fibers between the major bundles of collagen were disrupted (Fig. 12A). Photomicrographs of the ligament after being strained to 15% revealed widespread microscopic disruption and disorganization of collagen fibers at tensile loads 30% of those needed to cause a gross rupture of the ligament (Fig. 12B). These data indicate that, even though ligaments are subjected to loads within the linear range, microscopic failure can occur in fine fibers between the major bundles of collagen. The clinical significance of these data are currently unknown. Elongation to 20% strain showed ruptures of thick collagen fibers whose diameters were 5 to 10 μm. The ends of the fiber bundles were found to be coiled, possibly indicating a denaturation of the individual collagen fibers after tensile yielding and subsequent failure (Fig. 12C).

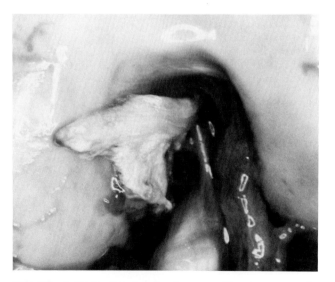

FIG. 10. A figure showing the "mop-end" appearance of a cruciate ligament after tensile separation within the substance rather than an avulsion injury. This mode of rupture inhibits a distinct visualization of ligament damage because of the multiple levels of injury within the substance. The ligament may appear intact until complete separation, as indicated.

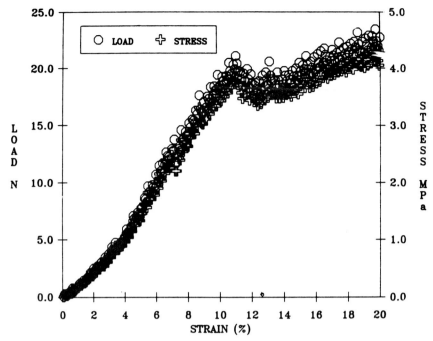

FIG. 11. The stress/load strain responses of a rabbit medial collateral ligament stretched to failure at low speed. Note the series of abrupt unloadings that occur at approximately 10.5%. Above 10.5%, microruptures occurred in thin collagen fibers (1 to 3 μm in diameter). The microfailures occur more frequently above 15% strain. (Contributed by H. Yahia and reproduced from ref. 75, with permission.)

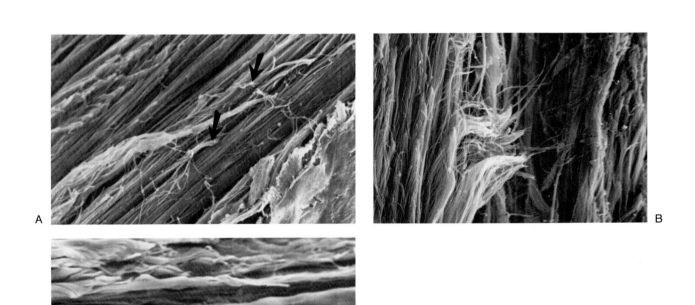

FIG. 12. Scanning electron micrographs of the strained medial collateral ligament. **A:** Disruption of thin collagen fibers between major bundles. **B:** Photomicrograph showing disruption of collagen fibers at strains well below the ultimate load of this ligament. **C:** Photomicrograph of the ligament strained to 20% showing rupture of collagen fiber bundles at 10 μm in diameter. (Approximately ×1,000) (Contributed by H. Yahia and reproduced from ref. 75, with permission.)

TIME-DEPENDENT FAILURE RESPONSES

Kennedy et al. (44) found that the maximum load tolerated by isolated human ACLs increased by 32%, on the average, for a fourfold increase in strain rate (12.5 to 50.0 cm/min). With animal models, the mechanisms of tensile failure for bone-ligament-bone preparations have been shown to be sensitive to the strain rate of loading (55). In studies by Noyes et al. (55) using the rhesus monkey, the mechanism of structural failure for the bone-ligament-bone preparation was via substance at 66% strain per second, whereas for a nominal strain rate of 0.66%/sec the primary mode was by avulsion of bone from the tibia. The maximum load and strain at failure were increased, on the average, 21.3% and 9.5%, respectively, in high- versus low-speed experiments.

Few studies have actually concentrated on the mechanisms of strain rate sensitivity (viscoelasticity) in the tensile failure properties of the ligament substance itself. This may be, in part, because of a relative insensitivity of the tensile response to strain rate (55) or the difficulty of performing controlled high-speed experiments (61). Before the onset of noticeable failure of collagen, the fibers are thought to be relatively straight. Earlier studies describing the mechanisms of viscoelasticity in ligaments and tendons implicated only the viscous forces associated with the uncrimping of collagen, as the fibers slide through the matrix of proteoglycans. Using an isolated RTT, Haut (32) documented that the sensitivity of tensile strength to strain rate was dependent on age and degree of maturation. High strain rates (720%/sec) delayed the onset of a tensile yielding process in collagen fibrils versus "low-speed" tests at 3.6%/sec. Changing the degree of covalent cross-linking in collagen at each age by the administration of a lathrogen to the animal's diet increased the sensitivity of tensile strength to strain rate, but age-dependent alterations were not affected (34). Selective digestion of proteoglycans in the matrix of the RTT did not alter the sensitivity of the failure properties to strain rate (33). Based on these data, with a unique tendon model, one might suggest that the viscoelastic (strain rate-sensitive) response during tensile failure is primarily due to collagen fibers themselves and therefore depends on the degree and character of the covalent cross-linkages in the fibrils. Clearly, this is an area of needed research emphasis.

THE MECHANICAL PROPERTIES OF SUBUNITS

The tensile failure properties of bone-ACL-bone preparations have also recently been shown to depend on flexion of the joint, especially when loaded along the tibial axis (22,71,72). This phenomenon is largely due to the recruitment of collagen fiber bundles in the ACL. That is, when the ACL is being stretched along its tibial axis, fewer collagen fiber bundles are being loaded simultaneously, especially as knee flexion increases. When stretched along the tibial axis, the tendency is for fiber bundles to successively be "peeled off" the tibia rather than avulsing abruptly at the tibia or failing abruptly by midsubstance tearing, as when using an anatomical ligament axis (72). Furthermore, because of its nonparallel bundles of unequal length, the force-deformation relationships of the ACL depend on flexion angle of the joint (Fig. 13). It is not hard, therefore, to imagine that during normal function of the knee some subunits (fascicles) are loaded more often than others and to varying degrees.

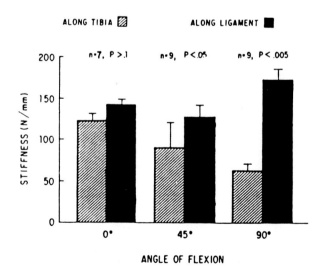
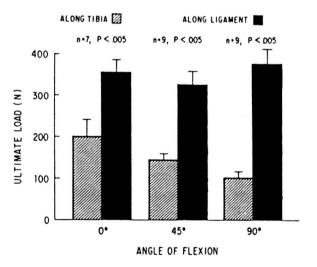

FIG. 13. Structural properties of the rabbit bone-ACL-bone preparation at three flexion angles. Note the increase in strength and stiffness of the preparation when it is stretched along its axis. This minimizes a "peeling-off" effect and more uniformly loads the individual bundles of collagen. (From ref. 71, with permission.)

Recent evidence suggests that the anteromedial bundle of the ACL supports the majority of the anteriorly directed load and that the posterolateral bundle remains slack at joint positions other than full extension (38,39). The anteromedial bundle probably appears more collagenous because of these enhanced stresses (73). The spatial variation in bundle morphology can be expected to translate into variations in the mechanical properties of the fasciculi. Guan and Butler (29) documented the tensile properties of anteromedial, anterolateral, and posterior bundles of the human ACL from five donors aged 27 ± 4 years. Significant differences were noted in the ultimate stress and failure strain energy density between the posterior and anteromedial bundles. These data help confirm the complex, inhomogeneous nature of the anterior cruciate ligament.

SUMMARY

There are a number of points that should be highlighted for future research. The readers are again referred to two recent review articles on the ACL by Butler (10,11). These articles describe many important areas of current and future research on the ACL not mentioned in this chapter. A point was made in the chapter that normal physiological responses of the ACL entail the nonlinear "toe" and early linear regions of tensile response. Although significant efforts are currently being expended on the morphological aspects of collagen in the ACL, we need to incorporate these data into more current, sophisticated microstructure-based models. The incorporation of the complex collagen fiber bundle morphology, as well as its interactions with matrix components, is essential in the development of these analytical tools. The influences of matrix proteoglycans and tissue water must be elucidated at injury-producing rates of loading. The documented inhomogeneities of the collagen fascicles and their complex geometry as they transverse the joint space will make this aspect a difficult, but needed, area of future research. Along these same lines, it will be critically important that we continue to study and document fully the morphological, anatomical, and biomechanical features of animal models, for it's via these models that advances in surgical reconstruction and more conservative approaches to rehabilitation will be realized. Another critically important aspect of our future effort should be the continued study of stress and motion on the healing response and morphology of the ACL and other musculoskeletal tissues.

ACKNOWLEDGMENTS

I thank Drs. H. Yahia and S. Belkoff for the figures they supplied. Dr. D. Butler was also very helpful in the assembly of pertinent reference information. I also acknowledge the help of Ms. Brenda Robinson and Ms. Tammy Haut in the preparation of this manuscript.

REFERENCES

1. Ahmed AM, Hyder A, Burke DL, Chan KH. (1987): *In-vitro* ligament tension pattern in the flexed knee in passive loading. *J Orthop Res*, 5:217–230.
2. Arnoczky SP. (1990): Animal models for knee ligament research. In: Daniel D, ed. *Knee ligaments: structure, function, injury, and repair.* New York: Raven Press, pp 401–417.
3. Belkoff SM, Haut RC. (1991): A structural model used to evaluate the changing microstructure of maturing rat skin. *J Biomech*, 24:711–720.
4. Belkoff SM, Haut RC. (1992): Microstructurally based model analysis of gamma-irradiated tendon allografts. *J Orthop Res*, 10:461–464.
5. Boltzmann L. (1874): Theorie der elastischen nachwirkung. *Sitzungsber Akad Wissenschaft II*, 70:275–306.
6. Boltzmann L. (1876): Zur theorie der eladtischen noachwirkung. *Ann Physik Chemie*, 7:624–654.
7. Burks RT, Haut RC, Lancaster R. (1989): Biomechanical and histological observations of the dog patellar tendon after removal of its central one-third. *Am J Sports Med*, 18:146–153.
8. Burks RT. (1990): Gross anatomy. In: Daniel D, Akeson W, O'Connor J, eds. *Knee ligaments: structure, function, injury and repair.* New York: Raven Press, pp 59–76.
9. Butler DL, Noyes FR, Grood E. (1980): Ligamentous restraint to anterior-posterior drawer in the human knee. *J Bone Joint Surg* [*Am*], 62A:259–270.
10. Butler DL. (1989): Anterior cruciate ligament: its normal response and replacement. *J Orthop Res*, 7:910–921.
11. Butler DL, Guan Y. (1991): Biomechanics of the anterior cruciate ligament and its replacements. In: Mow VC, Ratcliffe A, Woo SL-Y, eds. *Biomechanics of diarthrodial joints.* New York: Springer-Verlag, pp 105–154.
11a. Carlstedt, CA, Nordin M. Biomechanics of tendons and ligaments. In: Nordin M, VH Frankel, eds. *Basic biomechanics of the musculoskeletal system, 2nd edition.* Lea and Febiger, Philadelphia, p. 66.
12. Chen EH, Black J. (1980): Materials design analysis of the prosthetic anterior cruciate ligament. *J Biomed Mater Res*, 14:567–586.
13. Chimich L, Sterenberg D, Frank C, Shrive N, Marchuk L. (1989): Water content alters viscoelastic behavior of ligaments. *Trans Orthop Res Soc*, 14:186.
14. Cohen RE, Hooley CJ, McCrum NG. (1974): Mechanism of the viscoelastic deformation of collagenous tissue. *Nature*, 247:59–61.
15. Cohen RE, Hooley CJ, McCrum NG. (1976): Viscoelastic creep of collagenous tissue. *J Biomech*, 9:175–184.
16. Comminou M, Yannas. (1976): Dependences of stress-strain nonlinearity of connective tissue on the geometry of collagen fibers. *J Biomech*, 9:427–433.
17. Crowninshield R, Pope MH, Johnson RJ. (1976): An analytical model of the knee. *J Biomech*, 9:397–405.
18. Danylchuk KD, Finlay JB, Krcek JP. (1978): Microstructural organization of human and bovine cruciate ligaments. *Clin Orthop Rel Res*, 131:294–298.
19. DeDeyne P, Haut RC. (1991): The effects of gamma irradiation on patellar tendon allografts. *J Connect Tissue Res*, 27:51–63.
20. DeHaven K. (1980): Diagnosis of acute knee injuries with hemarthrosis. *Am J Sports Med*, 8:9–14.
21. Dortmans LJ, Sauren AA, Rousseau EP. (1984): Parameter estimation using the quasi-linear viscoelastic model proposed by Fung. *J Biomech Eng*, 106:198–203.
22. Figgie HE, Bahniuk EH, Heiple KG, Davy DT. (1986): The effects of tibial-femoral angle on the failure mechanics of the canine anterior cruciate ligament. *J Biomech*, 19:89–91.
23. Frank CB, Woo SL-Y. (1985): Clinical biomechanics of sports injuries. In: Nahum AM, Melvin J, eds. *The biomechanics of trauma.* Norwalk, CT: ACC, pp 181–203.
24. Frisen M, Magi M, Sonnerup L, Viidik A. (1969): Rheological

analysis of soft collagenous tissue: Part I. Theoretical considerations. *J Biomech,* 2:13–20.

25. Fukubayashi T, Torzilli P, Sherman M, Warren R. (1982): An *in vitro* biomechanical evaluation of anterior-posterior motion of the knee. *J Bone Joint Surg [Am],* 64A:258–264.

26. Fuss FK. (1991): Anatomy and function of the cruciate ligaments of the domestic pig *(Sus scrofa domestica): a comparison with human cruciates. J Anat,* 178:11–20.

27. Fung FBC. (1972): Stress-strain-history relations of soft tissues in simple elongation. In: Fung, Perrone, Anliker, eds. *Biomechanics: its foundations and objectives.* Englewood Cliffs, NJ: Prentice Hall, pp 181–208.

28. Gathercole LJ, Keller A. (1975): Light microscopic waveform in collagenous tissues and their structural implications. In: *Colston Papers,* No. 26. London: Butterworths, pp 153–187.

29. Guan Y, Butler D. (1990): Location-dependent variations in the material properties of anterior cruciate ligament subunits. *Adv Bioeng,* 17:5–7.

30. Haut RC, Little RW. (1969): The rheological properties of canine anterior cruciate ligaments. *J Biomech,* 2:289–298.

31. Haut RC, Little RW. (1972): A constitutive equation for collagen fibers. *J Biomech,* 5:423–430.

32. Haut RC. (1983): Age-dependent influence of strain rate on the tensile failure of rat-tail tendon. *J Biomech Eng,* 105:296–299.

33. Haut RC, DeCou JM. (1984): The effect of enzymatic removal of glycosaminoglycans on the strength of tendon. *Adv Bioeng ASME,* 48–49.

34. Haut RC. (1985): The effect of a lathyritic diet on the sensitivity of tendon to strain rate. *J Biomech Eng,* 107:166–174.

35. Haut RC, Powlison AC. (1990): The effects of test environment and cyclic stretching on the failure properties of human patellar tendons. *J Orthop Res,* 8:532–540.

36. Haut RC, DeDeyne P, Curcione PJ, Farquhar AL. (1990): Thermal stability and solubility of collagen in patellar tendons after gamma irradiation. In: Woo SL-Y, Wayne JS, MacKenna DA, eds. *Proceedings of the First World Congress of Biomechanics,* p 233.

37. Haut RC, Lancaster RL, DeCamp CE. (1992): Mechanical properties of the canine patellar tendon: some correlations with age and the content of collagen. *J Biomech,* 25:163–173.

38. Hollis JM, Marcin JP, Horibe S, Woo SL-Y. (1988): Load determination in ACL fiber bundles under knee loading. *Trans Orthop Res Soc,* 13:58.

39. Hollis JM, Horibe S, Adams DJ, Marcin JP, Woo SL-Y. (1989): Force distribution in the anterior cruciate ligament as a function of flexion angle. In: Torzilli PA, Friedman MH, eds. *Biomechanics Symposium.* New York: American Society of Mechanical Engineers, pp 41–44.

40. Jenkins RB, Little RW. (1974): A constitutive equation for parallel-fibered elastic tissue. *J Biomech,* 7:397–402.

41. Kastelic J, Galeski A, Baer E. (1978): The multicomposite structure of tendons. *Connect Tissue Res,* 6:11–23.

42. Kastelic J, Palley I, Baer E. (1980): A structural mechanical model for tendon crimping. *J Biomech,* 13:887–893.

43. Kellet J. (1986): Acute soft tissue injuries—a review of the literature. *Med Sci Sports Exerc,* 18:489–500.

44. Kennedy JC, Hawkins RJ, Willis RB, Danylchuk KD. (1976): Tension studies of human knee ligaments. *J Bone Joint Surg [Am],* 58A:350–355.

45. Lam T, Frank C, Shrive N. (1989): Ligament viscoelastic behavior changes with maturation. Presented at the 35th Annual Meeting of the Orthopaedic Research Society (p 187).

46. Lanir Y. (1978): Structure-strength relations in mammalian tendon. *Biophys J,* 24:541–554.

47. Lanir Y, Salant EL, Foux A. (1988): Physico-chemical and microstructural changes in collagen fiber bundles following stretch *in-vitro. Biorheology J,* 25:591–604.

48. Li JT, Armstrong CG, Mow VC. (1983): The effect of strain rate on mechanical properties of articular cartilage in tension. In: Woo SL-Y, ed. *1983 Biomechanics Symposium (ASME),* pp 117–122.

49. Lin HC, Kwan MK-W, Woo SL-Y. (1987): On the stress relaxation properties of anterior cruciate ligament. *Adv Bioeng,* 3:5–6.

50. Markolf KL, Mensch JS, Amstutz HC. (1976): Stiffness and laxity of the knee—the contributions of the supporting structure. *J Bone Joint Surg [Am],* 58A:583–593.

51. Morrison JB. (1970): The mechanics of the knee joint in relation to normal walking. *J Biomech,* 3:51–61.

52. Mow VC, Kuei SC, Lai WM, Armstrong CG. (1980): Biphasic creep and stress relaxation of articular cartilage in compression theory and experiments. *J Biomech Eng,* 102:73–84.

53. Myers BS, McElhaney JH, Doherty BJ. (1991): The viscoelastic responses of the human cervical spine in torsion: experimental limitations of quasi-linear theory, and a method for reducing these effects. *J Biomech,* 24:811–817.

54. Nigul I, Nigul U. (1987): On algorithms of evaluation of Fung's relaxation function parameters. *J Biomech,* 20:343–352.

55. Noyes FR, DeLucas JL, Torvik PJ. (1974): Biomechanics of anterior cruciate ligament failure: an analysis of strain-rate sensitivity and mechanisms of failure in primates. *J Bone Joint Surg [Am],* 56A:236–253.

56. Noyes FR, Grood ES. (1976): The strength of the anterior cruciate ligament in humans and rhesus monkeys. *J Bone Joint Surg [Am],* 58A:1074–1082.

57. Noyes FR. (1977): Functional properties of knee ligaments and alterations induced by immobilization. *Clin Orthop,* 123:210.

58. Noyes FR, Bassett RW, Grood ES, Butler DL. (1980): Arthroscopy in acute traumatic hemarthrosis of the knee: incidence of anterior cruciate tears and other injuries. *J Bone Joint Surg [Am],* 62A:687–695.

59. Noyes FR, Butler DL, Grood ES, Zernicke RF, Hefzy MS. (1984): Biomechanical analysis of human ligament grafts used in knee ligament repairs and reconstructions. *J Bone Joint Surg [Am],* 66A:344–352.

60. Panagiotacopulos ND, Pope MH, Krag MH, Block R. (1987): Water content in human intervertebral discs: Part I. Measurement by magnetic resonance imaging. *Spine,* 12:912–917.

61. Peterson RH, Woo SL-Y. (1986): A new methodology to determine the mechanical properties of ligaments at high strain rates. *J Biomech Eng,* 108:365–367.

62. Roy CS. (1880): The elastic properties of the arterial wall. *J Physiol,* 3:125–159.

63. Sheh MY, Butler DL, Stouffer DC, Kay MD. (1985): Correlation between structure and material properties in human ligaments and tendons. *Biomech Symp (ASME),* 17–20.

64. Viidik A. (1968): A rheological model for uncalcified parallel-fibered collagenous tissue. *J Biomech,* 1:3.

65. Viidik A. (1972): Simultaneous mechanical and light microscopic studies of collagen fibers. *Z Anat Entwicklungsgesch,* 136: 204–212.

66. Viidik A. (1980): Interdependence between structure and function in collagenous tissue. In: Viidik A, Vuust J, eds. *Biology of Collagen.* London: Academic Press, pp 257–280.

67. Vogel HG. (1976): Tensile strength, relaxation, and mechanical recovery in rat skin as influenced by maturation and age. *J Med,* 7:177–187.

68. Weber W. (1835): Uber die elasticitat der seidenfaden. *Ann Physik Chemie,* 34:247–257.

69. Woo SL-Y, Akeson WK, Jemmott GF. (1976): Measurements of nonhomogeneous directional mechanical properties of articular cartilage in tension. *J Biomech,* 9:785–791.

70. Woo SL-Y, Gomez MA, Akeson WH. (1981): The time and history dependent viscoelastic properties of the canine medial collateral ligament. *J Biomech Eng,* 103:293–298.

71. Woo SL-Y, Hollis JM, Roux RD, Gomez MA, Inque M, Kleiner JB, Akeson WH. (1987): Effects of knee flexion on the structural properties of the rabbit femur-anterior cruciate ligament-tibia complex (FATC). *J Biomech,* 20:557–563.

72. Woo SL-Y, Hollis JM, Adams DJ, Lyon RM, Takai S. (1991): Tensile properties of the human femur-anterior cruciate ligament-tibia complex. *Am J Sports Med,* 19:217–225.

73. Yahia L-H, Drouin G. (1988): Collagen structure in human anterior cruciate ligament and patellar tendon. *J Mater Sci,* 23:3750–3755.

74. Yahia LH, Drouin G. (1989): Microscopical investigation of canine anterior cruciate ligament and patellar tendon: collagen fascicle morphology and architecture. *J Orthop Res,* 7:243–251.

75. Yahia LH, Brunet J, Labelle S, Hilaire-Rivard C. (1990): A scanning electron microscopic study of rabbit ligaments under strain. *Matrix,* 10:58–64.

The Anterior Cruciate Ligament: Current and Future Concepts, edited by D.W. Jackson, et al.
Raven Press, Ltd., New York © 1993.

CHAPTER **6**

Knee Motions and Their Relations to the Function of the Anterior Cruciate Ligament

Mohamed Samir Hefzy and Edward S. Grood

Clinicians first described anterior cruciate ligament injuries over 100 years ago (33). A full understanding of knee kinematics is important in the diagnosis and management of injury to this ligament. In the past, there were differing clinical opinions about how this ligament functions in controlling knee motions (7) because of the subjective assessment methods utilized in early studies to determine the amount and type of abnormal motions that occur with ligamentous injuries. Since these early studies, researchers have conducted many studies to increase our understanding of ACL function and clarify the role of the ACL as a primary restraint to anterior translation. However, some disagreement remains over the function of this ligament as a restraint to other motions.

During the clinical examination, the diagnosis of a ligament disruption is based upon the demonstration of pathological knee motion. This requires the accurate measurement and description of this motion. Measurements of knee motion consist of determination of the relative motion between two rigid bodies, the femur and the tibia. In the past 20 years, there has been increased popularity in using 6 *df* instrumented spatial linkages (4,15–17,36,38) to measure indirectly the three rotations and the three translations between the femur and tibia.

The description of the relative motion between the femur and tibia was most commonly presented using the method of screws. However, this description is not readily understood by clinicians. Another description of the three-dimensional knee motions was introduced by Grood and Suntay (9) using the joint coordinate system method. This method describes knee motions in a way that relates to the commonly used clinical terms, thus facilitating communication between biomechanicians and physicians.

This chapter is divided in four parts. The first part includes a discussion on the use of the instrumented spatial linkage in measuring knee motions. The second part presents a summary of the two methods that have been employed to describe knee motions: the screw displacement axis (SDA) method and the joint coordinate system (JCS) method. The third part includes definitions of some terms for knee motion and position that we have found useful in describing ligament injury. The fourth part describes how changes in knee motions due to ligament section can provide an indication to ligament function and presents a summary of cadaveric ligament sectioning studies that serve as the basis of determining the function of the normal ACL.

THE USE OF INSTRUMENTED SPATIAL LINKAGES IN MEASURING JOINT MOTIONS

Accurate and reliable measurement of knee motions provides needed information for the understanding of knee kinematics. This understanding is important in the diagnosis of the joint disorders resulting from injury or disease, in the quantitative assessment of treatment, in the design of better prosthetic devices, and in the general study of locomotion.

Measurements of knee motion consist of the determination of the relative motion between two rigid bodies, the femur and the tibia. Many experimental techniques have been reported, either two-dimensional using con-

M. S. Hefzy: Biomechanics Laboratories, Department of Mechanical Engineering, University of Toledo, Toledo, Ohio; and Department of Orthopaedic Surgery, Medical College of Ohio, Toledo, Ohio 43606.

E. S. Grood: Noyes-Giannestras Biomechanics Laboratory, University of Cincinnati, Cincinnati, Ohio 45221.

ventional roentgenograms (5,40) or three-dimensional using high-speed photography (1), roentgen stereophotogrammetric methods (39), biplanar x-rays (36), electromagnetic devices (11,32), and exoskeletal linkage methods (4,15–17,36,38). Each of these methods has its advantages and limitations.

The exoskeletal linkage method consists of using a mechanical system for measuring joint motions. These devices are commonly referred to as "electrogoniometers" because potentiometers are used to monitor joint motions. Generally, electrogoniometers can be divided into three categories: (a) two-dimensional devices (14,24,37), (b) three-dimensional devices (13,15,18), and (3) spatial linkage devices (15–17,36,38). The two-dimensional devices, referred to as *planar electrogoniometers,* measure only one angular rotation. This type of device has been used to measure flexion and extension of the hip, knee, and ankle joints (14). The application of the planar devices is very limited because most joint motions are three-dimensional. Another limitation of these devices is that they were not self-aligning with the center of rotation of the joint.

The three-dimensional devices, referred to as *triaxial goniometers,* consist of three potentiometers that measure the rotations about three orthogonal axes at a joint. Triaxial goniometers are limited because they cannot measure total joint motion; they measure only rotations. Errors associated with cross-talk also occur when using these devices. Cross-talk is defined as the difference between the actual joint motion and the transducer measurements for the triaxial goniometer. Cross-talk occurs because the axes of the sensing potentiometers are not always parallel to the axes of motion being measured. In the triaxial goniometer cross-talk occurs primarily in the potentiometer that senses internal-external tibial rotation because it is attached to the tibia through a yoke that permits its orientation to vary with respect to the tibia (15).

The three-dimensional devices, known as 6 *df* instrumented spatial linkages, are capable of measuring the total motion of a joint. These devices were introduced by Kinzel et al. (15). Since then, their use has steadily grown to measure joint motions (15–17,36,38). In these devices none of the angles measured by the potentiometers give a direct measurement of any of the rotational or translational position parameters. Thus, the measured angles must be transformed into some other form. These calculations require computer analysis, which permits exact kinematic relations to be employed.

A typical instrumented spatial linkage (36) is shown in Fig. 1. The device consists of seven rigid links connected by six rotary potentiometers, which are used to measure the angles between the adjacent links. These measured angles and the known link geometries are used to construct a coordinate transformation between coordinate systems on adjacent links. However, due to tolerances of the linkage parameters, the system requires adopting a calibration scheme to refine the initial measurements of these parameters. Sommer and Miller (34) presented a calibration scheme for determining linkage parameters that minimize position measurement errors within a specified volume. They used a Levenberg-Marquardt algorithm to minimize the squared difference between known and calculated sets of motion parameters that related one linkage end to the other. Recently, Kirstukas et al. (17) pointed out that potential problems exist with this method. If the linkage is calibrated end to end rather than bone to bone, the predicted accuracy cannot be taken as a measure of the accuracy of the linkage in predicting bone position parameters. Furthermore, the calibration space used by Sommer and Miller (34) did not allow calibration of the linkage in the work space of the anatomical joint. The optimized linkage parameters were thus quite different from the actual parameters, and large measurement error could occur when the linkage is

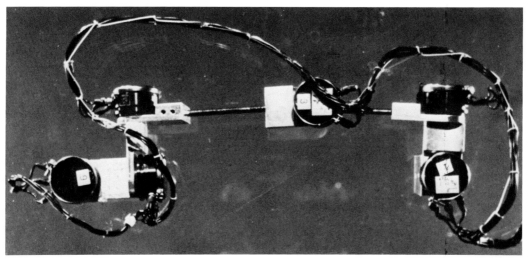

FIG. 1. A typical 6 *df* instrumented spatial linkage. Six rotary potentiometers are used to measure the angles between the rigid links.

used to measure joint motion. To overcome these problems, Kirstukas et al. (17) used a knee-like calibration device and developed a calibration algorithm where weighting was permitted so as to obtain a set of linkage parameters that is optimal for measuring certain anatomical position parameters.

In the analysis, link-to-link transformations are combined by successive matrix multiplications to obtain the transformation between linkage ends. There are two additional transformations, one between each end of the linkage and a coordinate system located in the adjacent bone. Two methods have been reported to measure these two transformations: biplanar x-rays as described by Suntay, et al. (36) or using the linkage as a three-dimensional coordinate digitizer to determine the spatial location of bony landmarks as described by Hefzy and Grood (10).

The transformation between the two bones forming the joint at any position, $[\mathbf{B}_{1-2}]$, is thus obtained by combining the transformation between linkage ends with the linkage end to bone transformations. In the knee, every point T on the tibia can be defined in terms of the femoral coordinate system as R_T or in terms of the tibial coordinate system as r_T. The following equation can thus be written:

$$(R_T) = [\mathbf{B}_{1-2}](r_T) \qquad [1]$$

where $[\mathbf{B}_{1-2}]$ is a square matrix of order 4 and is written in the form

$$[\mathbf{B}_{1-2}] = \begin{bmatrix} 1 & [0] \\ [O_T] & [R_1] \end{bmatrix} \qquad [2]$$

where $[0]$ is a null row vector of order 3, $[O_T]$ is the position vector of the origin of the tibial coordinate system relative to the femoral coordinate system, and $[R_1]$ is a rotation matrix defining the direction cosines of the tibial x, y, and z axes relative to the femoral coordinate system of axes.

A DESCRIPTION OF KNEE MOTION

The Screw Displacement Axis Method

The three-dimensional relative motion between two rigid bodies can be described as a rotation about and a

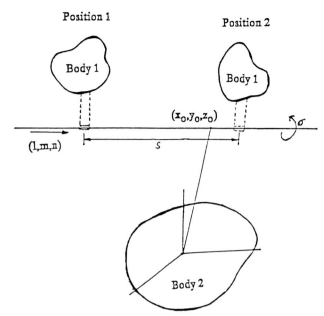

FIG. 2. The parameters required to define the general motion of Body 1 from Position 1 to Position 2 in terms of a screw motion; **s** is the translation and σ is the rotation along the screw axis.

translation along a uniquely defined axis, which is the screw displacement axis (35). Figure 2 illustrates the parameters required to define the general motion of Body 1 from Position 1 to Position 2 in terms of a screw motion. These parameters include the angle of rotation about the screw axis σ, the translation along the screw axis **s**, the coordinates of any point on the screw axis (x_0, y_0, z_0), and the direction cosines (l, m, n) of the screw axis with respect to a system of axes attached to the fixed body.

The coordinates of any point located on the moving body at Position 1 (x_1, y_1, z_1) are related to its coordinates at Position 2 (x_2, y_2, z_2) according to the following relation, which is given by

$$\begin{bmatrix} 1 \\ x_2 \\ y_2 \\ z_2 \end{bmatrix} = [\mathbf{B}]_{1-2} \begin{bmatrix} 1 \\ x_1 \\ y_1 \\ z_1 \end{bmatrix} \qquad [3]$$

where $[\mathbf{B}]_{1-2}$ is given as:

$$[\mathbf{B}]_{1-2} = \begin{bmatrix} 1 & 0 & 0 & 0 \\ sl - x_0(-V\sigma + V\sigma l^2) \\ \quad -y_0(-S\sigma n + V\sigma lm) & C\sigma & -S\sigma n & S\sigma m \\ \quad -z_0(S\sigma m + V\sigma ln) & +V\sigma l^2 & +V\sigma lm & +V\sigma ln \\ sm - x_0(S\sigma n + V\sigma lm) & S\sigma n & C\sigma & -S\sigma l \\ \quad -y_0(-V\sigma + V\sigma m^2) & +V\sigma lm & +V\sigma m^2 & +V\sigma mn \\ \quad -z_0(-S\sigma l + V\sigma_{mn}) \\ sn - x_0(-S\sigma m + Vln) & -S\sigma m & S\sigma l & C\sigma \\ \quad -y_0(S\sigma l + V\sigma mn) & +V\sigma ln & +V\sigma mn & +V\sigma n^2 \\ \quad -z_0(-V\sigma + V\sigma n^2) \end{bmatrix} \qquad [4]$$

where $V\sigma = (1 - \cos\sigma)$

Let us take the case where Body 1 (moving body) is the femur and Body 2 (fixed body) is the tibia. The transformations from Body 1 (femur) to Body 2 (tibia) at Positions 1 and 2, $[B_{1-2}]_1$ and $[B_{1-2}]_2$, respectively, are obtained using the electrogoniometer, as described in the previous section. Following the diagram shown in Fig. 3, the motion of Body 1 from Position 1 to Position 2 can be described by the transformation matrix $[B]_{1-2}$, which is calculated as

$$[B]_{1-2} = [B_{1-2}]_{2-1}[B_{1-2}]_1 \qquad [5]$$

Equating Eqs. 4 and 5, the parameters of the screw axis describing the motion of Body 1 (femur) from Position 1 to Position 2 with respect to Body 2 (tibia) are calculated in terms of b_{ij}, the elements of $[B]_{1-2}$, as follows:
The rotation angle

$$\text{Cos } \sigma = (b_{22} + b_{33} + b_{44} - 1)/2. \qquad [6]$$

The direction cosines of the screw axis

$$l = (b_{43} - b_{34})/(2 \text{ Sin } \sigma) \qquad [7.a]$$

$$m = (b_{24} - b_{42})/(2 \text{ Sin } \sigma) \qquad [7.b]$$

$$n = (b_{32} - b_{23})/(2 \text{ Sin } \sigma) \qquad [7.c]$$

The travel of the screw

$$\mathbf{s} = b_{21}l + b_{31}m + b_{41}n \qquad [8]$$

The coordinates of any point on the screw axis

$$x_0 = [b_{21} - \mathbf{s}l + a_1/\tan(\sigma/2)]/2. \qquad [9.a]$$

$$y_0 = [b_{31} - \mathbf{s}m + a_2/\tan(\sigma/2)]/2. \qquad [9.b]$$

$$z_0 = [b_{41} - \mathbf{x}n + a_3/\tan(\sigma/2)]/2. \qquad [9.c]$$

where

$$a_1 = b_{41}m - b_{31}n \qquad [10.a]$$

$$a_2 = b_{21}n - b_{41}l \qquad [10.b]$$

$$a_3 = b_{31}l - b_{21}m \qquad [10.c]$$

The Joint Coordinate System Method

A Description of the Joint Coordinate System

Grood and Suntay (9) introduced a convenient coordinate system to describe three-dimensional joint motion between two rigid bodies in a way that facilitates the communication among engineers and physicians. The purpose of a joint coordinate system is to allow the relative position between two bodies to be specified. This system is shown in Fig. 4, where it is used to describe the general motions between Body A and Body B.

As shown in Fig. 4, the geometry of each body is specified by a Cartesian coordinate system with origins located at O_A and O_B and a set of surfaces that describe its shape. The three axes that comprise the joint coordinate system are shown in Fig. 4. Two of the axes of this joint coordinate system are called *body fixed axes* and are embedded in the two bodies whose relative motion is to be described. The third axis of this system is called the *floating axis* and is the common perpendicular to the body fixed axes. The common perpendicular is referred to as the floating axis because it is not fixed in either body and moves in relation to both.

The components of the three-dimensional relative motion between Bodies A and B include three rotations

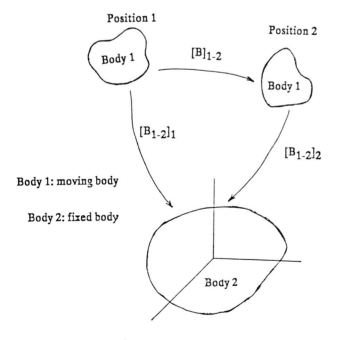

FIG. 3. The general motion of a moving body from Position 1 to Position 2.

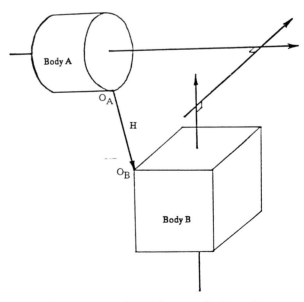

FIG. 4. A generalized joint coordinate system.

and three translations. Two of the relative rotations between the two bodies represent the spin of each body about its own fixed axis, while the other body remains stationary. The third relative rotation occurs about the floating axis. The relative translations between the two bodies are described by the relative position of two reference points, one located in each body as indicated by vector *H* in Fig. 4. The components of the translation vector taken along the direction of the three coordinate axes are the three translations.

The Application of the System to the Knee

In constructing the joint coordinate system for the knee or any other joint structure, it is necessary to specify (a) the Cartesian bony coordinate system fixed in each bone and (b) the body fixed axes of the joint coordinate system.

In most of the cadaveric ligament sectioning studies, the tibial bony coordinate system was established by taking the tibial mechanical axis as the Z axis. This axis passes midway between the two intercondylar eminences proximally and through the center of the ankle distally. The tibial Y axis was defined as the cross-product of the tibial Z axis with a medial-lateral line connecting the approximate center of each plateau. The third axis of the tibial coordinate system, the X direction, was obtained by completing a right-handed coordinate system. The origin of this bony system was located on the tibial mechanical axis, midway between the two intercondylar eminences.

The origin of the femoral bony coordinate system was defined as the center of the intercondylar notch. This point was located at the most distal point on the posterior surface of the femur in the intercondylar fossa, midway between the medial and lateral condyles. Two approaches have been utilized to establish this bony coordinate system. In the first method, it was established by assuming that it is parallel to the tibial bony coordinate system at full extension when the knee is intact and when no loads are applied to the tibia. In the second method, the femoral Z axis was taken as the femoral mechanical axis. This axis passes between the femoral origin and the center of the femoral head. The femoral Y axis was obtained by taking the cross-product of a vector parallel to the femoral mechanical axis and a vector connecting two points located in the frontal plane. These points were the most posterior points on the surface of the medial and lateral condyles. The femoral X axis was selected to form a right hand coordinate system.

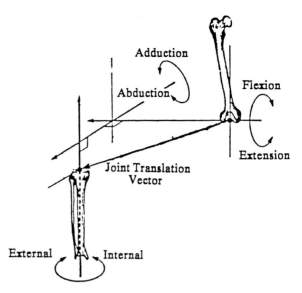

FIG. 5. The tibiofemoral joint coordinate system.

The tibiofemoral joint coordinate system is then constructed to describe the three-dimensional, 6 *df* tibiofemoral motions. This joint coordinate system is shown in Fig. 5 and consists of a fixed axis on the femur, a fixed axis on the tibia, and a floating axis that is perpendicular to these two fixed axes. The femoral fixed axis is taken as the femoral X axis; the tibial fixed axis is the tibial Z axis.

Tibiofemoral motions are described in terms of three rotations and three translations. These motions occur about the tibiofemoral joint coordinate system as shown in Fig. 5. Flexion-extension rotations occur about the femoral fixed axis, internal-external tibial rotations occur about the tibial fixed axis, and varus-valgus rotations occur about the floating axis.

Translations between the femur and the tibia are represented by the joint translation vector shown in Fig. 5. This vector is directed from the femoral origin to the tibial origin. Clinically, medial-lateral tibial thrust or shift, q_1, is the medial-lateral displacement of the tibial origin with respect to the femoral origin; anterior-posterior tibial drawer, q_2, is the displacement of the tibial origin along the floating axis; and joint distraction-compression, q_3, is the height of the femoral origin above (or below) the tibial transverse plane.

The rotational and translational clinical parameters describing joint motions are calculated using the coordinate transformation matrix between the tibial and femoral systems. Tibiofemoral rotations were calculated after rewriting $[\mathbf{R}_1]$ in the following form (9):

$$[\mathbf{R}_1]^{\mathrm{T}} = \begin{bmatrix} & -\cos\alpha\sin\tau & \sin\alpha\sin\tau \\ \sin\beta\cos\tau & -\sin\alpha\cos\beta\cos\tau & -\cos\alpha\cos\beta\cos\tau \\ & \cos\alpha\cos\tau & -\sin\alpha\cos\tau \\ \sin\beta\sin\tau & -\sin\alpha\cos\beta\sin\tau & -\cos\alpha\cos\beta\sin\tau \\ \cos\beta & \sin\alpha\sin\beta & \cos\alpha\sin\beta \end{bmatrix} \qquad [11]$$

where α is knee flexion, τ is tibial external rotation, and $\beta = (\pi/2 \pm \text{abduction})$; a positive sign indicates a right knee and a negative indicates a left one.

Mathematically, the three clinical translations are defined as the projections of the translation vector H along each of the axes of the joint coordinate system.

DEFINITIONS OF TERMS FOR THE DESCRIPTION OF KNEE MOTION AND POSITION

In a recently published article, Noyes et al. (27) stated that "a review of the literature of the knee reveals considerable discrepancies in the implied meanings of many terms." This problem is exacerbated when attempting to communicate the results of studies. The following is a list of terms we have found useful in describing the motion of the knee joint.

Position To define the position of a rigid body completely, one must specify the location of a point in the body with respect to a reference system and the orientation of the body. The orientation of a body refers to how it is rotated relative to other body segments. Applying this definition to the knee joint, Noyes et al. (27) suggested that the location of a point on the tibia with respect to a reference coordinate system on the femur can be described by three translational coordinates: anterior-posterior, medial-lateral, and proximal-distal. The orientation of the tibia with respect to the femur is described by the three angles of flexion-extension, abduction-adduction (varus-valgus), and internal-external rotation of the tibia.

Motion Noyes et al. (27) indicated that the motion of an object can be quantified just by describing the displacement (see later definition) between the starting and ending points of its path.

Displacement The displacement of a rigid body is the change in its position without regard to the path followed. From the early definition of position, the displacement of a rigid body is described by six quantities (6 *df*): three translations and three rotations.

Translation Translation is a type of motion of a rigid body in which all points in the body move along parallel paths. An equivalent definition is a type of motion of a rigid body in which all lines attached to it remain parallel to their original orientation. Translation of the knee is a term used in the orthopedic literature to describe the translation of the tibia using three quantities (3 *df*): medial-lateral translation, anterior-posterior translation, and proximal-distal translation.

Rotation Rotation is type of motion of a rigid body in which all points on the body move around an axis as a center; this axis is commonly referred to as the axis of rotation. Using the joint coordinate system (described

earlier), knee rotation is described using three quantities (3 *df*): flexion-extension rotation, internal-external rotation, and abduction-adduction rotation.

Motion of the knee can thus be described as the rotation and translation of the tibia. In practice, the translation of the tibia is measured by the translation of some reference point, arbitrarily chosen on the tibia. However, the amount of translation will depend on which point is selected because any associated rotation could cause a different motion for the reference point. Typically, this point is located midway between the medial and lateral margins of the joint.

KNEE MOTION VERSUS LIGAMENT FUNCTION: COUPLED MOTION AND PRIMARY AND SECONDARY RESTRAINTS

To understand how a ligament functions, you must know how a joint displacement occurs, what the displacement contributes to the resisting force, and how tension manifests itself in the ligament. Several experimental techniques have been employed to gain this knowledge, including the flexibility and the stiffness methods. These two methods use selective cutting of ligaments to determine their specific contribution to the stability of the knee and involve two loading modes: either applying specific forces and moments to the joint or applying specific displacements and rotations. These two loading modes are just different conditions imposed on the secondary degrees of freedom.

The secondary degrees of freedom represent the coupled motions. Coupled motions often occur during the clinical examination. Coupled motions are different from primary motions. For example, tibial internal-external rotations resulting from tibial torques are primary motions, whereas tibial internal-external rotations resulting from the application of anterior force to the tibia are coupled motions.

With the flexibility method, a load is applied and the resulting joint displacement is measured (23). A ligament is then severed and the altered motion (i.e., laxity) is determined. In this type of test, the secondary degrees of freedom (coupled motions) are unconstrained. However, the change in motion depends on the order in which the ligaments are cut because the remaining intact ligaments control the joint motions, not the cut ligament. Thus, the amount of laxity is determined by the order of cutting because this order determines which ligaments control joint motion.

With the stiffness method, ligament function is quantified by measuring the ligament's restraining force during precisely controlled displacements (3,8). The controlled displacements are accomplished by constraining all joint motions except the one of interest. The reduction in restraining force that occurs after cutting a ligament defines its contribution. The results obtained by using this method are independent of the order used to cut the ligaments because the joint displacement is precisely controlled and reproduced from test to test. Because the joint displacement controls the amount of ligament stretch, it controls the force developed in the ligament. Reproducing the displacement results in reproducing the force in each ligament. This means that, even after a single ligament is sectioned, the contributions of the remaining ligaments are not affected; that is, the independence of cutting order allows all ligaments to be studied in each knee. The ligaments are ranked based on the percentage of the total restraining force that each provides.

The stiffness method directly measures ligament function, but only for the specific joint displacements applied. Unlike the flexibility method, the stiffness method constrains the coupled motions. As a result, the ligament forces measured are larger than those measured in a comparable flexibility test appropriate for unconstrained coupled motions.

The data obtained using the flexibility or stiffness method are presented using force-displacement curves, also called response curves. A typical response curve for an anterior-posterior drawer test is shown in Fig. 6 using the data of Markolf et al. (23). The force in Newtons is shown on the vertical axis; the displacement in millimeters is shown on the horizontal axis. An important feature of the response curve is the establishment of the joint position that divides the curve into two parts, anterior and posterior. Often called the neutral position, this joint position has been defined slightly differently by each investigator.

Butler et al. (3) introduced the concept of primary and secondary restraints to motion in a specific direction.

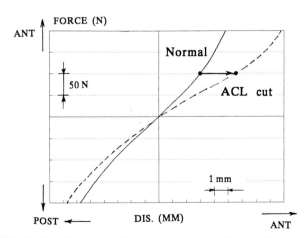

FIG. 6. A typical force-displacement curve obtained by using the flexibility method for an anterior-posterior drawer test. The anterior displacement increases after cutting the ACL for anterior drawer.

Resecting a primary restraint results in an increase in joint motion. Isolated sectioning of a secondary restraint will not alter joint motion; however, disruption of a secondary restraint in the absence of a primary restraint will alter joint motion.

Figure 6 shows that, when the ACL is severed, no significant differences exist between the posterior response curves for injured and normal knees. Because no difference exists, we know that this ligament does not provide the primary restraints for posterior instability. Conversely, there are marked differences between the anterior response curves, which indicates that this ligament provides the primary restraints for anterior instability. A ligament may function as a primary restraint to one of the six components of the motion and as a secondary restraint to another component of the motion.

THE PRIMARY FUNCTION OF THE NORMAL ANTERIOR CRUCIATE LIGAMENT

There is nearly universal agreement that substantial increases in anterior knee displacement occur after an ACL rupture and that the ACL functions as the primary restraint to limit anterior tibial displacements (6,12,21, 28). Because this ligament offers no restraint to posterior tibial displacements, it provides no resistance to posterior drawer (2,3,6,21,22,26,28,30).

Experimentally, measurements of anterior-posterior displacement are affected by whether the tibia is constrained to prevent tibial rotations or allowed to rotate freely. Fukubayashi et al. (6) reported that anterior-posterior tibial displacements were 30% higher when free tibial rotations were allowed.

Furthermore, when attempting to compare the results of different studies and to present a coherent summary, one must understand how these results have been normalized. For instance, Fukubayashi et al. (6) and Levy et al. (19) reported that the maximum and minimum increases in the anterior displacement after cutting of the ACL occur at 45° and 0° of knee flexion, respectively. On the other hand, Markolf et al. (21) reported that isolated section of the ACL produced the greatest increase in anterior laxity at full extension. Their results thus seem contradictory with those reported by Fukubayashi et al. (6) and Levy et al. (19). However, two methods were used to present these results. Although Fukubayashi et al. (6) and Levy et al. (19) reported values for the increased anterior displacement (in millimeters) that occurs after cutting of the ACL, Markolf et al. (21) presented ratios of the values for laxity to the comparable values determined before sectioning of the ACL. Careful study of the data of Markolf et al. (21) shows that the maximum increase in the value of the anterior laxity after cutting of the ACL occurs at 20° of flexion and not at full extension.

THE SECONDARY FUNCTION OF THE NORMAL ANTERIOR CRUCIATE LIGAMENT

Primary-Secondary Function: Internal Tibial Rotations

The literature contains ambiguous results concerning the role of the ACL in restraining tibial rotation (12,20,21). This ambiguity reflects variations in loading conditions and experiments used in those studies. For instance, some authors used larger torsional moments than others. Seering et al. (29) used torques ranging from 34 Newton-meters (N-m) to 47 N-m; Wang et al. (41) used torques up to 5 N-m; and Markolf et al. (21) applied torques of 1 to 8 N-m. Also, results depend on whether joint compression is allowed during testing.

Based on the data available in the literature (21,22, 29,30), the ACL is considered to function as a primary-secondary restraint to internal rotation. The effects of this ligament in restraining rotation are larger at full extension. During internal rotation and at full extension, the taut ACL fibers wrap around the posterior cruciate ligament, thereby exerting a resistance to internal tibial torques. Injury to the ACL is thus expected to decrease this resistance. Shoemaker and Markolf (30) reported that, when response curves were determined at 0° and 20° of flexion, secondary section of the ACL—after section of the medial collateral ligament—produced greater increases in total torsional laxity than did isolated section of the ACL.

Secondary-Secondary Function: Varus-Valgus Angulations and External Tibial Rotations

Grood et al. (8) reported that the ACL acts as a secondary restraint to medial and lateral openings at full extension. Grood et al. (8) also reported that the contribution of the ACL to lateral restraints (restraints to varus opening) was somewhat larger than its contribution to the medial restraints, both contributions being larger at extension than at 25° of flexion. Yet Nielsen et al. (25) reported that cutting the ACL caused slight varus instability, which was maximal at 30° of flexion. Markolf et al. (21), with no breakdown between varus and valgus angulation, reported that the increase in varus-valgus laxity after cutting the ACL was small and was detected only at full extension. Also, they reported that this laxity increased 2.0 to 3.0 times after they sectioned the lateral collateral ligament alone or in combination with the ACL at full extension and increased 3.2 to 4.6 times after they sectioned the medial collateral ligament alone or in combination with the ACL at full extension.

Grood et al. (8), Nielsen et al. (25), and Markolf et al. (21) suggested that the ACL functions as a secondary-secondary restraint to varus-valgus angulation at full extension beyond that provided by the primary stabilizers, the medial and lateral collateral ligaments.

It is also thought that the ACL provides a secondary-secondary restraint to external tibial rotation (31). Nielsen and Helmig (26) indicated that coupled external rotations associated with anterior-posterior loading increased markedly in the flexed position after the further cutting of the ACL in knees with resected medial collateral ligaments.

REFERENCES

1. Blacharski PA, Somerset JH. (1975): A three-dimensional study of the kinematics of the human knee. *J Biomech*, 8:375–384.
2. Brantigan OC, Voshell AF. (1941): The mechanics of the ligaments and menisci of the knee joint. *J Bone Joint Surg*, 23:44–46.
3. Butler DL, Noyes FR, Grood ES. (1980): Ligamentous restraints to anterior-posterior drawer in the human knee. *J Bone Joint Surg [Am]*, 62A:259–270.
4. Chao EY. (1978): Experimental methods for biomechanical measurement of joint kinematics. In: *CRC Handbook of Bioengineering in Medicine and Biology,* Cleveland, Ohio: CRC Press, No. 1, pp 385–411.
5. Frankel VH, Burstein AH. (1970): *Orthopaedic Biomechanics.* Philadelphia: Lea & Febiger.
6. Fukubayashi T, Torzilli PA, Sherman MF, Warren RF. (1982): An *in-vitro* biomechanical evaluation of anterior-posterior motion of the knee, tibial displacement, rotation and torque. *J Bone Joint Surg [Am]*, 64A:258–264.
7. Girgis FG, Marshall JL, Monajem ARS. The cruciate ligaments of the knee joint: anatomical, functional and experimental analysis. *Clinical Orthopaedics and Related Research,* No. 106, Jan–Feb., 1975, pp. 216–231.
8. Grood ES, Noyes FN, Butler DL, Suntay WJ. (1981): Ligamentous and capsular restraints preventing straight medial and lateral laxity in intact human cadaver knees. *J Bone Joint Surg [Am]*, 63A:1257–1269.
9. Grood ES, Suntay WJ. (1983): A joint coordinate system for the clinical description of three-dimensional motions: application to the knee. *J Biomech Eng,* 105:136–144.
10. Hefzy MS, Grood ES. (1986): Sensitivity of insertion locations on length patterns of anterior cruciate ligament fibers. *J Biomech Eng,* 108:73–82.
11. Hefzy MS, Zoghi M, Jackson WT, DiDio LJA. (1988): A method to measure the three-dimensional patello-femoral tracking. *Adv Bioeng,* Nov–Dec:47–49 BED, Vol. 8.
12. Hsieh H-H, Walker PS. (1976): Stabilizing mechanisms of the loaded and unloaded knee joint. *J Bone Joint Surg [Am]*, 58A:87–93.
13. Johnston RC, Smidt GL. (1969): Measurement of hip joint motion during walking: evaluation of an electrogoniometric method. *J Bone Joint Surg [Am]*, 51A:1083–1094.
14. Karpovich PV, Karpovich GP. (1960): Electrogoniometer study of joints. *US Armed Forces Med J,* 11:424.
15. Kinzel GL, Hillberry BM, Hall AS Jr, Sickle V, Harvey WM. (1972): Measurement of the total motion between two body segments: II. Description of application. *J Biomech,* 5:283–293.
16. Kirstukas SJ, Lewis JL, Erdman AG. (1992): 6R instrumented spatial linkages for anatomical joint motion measurement—Part 1: design. *J Biomech Eng,* 114:92–100.
17. Kirstukas SJ, Lewis JL, Erdman AG. (1992): 6R instrumented spatial linkages for anatomical joint motion measurement—Part 2: calibration. *J Biomech Eng,* 114:101–110.
18. Lamoreux LA. (1971): Kinematic measurements in the study of human walking. *Bull Prosth Res,* 3:10–15.
19. Levy IM, Torzilli PA, Warren RF. (1982): The effect of medial meniscectomy on anterior-posterior motion of the knee. *J Bone Joint Surg [Am]*, 64A:883–888.
20. Lipke JM, Janecki CJ, Nelson CL, McLeod P, Thompson C, Thompson J, Haynes DW. (1981): The role of incompetence of the anterior cruciate and lateral ligaments in anterolateral and anteromedial instability. *J Bone Joint Surg [Am]*, 63A:954–960.
21. Markolf KL, Mensch JS, Amstutz HC. (1976): Stiffness and laxity

of the knee—the contributions of the supporting structures. A quantitative *in vitro* study. *J Bone Joint Surg [Am]*, 58A:583–594.

22. Markolf KL, Bargar WL, Shoemaker SC, Amstutz HC. (1981): The role of joint load in knee stability. *J Bone Joint Surg [Am]*, 63A:570–585.

23. Markolf KL, Kochan A, Amstutz HC. (1984): Measurement of knee stiffness and laxity in patients with documented absence of the anterior cruciate ligament. *J Bone Joint Surg [Am]*, 66A:242–253.

24. McLeod PC, Kettelkamp DB, Srinivasan V, Henderson OL. (1975): Measurement of repetitive activities of the knee. *J Biomech*, 8:269–273.

25. Nielsen S, Ovesen J, Rasmussen O. (1984): The anterior cruciate ligament on the knee: an experimental study of its importance in rotatory knee instability. *Arch Orthop Trauma Surg*, 103:170–174.

26. Nielsen S, Helmig P. (1985): Instability of knees with ligament lesions: cadaver studies of the anterior cruciate ligament. *Acta Orthop Scand*, 56:426–429.

27. Noyes FR, Grood ES, Torzilli PA. (1989): Current concepts review: the definitions of terms for motion and position of the knee and injuries of the ligaments. *J Bone Joint Surg [Am]*, 71A:465–472.

28. Piziali RL, Seering WP, Nagel DA, Schurman DJ. (1980): The function of the primary ligaments of the knee in anterior-posterior and medial-lateral motions. *J Biomech*, 13:785–794.

29. Seering WP, Piziali RL, Nagel DA, Schurman DJ. (1980): The function of the primary ligaments of the knee in varus-valgus and axial rotation. *J Biomech*, 13:785–794.

30. Shoemaker SC, Markolf KL. (1985): Effects of joint load on the stiffness and laxity of ligament-deficient knees: an *in vitro* study of the anterior cruciate and medial collateral ligament. *J Bone Joint Surg [Am]*, 67A:136–146.

31. Shoemaker SC, Daniel DM. (1990): The limits of knee motion: *in vitro* studies. In: Daniel DM, Akeson WH, O'Connor JJ, eds. *Knee ligaments: structure, function, injury and repair*. New York: Raven Press, pp 153–161

32. Sidles JA, Larson RV, Garbini JL, Downey DJ, Matsen FA III. (1988): Ligament length relationships in the moving knee. *J Orthop Res*, 6:593–610.

33. Snook GA. (1983): A short history of the anterior cruciate ligament and the treatment of tears. *Clin Orthop*, 172:11.

34. Sommer HJ III, Miller NR. (1981): A technique for the calibration of instrumented spatial linkages used for biomechanical kinematic measurements. *J Biomech*, 14:91–98.

35. Suh CH, Radcliff CW. (1978): *Kinematics and mechanisms design*. New York: John Wiley.

36. Suntay WJ, Grood ES, Hefzy MS, Butler DL, Noyes FR. (1983): Error analysis of a system for measuring three-dimensional joint motion. *J Biomech Eng*, 105:127–135.

37. Tata JA, Quanbury AO, Steinke TG, Grahame RE. (1978): A variable axis electrogoniometer for the measurement of single plane movement. *J Biomech*, 11:421–425.

38. Townsend MA, Izak M, Jackson RW. (1977): Total motion knee goniometry. *J Biomech*, 10:183–193.

39. Van Dijk R, Huiskes R, Selvik G. (1979): Roentgen stereophotogrammetric methods for the evaluation of the three-dimensional kinematic behaviour and cruciate ligament length patterns of the human knee joint. *J Biomech*, 12:727–731.

40. Walker PS, Skoji H, Erkma MJ. (1972): The rotational axis of the knee and its significance to prosthesis design. *Clin Orthop Rel Res*, 89:160.

41. Wang CJ, Walker PS, Wolf B. (1973): The effects of flexion and rotation on the length patterns of the ligaments of the knee. *J Biomech*, 6:587–596.

The Anterior Cruciate Ligament: Current and Future Concepts, edited by D.W. Jackson, et al. Raven Press, Ltd., New York © 1993.

CHAPTER 7

The Estimation of Anterior Cruciate Ligament Loads *In Situ:* Indirect Methods

J. Marcus Hollis and Savio L-Y. Woo

A thorough understanding of the biomechanics of the anterior cruciate ligament on both a structural level and a fiber bundle level is essential to better address some of the problems associated with ligament replacement. As has been described in previous chapters, the ACL is not a linear arrangement of fibers but a group of fibers that have different orientations, lengths, and properties in different areas. The more complex nature of the ligament can be appreciated from a biomechanical viewpoint once the loading and function of the ligament is examined on a smaller scale. This chapter presents research conducted to determine the loads on the ACL and, perhaps more importantly, the load distribution across the ACL and the effect of flexion angle on this distribution.

FORCE MEASUREMENT BY INDIRECT METHODS

Force in the ACL has been studied using a variety of direct methods including buckle force transducers, bone strain sensors, and insertion bone block force transducers. The method described in this chapter is an indirect approach to measuring the force in the ACL, so called because the force is not measured directly but calculated from kinematic and joint force measurements.

The method developed to determine the force in the ACL consisted of six steps, as outlined in Fig. 1. First, the knee specimen was prepared, a kinematic linkage device was attached to the knee joint to measure the relative

J. M. Hollis: Department of Orthopaedic Surgery, University of Arkansas for Medical Sciences, Little Rock, Arkansas 72205.

S. L-Y. Woo: Musculoskeletal Research Center, Department of Orthopaedic Surgery, University of Pittsburgh School of Medicine, Pittsburgh, Pennsylvania 15261.

motion of the tibia to the femur, and then the specimen was mounted to a frame for applying external loads.

Second, loads were applied to the knee joint, and the 6 *df* motion of the knee specimen was measured and recorded on a computer. The 6 degree-of-freedom (DOF) measured were three translations corresponding to anterior-posterior (A-P), proximal-distal, and medial-lateral and three rotations corresponding to varus-valgus (V-V) rotation, tibial axial rotation, and flexion-extension. A 6 DOF spatial kinematic linkage device was designed to measure knee motion (Fig. 2). The translations were measured using linear variable differential transducers (LVDTs). The tibial axial and the V-V rotations were measured with two rotary variable differential transducers (RVDTs), and the flexion angle was measured with a rotary variable capacitive transducer with a range of 130°. In the 6 DOF kinematic linkage, the translations occurred through three sets of linear bearings, set in aluminum blocks, which rolled along a set of two parallel linear shafts. The shafts were held rigid at either end by aluminum blocks. The rotational degrees of freedom for the linkage were provided by shafts held in axial alignment by pairs of rotary bearings.

Third, an anterior draw test was performed with only the ACL intact to obtain a load versus length curve for the ACL. Next, the insertion sites of the ACL were located and digitized.

The relative motion of the tibial versus femoral insertion sites was calculated for the previously measured knee motion to yield the ACL length versus knee loading. Finally, the *in situ* load in the ACL was calculated by combining the length-versus-knee-loading data with the load-length relationships determined for both the anterior and posterior portions of the ACL.

The following assumptions were made in calculating the loads in the ACL and its length: (a) The ACL is com-

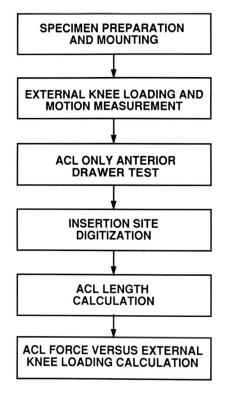

FIG. 1. Flow chart of steps used to determine the *in situ* forces in the ACL during external knee loading.

posed of discrete fiber bundles. This assumption is based on the bundle structure of the ACL, which has been well documented by other investigators (7). Norwood and Cross (17), in a study of the function and anatomy of the ACL, showed the ligament to be made up of three bundles, the anteromedial, intermediate, and posterolateral. (b) The bundles are oriented in a straight line running from the tibial to the femoral insertion site. Thus, lengths were calculated based on a straight line distance from tibial to femoral insertion site, and any deviation from a straight line by the ACL bundle would therefore not be accounted for, leading to an underestimation of the actual length.

The A-P loading was applied by a knee apparatus (Fig. 3). The force was provided by an Instron testing machine cross-head acting through the load cell that was used to measure the applied load. The force was applied perpendicular to the tibia in the anterior-posterior direction. The load was applied to the tibia through a rotary bearing that allowed the tibia to rotate about its longitudinal axis during testing. Five DOF motion was possible with only the knee flexion angle being fixed. The center of rotation of the tibia in V-V rotation was not constrained by the loading device because translation was allowed in the plane of the moment application. The translation was provided by three sets of orthogonally aligned linear

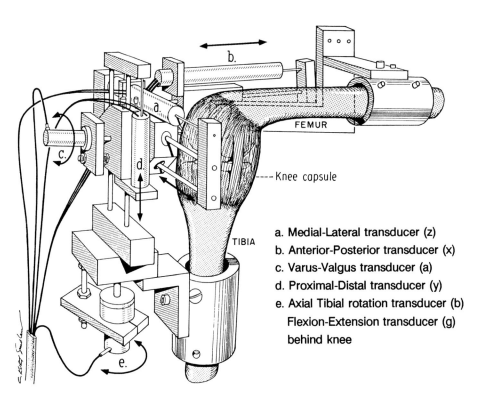

a. Medial-Lateral transducer (z)
b. Anterior-Posterior transducer (x)
c. Varus-Valgus transducer (a)
d. Proximal-Distal transducer (y)
e. Axial Tibial rotation transducer (b)
   Flexion-Extension transducer (g)
   behind knee

FIG. 2. Kinematic linkage device designed to measure the three translational and three rotational degrees of freedom of a knee.

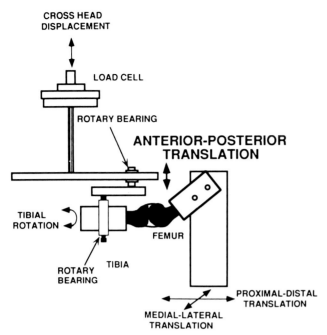

FIG. 3. Schematic diagram showing the loading device used to apply external loads to the knee. Five degrees of freedom of knee motion are allowed during anterior-posterior and varus-valgus loading on the knee.

shafts with linear ball bearings that provided low friction and smooth motion. Rotation about the two free axes was provided by rotary bearings, one aligned along the longitudinal axis of the tibia and the other along the axis of force application, perpendicular to the tibia. Tibial-axial and V-V rotations, as well as medial-lateral, proximal-distal, and A-P translations, were allowed.

THE EXPERIMENTAL PROCEDURE

Human knee specimens from donors (average age, 36 years; range, 23 to 46 years) were tested. The knee specimens were obtained frozen (not embalmed) and were thawed before testing. All muscle and other soft tissue was dissected away except for the knee joint capsule, ligaments, and intraarticular structures. The femur and tibia were then cut to 25 cm distal to the knee joint and placed into thick-walled aluminum cylinders with bolts. The 6 DOF kinematic linkage system was bolted to these cylinders for measurement of the relative 6 DOF tibial motion with respect to the femur in three dimensions, as shown in Fig. 2. The knee was placed in the loading apparatus, and a ±100 N A-P load was applied to the specimen. After five cycles of specimen preconditioning, the kinematic parameters were recorded for one cycle. The knee was then repositioned at another flexion angle and the test repeated. Tests were performed at 0°, 30°, 45°, and 90° of knee flexion. The data points were stored in the computer. The anterior draw test was repeated

with the loading device adjusted such that only A-P motion was allowed.

Next, all soft tissue except for the ACL was dissected from the knee. Markers were placed in the tibial insertion site of the ACL, and then the fibers that inserted in the tibia at the location of the markers were traced up to their femoral insertions and markers were placed at these locations. The ACL marker locations are shown in Fig. 4.

A load versus length curve was then obtained for the ACL specimens by loading the knee in anterior drawer with only the ACL intact. For this test, all motions of the loading device were fixed in a location recorded for the intact joint except for the A-P direction, which was left free. The loading was repeated with only the anterior portion of the ACL intact and the posterior portion dissected. This provided data for the load versus length curves for the total ACL and both the anterior and the posterior portions. The load versus length curve for the posterior portion could be obtained by subtracting the stiffness values of the anterior portion of the ACL from the stiffness values of the whole ACL. Upon completion of the knee loading and recording of the knee motion, the length of the ACL for the measured knee motion was calculated. To accomplish this, the insertion sites of the ACL were digitized (i.e., the coordinates of the insertion sites were obtained). The position of the tibia with respect to the femur was fixed and recorded with the linkage system. The linkage was then detached from the tibia. A pointer was placed on the detached end of the kinematic linkage, and the coordinates of the tibial and corresponding femoral insertion site markers were digitized.

KINEMATIC CALCULATIONS

Kinematic methods were used in this study to find the location of both the tibial and the femoral insertion sites of the ACL during joint motion. The insertion site markers were digitized, and the coordinates of these markers were calculated for the knee motion, recorded during the application of knee loading. A coordinate transformation strategy allowed the coordinates of a point, such as an insertion site, defined in one coordinate system (e.g., fixed with respect to the tibia) to be found for the same point but defined with respect to a second coordinate system (e.g., fixed with respect to the femur).

Two coordinate systems were defined: System Ot, which was fixed with respect to the tibia (Fig. 4), and System Of, fixed with respect to the femur. The coordinate system Ot was related to Of by a series of six transformations corresponding to the 6 DOF measured by the kinematic linkage connecting the tibia and femur. The coordinates of a point in one of the coordinate systems could be transformed into the coordinates for the same point referred to the other coordinate system by a "coordinate transformation matrix." This matrix was multi-

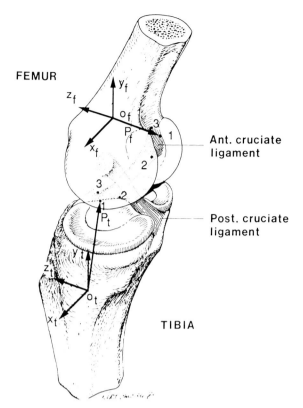

FEMUR

Ant. cruciate
ligament

Post. cruciate
ligament

TIBIA

FIG. 4. Femur and tibia with cruciate ligaments to show the typical position of pairs of markers.

plied by the position vector in one coordinate system to yield the coordinate vector in the other coordinate system.

The rotation and translation DOF were considered separately for simplicity. The equation for coordinate transformation of a point of interest could then be written in one form as $c2 = [T][R]c1$, where $c1$ was the position vector for the point in the initial coordinate system and $c2$ was the position vector for the same point in the final coordinate system. The transformation matrix for a general rotation ([R]) of one coordinate system with respect to another was adapted from Beggs (2).

The series of transformations was described by multiplication, in the proper order, of the individual transformation matrices for the individual transformations that comprise the transformation series, that is, $[R]1,4 = [R]3,4 \ [R]2,3 \ [R]1,2$ where the subscripts refer to intermediate coordinate systems. The requirement for this application was a coordinate transformation matrix $[Wf,t]$ that would transform a coordinate vector (Pt) in the tibial coordinate system (Ot) to the coordinate vector (Pf) for the same point in the femoral coordinate system (Of). Five more intermediate coordinate systems, 01 through 05, were defined as the coordinate systems fixed with respect to the links between the six position transducers of the kinematic linkage. The coordinate transformation matrix $[Wf,t]$ could be determined by multiplying the six individual transformation matrices for the six motions measured from the kinematic linkage transducers together.

$$[WF,t] = [W0,6]$$

$$= [R5,f][T4,5][T3,4][R2,3][T1,2][Rt,1] \quad \text{Eq. 1}$$

where: Rt,1 = tibial axial rotation; T1,2 = proximal distal translation; R2,3 = varus valgus rotation; T3,4 = medial lateral translation; T4,5 = A-P translation; R5,f = flexion-extension.

To find the transformation matrix that describes the entire motion from one end of the linkage to the other, Eq. 1 was expanded to yield

$$[Wt,f] = \begin{bmatrix} 1 & 0 \\ -Sg\ Dy\ Ca - Dx\ Cg & Cg\ Cb + Sg\ Sb\ Sa \\ -Dy\ Ca\ Cg + Sg\ Dx & -Sg\ Cb + Sb\ Sa\ Cg \\ Sa\ Dy - Dz & Sb\ Ca \end{bmatrix}$$

$$\begin{bmatrix} 0 & 0 \\ Sg\ Ca & Sg\ Sa\ Cb - Sb\ Cg \\ Cg\ Ca & Sa\ Cg\ Cb + Sg\ Sb \\ -Sa & Cb\ Ca \end{bmatrix} \quad \text{Eq. 2}$$

where: Sg = Sin g; Cg = Cos g; and Dx, Dy, Dz are the total offset between the rotation axis.

This matrix was then multiplied by the column vector containing the coordinates of a point in the tibial coordinate system, $[Pt] = [1,Xt,Yt,Zt]T$, and the coordinates for this point referenced to the femoral coordinate system, $[Pf] = [1,Xf,Yf,Zf]T$, were obtained.

$$[Pf] = Wt,f][Pt] =$$

$$\begin{bmatrix} 1 \\ (-Sg\ Dy + YT\ Sg)Ca + (XT\ Cg + ZT\ Sg\ Sa)Cb + (-Dx - ZT\ Sb)Cg + XT\ Sg\ Sb\ Sa \\ (-Dy + YT)Cg\ Ca + (ZT\ Sa\ Cg - XT\ Sg)Cb + XT\ Sb\ Sa\ Cg + Sg\ Dx + ZT\ Sg\ Sb \\ (ZT\ Cb + XT\ Sb)Ca + Sa\ Dy - Dz - YT\ Sa \end{bmatrix} \quad \text{Eq. 3}$$

Thus, the position of any point tibial coordinate system for which the coordinates were known could be determined with respect to the femoral coordinate system.

For determination of this position vector for all ACL insertion-site marker locations, these sites were digitized as previously described. The location vector of the insertion-site markers was determined by placing the end of the pointer at these locations sequentially and recording the position of the tibial end of the linkage. The position of these points in the femoral coordinate system was then calculated using Eq. 3 and the previously measured geometry of the pointer as the position vector in the tibial coordinate system (**Pt**). Next, the position vector of these points in the tibial coordinate system was calculated using the inverse of the transformation given by Eq. 2 and the parameters *a, b, g, DX, DY,* and *DZ* as recorded for the tibia after it was fixed with respect to the femur and before the linkage was detached from it. The coordinates of the tibial insertion sites in the tibial coordinate system were required for the later calculations.

Using the series of parameters (*a, b, g, DX, DY, DZ*) measured during the knee motion in Eq. 3 and position vectors of the tibial insertion-site marker in the tibial coordinate system, the coordinates of these points in the femoral coordinate system were calculated. The position vectors of the tibial insertion-site markers were then subtracted from the position vectors of the femoral insertion-site markers, and this difference was used as the measure of ACL length.

RESULTS

Knee Motion

The use of the spatial kinematic linkage system provided an accurate measure of both the knee motion and the position of the ACL insertion sites. Application of an A-P load produced perceptible A-P tibial translation and axial-tibial rotation but not significant medial-lateral translation, proximal-distal translation, nor V-V rotation. The average A-P knee translation (measured as the total peak-to-peak A-P displacement of the knee) changed with flexion angle. The total A-P translation averaged 6.6 mm at 0°, 10.0 mm at 30°, 9.7 mm at 45°, and 6.9 mm at 90° of knee flexion. The tibia rotated internally with anterior loading and externally with posterior loading. The total axial-tibial rotation during A-P loading for the four angles of knee flexion increased with

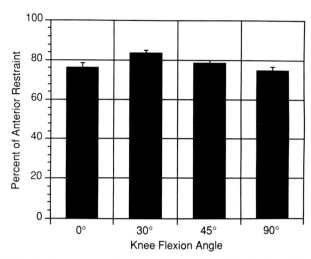

FIG. 6. Percentage of anterior restraint provided by the ACL.

increasing flexion angle from 0° to 45° of flexion averaging 4.5°, 11.9°, 14.2°, and 13.0°, respectively, at 0°, 30°, 45°, and 90° of knee flexion.

Anterior Cruciate Ligament Length

The relative lengths of the anterior and posterior portions of the ACL were significantly different, with the anterior bundle being longer. These two portions also had different patterns of length change with each increase in the flexion angle. The anterior portion lengthened with increases in flexion angle, whereas the posterior portion was longest at 0° of flexion and decreased in length with each increase in flexion angle. These trends for the anterior portion and posterior portion were present in each specimen. Under A-P loading, length change of the anterior portion of the ACL averaged 0.71, 1.26, 1.31, and 1.63 mm, respectively, at 0°, 30°, 45°, and 90°

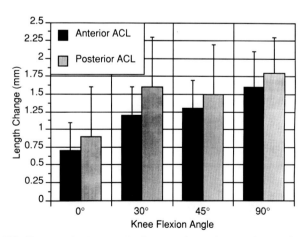

FIG. 5. Length changes in the anterior and posterior portions of the ACL for 100-N anterior loading of knee.

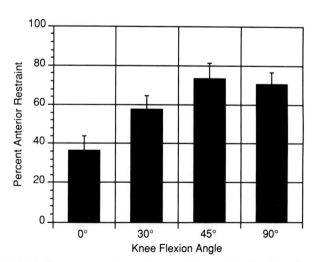

FIG. 7. Percentage of anterior restraint provided by the anterior portion of the ACL.

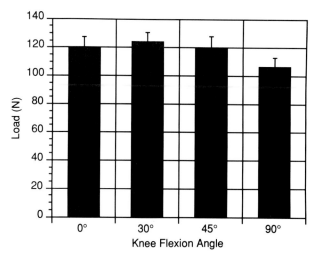

FIG. 8. Force in the ACL during a 100-N anterior draw test.

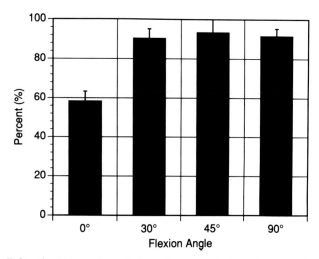

FIG. 10. Percentage of ACL force carried by the anterior portion.

of knee flexion (Fig. 5). Length change was smallest at 0° of flexion.

Anterior Cruciate Ligament Load

The results of the anterior draw test with the flexion angle only fixed showed that the ACL supplied 76.2 ± 2.3, 83.5 ± 1.3, 78.3 ± 1.8, and 74.8 ± 1.7% of the restraint to anterior draw at flexion angles of 0°, 30°, 45°, and 90°, respectively (Fig. 6). Of this constraint, most was borne by the anterior portion except at 0° of flexion (36.5 ± 2.3, 57.8 ± 1.5, 73.5 ± 2.6, and 70.5 ± 2.3% at flexion angles of 0°, 30°, 45°, and 90°, respectively) (Fig. 7). There was a trend toward the anterior portion of the ACL carrying higher loads at larger angles of flexion.

During external application of the 100-N anterior knee load, the *in situ* ACL load was 120 ± 7.5, 124 ± 7, 120 ± 8, and 107 ± 6 N at flexion angles of 0°, 30°, 45°,

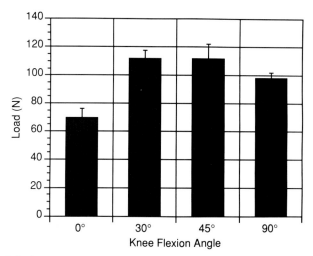

FIG. 9. Force in the anterior portion of the ACL during a 100-N anterior draw test.

and 90°, respectively (Fig. 8). The effect of flexion angle on ACL load was found to be significant using a one-way analysis of variance test. The anterior portion of the ACL carried the lowest percentage of the load at 0° of knee flexion with values of 70 ± 6 N, 112 ± 6 N, 112 ± 10 N, and 98 ± 4 N at flexion angles of 0°, 30°, 45°, and 90°, respectively (Fig. 9). Looking at the percentage of restraint at the different flexion angles, the anterior portion resists 58% at 0° flexion but carries almost all of the load at higher flexion angles (Fig. 10). During passive flexion the load in the anterior portion was less than 10 N. The load in the posterior portion of the ligament was calculated to be 50 N, 12 N, 8 N, and 9 N at the corresponding four flexion angles. This result shows that the posterior portion of the ACL plays a role in knee stability at 0° of flexion.

DISCUSSION

Comparison of Results with Other Studies

The knee kinematic data agree well with the data reported from other studies. Grood et al. (8) determined the laxity of the knee at different flexion angles using A-P loads of 100 N and V-V moments of 20 N-m. They reported that the A-P laxity was highest at 30° of flexion. Fukubayashi et al. (6) measured the A-P laxity and tibial rotation of knee joints, finding A-P laxity to be 13 mm at 30° and less at 0° and 45° for an applied load of +100 N. Tibial rotation was 20° with A-P loading at 90° of flexion and 8° at 0° of flexion. Maximal internal rotation occurred between 30° and 45° of knee flexion. These values are comparable with the values measured in the present study.

Previous experiments have been able to yield very little data on the distribution of the forces among the ACL bundles. Girgis et al. (7) observed that the posterior portion of the ACL is lax in the flexed knee and that the anterior portion is relatively taut throughout flexion. This observation is consistent with our results for the posterior portion, but we found that the anterior portion increased in length with flexion from full extension. France et al. (5) estimated the force in the posterior and anterior portions of the ACL using strain gauges placed on the bone at the ACL insertion site. The preliminary results of that study agree with those of the present study, suggesting that the force in the ACL was concentrated in the posterior portion at 0° of flexion, evenly distributed at 30° of flexion, and concentrated in the anterior portion of the ligament at 45° of flexion.

The forces in the anterior portion at 45° calculated in the present study were higher than the 70 N value reported by Ahmed et al. (1), who used their buckle force transducer. Butler et al. (3) showed that the ACL contributes 67% to 85% of the force that resists anterior drawer of 1 to 5 mm. The load calculated in the present study would be close to that found in Butler's study, depending on the exact orientation of the portion of the ACL resisting the load. Markolf et al. (13) measured both the magnitude and the direction of the force at the tibial insertion of the ACL with a unique load-cell attached to a bone plug containing this insertion. Our results confirm their findings that the ACL carries most of the anterior force applied to the tibia and that the *in situ* loads on the ACL exceed the applied anterior knee load. However, Markolf et al. could not measure the contributions of different portions of the ACL.

The Function of Different Portions

The most significant finding from these tests is the force distribution within the ACL. The ACL is a complex structure, and different portions of this ligament function at different flexion angles. This finding has important implications regarding the structural properties of the ACL and the biomechanical properties that a substitute for the ACL would require to emulate the natural ACL.

The Implications Regarding ACL Injury

In ACL biomechanics, the stress distribution is important for understanding the structural properties of the ACL. The maximum load that the ACL can withstand is limited by the maximum stress that any small group of fibers can withstand. This study demonstrated an uneven distribution of the force in the ACL. Therefore, the maximum stress that exists in the ACL cannot be determined by dividing the total force carried by the ligament by the cross-sectional area. Concentration of the force in either the anterior or the posterior portion of the liga-

ment, with certain degrees of flexion, is a factor in ACL failure at loads below that which could be achieved with a uniform stress distribution. Our finding that the loads in the ligament were more uniform at 30° of flexion than at the greater flexion angles could well explain the results of some of the recent studies conducted in our laboratory on the porcine and the human ACL (9–11,18). Those studies showed that the ultimate load in the ligament is greater at 30° of flexion than at 90° of flexion. Thus, calculation of the maximum stress level in an ACL made by considering the ACL a simple, one-dimensional structure would be inaccurate.

The ACL has been reported to be a less significant restraint of axial-tibial rotation when the knee is flexed (14,15). Nevertheless, we noted that limiting knee motion to A-P translations only led to longer anterior portions of the ACL, even at higher angles of flexion. These results suggest that a rupture of the anterior portion of the ACL is more likely when knee loading coincides with limited axial-tibial rotation. This situation could occur when the foot is planted or secured in a ski binding. In unconstrained anterior loading of the knee, axial-tibial rotation may serve to unload the anterior portion of the ACL and more evenly distribute the load between the anterior and posterior portions.

The Implications for Replacement Design

Our results showed that the anatomy and location of the ACL present a unique structure and function that may be difficult to replace with a single-stranded structure. It may be more appropriate to replace the ligament with a graft with multiple strands that would function at different flexion angles. These issues should be considered when choosing a replacement graft and procedure. Some clinical trials have been conducted using double tendon grafts, one in the place of the posterolateral anatomical portion of the ACL and one in the place of the anteromedial portion, as reported by Mott (16) and Zariczny (19). These procedures used the semitendinosus tendon, which was placed through one hole in the femur and two holes in the tibia. Multiple-strand prosthetic ligaments also have been developed. In a study by Chen, results using a two stranded prosthetic ligament in a canine model were superior to results in other reported studies of single-strand devices (4).

FUTURE DIRECTIONS

The Potential Use of the Method

The significant difference in force in the fiber bundles and the significant change in ACL force distribution with changes in flexion, which were demonstrated in this study, show the importance of determining the force in the bundles independently. The successful application of this method to the ACL demonstrates its potential usefulness, which could be utilized for other studies. Investigation of ligament substitutes is also an obvious application of this method. For example, knee kinematics and the load could be compared in the natural ACL and ACL replacement grafts. However, the attachment of the prosthesis to the bone could be difficult to simulate because bone ingrowth and/or soft tissue provide fixation for the graft *in vivo*. In addition, different specimens would be needed for the normal ACL and prosthetic ACL tests if the loads are to be determined in the normal ACL because the bone must be dissected away with the normal ligament for the load-length tests. Whether a multistrand ACL replacement could more accurately reproduce the function of the ACL than can a single patellar tendon autograft is not known but could be investigated with a method similar to that used in the present study. Simultaneous evaluation of the force in the tendon graft and the knee kinematics would provide a basis for comparing different reconstruction techniques. The other ligaments of the knee could be studied using variations of this protocol. The posterior cruciate ligament and lateral collateral ligament, with their well-defined insertion sites, would be more appropriate for such a study than would the medial collateral ligament, which has a rather long and ill-defined tibial insertion.

Improvements in the Method

This study has demonstrated that the method can provide an estimate of the load in the ACL fiber bundles using a simple structural model. Future refinement of this technique could produce improvement in several areas. A necessary future direction in studying the role of the ACL in normal knee kinematics is the more precise reproduction of the knee position after partial dissection of the knee. In this study we avoided the problem of accurate fiber alignment in the ACL after incremental dissection by applying anterior load to a knee that was allowed only anterior translation of the tibia. Although this approach allows rigorous investigation of the load distribution within the ACL, it currently does not allow for complex motions.

The quantitative data obtained in this study should be useful in defining ACL function as it changes with knee motion and applied loading and should lead to suitably more complex replacements or reconstruction techniques. The load and load distribution in the ACL during fully unconstrained knee motions with a more accurate scheme of tibial manipulation are under investigation. A new testing device has been developed (12) to improve the alignment of the ACL during the test to determine the load versus length curve. This device enables the relative position of the two bones to be defined

precisely in all 6 *df* in any position. When this device is used in conjunction with a 6 *df* spatial kinematic linkage, a position recorded with the linkage later can be reproduced in the joint with very high accuracy. Tests will be performed with this device to determine the force in the ACL for a larger variety of joint loadings, including axial-tibial rotation, V-V moments, and these loadings combined with A-P drawer.

The Advantages and Disadvantages of the Method

The advantages of the method used in this chapter are that (a) it enables the determination of loads in different portions of the ACL simultaneously, (b) the evaluation can be conducted while the knee is intact, and (c) the contribution of the ACL to the stiffness of the joint motion of the knee can be determined while the knee is unconstrained, with only the flexion angle fixed.

Disadvantages of the method used in this study are that the method is limited by the need to reproduce the position of the ACL insertions between *in situ* tests and the load versus length tests (ACL-only test). This implies that, for a different loading, such as tibial rotation, the load versus length curve when generated by anterior loading may not be sufficiently accurate for determining the load. The ACL could be at a different orientation and therefore have subunits coming into play at different lengths as compared to another orientation.

The Limits on Results and the Conclusions of the Study

The results of this study are from tests performed with several constraints and limitations: (a) there are no muscle forces acting across the joint, (b) there is no weight load on the joint, (c) the loading is restricted to the anterior direction and does not include axial tibial rotation torque, medial-lateral force, and varus-valgus moment. The implication of these limitations is that there may be some loading situations in which the distribution of forces in the ACL is different from that seen for anterior loading. This possibility has not been investigated. The trend that the posterior portion of the ACL carries a portion of the load at full extension is expected to be similar for other loading conditions.

REFERENCES

1. Ahmed AM, Hyder A, Burke DL, Chan KH. (1987): *In-vitro* ligament tension pattern in the flexed knee in passive loading. *J Orthop Res,* 5:217–230.
2. Beggs JS. (1983): *Kinematics.* Washington, DC: Hemisphere Publishing, p 37.
3. Butler DL, Noyes FR, Grood ES. (1980): Ligamentous restraints to anterior-posterior drawer in the human knee. *J Bone Joint Surg* [*Am*], 62A:259–270.
4. Chen E. (1991): *The design and evaluation of a canine anterior*

cruciate ligament prosthesis [Dissertation]. New Brunswick, NJ: Rutgers University.

5. France PE, Daniels AU, Goble ME, Dunn HK. (1983): Simultaneous quantitation of knee ligament forces. *J Biomech,* 16:553–564.

6. Fukubayashi T, Torzilli PA, Sherman MF, Warren RF. (1982): An *in vitro* biomechanical evaluation of anterior-posterior motion of the knee. *J Bone Joint Surg [Am],* 64A:258–264.

7. Girgis FG, Marshall JL, Al Monajem ARS. (1975): The cruciate ligaments of the knee joint: anatomical, functional and experimental analysis. *Clin Orthop Rel Res,* 106:216–231.

8. Grood ES, Stowers SF, Noyes FR. (1988): Limits of movement in the human knee. *J Bone Joint Surg [Am],* 70A:88–97.

9. Hollis JM, Lee EB, Ballock RT, Gomez MA, Woo SL-Y. (1986): The effect of loading direction on the failure properties of the femur-anterior cruciate ligament-tibia complex. *Adv Bioeng,* 12:168–169.

10. Hollis JM, Lee EB, Ballock RT, Inoue M, Gomez MA, Woo SL-Y. (1987): Variation of structural properties of the anterior cruciate ligament as a function of loading direction. *Trans Orthop Res Soc,* 12:196.

11. Hollis JM, Lyon RM, Marcin JP, Horibe S, Lee EB, Woo SL-Y. (1988): Effect of age and loading axis on the failure properties of the human ACL. Presented at the 34th Annual Meeting of the Orthopaedic Research Society, Atlanta, GA, February 1–4.

12. Hollis JM. (1988): *Development and application of a method for determining the* in situ *forces in anterior cruciate ligament fiber bundles* [Dissertation]. San Diego, CA: University of California.

13. Markolf KL, Gorek JF, Kabo JM, Shapiro MS. (1990): Direct measurement of resultant forces in the anterior cruciate ligament. *J Bone Joint Surg [Am],* 72A:557–567.

14. Markolf KL, Mensch JS, Amstutz HC. (1976): Stiffness and laxity of the knee—the contributions of the supporting structures. *J Bone Joint Surg [Am],* 58A:583–593.

15. McMaster NC. (1975): Isolated posterior cruciate ligament injury: Ligament review and case reports. *J Trauma,* 15:1025–1029.

16. Mott WH. (1983): Semitendinous anatomic reconstruction for cruciate ligament insufficiency. *Clin Orthop Rel Res,* 172:90–92.

17. Norwood LA, Cross MJ. (1979): Anterior cruciate ligament: functional anatomy of its bundles in rotary instabilites. *Am J Sports Med,* 7:23–26.

18. Woo SL-Y, Hollis JM, Adams DJ, Lyons RM, Takai S. (1991): Tensile properties of the human femur-anterior cruciate ligament-tibia complex: the effects of specimen age and orientation. *Am J Sports Med,* 19(2).

19. Zariczny B. (1987): Reconstruction of the anterior cruciate ligament of the knee using a doubled tendon graft. *Clin Orthop Rel Res,* 220:162–175.

The Anterior Cruciate Ligament: Current and
Future Concepts, edited by D.W. Jackson, et al.
Raven Press, Ltd., New York © 1993.

CHAPTER 8

The Measurement of Anterior Cruciate Ligament Loads: Direct Methods

Jack L. Lewis, William D. Lew, and Keith Markolf

The anterior cruciate ligament is well recognized as a key structure in providing stability to the knee. Forces experienced by the ACL and its replacement grafts influence injury, repair, and remodeling of these tissues. Overloading the ACL or an ACL graft can cause rupture; underloading can cause atrophy and weakening. Knowledge of the forces in the natural ACL is important for guiding treatment in repair and healing of the ACL and for basic understanding of articulating joints. Knowledge of the forces in the ACL is also important, in the design of ACL replacements, for determining the appropriate materials and in the tailoring of surgery and rehabilitation techniques to achieve optimum loads for graft remodeling.

In spite of this importance, however, there is limited information available on forces in the ACL. Direct measurement of ACL force has presented a formidable challenge to biomechanical investigators, and it is fair to say that no perfect method presently exists to measure directly the total force generated in the natural ACL.

For in vitro testing, there have been several direct methods proposed, with varying success and range of application. Two accepted methods for direct force measurement involve the use of buckle transducers (1,8,10), or force transducers mounted external to the joint (11). These approaches form the basis of this chapter.

As mentioned above, different techniques have been utilized. For completeness, a short summary of several of these is provided. The use of strain gauges bonded to bone near the ligament insertion sites was reported by France et al. (5). These gauges sense deformation of the bone, and their output is calibrated by direct pull on the ligament. The primary disadvantage of this method is that the strain gauges also respond to tibiofemoral con-

tact forces, thereby altering the measurement of the ligament forces.

A conceptually simpler approach to estimating in vitro forces in the natural ligament involves the substitution of a steel cable for the resected natural ACL. With this technique, the cable is attached to a tibial load cell assembly that contains a rubber washer for the adjustment of the overall stiffness of the construct to that of a normal bone-ACL-bone preparation. Direct measurements of cable force have been recorded for applied anterior tibial force (2).

Another approach is to replace the resected ligament with a synthetic substitute. In a cadaveric study using the Gore-Tex ligament [a multistranded polytetrafluoroethylene (PTFE) prosthesis], a load cell was connected to the tibial eyelet of the device and direct measurements of ligament force were recorded as the knee was loaded manually by passive flexion/extension, anterior tibial force, and tibial torque (12). There was wide scatter in the force levels recorded when the knee was extended passively. Internal rotation of the tibia with the knee at full extension was identified as a mode that highly loaded the ligament substitute and, therefore, would also load the ACL. More recently, a similar technique using a braided polyethylene ACL substitute (Richards) was employed to examine ligament force data during straight anterior tibial loading (4).

This chapter concentrates on methods in which force in the ACL is measured directly, rather than through indirect methods such as force predictions from kinematics. Surface strain measurement will not be addressed, since this will be covered in other chapters. Because most published reports of direct measurement of forces in the ACL have utilized human cadaver knees, the present focus will be on in vitro approaches. Work on in vivo force measurement in animals is under way in several laboratories, and this will be covered briefly, as results have not yet appeared in the literature. As the two most frequently used in vitro techniques have been buckle

J. L. Lewis and W. D. Lew: Department of Orthopaedic Surgery, University of Minnesota, Minneapolis, Minnesota 55455.
K. Markolf: Division of Orthopaedic Surgery, University of California at Los Angeles, Los Angeles, California 90024.

transducers and external force transducers, these two methods will be described here in detail.

THE BUCKLE TRANSDUCER TECHNIQUE

Description

Buckle-type transducers were introduced by Salmons (13) in 1969 for measuring forces in tendons of animals. Lewis and Fraser (6) applied a buckle transducer of modified design to ligaments in human cadaver knees. These transducers have been used in studies by various investigators since then. The transducer used by Lewis and colleagues on ligaments consists of a rectangular frame with a removable cross-bar (Fig. 1). Strain gauges are mounted on the frame. To install a buckle on a ligament, one manipulates the ligament and the cross-bar through the inner portion of the frame, so that the cross-bar becomes seated upon the frame, yet under the ligament. When installed, the ligament undergoes a slight deflection from its normal path. When the ligament experiences tension, it tends to straighten itself, which deforms the frame and produces a response in the strain gauges. A buckle transducer installed on an ACL is shown in Fig. 2. Ligament force is calibrated to transducer output by pulling directly on the ligament with known loads.

The advantages of the transducer are that (a) it can be applied directly on the ligament; (b) it is a direct force transducer, rather than a strain transducer (if no force is generated, there is no output), and (c) it is rugged enough to withstand the practical demands of cadaver testing. The disadvantages include (a) the potential for impingement with bone, causing spurious output; (b) viscoelastic creep of the tissue within the buckle, causing change in the calibration constant; (c) variation of the stress distribution in the tissue within the transducer, causing change in the calibration constant; and (d) a small amount of ligament shortening when the transducer is installed on the natural ACL, which can change the dis-

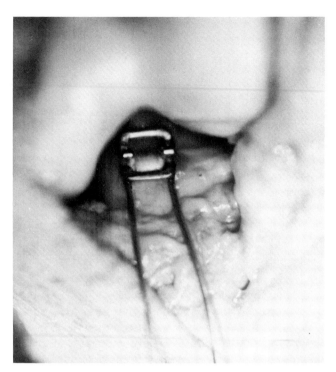

FIG. 2. A buckle transducer on an *in vitro* ACL. (From ref. 5a, with permission.)

tribution of loads within the joint. This latter problem does not occur with ACL grafts because the transducer is installed before fixing the graft.

The potential problems with the buckle transducers have been dealt with in several ways. Lewis et al. removed bone that may impinge on the transducer (8,10). This bone removal has the potential to alter the distribution of loads within the joint. This, however, has not seemed to be a problem because the bone removed does not normally impinge on the ACL when no buckle transducer is present. Also, bone removal may potentially alter the kinematics of the joint; however, this effect has been shown to be minimal (8). Ahmed et al. (1) avoided the impingement problem by not testing the joint near extension, where bony contact is most likely to occur. Tissue creep can cause the calibration to change by up to 50% for a constant load applied over 3 min (8). This can be minimized by preconditioning the buckle transducer *in situ* before calibrating and by measuring the ligament force as soon as possible after loading the joint (8,10). The change in calibration with altered stress distribution is most evident when the entire ACL is within the buckle and the ACL is loaded at different joint flexion angles. For example, changes of over 50% can occur in the calibration constant for the buckle on the entire ACL between full extension and 90° flexion. This problem can be minimized by calibrating the ligament and buckle at each flexion angle tested, although there may still be some changes for large motions at a given flexion angle, such as axial rotations. Discussion of error sources in the

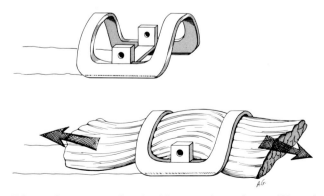

FIG. 1. Schematic of a buckle transducer frame (**A**) and cross-bar (**B**). (From ref. 5a, with permission.)

use of buckle transducers and ways to minimize these errors are contained in References 1, 8, and 10.

Current Estimates of *In Vitro* Forces in the ACL Using Buckle Transducers

There have been several studies of the forces in the intact ACL in cadaver joints using buckle transducers. Lewis et al. (7) measured force in the anteromedial band of the ACL during the application of a variety of external load states to seven specimens. The buckle transducers were installed on the anteromedial band of the ACL, bone was removed from the lateral region of the intercondylar notch to prevent impingement, and external loads were applied manually to the tibia using a spring scale. Results showed that the ACL carried force in hyperextension and during applied anterior tibial load, internal rotation, and varus moments near full extension. There were negligible ACL forces at 90° flexion for any of these external loading states. Little or no force in the ACL was observed for applied posterior tibial load, external rotation, or valgus moment. The largest ACL forces occurred for internal rotation moments of 3.7 N-m at extension (approximately 100 N). For an anterior tibial load of 45 N at extension ACL forces were approximately 60 N.

Ahmed et al. (1) measured forces on the anteromedial band of the ACL using buckle transducers in 30 human cadaver knees to determine applied anterior tibial force and tibial torque. Rather than remove bone to prevent buckle transducer impingement near extension, these investigators limited testing to between 40° and 90° of flexion. They measured ligament forces as a function of applied joint displacement and then measured load versus displacement response of the joint separately. They measured ACL forces of approximately 70 N for 5 mm of anterior tibial displacement (which required 100 N of anterior tibial load) at both 40° and 90° of flexion. The ACL force was reduced by an axial compressive preload of 900 N. The anteromedial band of the ACL was loaded in internal rotation, but not in external rotation, at 40° flexion only. Ligament forces in rotation were highly variable, but average ACL forces at 40° were approximately 4 N at 2 N-m and 20 N at 8 N-m.

The results of these two studies are in qualitative agreement. It is difficult to compare quantitative results in much detail because most test conditions varied. However, comparisons can be made for states that were similar. As estimated from published graphical data, at 45° and 45 N of anterior tibial load, Lewis et al. (7) measured approximately 30 N in the anteromedial band of the ACL; Ahmed et al. (1) recorded 35 N for the same load at 40°. Lewis reported approximately 40 N in the anteromedial band at 45° due to a 3.7 N-m internal rotation torque; Ahmed et al. reported approximately 10 N at 40°

for the same torque. Both studies noted large interspecimen variability in ACL force.

In a second study by Lewis et al. (9), the forces in the intact ACL were measured with the entire ACL placed within the buckle transducer. For a 90 N anterior tibial load, ACL forces were 100 N at extension and 30 N in flexion. This was similar to the earlier study in which only the antero-medial band was instrumented, except that there was now a load measured in flexion. This probably reflected the load carried by the posterolateral band, which was not measured in the earlier study.

THE IN-LINE EXTERNAL FORCE TRANSDUCER TECHNIQUE

Description

A new and unique experimental technique was developed for direct measurement of the resultant force in the natural ACL in cadaver specimens. This technique involves mechanical isolation of a bone plug (containing the ACL's tibial insertion) that has been fixed onto a specially designed miniature load cell. The three components of ACL force measured by the load cell as external loads are applied to the tibia. The advantages of this method are that (a) the ligament fibers themselves are not altered in any way during the measurement, (b) the base of the ligament remains in its precise anatomical location with respect to the tibia, and (c) the total resultant force within the ligament is recorded directly (as opposed to localized measurements in specific bands of the ligament).

In this procedure, a guide hole drilled in the tibia exits at the center of the insertion of the ACL in the tibial plateau; this hole is approximately in line with the fibers of the ACL. Using a series of cannulated drills and a cylindrical reamer, a sector of cancellous bone beneath the ACL is partially isolated. Before complete mechanical isolation of a bone cap containing the tibial insertion fibers of the ACL, six miniature wood screws are fixed to its undersurface. The cancellous bone and protruding screw heads are incorporated into an acrylic cylinder containing a steel core. This core is connected by an attachment screw to the shaft of a specially designed miniature load cell. The base of the load cell is attached by a hex head bolt to a mounting plate, which in turn is incorporated into a large acrylic mass surrounding screws fixed into the tibial shaft. After final mechanical isolation of the bone cap with a special coring cutter, all ligament force passes directly through the load cell. A schematic diagram of the load cell installed on a tibial specimen is shown in Fig. 3.

The load cell has two pairs of strain gauges bonded to the base of its shaft in half-bridge configurations to measure the two orthogonal components of force acting per-

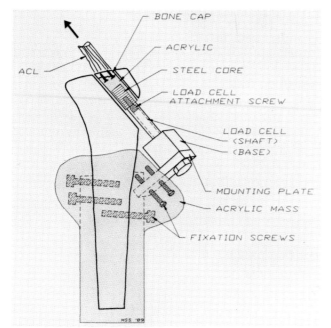

FIG. 3. Schematic view of the load cell-bone plug construct. The shaft of the load cell is attached by an internal screw to a steel core embedded within a cylinder of acrylic. The proximal end of this acrylic mass also incorporates small wood screws inserted into the undersurface of a mechanically isolated bone cap that contains the base of the tibial attachment of the anterior cruciate ligament. The base of the load cell is secured by a hex head bolt to a metal plate. A large acrylic mass incorporates this plate, the potted tibial shaft, and screws within the plate and potted tibia into a solid structural base. All force generated by the ligament passes through the load cell to the tibia through this acrylic mass. (From ref. 11, with permission.)

pendicular to the shaft axis. The component of force acting along the axis of the shaft is measured by four strain gauges bonded to the inner and outer surfaces of circular cutouts in the rectangular portion of the transducer. Before each test session, the load cell is calibrated in the three mutually perpendicular directions by hanging weights at its tip; transverse force calibrations incorporate the actual distance from the ACL insertion to the tip of the load cell. The three components of force are referred to an origin located at the geometric center of the ACL attachment on the surface of the tibia. As the ligament is loaded during testing, the force components and resultant data are recorded using a computerized data acquisition system.

Sources of Error Associated with the Technique

As with any measurement system, there are sources of error associated with the recorded force values. The first source of error is within the load cell itself. The maximum error in the resultant force vector (principally due to slight errors in gauge alignment and minor distortion strains in the axial gauges generated by transverse force compo-

nents) is typically 10% for the extremes of the angles of ACL pull generated in these experiments. For angles of pull more closely aligned with the long axis of the load cell, the error in the resultant force is less than 3%.

A second source of error in these experiments relates to motion of the isolated ligament base with respect to the tibial plateau. The ligament force acts over a long lever arm with respect to the fixed base of the load cell, creating an inherently flexible cantilever beam support structure. Therefore, the isolated bone plug does not remain absolutely centralized with respect to the coring hole in the tibial plateau and in fact is displaced posteriorly with respect to the tibial plateau as anterior force is applied to the tibia. If the anterior cruciate ligament were the only structure undergoing strain during anterior tibial displacement, then motion of the bone plug would introduce no error in the force measurements under similar loading states. However, if other structures are also capable of generating significant resistive force as they are strained during the loading tests, motion of the bone plug relative to the tibia would generate increased strain and load sharing in these secondary tissues. This could cause the recorded ligament force values to be artificially low. At present there is no available solution for eliminating this source of error. Based upon anterior-posterior testing, however, a 1% to 9% underestimation of the ACL force has been calculated from straight anterior tibial loading, which is arguably the worst case scenario because the direction of ligament fiber loading is transverse to the load cell axis.

Another potential source of error relates to contact of the bone plug with the perimeter of the tibial tunnel hole as ligament force is applied. If contact occurs, it is easily detected. Typically, one bending component of load cell force changes abruptly (stops increasing) when a certain level of applied load is attained. If this happens, the gap between the bone plug and tibial hole is widened until the problem is eliminated. Similarly, contact of a femoral condyle with the isolated tibial bone cap can be detected by a sudden change in the axial component of load cell force (which is typically driven into compression). If this occurs, a small portion of the femoral condyle is trimmed away to eliminate the impingement. One final limitation of the technique relates to the necessity for good quality cancellous bone at the tibial bone plug. If the bone is weak, the wood screws pull out from the bone and fixation of the bone plug to the load cell is lost. This often precludes use of specimens from elderly donors, especially women, whose bone may osteoporotic.

Current Estimates of ACL Force Using the In-Line External Force Transducer Technique

Detailed results of direct force measurements using this technique on 18 cadaver knees can be found in reference 11; important findings are summarized here.

Passive Knee Flexion/Extension

Passive knee extension (and especially hyperextension) loaded the ACL in all specimens (Fig. 4); ligament forces at full extension ranged from 16 to 87 N and from 50 to 241 N at 5° of hyperextension. Application of a 200-N quadriceps tendon pull increased ACL force, especially beyond 10° of flexion, where negligible force is generated in the intact state (Fig. 4). From these results it was concluded that active quadriceps extension in the 0° to 45° range would not be advisable if one wished to limit forces in a repaired or substituted ACL; hyperextension should clearly be avoided.

Internal-External Tibial Rotation

Internal tibial rotation always generated greater ACL force than did external rotation (Fig. 5). Ligament forces from 10 N-m of applied torque were highest in hyperextension, where loads ranged from 133 to 370 N; tibial torque applied to a hyperextended knee is a common mechanism for injury to the ACL.

Varus-Valgus Tibial Rotation

Ligament force was generated for applied varus and valgus moments (Fig. 6). ACL forces in both cases were highest in full extension and would be expected to be even higher if the knee was forced into hyperextension. Ligament forces from 15 N-m of applied varus moment at full extension ranged from 94 to 177 N. Transverse blows to the knee with the joint in full extension or slight flexion (such as a clipping injury in football) would be expected to generate high ACL forces.

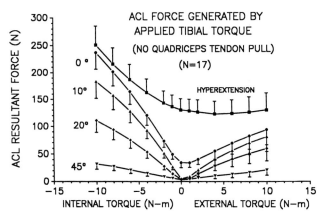

FIG. 5. Mean curves of anterior cruciate ligament force generated by the application of internal and external tibial torque. Error bars indicate the 95% confidence interval for the mean. The *curve* labeled *hyperextension* represents specimens with an applied extension moment of 10 N-m. All mean curves shown are significantly different from one another. (From ref. 11, with permission.)

Anterior Tibial Translation

The ACL force generated from an applied anterior tibial load was slightly higher than the magnitude of the applied load itself, confirming that this ligament is indeed the primary restraint to anterior tibial translation. Under 925 N of tibiofemoral contact load, the resultant ACL force from an applied anterior tibial force was decreased an average of 36% at 0° flexion and 46% at 20° of flexion.

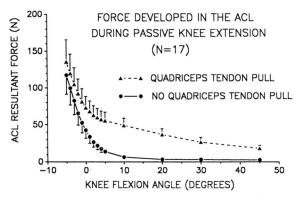

FIG. 4. Mean curves of anterior cruciate ligament force versus knee flexion angle for specimens during manual knee extension against gravity (*solid curve*), and for specimens extended slowly against tibial resistance by an applied 200-N quadriceps tendon pull (*dashed curve*). Error bars indicate the 95% confidence interval for the mean. The effects of quadriceps tendon pull are diminished as the knee is hyperextended. (From ref. 11, with permission.)

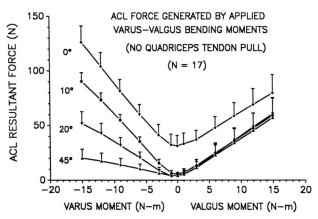

FIG. 6. Mean curves of anterior cruciate ligament force generated by the application of varus and valgus bending moments to the tibia. Error bars indicate the 95% confidence interval for the mean. For an applied varus moment, ligament force levels are significantly different between flexion angles. Beyond 10° of flexion, the anterior cruciate ligament force generated by an applied valgus moment is unchanged. The slopes of all mean valgus curves shown are equivalent. (From ref. 11, with permission.)

IN VIVO MEASUREMENTS

At this time, the authors are not aware of any published reports of *in vivo* measurement of ACL forces using direct methods. However, there are several transducers used or in development that are intended for this purpose. Lewis et al. (7) used buckle transducers to measure forces in the medial collateral ligament of the canine stifle joint and are currently using them to measure forces in an ACL graft in the goat. Grood, Butler, and coworkers (3) developed a transducer for installation within the ligamentous substance, which they call an implantable force transducer (IFT). This transducer is a curved metal sheet with strain gauges mounted on it. When present in a loaded ligament, the ligament tissue compresses the sheet and causes strain in the gauges. The transducer is calibrated by direct pull on the ligament. These investigators have reported *in vivo* force data from such a transducer implanted into the patellar tendon of a goat (3) and are currently using it in the ACL of the functioning goat. Similar *in vivo* measurements performed in humans will be critical to the evaluation and interpretation of published human data.

SUMMARY

We have discussed two *in vitro* measurement techniques for directly recording forces in the ACL during human cadaver testing. Both methods have potential sources of error, but the errors are sufficiently small to allow meaningful measurements of ACL forces. ACL forces have been reported during externally applied loading conditions; active and passive muscle constraints are necessarily absent. Muscle action undoubtedly has a major effect on the ACL forces, but the effects are unknown. Researchers are beginning to attempt measurements of ACL forces in living animals. Comparing these results with equivalent tests on animal cadavers should provide guidance as to the relevance to living humans of the extensive testing on human cadaver specimens.

REFERENCES

1. Ahmed AM, Hyder A, Burke DL, Chan KH. (1987): *In vitro* ligament tension pattern in the flexed knee in passive loading. *J Orthop Res,* 5:217–230.
2. Bylski-Austrow Dl, Grood ES, Hefzy MS, Holden JP, Butler DL. (1990): Anterior cruciate ligament replacements: a mechanical study of femoral attachment location, flexion angle at tensioning, and initial tension. *J Orthop Res,* 8:522–531.
3. Cummings JF, Holden JP, Grood ES, Troble RR, Butler DL, Schafer JA. (1991): *In vivo* measurement of patellar tendon forces and joint position in the goat model. *Trans Orthop Res Soc,* 16:601.
4. Fleming B, Beynnon B, Howe J, McLeod W, Pope M. (1992): Effect of tension and placement of a prosthetic anterior cruciate ligament on the anteroposterior laxity of the knee. *J Orthop Res,* 10:177–186.
5. France EP, Daniels AU, Goble EM, Dunn HK. (1983): Simultaneous quantitation of knee ligament forces. *J Biomech,* 16:553–564.
5a. Hanley P, Lew WD, Lewis JL, Hunter RE, Kirstukas S, Kowalczyk C. (1989): Load sharing and graft forces in anterior cruciate ligament reconstructions with the ligament augmentation device. *Am J Sports Med* 17(3):414–422.
6. Lewis JL, Frasier G. (1979): On the use of buckle transducers to measure knee ligament forces. In: *Proceedings of the 1979 ASME Biomechanics Symposium,* pp 71–74.
7. Lewis JL, Lew WD, Shybut GT, Jasty M, Hill JA. (1985): Biomechanical function of knee ligaments. In: Finerman G, ed. *Symposium on sports medicine: the knee.* St Louis, MO: CV Mosby, pp 152–168.
8. Lewis JL, Lew WD, Schmidt J. (1988): Description and error evaluation of an *in vitro* knee joint testing system. *J Biomech Eng,* 110:238–248.
9. Lewis JL, Lew WD, Hill JA, Hanley P, Ohland K, Kirstukas S, Hunter RE. (1989): Knee joint motion and ligament forces before and after ACL reconstruction. *J Biomech Eng,* 111:97–106.
10. Lewis JL, Lew WD, Schmidt J. (1982): A note on the application and evaluation of the buckle transducer for knee ligament force measurement. *J Biomech Eng,* 104:125–128.
11. Markolf KL, Gorek JF, Kabc JM, Shapiro MS. (1990): Direct measurement of resultant forces in the anterior cruciate ligament—an *in vivo* study performed with a new experimental technique. *J Bone Joint Surg [Am],* 72A:557–567.
12. More RC, Markolf KL. (1988): Measurement of stability of the knee and ligament force after implantation of a synthetic anterior cruciate ligament: *in vitro* measurement. *J Bone Joint Surg [Am],* 70A:1020–1031.
13. Salmons S. (1969): The 8th International Conference on Medical and Biological Engineering—meeting report. *Biomed Eng,* 4:467–474.

The Anterior Cruciate Ligament: Current and Future Concepts, edited by D.W. Jackson, et al. Raven Press, Ltd., New York © 1993.

CHAPTER 9

The Measurement of Anterior Cruciate Ligament Strain *In Vivo*

Bruce D. Beynnon, Braden C. Fleming, Malcolm H. Pope, and Robert J. Johnson

The anterior cruciate ligament is the most frequently totally disrupted ligament within the knee (38). A surprising proportion of active young people sustain the injury, the consequences of which are potentially debilitating (43).

The management of the acute ACL injury and the reconstruction of the ACL in the ADL-deficient knee has become synonymous with orthopedic sports medicine. Many competitive athletes have markedly compromised their careers because of limitations in our ability to diagnose, treat, and rehabilitate ACL injuries. Although the function of the ACL has been studied *in vitro,* some of these data are contradictory. Further work is needed to define the characteristics and behavior of the normal ACL so that damage to this structure can be diagnosed and treated effectively. Such data can improve knee rehabilitation programs and reconstructive surgery using autogenous tissues or may be used in the design and development of prosthetic ligaments. In addition, the data may be used as input to or verification of mathematical knee models.

The clinical diagnosis of ACL injuries is not straightforward because several structures are often involved. For diagnosis of the instabilities of the knee, numerous laxity tests have been proposed (25,35–37,48,49,55). These methods combine various standard motions of the knee, such as flexion with anterior-posterior translation, internal/external tibial rotation, and valgus moments. Posterolateral instability is normally diagnosed by the tests described by Jacob (37) and Noyes et al. (55). Despite the development of instrumented knee testing,

clinicians evaluate the integrity of the ACL manually by subjectively measuring the anterior excursion of the tibia relative to the femur with the knee flexed at 30° (Lachman test) or at 90° (anterior drawer test). Large inter- and intraobserver errors in clinical laxity testing have been reported (23,52,56). Similar errors were found evaluating various commercial machines (22–24,30,47,61). For these reasons we believe that work is still needed to understand fully the frequently utilized clinical tests. In spite of the attempts by some clinicians to classify injuries, specific diagnoses remain equivocal, and more basic studies are undoubtedly required. In previous *in vitro* work, Arms et al. (4) calculated the ACL strains when a Lachman or anterior drawer test is used, but *in vivo* data are necessary to understand the relationship between the clinical test and the ligament strain biomechanics.

Once the clinician has encountered the diagnostic problem of evaluating the integrity of the injured ligament, there remains the challenge of treatment and subsequent rehabilitation. Classically, after reconstruction procedures the joint has been immobilized for 6 weeks or more while tissues heal and joint inflammation diminishes. Innumerable investigations have documented the deleterious effects of knee immobilization on leg muscles, articular cartilage, periarticular bone, ligaments, and capsular structures (28,40–42,44,54). Yet it is possible that early unprotected motion may result in permanent elongation, if not destruction, of repaired or reconstructed ligaments, grafts, or capsular tissues. Thus, many advocate immobilization immediately after ACL reconstructions, whereas others believe that early mobilization of such reconstructions avoids many of the disadvantages while not significantly endangering the healing tissues (60).

Johnson (38) expressed concern about the potentially dangerous effect of quadriceps activity on recently re-

B. D. Beynnon, B. C. Fleming, M. H. Pope, and R. J. Johnson: McClure Musculoskeletal Research Center, Department of Orthopaedics, University of Vermont Medical School, Burlington, Vermont 05405.

paired or reconstructed ACLs. Rehabilitation recommendations were based on *in vitro* experimentation (1,3–6). The ACL strain was reported to be high enough potentially to cause damage to recently repaired or reconstructed ligaments (4,6). Consequently, the avoidance of early quadriceps contractions was advised between the limits of 60° of flexion and full extension after reconstruction of the ACL. Others advocated early quadriceps and hamstring exercises (38). Several investigators reported no evidence of damage to their reconstructions using early exercise programs (60). Thus, it seems that these issues have been incompletely studied, and the role of muscle contraction in clinical rehabilitation remains to be defined.

The above discussion demonstrates the controversy and thus the need to establish a scientific basis for the various means of protection and mobilization of the knee after ACL reconstruction. The biomechanical function of the knee ligaments has been studied by using either modeling or experimental investigation techniques. This chapter presents a review of the different biomechanical approaches used for measuring strain in the ACL, along with a summary of some of the more important findings as they pertain to the clinical environment.

STRAIN MEASUREMENT

Several investigators have measured ACL displacement patterns, enabling calculation of strain pattern, in an attempt to understand the effect of knee joint position and muscle activity on ligament biomechanics (4,5,45,46,57,66). Most of this work has been carried out *in vitro,* and some of the results are conflicting.

Edwards et al. (21), Kennedy et al. (46), and Brown et al. (11) utilized mercury-filled strain gauges to measure the length of ligaments at various angles of knee flexion. Other investigators (7,29,34,53,69) constructed various kinds of strain transducers to measure strain in various biological materials. Mutchler et al. (53) used a U-shaped metallic strain gauge to measure strain in the MCL. White and Raphael (69) used a stainless steel-backed metallic strain gauge for *in vitro* measurements of the MCL, but it is not clear that this allowed accurate strain measurement in the tissue.

Butler et al. (13) and Woo et al. (70,71) developed optical techniques for the mapping of surface strains in various tissues. Butler et al. (13) used high-speed cameras to record the movements of surface markers and to measure local deformations along the length of the ligament. These techniques are an ideal method for monitoring surface strains without contact or invasion of the ligament substance, particularly during high rate tests. Both the structural and the material behavior of soft tissue structures can be simultaneously measured with op-

tical techniques. Structural properties of soft tissue structures are characterized to describe the behavior of the bone-soft tissue-bone preparation. For the anterior cruciate ligament this includes measurement of the insertion site and midsubstance behavior (72). Material properties are characterized to describe the behavior of the ligament substance isolated from the insertion site effects (71). Weiss et al. (68) recently used an optical technique to measure longitudinal and transverse ligament strain, providing valuable data for analytic model applications. However, optical techniques may not be useful for out-of-plane movements or for ligaments such as the cruciates, which cannot be directly viewed *in situ.* They also suffer from the theoretical disadvantage that the tissue of interest has to be exposed to a nonphysiological state.

Measurement of cruciate ligament subbundles dissected from human cadaver specimens has revealed that spatial variations in strain values exist along the length of the cruciate ligaments, with greater magnitudes occurring at the insertion sites (12,15). In a later investigation Butler et al. (14) revealed that anterior ACL subbundles have significantly larger strain energy density and stress values at failure in comparison to the posterior ACL subbundles. All ACL subbundles were reported to have similar maximum strain values at failure, indicating that each subbundle fails by a strain-dependent mechanism (14). Woo et al. (72) evaluated isolated ACLs and demonstrated that the structural properties are dependent on the alignment of the specimen during failure loading.

Other workers have calculated strain by measurement of the change of ligament attachment length under various loads. For example, Wang et al. (66) measured the three-dimensional coordinates of pins stuck in a cadaver joint at the palpated origin and insertion points of the major knee ligaments. They recorded the relationship between torque and angular displacement with relative motion between the femur and the tibia. After excision of certain ligaments, the tests were then repeated to determine the contribution of these elements to torsional restraint. According to Wang and associates (66), the ACL increases in strain with knee flexion, starting at 0% in full extension and reaching 10% at 120° of flexion. These results are in contradiction to the findings of Kennedy et al. (46), who found that a minimum ACL length occurs between 30° and 40° of knee flexion. In the most extensive and elegant studies, Sidles et al. used a three-dimensional digitizer to compute ligament length patterns (62). This investigation presented the locations of anterior and posterior cruciate sites that displayed a minimum change in length, termed *near isometric,* for motion of the knee joint.

In a slightly different approach, Trent et al. (65) used pins embedded in the ligament attachments and measured the displacement of one pin relative to the other. In addition, they located the instant centers of transverse rotation. They found the anterior fibers of the ACL to be nearly constant in length with knee flexion ranging between 0° and 60° and at a minimum at 75°. Warren et al. (67) also used pins placed at ligament origins but measured displacements with a radiographic technique.

The pins or other markers that are used as locators of ligament origin generally estimate average ligament strain and can give confusing results due to the changes in strain between the midsubstance and the ligament insertion sites and the difficulty in choosing the center of a ligament insertion.

Previous investigation performed at the University of Vermont focused on the measurement of ACL displacement in the *in vitro* environment using the Hall effect strain transducer (HEST) (Microstrain Co., Burlington, Vermont) (4). This approach allows the measurement of ACL displacement over a known gauge length and thus computation of strain (1,4,5,57). Evaluation of clinical ACL examination techniques found that the Lachman test does not result in as much positive ACL strain as does the drawer test *in vitro* (4). Rehabilitative activities were also investigated by simulating quadriceps function while ACL strain was measured. Simulated isometric contraction of the quadriceps increased ACL strain significantly above the normal resting level between 9° and 45° of knee flexion (4). Isometric contractions at flexion angles greater than 60° actually decreased ACL strain below the normal resting level (4). During the eccentric quadriceps contraction, at flexion angles greater than 70°, the pattern of strain was very similar to the normal passive range of motion pattern.

Henning et al. (29) were the first to study ACL elongation *in vivo*. Their technique necessitated an arthrotomy and the removal of bone from the tibia. The data were obtained from only two patients, problems of accuracy were reported, and no statistical analysis was possible because of the sample size. Rosenberg and Rasmussen (58) estimated tension in the ACL through an arthroscopic approach. There were many limitations in the accuracy of the technique and only the anterior drawer and the Lachman tests were evaluated.

The studies performed by Arms et al. (1,3–6) and Henning et al. (29) suggest that muscle tone and contraction patterns, as well as knee flexion angle, affect ACL behavior. Therefore, this indicates that ACL strain may be quite different *in vivo* in comparison to the *in vitro* situation, where there is no resting muscle tone and the muscle contraction patterns are different. Understanding normal function of the ACL is useful in attempting to recreate similar function with an ACL reconstruction procedure. In addition, to determine the effects of rehabilitation exercises on the ACL graft, one must first fully understand the effects on the normal ACL. This has directed research at the University of Vermont toward the characterization of ACL strain biomechanics *in vivo*. These *in vivo* investigations have been designed with the objective of providing data invaluable to the clinical management of injured patients with ACL problems.

ANTERIOR CRUCIATE LIGAMENT STRAIN MEASUREMENT *IN VIVO*

Transducer Design

The goal of the transducer design effort was to develop a device capable of measuring displacement in the *in vivo* environment of the ligamentous unit, having the sensitivity to measure displacement within small segments of the ligament, and being arthroscopically implantable. For the series of *in vivo* experiments described herein, the HEST previously used by Arms et al. (4) *in vitro* but adapted for this *in vivo* application was used. The current design configuration is shown in Fig. 1. The HEST works by the nearly frictionless sliding of a cylindrical, stainless steel-encased magnetic core within a stainless steel tube. A Hall effect generator is bonded to the outer tube. Barbs on the end of each tube are the attachment points of the device to the ligamentous tissue. The HEST device produces a voltage linearly proportional to the strength of a magnetic field. Therefore, the sensitivity of the transducer is dependent primarily on the perpendicular component of the magnetic field present. The maximum hysteresis of the HEST varies by 0.2% of full scale (FS) over its functional range, and the nonrepeatability is a maximum of 0.1% FS. The sensors are completely biocompatible, rugged, and moisture resistant and are easily sterilized by standard ethylene ox-

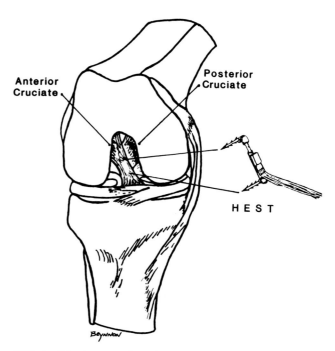

FIG. 1. Attachment orientation on the Hall effect strain transducer. (From ref. 8, with permission.)

ide gas sterilization techniques. A summary of the device characteristics and the detailed HEST specifications was presented by Arms (2).

The body of the HEST consists of a tube that slides within a tube and is highly compliant because it has minimal frictional contact forces between the sliding tubes. A force less than 0.5 g elongates or contracts the HEST. The ligament displacement can, therefore, be measured with minimal influence on the normal behavior of the tissue. It is compliant enough to measure both shortening and lengthening of ligaments. Unlike buckle gauges, the HEST does not distort or "prestrain" the ligament. The long axis of the HEST is aligned collinear with the ligament's fiber bundles. This alignment assures that the natural elongation pattern of the ligament is recorded.

The HEST has been calibrated against a linear variable differential transformer (LVDT) in a Materials Testing System (MTS Corp., Minneapolis, Minnesota) and a micrometer (Starrett Corp., Acton, Massachusetts). It was demonstrated that the voltage output from the HEST was linearly related to its elongation (1,2). Implantation experiments in cadaver ligaments have shown that the HEST gives repeatable output for the same test of strain when it is attached to a ligament, removed, and reattached (1). There was no statistical difference between ligament strain measured by the HEST and that measured with optical techniques (1).

Transducer Implantation

Great care was taken throughout the development of the *in vivo* experimental technique to assure that there was complete protection for the human subject. Both the HEST and the insertion tool were tested in the laboratory and in cadavers so that failure of the device would be unlikely. In the unlikely event of device failure, it was established in the human cadaveric specimens that the components could be readily removed with standard arthroscopic tools. The electrical safety of the equipment was independently inspected. Before performing our studies, we obtained approval from the Human Research Committee. Full informed consent was obtained for each patient, and no monetary compensation was given.

The clinical follow-up data on the initial five study patients were presented by Howe et al. (33). All were candidates for exploratory arthroscopy or arthroscopic meniscectomy. Those suspected of having ACL injuries were excluded. The ACL and other knee structures were carefully inspected for abnormalities, and any potential study patient who had ligamentous instability of any of the four major ligaments (anterior cruciate, posterior cruciate, medial collateral, or lateral collateral) was excluded. Those with cardiovascular problems, previous knee surgery, or current debilitating diseases were ex-

cluded. Patients were also excluded if they had any form of arthritis or other pathological condition that would affect the normal kinematics and/or stability of the knee. Thus, these data are representative of the healthy population with normal ACLs. The extra operative time required to perform the experiment, usually an hour in duration, did not constitute a significant risk, and no extra cost was incurred by the patient. Both the surgical and the experimental procedures were performed under local anesthesia [a mixture of bupivacaine (Marcaine) and 2-chloroprocaine hydrochloride (Nesacaine)].

After the routine surgical procedure was complete, the HEST was prepared for insertion. For HEST introduction into the joint, a sleeve 9 mm in diameter was placed in the anterior lateral portal of the knee and the arthroscope was positioned in the anterior medial portal. The HEST was mounted on the end of an insertion instrument, and both were introduced into the knee through the 9-mm sleeve. Before ligamentous attachment, the HEST barbs were aligned collinear with the fiber bundles of the anteromedial band, and then the barbs were engaged into the AMB by pushing along the axis of the insertion tool. This procedure ensured that elongation of the AMB was duplicated by elongation of the compliant HEST. Once the barbs were embedded into the AMB, the insertion tool was disengaged and withdrawn through the sleeve. The sleeve was then removed, and the knee joint was passively extended to allow observation of the orientation of the HEST relative to the femoral notch. If the HEST impinged against the roof of the intercondylar femoral notch, the knee extension angle would be limited during testing to prevent this from occurring. The perfusate was then evacuated from the joint and the arthroscope removed. Portals were closed with staples and dressed in a sterile fashion. Output wires from the HEST and removal sutures attached to the HEST within the joint were allowed to course through the lateral portal and run along the lateral aspect of the patient's thigh.

The Calculation of Strain

The HEST is a highly compliant displacement transducer; consequently, its application provides the advantage of measuring the ACL displacement pattern without loading or stretching the ligamentous tissue. The ACL may exhibit marked laxity and become slack or unloaded under some joint loading conditions (31,32,50). For example, when a posterior shear force is applied across the knee joint during the Lachman test, the ACL is palpably slack and, as the posterior shear load is released and an anterior load is applied, the ACL becomes taut or is a load-bearing structure. Therefore, the HEST will measure displacement when the ACL is either palpably slack or taut. To differentiate between slack and taut states, we have chosen to calculate strain with a reference length based on the slack-taut transition state of the ACL. This reference was evaluated in two study patients. A procedure was defined that used simultaneous arthroscopic visualization and palpation of the AMB, with a barbed probe embedded next to the HEST, while anterior-posterior shear loading was applied to the tibia relative to the femur in 30° of knee flexion with a custom-designed load cell (9). The investigator palpated the AMB by gently pulling on the probe, arthroscopically observed this portion of the ligament tent, and simultaneously applied shear load across the tibiofemoral joint in a continuous fashion (Fig. 2). As the shear load was applied in an anterior direction, the investigator was able to detect and arthroscopically visualize a transition in the AMB. This transition was defined as the palpated slack-taut transition and was documented by the investigator closing a switch at the point of the palpated transition. This enabled correlation of applied shear load with the HEST length, defined as reference length L_0, at which the transition occurred (Fig. 3). This reference was used in the calculation of strain. When the ligament elongates beyond this point, it is defined by positive strain values (or is in a load-bearing state), and when the ligament contracts and becomes smaller it is considered unstrained (or is in a slack, non-load-bearing state) (9).

The use of this reference provides more meaning to the interpretation of the *in vivo* strain data and is different from previous *in vitro* studies that arbitrarily chose

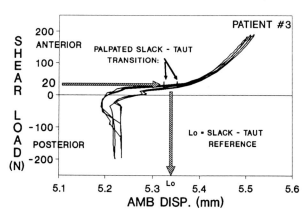

FIG. 3. *In vivo* anterior-posterior shear loading at 30° of flexion (Lachman test). Shear load (N) versus ACL anteromedial bundle displacement (mm). (From ref. 9, with permission.)

the length of the AMB with the knee in full extension (0°) as a reference for strain calculation (4,57). The choice of a load-bearing strain reference is based on the following three observations: (a) The applied A-P shear load versus HEST displacement relationship produced a hysteresis loop pattern with two characteristic regions (Fig. 3). The region of the curve to the right of the inflection point is closed and repeatable, indicating a taut AMB, whereas the region to the left of the inflection point is open and repeatable and is characteristic of a slack structure. (b) The applied anterior shear load at the inflection point of this curve consistently measured 20 N of force across all patients. This force corresponds to the force that must be applied to offset the gravity load on the tibia as it is held over the edge of the operating table. Static equilibrium of forces in the sagittal plane would predict that an anterior shear force equal in magnitude but opposite in direction must be applied to overcome the posterior shear force due to the weight of the tibia, just before the ACL becomes a restraint to an increased magnitude of anterior shear load. (c) Simultaneous A-P shear loading and palpation of the AMB found the slack-taut transition to occur at the inflection point of the applied A-P load versus HEST displacement relation. Based on these three observations, the HEST displacement value at the inflection point of the applied A-P shear versus HEST displacement relation, performed at 30° of flexion, was used as a reference length for the calculation of strain.

DISCUSSION

The Lachman (A-P shear applied at 30°) and drawer (A-P shear applied at 90°) clinical examination techniques were evaluated by measuring ACL strain while applying anterior/posterior shear across the knee (Fig. 2) (9). This study has revealed that, for a similar load magnitude of 150 N, anterior shear testing at 30° produces

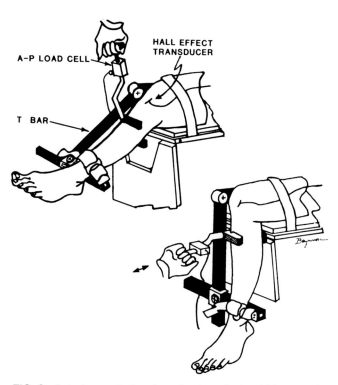

FIG. 2. Anterior-posterior shear load applied at 30° and 90° of knee flexion. (From ref. 9, with permission.)

more strain than does shear testing at 90° (Fig. 4). This finding is in contrast to the earlier *in vitro* studies performed by Arms et al. (4). The reasons for the dissimilarity between results are attributed to the *in vitro* work not making comparisons of strain values at similar shear load magnitudes and an arbitrary choice of reference length for the calculation of strain. This arbitrary choice of reference combined the strained and unstrained states of the ligament into one value and therefore the actual values of the strained ligament were not compared. Henning et al. (29) directly measured the displacement pattern of the AMB *in vivo* under anterior shear load conditions and also demonstrated that the Lachman test produced greater elongation of the AMB in comparison to the anterior drawer test. Torzilli et al. (64) used an *in vivo* radiographic approach to demonstrate that the drawer test produces inconsistent results in patients with documented ACL ruptures. These *in vivo* results are in agreement with previously published studies that used either instrumented knee laxity testing or clinical impressions to assess the behavior of the ACL under clinical examination conditions. Markolf et al. (51) measured the force-displacement response of the tibiofemoral joint *in vitro* and found the normal joint laxity to be a minimum at full extension and 90° of flexion and a maximum at 20° of flexion. This finding suggests that clinical evaluation of the ACL might best be performed at a flexion angle of 20°, where an appreciation of the largest magnitude of A-P laxity may be gained. Daniel et al. (18) chose a knee flexion angle of 20° to perform evaluation of the ACL with the KT-1000 arthrometer. Jacob (37), Johnson and Eriksson (39), and Torg et al. (63) argued that the Lachman test is the clinical examination of choice to evaluate the integrity of the ACL. Direct measurement of ACL strain *in vivo* has quantitatively described why the Lachman test is a more sensitive evaluation of ACL integrity in comparison to the drawer test (9). This study revealed that the Lachman test produced more AMB strain in comparison to the drawer test. This may be due to secondary structures (active musculature, posterior capsule, meniscus) that resist motion at 90° of flexion, while these structures provide less resistance to anterior translation of the tibia at 30°, requiring the AMB to provide the resistance to externally applied loading. In addition, the Lachman evaluation allows the examiner to measure the movement of the tibia subjectively in relation to the femur where the primary restraint is undergoing a maximal change in length.

The effect of isometric quadriceps activity on ACL strain was also investigated *in vivo* (9) (Fig. 5). There was no significant change in AMB strain during isometric contraction when the knee was maintained at a flexion angle of 90° (Fig. 6). At this flexion angle, across all patients, the AMB remained at its resting state as quadriceps activity was increased. Isometric quadriceps strengthening should, therefore, be safe in the ACL-injured or reconstructed knee if the joint is maintained at 90° of flexion. At 30° of knee flexion, isometric quadriceps activity produced a large increase in AMB strain and should be carefully controlled, especially during the early stages of rehabilitation, where graft fixation may be tenuous (Fig. 6). Grood et al. (27) found that leg extension exercises (in the range of 0° to 30°) produce loadings that are potentially destructive to the repaired or reconstructed ACL in an *in vitro* model. The knee flexion angle at which isometric quadriceps activity produces an increase in AMB strain and may become unsafe for the injured or reconstructed ligament is somewhere between 90° and 30° and remains to be delineated. At present we are performing an *in vivo* investigation to determine the "safe zone" where isometric quadriceps muscle activity and joint position do not detrimentally strain the ligament.

The effect of passive range of knee motion (PROM)

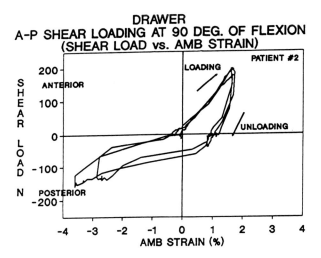

DRAWER
A-P SHEAR LOADING AT 90 DEG. OF FLEXION
(SHEAR LOAD vs. AMB STRAIN)

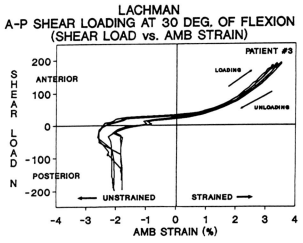

LACHMAN
A-P SHEAR LOADING AT 30 DEG. OF FLEXION
(SHEAR LOAD vs. AMB STRAIN)

FIG. 4. *In vivo* ACL anteromedial bundle strain pattern for anterior-posterior shear loading at 30° and 90° of knee flexion. (From ref. 9, with permission.)

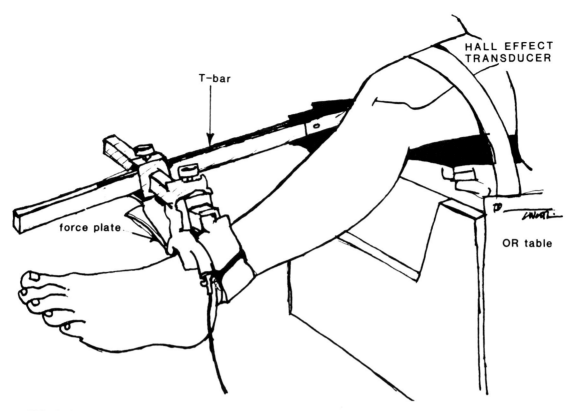

FIG. 5. Isometric quadriceps contraction at 30° and 90° of knee flexion. (From ref. 9, with permission.)

on ACL strain was investigated (9) by instructing the patient to relax all leg musculature while the investigator coursed the tibia through a continuous range of motion. This study revealed that the AMB reaches positive strain values as the joint is brought into extension and remains at, or below, the zero strain level between the limits of 11.5° and 110° of extension using heel support loading. Therefore, continuous passive motion (CPM) of the knee between these limits should be safe for an ACL graft immediately after surgery, when the leg is supported near the ankle throughout flexion/extension motion without applied varus/valgus loading, internal/external torques, or anterior shear forces. The limits near extension (10°), however, can cause small magnitudes of strain (1% or less). This should be viewed as a relatively mild constraint to the use of continuous passive motion in a rehabilitation program.

The *in vivo* PROM investigations (9) and previous *in vitro* studies used similar methods and presented data indicating that the AMB does not remain an "isometric" or constant length structure as the knee is brought through PROM (1,4,59). The method used to perform the PROM activity is similar to that used intraoperatively by the orthopedic surgeon making predictive ACL reconstruction tunnel placement measurements with compliant displacement transducers ("isometers"). Our *in vivo* data for this activity may serve as important standards against which isometer measurements, of poten-

tial reconstruction tunnel placement sites, may be accepted or rejected (9).

Active range of motion (AROM) flexion-extension of the knee performed by the patient consistently produced a positive region of strain values between full extension and 48° and an unstrained region between 48° and 110° of flexion (9). AROM rehabilitation programs may now be prescribed with the two flexion angle regions adapted to the clinician's requirements. In the unstrained region, quadriceps activity associated with AROM did not pro-

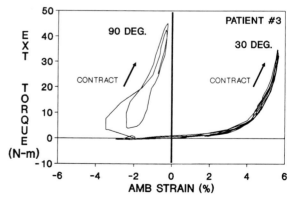

FIG. 6. *In vivo* ACL anteromedial bundle strain pattern for isometric quadriceps contraction at 30° and 90° of flexion. Quadriceps-induced extension torque (N-m) versus anteromedial bundle strain. (From ref. 9, with permission.)

duce significantly different AMB strain values in comparison with PROM. This suggests that AROM between the limits of 50° and 100° may be performed safely immediately after ACL reconstruction. The AROM activity may then move to the positive strain region as the graft and fixation construct will tolerate. The maximum AROM strain values were greater (ranging between 4.1% and 1.5%) in comparison with maximum PROM strain values. Further investigation is required to determine if the AROM strain values in the positive strain region are large enough in magnitude to produce permanent stretching out of the reconstructed tissue or the fixation construct.

This study illustrates that both muscle activity and knee position determine AMB strain at rest and with joint motion (9). It seems that the AMB is strained between the limits of full extension and 48° for AROM. These findings are consistent with Henning et al.'s (29) *in vivo* study of two patients with injured ligaments.

Qualitative comparison between the *in vivo* PROM passive data (9) and the *in vitro* data reported by Arms et al. (4) and Sapega et al. (59) shows similarities in patterns. There are differences, however, between the strain values or calculated changes in length. We found that the AMB reaches a mean peak strain value of 0.1% at 10° of extension, whereas the data presented by Arms et al. (4) and Sapega et al. (59) remained unstrained as the joint was extended. For AROM, there are also differences between our findings and the *in vitro* work of Arms et al. (4). They described a 3% mean peak AMB strain value at 10° of flexion and a transition between strained and unstrained values at 35° of flexion (4). We reported a similar mean peak AMB strain of 2.8%; however, this occurred at 20°, while the strained-unstrained transition occurred at 48° of knee flexion (9). There are a number of possible explanations for the differences between the *in vivo* and *in vitro* findings. First, the reference for strain calculation is carefully defined in our *in vivo* work. This enabled us to differentiate between the strained and unstrained conditions of the AMB. Second, the *in vitro* experiments were made in cadaver specimens, where the compliance of the soft tissues was undoubtedly different from that in the *in vivo* study. This is not only due to the changes postmortem but also due to the changes accompanying age, since the cadaver subjects had an average age of 56.9 years while subjects for the *in vivo* study ranged in age between 18 and 35 years. In the cadaver experiments, the operative approach was different in comparison to that used *in vivo*. A medial parapatellar incision was used to expose the knee joint, and the extensor mechanism was longitudinally divided up to 5 cm proximal to the patella. Next, the intercondylar notch was enlarged if necessary to avoid impingement of the HEST as the knee was extended (the HEST was larger when cadaver specimens were tested), but the attachments of the cruciate ligaments were left unaltered. The ligamentum mucosum was transected and the synovial sheath overlying the ACL was carefully removed. Before strain measurement, the capsule was repaired. In contrast, the *in vivo* experiments required only the entrance of the arthroscope. The stab wounds from the HEST in the AMB were all that were necessary, and both the intercondylar notch and ligamentum mucosa were not disturbed.

Perhaps the most important difference between the *in vivo* and *in vitro* studies was the function of the muscles and their tendinous attachments. It is the subjective assessment of clinicians that the cadaveric knee does not seem to have the same kinematics as that of the live subject. More definitively, practical experience demonstrates that normal muscle activity protects the knee from harm. The primary function of the quadriceps mechanism is clearly to extend the knee but, just as importantly, it also controls flexion by antagonizing gravity and the hamstring muscle group. The quadriceps insert through the patellofemoral mechanism into the tibial tubercle and are oriented anterior to the transverse axis of knee rotation. This allows the quadriceps to assist in the prevention of posterior subluxation of the tibia relative to the femur, working synergistically with the posterior cruciate ligament between extension and 70° of flexion. Daniel and associates (17,19,20) reported that, beyond approximately 70°, the quadriceps' role reverses and it becomes the protagonist of the ACL. This finding was supported by the *in vitro* work of Arms et al. (4), who found that the ACL strain was reduced if a simulated quadriceps contraction was performed in the flexion range (70° to 120°). Our *in vivo* work (9) did not find this effect, although the strain values remained at low or unstrained levels.

FUTURE RESEARCH DIRECTIONS

Recent experimental investigations have described the complex morphometry of the ACL and have emphasized that this structure comprises subbundle units. *In vivo* studies as described herein have shown that the strain values along each subbundle are dependent not only on joint position, but also on the magnitude of knee joint loading. Tensile failure testing has revealed divergent values of maximum stress values and strain energy density for isolated ACL subbundles taken from anterior and posterior portions of the ACL. Investigation of the individual ACL subbundle units *in situ* during simulated rehabilitation activities has shown that each subbundle demonstrates a different displacement pattern and consequently has varied strain behavior. Therefore, it may not be adequate to consider the ACL as a single structure and only study the resultant ACL load. Experimental and analytical investigation of the ACL should consider this complex structure to have a stress and strain distribution across a transverse cross-section, which will vary along the length of the ACL, with higher magnitudes of strain near the ligament insertions.

Analytic models of the cruciate ligaments, such as that developed by the authors (8), have investigated the subbundle structure of the cruciate ligaments and their complex interaction with the tibiofemoral joint. However, further work is needed to include the patellofemoral articulation. Experimental measurements of model input parameters such as joint geometry, ligament insertion positions, initial subbundle strain values, and ligament element load-displacement or stress-strain response must be made on an individual knee specimen. Since there is a wide variation in the kinematic behavior between different human knees, modeling efforts must acquire all input parameters from a knee joint while, on the same specimen, experimental studies should be performed for validation of the model. Model validation and parameter optimization algorithms that will match experimental measures with model predictions in 6 *df* must be developed. A fully validated model of an individual knee joint may then be applied to study injury mechanisms, soft tissue reconstruction procedures, or commonly prescribed rehabilitation activities. Analytic models may also be used to study the interaction between the ACL and joint kinematics at a selection of applied joint loadings or knee positions. Similar studies could be performed for different cruciate ligament graft materials, intraarticular positions, and initial tension values at fixation.

Experimental investigations of the ACL should consider its complex subbundle structure and fully characterize the strain or stress distribution. To accomplish this task, one should measure strain and either force or stress along the discrete subbundle regions of the ACL. The *in vivo* strain measurements as described in this chapter have accomplished this task through highly specific measurements; however, these studies have focused only on the anteromedial portion of the ACL (8–10). Other regions of the ACL, including the mid and posterior subbundles and the insertion sites, also should be investigated *in vivo* to describe this structure fully. Promising advances in transducer development have been made to accomplish this task (10,16,26). Beynnon et al. (10) developed a sensor to measure local strain and force simultaneously in soft tissue (Fig. 7). Data from the sensor can be used to determine an absolute zero reference force in the instrumented soft tissue (10). This may prove to be the optimal means of referencing soft tissue strain measurements. A potential advantage of this measurement system is found in the capability of simultaneously measuring different regions of the ACL (i.e., anteromedial and posterolateral bundles) rather than mechanically constraining the different fiber bundles into one group and measuring a mechanically averaged ligament force. Continued work is needed to make the sensors smaller,

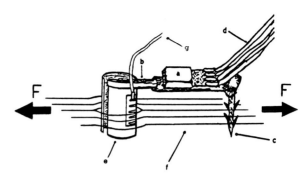

FIG. 7. The combined force and Hall effect strain transducer. A schematic view of the device is presented as it would look implanted in soft tissue under an applied tensile load (*F*). The components are as follows: *a*, Hall effect generator; *b*, inner tube that houses a magnet; *c*, barb for attachment to soft tissue; *d*, electrical connection to Hall effect generator; *3*, the split tube soft tissue force sensor; *f*, midsubstance of soft tissue; *g*, electrical connection to the force sensor. (From ref. 10, with permission.)

less invasive, and applicable for chronic use *in vivo*. All current transducer designs that have been applied to soft tissue structures are constrained to measure uniaxial behavior. The ACL and most soft tissue structures deform in three dimensions. Therefore, investigation of the ACL may be incomplete if transducers are applied that make a mechanically constrained uniaxial measurement or if the data from the sensor are presented with the assumption that the ligament behaves only as a one-dimensional structure. New multiaxis sensors need to be designed.

Analytic models of the knee, soft tissue transducers, and three-dimensional digitizers should be combined to study the normal ACL and applied to aid the surgeon with cruciate ligament reconstruction procedures. For example, in the intraoperative environment the surgeon could select potential attachment regions for a cruciate ligament reconstruction. The analytic model could then simulate common activities of daily living and predict the kinematic response of the knee. The surgeon could then determine if the kinematic response was within normal limits and either accept or reject the potential position of the ACL replacement. Similarly, the model could then be applied to predict the initial graft tension required to restore knee kinematics, such as A-P laxity, and recommend safe rehabilitation activities for specific patients.

REFERENCES

1. Arms SW. (1984): *Knee ligament strain* [Thesis]. University of Vermont, Burlington, VT.
2. Arms SW. (1989): Miniature Hall effect displacement sensors for medical applications. Presented at the Sensors Exposition International, Cleveland, OH, September 12–14.
3. Arms SW, Beynnon BD, Fischer RA, Miller LM, Pope MH, Renström P, Johnson RJ. (1987): The biomechanics of ACL reconstructions in the canine model. In: *Proceedings of the 33rd* Annual

Meeting of the Orthopaedics Research Society, San Francisco, January, p 101.

4. Arms SW, Pope MH, Johnson RJ, et al. (1984): The biomechanics of anterior cruciate ligament rehabilitation and reconstruction. *Am J Sports Med,* 12:8–18.

5. Arms SW, Pope MH, Renström P, Johnson RJ. (1986): The determination of zero strain within the anteromedial fibers of the ACL. Presented at the 32nd Annual Meeting of the Orthopaedic Research Society, New Orleans, February.

6. Arms SW, Pope MH, Johnson RJ, Renström P, Fischer RA, Jarvinen M, Beynnon BD. (1990): Analysis of ACL failure strength and initial strains in the canine model. In: *Proceedings of the 36th Annual Meeting of the Orthopaedics Research Society, New Orleans, February,* p. 524.

7. Bass P, Wiley JN. (1972): Contractile force transducer for recording muscle activity in unanesthetized animals. *J Appl Physiol,* 32:567.

8. Beynnon BD. (1991): *The in-vivo biomechanics of the anterior cruciate ligament: reconstruction and application of a mathematical model to the knee joint* [Dissertation]. Burlington: University of Vermont.

9. Beynnon BD, Howe JG, Pope MH, Johnson RJ, Fleming BC. (1992): The measurement of anterior cruciate ligament strain in-vivo. *Int Orthop,* 16:1–12.

10. Beynnon BD, Stankewich CJ, Fleming BC, Pope MH, Johnson RJ. (1991): The development and initial testing of a new sensor to simultaneously measure strain and pressure in tendons and ligaments. In: *Transactions of the Combined Meeting of the Orthopaedics Research Societies of the USA, Japan, and Canada, Banff, Alberta, Canada, October 21–23,* p 104.

11. Brown TD, Sigal L, Njus GO, Njus NM, Singerman RJ, Brand RA. (1986): Dynamic performance characteristics of the liquid metal strain gauge. *J Biomech,* 19:165–173.

12. Butler DL. (1989): The anterior cruciate ligament: its normal response and replacement. *J Orthop Res,* 7:910–921.

13. Butler DL, Grood ES, Zernicke RR, Hefzy MS, Noyes FR. (1983): Non-uniform surface strains in young human tendons and fascia. Presented at the 29th Orthopaedic Research Society Meeting, Anaheim, CA, February.

14. Butler DL, Guan Y, Kay MD, Feder SM, Cummings JF. (1991): Location-dependent variations in the material properties of the anterior cruciate ligament subunits. *Trans Orthop Res Soc,* 16:234.

15. Butler DL, Sheh MY, Stouffer DC, Samaranayoke VA, Levy MS. (1990): Surface strain variation in human patella tendon and knee cruciate ligaments. *J Biomech Eng,* 112:38–45.

16. Cummings JF, Holden JP, Grood ES, Wroble RR, Butler DL, Schafer JA. (1991): In-vivo measurement of patellar tendon forces and joint position in the goat model. *Proc Orthop Res Soc,* 16:601.

17. Daniel D, Akeson WH, O'Conner JJ. (1990): *Knee ligaments: structure, function, injury, and repair.* New York: Raven Press.

18. Daniel D, Malcolm L, Losse G, Stone M, Sachs R, Barks R. (1985): Instrumented measurement of anterior laxity of the knee. *J Bone Joint Surg [Am],* 67A:720–725.

19. Daniel D, Robertson D, Flood D, Biden E. (1987): The anterior cruciate deficient knee: new concepts in ligament repair. Fixation of soft tissue. St Louis, MO: CV Mosby, pp 114–126.

20. Daniel D, Sachs R, Stone M, Penner D. (1986): The quadriceps active test: to diagnose a posterior cruciate ligament disruption. Presented at the 53rd Annual Meeting of the American Association of Orthopaedic Surgeons, New Orleans, February.

21. Edwards RG, Lafferty JF, Lange KD. (1970): Ligament strain in the human knee. *J Basic Eng,* 92:131–136.

22. Emery M, Moffroid M, Boerman J, Fleming B, Howe J, Pope M. (1988): Reliability of force/displacement measures in a clinical device designed to measure ligamentous laxity at the knee. *J Orthop Sports Phys Ther,* 5:441.

23. Fleming BC, Johnson RJ, Shapiro E, Fenwick J, Howe JG, Pope MH. (1990): Clinical versus instrumental knee testing. *Clin Orthop Rel Res,* September, 282.

24. Forster IW, Warren-Smith CD, Tew M. (1989): Is the KT-1000 knee ligament arthrometer reliable? *J Bone Joint Surg [Br],* 71B:843–847.

25. Galway RD, Beaupre A, MacIntosh DL. (1972): The lateral pivot shift: A clinical sign of symptomatic anterior cruciate insufficiency. *J Bone Joint Surg [Br],* 54B:762–763.

26. Glos DL, Holden JP, Butler DL, Grood ES. (1990): Pressure versus deflected beam force measurement in the human patellar tendon. *Trans Orthop Res,* 15:490.

27. Grood ES, Suntay WJ, Noyes FA, Butler DL. (1984): Biomechanics of the knee-extension exercise. *J Bone Joint Surg [Am],* 66A:725–733.

28. Häggmark T, Eriksson E. (1979): Cylinder or mobile cast brace after knee ligament surgery: a clinical analysis and morphological and enzymatic study of changes in the quadriceps muscle. *Am J Sports Med,* 7:48–56.

29. Henning CE, Lynch MA, Glick KR. (1985): An *in vivo* strain gauge study of the anterior cruciate ligament. *Am J Sports Med,* 13:22–26.

30. Highgenboten CL, Jackson A, Meske N. (1989): Genucom, KT-1000, and Stryker knee laxity measuring device comparisons. *Am J Sports Med,* 17:743.

31. Hollis JM. (1988): *Development and application of a method for determining the in-situ forces in anterior cruciate ligament fiber bundles* [Dissertation]. San Diego: University of California.

32. Hollis JM, Marcin JP, Horibe S, Woo SL-Y. (1988): Load determination in ACL fiber bundles under knee loading. *Trans Orthop Res Soc,* 13:58.

33. Howe JG, Wertheimer CM, Johnson RJ, Nichols CE, Pope MH, Beynnon BD. (1990): Arthroscopic strain gauge measurement of the normal anterior cruciate ligament. *Arthroscopy,* 6:198–204.

34. Huble KH, Follick MF. (1976): A small strain gauge for measuring intestinal mobility in rats. *J Diagn Dis,* 21:1075–1078.

35. Hughston JC, Andrews JR, Cross MJ, Moschi A. (1976): Classification of knee ligament instabilities: Part 1. The medial compartment and cruciate ligaments. *J Bone Joint Surg [Am],* 58A:159–172.

36. Hughston JC, Andrews JR, Cross MJ, Moschi A. (1976): Classification of knee ligament instabilities: Part 2. The lateral compartment. *J Bone Joint Surg [Am],* 58A:173–179.

37. Jacob RP. (1981): Observations on rotary instability of the lateral compartment of the knee. *Acta Orthop Scand,* 52[Suppl 1]:1–31.

38. Johnson RJ. (1982): The anterior cruciate: a dilemma in sports medicine. *Int J Sports Med,* 3:71–79.

39. Johnson RJ, Eriksson E. (1982): Rehabilitation of the unstable knee. In: Frankel V, ed. *AAOS instructional course lectures.* St. Louis: CV Mosby, vol 31, pp 114–125.

40. Jozsa L, Jarvinen M, Kannus P, Reffy A. (1987): Fine structural changes in the articular cartilage of the rat's knee following short-term immobilization in various positions: a scanning electron microscopical study. *Int Orthop,* 11:129–133.

41. Jozsa L, Reffy A, Jarvinen M, Kannus P, Lehto M, Kvist M. (1988): Cortical and trabecular osteopenia after immobilization—a quantitative histological study in rats. *Int Orthop,* 12:169–172.

42. Jozsa L, Thöring J, Jarvinen M, Kannus P, Lehto M, Kvist M. (1988): Quantitative alterations in intramuscular connective tissue following immobilization: an experimental study in rat calf muscle. *Exp Mol Pathol,* 49:267–278.

43. Kannus P. (1988): *Conservative treatment of acute knee distortions —long term results and their evaluation methods* [Dissertation]. Tampere, Finland: University of Tampere. *Acta Univ Tamperensis Ser A,* 250:1–110.

44. Kennedy JC. (1982): Symposium: current concepts in the management of knee instability. *Contemp Orthop,* 5:59–78.

45. Kennedy JC, Hawkins RJ, Willis RB, Danylchuck KD. (1976): Tension studies of human knee ligaments, yield point, ultimate failure and disruption of the cruciate and tibial collateral ligaments. *J Bone Joint Surg [Am],* 58A:350–355.

46. Kennedy JC, Haskins RJ, Willis RB. (1977): Strain gauge analysis of knee ligaments. *Clin Orthop Rel Res,* 129:225–229.

47. King JB, Kumar SJ. (1989): The Stryker knee arthrometer in clinical practice. *Am J Sports Med,* 17:649–650.

48. Losee RE, Ennis T, Johnson R, et al. (1978): Anterior subluxation of the lateral tibial plateau: a diagnostic test and operative review. *J Bone Joint Surg [Am],* 60A:1015–1030.

49. MacIntosh DL, Galway HR. (1972): The lateral pivot shift: a symptomatic and clinical sign of anterior cruciate insufficiency. Presented at the Annual Meeting of the American Orthopaedics Association.

50. Markolf KL, Gorek JF, Kabo M, Shapiro MS. (1990): Direct measurement of resultant forces in the anterior cruciate ligament: an

in-vitro study performed with a new experimental technique. *J Bone Joint Surg [Am]*, 72A:557.

51. Markolf KL, Graff-Radford A, Amstutz HC. (1978): *In vivo stability—a quantitative assessment using an instrumented clinical testing apparatus. J Bone Joint Surg [Am]*, 60A:664–674.

52. Marks J, Palme M, Burke M, Smith P. (1978): Observer variations in the examination of knee joints. *Ann Rheum Dis*, 37:376.

53. Mutchler W, Burri C, Claes L. (1979): *A new possibility of measuring absolute stress and strain of ligaments.* Department of Traumatology, University of Ulm, West Germany.

54. Noyes FR. (1977): Functional properties of knee ligaments and alterations induced by immobilization. *Clin Orthop Rel Res*, 123:210–242.

55. Noyes FR, Grood ES, Butler DL, et al. (1980): Clinical laxity tests and functional stability of the knee: biomechanical concepts. *Clin Orthop*, 146:84–89.

56. Pope MH, Johnson R, Kristiansen T, Lavalette R. (1987): Variations in the examinations of the medial collateral ligament. *Clin Biomech*, 2:71–73.

57. Renström PA, Arms SW, Stanwyck TS, Johnson RJ, Pope MH. (1986): Strain within the anterior cruciate ligament during hamstrings and quadriceps activity. *Am J Sports Med*, 14:83–87.

58. Rosenberg TD, Rasmussen GL. (1984): The function of the anterior cruciate ligament during anterior drawer and Lachman's testing. *Am J Sports Med*, 12:318–321.

59. Sapega AA, Moyer RJ, Schneck C, Komalahiranya N. (1990): Testing for isometry during reconstruction of the anterior cruciate ligament. *J Bone Joint Surg [Am]*, 72A:259–267.

60. Shelbourne KD, Nitz P. (1990): Accelerated rehabilitation after ACL reconstruction. *Am J Sports Med*, 18:292–299.

61. Sherman O, Markolf K, Weibel W, Ferkel R. (1984): Instrumented testing of normal and ACL-deficient knees: a comparison of two devices. *Trans Orthop Res Soc*, 10:275.

62. Sidles JA, Larson RV, Garbini JL, Downey DJ, Matsen FA. (1988): Ligament length relationships in the moving knee. *J Orthop Res*, 6:593–610.

63. Torg J, Conrad W, Kalen V. (1976): Clinical diagnosis of ACL instability. *Am J Sports Med*, 4:84–92.

64. Torzilli P, Greenberg R, Hood R, Pavlov H, Insall J. (1984): Measurement of anterior-posterior motion of the knee in injured patients using a biomechanical stress technique. *J Bone Joint Surg [Am]*, 66A:1438–1442.

65. Trent PS, Walker PS, Wolf B. (1976): Ligament length patterns, strength and rotational axes of the knee joint. *Clin Orthop*, 117:263–270.

66. Wang CJ, Walker PS, Wolf B. (1973): The effects of flexion and rotation on the length patterns of the ligaments of the knee. *J Biomech*, 6:587–596.

67. Warren LF, Marshall JL, Girgis F. (1974): The prime static stabilizer of the medial side of the knee. *J Bone Joint Surg [Am]*, 56A:665–674.

68. Weiss JA, France EP, Bagley AM, Bomstrom GL. (1992): Measurement of 2-D strains in ligaments under uniaxial tension. *Trans Orthop Res Soc*, 17:662.

69. White AA, Raphael IG. (1972): The effect of quadriceps loads and knee position on strain measurements of the tibial collateral ligament. *Acta Orthop*, 43:176.

70. Woo SL-Y, Gomez MA, Woo YA, Akeson WH. (1982): Mechanical properties of tendons and ligaments: 1. Quazi-static and nonlinear viscoelastic properties. *Biorheology*, 19:385–396.

71. Woo SL-Y, Gomez MA, Akerson WH. (1983): Mechanical properties along the medial collateral ligament. In: *Transactions of the 29th Annual Meeting of the Orthopaedic Research Society*, Anahiem, CA, p. 7.

72. Woo SL-Y, Hollis MJ, Adams DJ, Lyon RM, Takai S. (1991): Tensile properties of the human femur-anterior cruciate ligament-tibia complex: the effects of specimen age and orientation. *Am J Sports Med*, 19:217–225.

The Anterior Cruciate Ligament: Current and
Future Concepts, edited by D.W. Jackson, et al.
Raven Press, Ltd., New York © 1993.

CHAPTER 10

Joint Kinematics in Muscle-Stabilized Knees

Kenton R. Kaufman, Dale M. Daniel, and Savio L-Y. Woo

Although the biomechanical response of the human knee has been the subject of numerous *in vitro* investigations, many of these investigations have dealt exclusively with the response to static joint loads. However, for the clarification of knee biomechanics and for the design of knee prosthetic ligaments, it is equally important to determine characteristics such as the spatial displacement between the joint members, passive soft tissue stress, and articular surface stress corresponding to dynamic functional activities. Experiments on whole cadaver joints are often the most direct way of assessing changes in the mechanics of the knee. Brantigan and Voshell (10) began the modern era of *in vitro* knee testing by clamping a cadaver femur to a plank and applying loads to the distal tibia. They performed studies to identify the contributions of various ligamentous structures to knee stability. Since then, such tests have become a common method in the study of the mechanics of the knee.

The design of a joint simulator requires a compromise between the degree of complexity required and the amount of time and money expended. Ideally, a dynamic loading simulator should be capable of applying to a joint specimen all the external forces (ground reaction, inertia, gravity) that affect the internal joint forces (muscle, ligament, articular surface) in a manner such that their time histories correspond to the functional activity under simulation. Moreover, the method of application of the forces should not constrain the resultant response of the joint. The design of such a simulator is a formidable task. *In vitro* evaluation of the dynamic response characteristics of the knee requires a loading pattern that is close enough to physiological conditions to provide meaningful data. Thus, it is important to understand the features of various experimental methods that have been utilized for *in vitro* examination of knee joint mechanics. In this chapter we discuss the philosophy behind testing of cadaver joints and examine typical types of tests that are used. We then provide results of knee joint kinematics in the quadriceps-stabilized state.

IN VITRO EXPERIMENTAL KNEE MODELS

Tests on cadaver knee joints have been performed for the following reasons: (a) to determine the range of movement of the bones in the presence of various external loads, (b) to determine the role of muscles, ligaments, and articular surfaces in controlling and limiting the movement of bones relative to each other, and (c) to understand the transmission of load across the articular surface. If these objectives are to be fully met, it is necessary that the movement of the bones relative to each other should be measured and that the loads applied should be measured so that the resultant joint force and moment transmitted at the joint can be determined. Only then can the complete mechanical circumstances of the experiment be fully defined. Tests on cadaver joints can be divided into two categories based on the absence or presence of a joint compressive force. Tests that include a joint compressive force achieve the force through either direct axial force or through muscle stabilization.

Tests Without Joint Compressive Forces

The initial tests on the knee joint were performed by Brantigan and Voshell (10) in 1941. They clamped the femur to a plank and applied medial or laterally directed loads to the distal end of the foot (Fig. 1). Markolf et al. (32) used a similar method of fixing the femur. Force "handles" were used to apply measured loads to the tibia (Fig. 2). Neilsen et al. (38) used a similar arrangement to

K. R. Kaufman: Children's Hospital and University of California, San Diego, California 92020.

D. M. Daniel: Kaiser Permanente and University of California, San Diego, California 92020.

S. L-Y. Woo: Musculoskeletal Research Center, Department of Orthopaedic Surgery, University of Pittsburgh School of Medicine, Pittsburgh, Pennsylvania 15261.

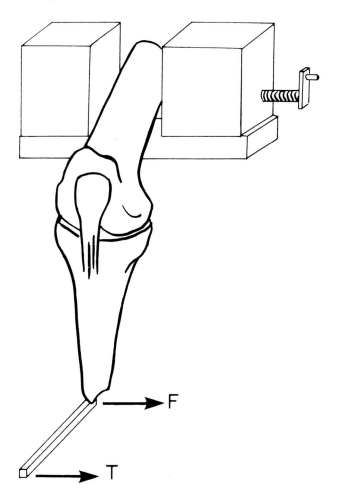

FIG. 1. The testing rig used by Brantigan (10). The femur was clamped to a rigid base, and forces at *F* or *T* were applied. Force *F* acts to abduct or adduct the joint. Force *T* is intended to produce tibial torsion. (From Biden and O'Connor, ref. 5, with permission.)

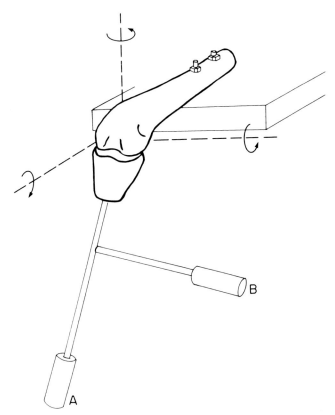

FIG. 2. Test rig used by Markolf (32). The force handles at *A* and *B* can be manipulated to simulate various clinical tests. Forces are well defined in this device, but no muscle action can be simulated. (From Biden and O'Connor, ref. 5, with permission.)

measure the response of the knee to sectioning of the medial collateral ligament and the anterior cruciate ligament. These tests reported the now familiar pattern of an initially compliant (lax) zone followed by one of increasing stiffness as the structures of the knee tightened and limits of knee motion were approached. Wang and Walker (54) used the terms *primary laxity* and *secondary laxity* to distinguish between the compliant and stiff zones.

Fukubayashi et al. (19) and Sullivan et al. (51) also simulated the drawer test. In the tests described by Fukubayashi et al. (19) (Fig. 3A), the device used to hold the knee between the fixed and moving heads of the testing machine allowed the bones 4 *df* "preventing unphysiologic compression caused by apparatus constraints." One of their findings was that up to 1.4 N-m of external and 1.2 N-m of internal tibial torque were produced as an adjunct to the anterior posterior forces. Sullivan et al. (51) in a follow-up paper described a modified rig having

5 *df* (Fig. 3B) and found that the lack of allowance for medial-lateral motion in the test rig reported in the first paper caused tibial torques considerably different from those observed in the rig with less constraint. This work points out the importance of recognizing constraint in devices that do not allow completely "free motion" to the joint.

It is rare for any anatomical movement to require only 1 *df*. Knee flexion is associated primarily with rotation about a mediolaterally directed axis. However, the tibia also rotates about the long axis of the tibia and the tibia also translates along the anterior-posterior direction as flexion occurs. Motions such as these are referred to as "coupled motions." Equally, it is rare that the external loads are such that only one component of force or moment is transmitted across the joint. For example, an external load that tends to extend the knee joint requires a flexion moment at the knee (Fig. 4). This external load also pushes the surfaces of the bones together, and is counteracted by a joint compressive force. Further, the external force slides the tibia on the femur, which is resisted by an internal shear force. As a second example, an external load applied to the tibia in the anterior direction

A

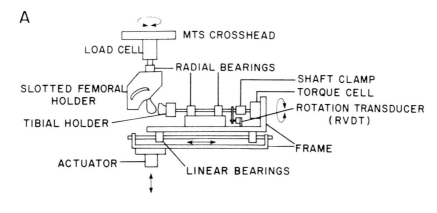

B

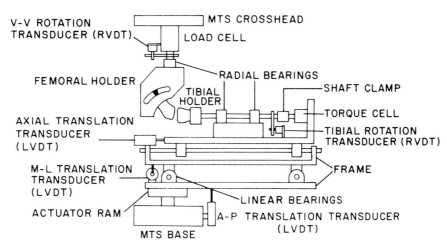

FIG. 3. A: A 4 *df* test rig used by Fukubayashi (19). **B:** A 5 *df* test rig used by Sullivan (51). The 4 *df* system suppresses both flexion-extension and mediolateral motion. Significantly different effects between test rigs were observed in experiments. Because most motions consist of a combination of the six basic motions, suppressing one is likely to affect the others. In both rigs, flexion is resisted by the device. No muscle action is simulated. (From Biden and O'Connor, ref. 5, with permission.)

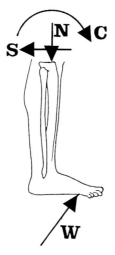

FIG. 4. An extending load *W* balanced at the knee by a flexing moment *C*, a compressive force *N*, and a shear force *S*. (From Biden and O'Connor, ref. 5, with permission.)

usually produces a coupled motion (Fig. 5). As shown in Fig. 5A, an anteriorly directed force that is applied to the tibia lateral to the axis of tibial rotation produces internal rotation as well as anterior translation of the tibia relative to the femur. In Fig. 5B, the force is applied medial to the rotation axis and produces external rotation as well as translation. Only when the load is applied through the axis and has zero moment about the axis, is the resulting motion one of pure translation without coupled rotation (Fig. 5C). Therefore, qualitative as well as quantitative differences have occurred during cadaver testing because of different designs of apparatus that do not permit or allow coupled motions to occur.

Tests with Joint Compressive Force

A number of studies have used testing machines to apply compressive load between the bones without at-

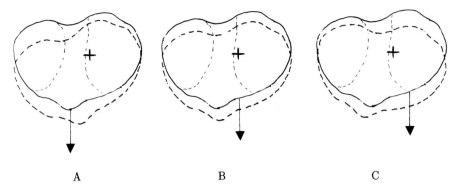

FIG. 5. A: Anterior force applied to the tibia lateral to axis of rotation produces internal rotation as well as anterior translation. **B:** Anterior force applied through axis of rotation produces only anterior translation. **C:** Anterior force applied medial to axis of rotation produces external rotation as well as anterior translation. (From Biden and O'Connor, ref. 5, with permission.)

tempting to simulate muscle action. Wang and Walker (54) used a compression-torsion machine allowing 2 *df* to study the effects of compressive load on the rotary laxity of the knee. They showed that compressive load decreased the laxity of the knee. In a later paper, Hsieh and Walker (23) found a similar influence of compressive load on anterior-posterior stability.

Another device that attempted to account for the tibiofemoral contact force was used by Markolf et al. (33) and Shoemaker and Markolf (47). This experimental setup allowed the bones complete freedom of movement but large loads could be applied across the knee at a variety of flexion angles in such a way that the load always

passed through the "center" of rotation of the joint and hence produced no moment that required additional muscle forces for stability (Fig. 6). They showed that the compressive load increased the anterior-posterior, medial-lateral, varus-valgus, and torsional stiffness and reduced the corresponding laxity of the knee. Blankevoort (7) used a 6 *df* rig to define the envelope of passive knee joint motion. In the presence of compressive force without simulated muscle action, it was necessary to clamp the bones and remove the freedom to flex or extend the knee in order to hold different positions of flexion.

MUSCLE-STABILIZED TESTING

One of the basic requirements of a knee simulator is that it simulate dynamic functional activities. The joint should remain entirely unconstrained. The applicability of tests that apply large tibiofemoral contact forces and restrain motion is questionable. During physiological loading, large contact forces and large muscle forces occur simultaneously. Large muscle forces act through short lever arms at the knee to balance the effects of small external loads acting through large lever arms along the leg. Large tibiofemoral contact forces are needed to balance the large muscle forces that result. Studies of joint mechanics are likely to have clinical relevance only if both muscle and contact forces are present simultaneously. A successful knee joint simulator should encompass the motions and forces of daily living.

The forces produced in the knee joint during activities of daily living can be approximated in a knee simulator by reproducing the forces acting across the knee. Physiological joint loading can be obtained by applying muscle forces required to perform specific activities. By ensuring that all forces cross the joint at anatomical locations and in anatomical directions, reasonable life-like simulation can be obtained. The fundamental motions of daily liv-

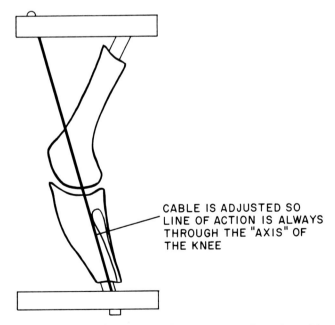

CABLE IS ADJUSTED SO LINE OF ACTION IS ALWAYS THROUGH THE "AXIS" OF THE KNEE

FIG. 6. Markolf (33) developed a test rig that allowed considerable freedom of motion to the joint without requiring simulated muscle action. To do this, his rig adjusts so that compression is always applied along the axis of the tibia. Hence, the force has no lever-arm, and the joint does not flex or extend. (From Biden and O'Connor, ref. 5, with permission.)

TABLE 1. *Maximum quadriceps force for various activities*

Author	Activity	Knee angle (degrees)	Force (Newtons)
Reilly & Martens, 1972 (43)	Walking	8	608
Morrison, 1969 (36)	Up ramp	—	783
	Walking	—	850
Ericson & Nisell, 1987 (18)	Cycling	90	900
Reilly & Martens, 1972 (43)	Leg raise	0	1,130
Morrison, 1969 (36)	Down stairs	—	1,690
	Down ramp	—	1,913
	Up stairs	—	1,926
Reilly & Martens, 1972 (43)	Stair descent	60	2,205
	Stair climbing	60	2,450
	Deep knee bend	100	2,940
Wahrenberg et al., 1978 (53)	Kicking a ball	100	3,633
Kaufman et al., 1991 (25)	Isokinetic, 180°/sec	54	3,730
Smidt, 1973 (49)	Isometric	90	4,549
Kaufman et al., 1991 (25)	Isokinetic, 60°/sec	56	4,695

ing include level walking, stair ascent and descent, and rising from a chair. It is recognized that during some of these activities, muscle groups other than the quadriceps play an important role in knee joint loading. However, the quadriceps supplies the dominant muscle force across the knee joint during the activities to be simulated. Therefore, a simplified simulator of the knee, incorporating the quadriceps muscle, will provide meaningful data. The amount of force in the quadriceps has been estimated for several activities of daily living (Table 1). A knee joint testing machine should attempt to replicate these forces. The quadriceps has been frequently used to provide simulated muscle action during knee testing. The quadriceps has been selected because quadriceps action is important in day-to-day activities and also because the arrangement of the quadriceps, patella, and patellar tendon make it possible to provide reasonably lifelike simulation of muscle action simply by pulling on the quadriceps tendon. A similar goal for a knee testing machine would be to duplicate the net knee moment obtained for various activities of daily living (Table 2). These moments could be obtained by either application of loads through the quadriceps tendon alone or in combination with loads through the hamstrings.

A number of researchers have used a muscle-stabilized arrangement where the leg is fixed in a horizontal posi-

TABLE 2. *Maximum knee moment for various activities*

Author	Activity	Knee angle (degrees)	Moment (N − m)
Ericson & Nisell, 1986 (18)	Cycling	90	25
Cavanagh & Gregor, 1975 (12)	Walking (swing)	20	25
Winter, 1980 (55)	Walking	—	45
Bresler & Frankel, 1950 (11)	Walking	20	47
Morrison, 1968 (35)	Walking	—	51
Andriacchi et al., 1980 (1a)	Up stairs	65	54
Boccardi et al., 1981 (8)	Walking	—	60
Radcliffe, 1962 (42)	Walking	20	61
Schuldt et al., 1983 (44)	Rising from squat	105	70
Kelley et al., 1978 (27)	Rising from chair	90	110
Smidt, 1973 (49)	Isometric	45	119
Kaufman et al., 1991 (26)	Isokinetic, 180°/sec	50	139
Andriacchi et al., 1980 (1a)	Down stairs	60	147
Kaufman et al., 1991 (26)	Isokinetic, 60°/sec	54	161
Nisell, 1985 (39)	Isokinetic, 180°/sec	65	181
Wahrenberg et al., 1978 (53)	Kicking a ball	100	182
Nisell, 1985 (39)	Isometric extension	90	198
Winter, 1983 (56)	Jogging	50	210
Lindahl et al., 1967 (30)	Isometric extension	60	225
Nisell, 1985 (39)	Parallel squat	120	455
Zernicke et al., 1977 (60)	Tendon rupture	90	550

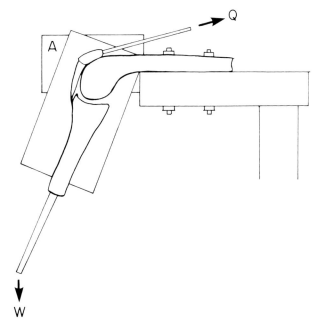

FIG. 7. Malcom (31) and Grood (21) used similar test rigs. In both cases the femur is clamped to a table and a weight *W* is applied distal to the joint. The knee is held in equilibrium by a force *Q* applied to the end of the quadriceps tendon. In the Malcom experiment, relative orientation of the femur and tibia was determined by having a plate *A* attached to the femur and a card attached to the tibia. By marking the card through holes drilled in plate *A,* the relative orientation of the bones could be documented. This method has some sensitivity to motions outside the sagittal plane, but they are difficult to interpret. (From Biden and O'Connor, ref. 5, with permission.)

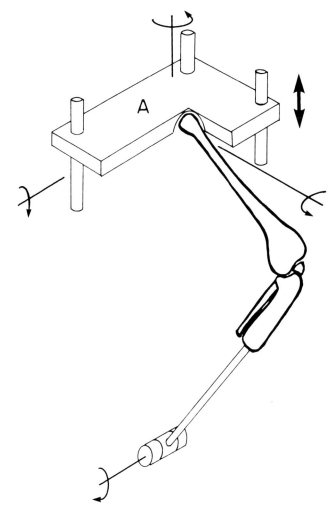

FIG. 8. Perry (41) used this rig to measure quadriceps force as a function of flexion angle. Four degrees of freedom (three rotations plus up-and-down motion) are allowed at the hip, and a fifth degree of freedom (rotation of the ankle) is allowed as well. Equilibrium is maintained by pulling on a strap attached to the quadriceps tendon. This rig appears to have 5 *df,* but in fact both tibial rotation and abduction-adduction are suppressed because the tibia is constrained to move in a single plane. Flexed knee stance under a vertical load at the hip involves only minor abduction-adduction or rotatory effects, and these have little effect on quadriceps tension. (From Biden and O'Connor, ref. 5, with permission.)

tion. Malcom and Daniel (31) and Grood et al. (21) attached the femur to a test bench and simulated leg extension exercise (Fig. 7). Using different techniques, they found that the ACL was active in early flexion in association with quadriceps action. Grood and colleagues (21) showed that ACL sectioning produced additional anterior laxity. Harding et al. (22) attached the tibia vertically to a base, extended the femur using a rod in the medullary canal, and attached a dead weight load to the end. They stabilized the knee using a strap attached between the quadriceps tendon and the femur. Goodfellow (20) used the apparatus to study the kinematics of the patello-femoral joint.

Other researchers have used vertically loaded, muscle-stabilized test rigs. Shaw and Murray (45) used a hydraulically activated cable to simulate quadriceps muscle action in a cadaver specimen. The cable was attached via a pulley to the tibia rather than through the patellar mecha-

nism. Perry (41) placed knees in a simulated, flexed knee stance and then attached a tensile force transducer to the quadriceps tendon and placed a compressive force transducer under the tibial plateau. Vertical load was applied at the hip and quadriceps force needed to stabilize the limb in different positions of flexion was measured (Fig.

FIG. 10. A: The original Oxford rig. **B:** The Oxford rig with modification to allow offset of the hip. The Oxford rig allows 6 *df* to the knee. The two rotations at the hip and three rotations at the ankle act like a pair of ball-and-socket joints, and the slider allows height to change as the knee flexes. Simulated muscle action is required for equilibrium except at full extension where the load passes down the tibial axis, producing no flexing or extending moment.

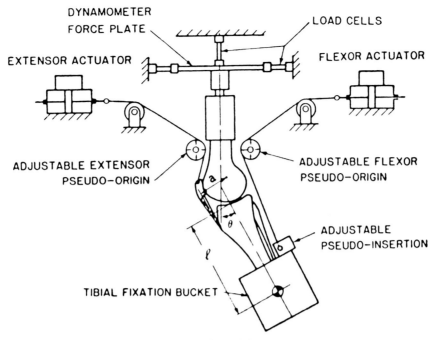

FIG. 9. Ahmed used a knee simulator that reproduces joint dynamic loads by controlling the tension in two flexible cables that act as lumped muscle group equivalents (1).

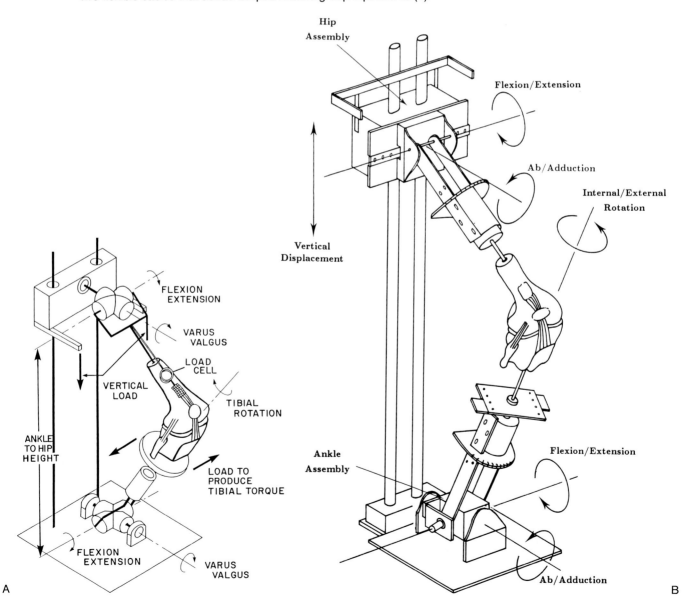

8). Perry's test apparatus was over constrained by 1 *df*. The lower tibia was attached to the base using a simple hinge that constrained it to move in a plane without any possibility for tibial rotation. However, such constraint is unlikely to affect the relationship between quadriceps force and load, and the results obtained with this 5 *df* system are consistent with those found with 6 *df* devices.

Zachman et al. (59) designed a sophisticated testing machine that utilized four activators to produce loads across the knee joint. Flexion, vertical load, torque about the vertical axis, and abduction-adduction of the tibia relative to the femur were controlled by separate hydraulic servo-control loops. Szklar and Ahmed (52) designed a simple knee simulator that reproduced joint dynamic loads by controlling the tension in two flexible cables that acted as lumped muscle group equivalents (Fig. 9). The muscle groups were the knee flexors and extensors.

The two cable tensions were controlled individually to achieve flexion-extension motion while their simultaneous action was used to control the joint compressive force. These actions were achieved without constraining the natural conjunct and passive motions of the specimens.

O'Connor and colleagues from Oxford (4,6,9) used a rig that also simulated flexed knee stance (Fig. 10). The Oxford rig differs from that used by Perry (41) by allowing the bone 6 *df* so that their movements upon each other were constrained only by the structures of the knee. These test devices allowed the knee to be loaded in flexion with stability maintained by pulling on the quadriceps tendon through a load cell. The advantage of this experimental setup is that it simulates standing with the knees bent, riding a bicycle, climbing stairs, and the early stance portion of gait.

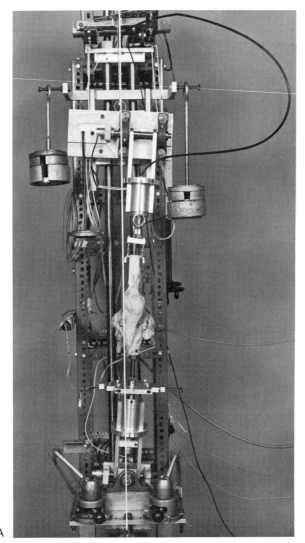
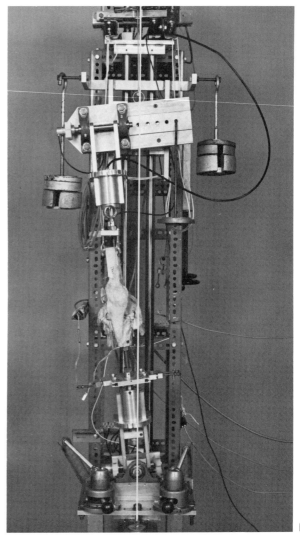

A

B

FIG. 11. A: Hip slider positioned so that the vertical plane through hip and ankle passes through the lateral compartment of the knee. **B:** Hip slider positioned so that the vertical plane through centers of hip and ankle passes medial to the knee. (From Biden and O'Connor, ref. 5, with permission.)

THE OXFORD KNEE TEST RIG

The Oxford knee rig has been used extensively in our laboratory for tests of quadriceps-stabilized knees. This device allows 6 *df* to the knee while simulating flexed knee stance. The specimen is prepared with about 20 cm of bone above and below the joint line. The threaded rods are fixed in the intramedullary cavities of both bones. The threaded rods are used to attach the specimen to the "hip" and "ankle" of the apparatus. The ankle assembly comprises three sets of rotary bearings that allow flexion-extension, abduction-adduction, and internal-external rotation of the tibial link. The axes of the three bearings intersect at a fixed point, the center of the "ankle." The "hip" assembly comprises two sets of rotary bearings, allowing ab/adduction and flexion-extension to the femoral link. The axes of these bearings intersect at a point vertically above the "ankle" simulating the center of the "hip." Linear bearings running along two vertical rods guide vertical movement of the

hip relative to the ankle. The lengths of the tibial and femoral links are adjusted to simulate physiological dimensions (15). The moving parts of the apparatus are counterbalanced with the specimen in place. Hence, the "leg" can then remain placed in any position of flexion. A vertical load is applied by hanging weights onto the hip assembly. Collapse of the system is prevented by means of tension in a strap attached to the quadriceps tendon. The specimen is flexed by a servo-electric motor that lengthens the strap attached to the quadriceps tendon. The simulation of muscle force necessary to stabilize the leg in the presence of a vertical load is measured by a strain gauged load cell that is attached in series to a strap, which is sutured to the quadriceps tendon.

A sliding hip assembly is used to adjust for the mechanical axis of the limb in the coronal plane (Fig. 11). The femoral link that attaches to the hip assembly is allowed to move medially or laterally. This permits the plane of knee flexion to be rotated about the ankle. When the slider is fixed so that the tibia lies in a vertical

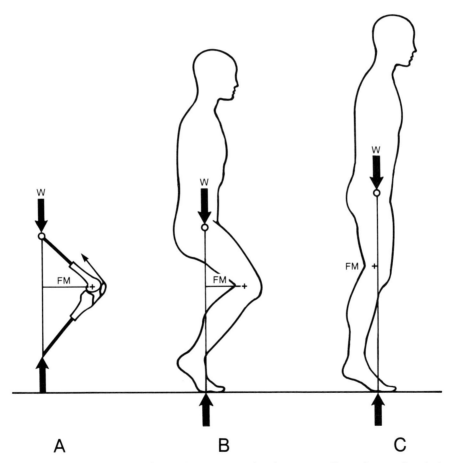

FIG. 12. The Oxford rig simulates flexed knee stance but is not exactly analogous to what occurs in everyday life. For instance, if Diagram **A** (representing the rig) and Diagram **B** (representing stance) are compared, it is easy to see that shifts in trunk position or where load (*W*) passes through the foot will influence the flexing moment (*FM*) at the knee. In the Oxford rig, load is applied through the center of the hip, and thus the moment arm is usually longer than normal. Another situation occurring in everyday life is depicted in **C**. When one stands with knees extended and shifts one's weight onto the balls of the feet, body weight passes anterior to the knee flexing axis (+) and produces an extending moment. This situation cannot occur in the Oxford rig. (From Biden and O'Connor, ref. 5, with permission.)

plane, this arrangement simulates the natural valgus angle of the femur (Fig. 11A). In other positions, it is possible to allow the plane of the limb to be set at any desired angle relative to the vertical load. For instance, to simulate single leg stance (Fig. 11B) the line of action passes medial to the knee (2).

Five rotary variable differential transformers (RVDTs) (Schaevitz, Pennsauken, New Jersey) are used to measure rotations at the five sets of rotary bearings. A linear variable differential transformer (Schaevitz, Pennsauken, New Jersey) is used to measure the vertical position of the hip assembly. These transducers give an output voltage proportional to position. Their accuracy is ±0.5°. The signals are recorded by an analog-digital convertor (Data Translation) and recorded by a Microvax II computer (Digital Equipment Corporation, Maynard, Massachusetts). Records of experiments are stored on computer disk.

There are several advantages of the Oxford knee rig. First, it permits complete 6 *df* of knee motion while providing a simulated muscle action for equilibrium (Fig. 10). Second, the Oxford rig allows a torque to be applied to the tibia to permit constrained external and internal loads to be applied to the tibia in conjunction with the muscle loads. Third, the location of the load in the coronal plane can be adjusted to vary the mechanical axis of

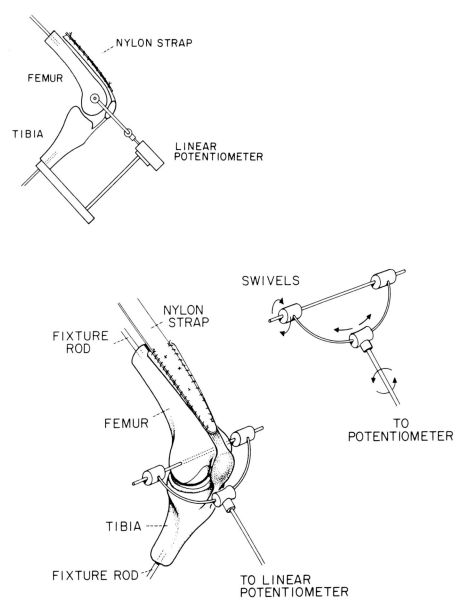

FIG. 13. Schematic of device used to measure anterior tibial translation. The potentiometer is rigidly mounted to the threaded tibial rod and also attached to the semicircular linkage. The linkage is attached to a Steinmann pin that has been drilled through the femoral condyles. The linkage is allowed to rotate in all planes.

the knee, thereby permitting the simulation of single limb stance during gait.

There are also some limitations to the Oxford rig. First, when simulating muscle action, the magnitudes of the loads that can be applied are limited by the strength of the attachment to the muscle tendon. This limits the amount of load that can be applied to the quadriceps tendon to about 1500 N. Second, the leverage of the vertical hip load about the knee (Fig. 12A) is larger than under normal physiological situations where the load passes anterior to the ankle, through the ball of the foot, and anterior to the hip joint secondary to hip flexion (Fig. 12B). Thus the force line passes closer to the knee joint. In fact, near extension, the load through the foot can pass in front of the knee requiring flexor action for equilibrium (Fig. 12C). The simulated quadriceps forces measured in the rig at higher flexion angles are therefore larger in proportion to the applied load than is true under normal flexed knee stance. Third, the rig as presently designed does not easily permit physiological simulation of hamstrings-quadriceps co-contraction loads. The simulated contraction of the hamstrings has to be held at a constant value, which may overemphasize the hamstrings at certain flexion angles and underemphasize them at other flexion angles.

IN VITRO MUSCLE-STABILIZED KINEMATIC STUDIES

Functionally, knee stability is dependent upon interactions between ligamentous structures, muscle forces, and joint surface geometry which are resisting external loads. Many biomechanical studies have concentrated on these factors individually. In these experiments, forces were applied and the motions that resulted were measured while the joint was maintained in a static, flexed position (19,32,51,54). The effects of axial compressive force on limits of knee motion have also been reported at static flexion positions (32,46). The advent of material testing devices further allowed documentation of knee motion throughout a range of flexion (57). However, simulated joint compressive forces and muscle action were not considered.

The Oxford knee rig has been used to measure quadriceps forces, anterior-posterior tibial displacement, and internal-external tibial rotation of the vertically oriented, intact, and anterior cruciate ligament sectioned knee. Anterior-posterior tibial translation was measured directly with a linear potentiometer mounted rigidly to the tibia and connected through a semicircular link to a Steinmann pin that had been drilled through the femoral condyles (Fig. 13). Additional tests have evaluated the synergistic relationship between the ACL and hamstring muscle activity. The hamstring load was applied equally

to the medial and lateral hamstring tendons by a yoke that attached to two wire cables that passed over the hip assembly of the Oxford Rig (Fig. 14). On the lateral side the strap was attached to the biceps femoris tendon. On the medial side, the end of a strap was sutured to the semimembranosus tendon and the other end to the semitendinosus tendon. Further, the rig has been utilized to study the effects of tibial rotational torque on tibial rotation. A rotational torque was applied through pulleys placed on the medial and lateral aspects of the tibia and orientated orthogonally to the longitudinal axis of the tibia (Fig. 15).

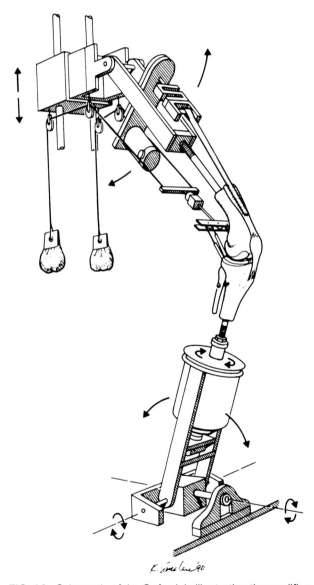

FIG. 14. Schematic of the Oxford rig illustrating the modification for applying a load to hamstrings in addition to the load on quadriceps. The hamstring apparatus has straps attached to the medial and lateral hamstring tendons, which then go through a yoke and attach to wires. The wires are looped over pulleys attached to the hip slider mechanism and are loaded with weights.

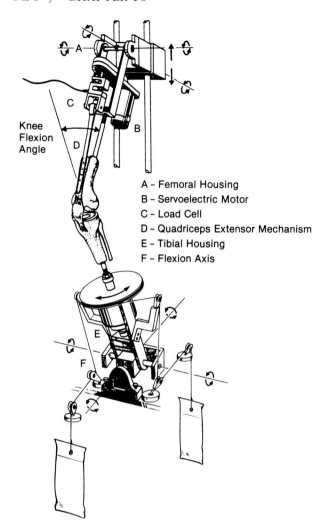

FIG. 15. Schematic of the Oxford rig illustrating the modifications to apply a constant tibial torque in addition to the quadriceps load. Wires are attached to a pulley that is mounted on the tibial shaft. The wires are looped over pulleys and are loaded with weights. The pulleys are mounted so that the wires always pull at right angles to the long axis of the tibia. The wires are loaded with equal weights, which results in a rotational torque being applied to the tibia throughout the flexion range of the knee.

A – Femoral Housing
B – Servoelectric Motor
C – Load Cell
D – Quadriceps Extensor Mechanism
E – Tibial Housing
F – Flexion Axis

Knee Moment

The application of a weight to the hip joint of the Oxford knee rig results in a flexion moment about the knee joint center. This moment is counteracted by the moment produced by the quadriceps force. The moment at the knee is minimum at full extension and increases as the flexion angle increases (Fig. 16). The peak moment resulting from the application of a 45 N hip load is 32 ± 4 N-m. The magnitude of this moment compares favorably with several activities of daily living (Table 3). It is 28% greater than cycling or the swing phase of walking. The knee moment in the Oxford Rig is 52% to 71% of the knee moment obtained during the stance phase of gait,

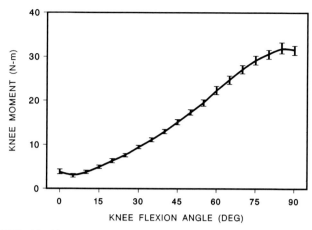

FIG. 16. Knee moment generated when a 45 N load is applied to the hip joint of the Oxford Knee Rig.

59% of that obtained during stair climbing, and 46% of the moment during rising from a squat position. Therefore, even though the hip load (45 N) seems low in comparison with the weight of the upper body, the difference in lever arm of this load to the knee joint center (Fig. 12) results in a knee moment that is close to those experienced during activities of daily living.

Quadriceps Force

The Oxford knee rig provides the ability to directly measure the quadriceps force as the knee is flexed and extended. The quadriceps force sufficient to extend the intact knee against a 45 N hip load varies with flexion angle (Fig. 17). At full extension, the quadriceps force is minimum, whereas at increasing flexion angles the quadriceps force increases. The quadriceps force generated in the anterior cruciate ligament deficient state is no different than that measured in the intact state (48). Addition of a hamstring load has no effect on quadriceps load (Fig. 18) (34). The peak quadriceps force resulting from the application of a 45 N hip load is 831 ± 97 N (Fig. 17). This loading condition is approximately equivalent to that experienced during cycling, level walking, or walking up a ramp (Table 4). In addition, it is 35% to 50% of the quadriceps load obtained during stair ascent or descent.

TABLE 3. *Comparison of knee moment for various activities to Oxford knee rig*

Activity	Magnitude (%)
Cycling	128
Walking (swing)	128
Walking (stance)	52–71
Up stairs	59
Squat	46
Down stairs	22

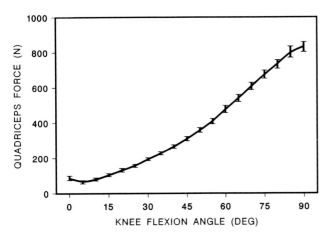

FIG. 17. Quadriceps force generated as the intact knee is extended from 100° to 0° flexion against a 45 N hip load.

TABLE 4. Comparison of quadriceps force for various activities to Oxford knee rig

Activity	Magnitude (%)
Walking	98–137
Up ramp	106
Cycling	92
Down stairs	38–49
Up stairs	34–43

Anterior Tibial Displacement

Anterior tibial displacement has been measured in the quadriceps-absent state as a function of externally applied anterior-posterior load and varying knee flexion angle (48). Maximum femoral rollback occurred in all knees at 90° flexion, whereas the minimum value occurred at 0° flexion (Fig. 19). The average femoral rollback was 24.8 ± 1.8 mm. This large displacement represents the magnification of the normal femoral rollback encountered due to placing the pin anterior to the center of rotation of the knee. The reference point for measurement of A-P displacement was purposely placed anterior to the center of knee rotation to avoid binding the medial collateral ligament and periarticular tissue. Nevertheless, this measurement technique provides a good baseline for

detecting changes in joint kinematics caused by changes in muscle action or ligament disruption, since each specimen serves as its own control. When a 90 N force was applied to the tibia in the anterior and posterior directions, the envelope of passive A-P displacement was defined. Comparison of the ACL intact and sectioned states demonstrates that anterior displacement is increased at all flexion angles in the quadriceps absent state.

Anterior tibial displacement in the quadriceps-stabilized state is significantly different than that seen in the quadriceps absent state (Fig. 20) (48). This effect is highly dependent upon the knee flexion position. At high flexion angles, no difference is observed in the anterior displacement due to quadriceps force. As the knee is extended, anterior tibial displacement in the quadriceps-stabilized state increases beyond that seen in the quadriceps absence state. The largest difference (3.5 mm) is seen between 40° and 25° of flexion. The change in anterior displacement decreases slightly as the knee approaches full extension. The addition of a hamstring load causes a significant reduction in the amount of anterior displacement (Fig. 21) (34).

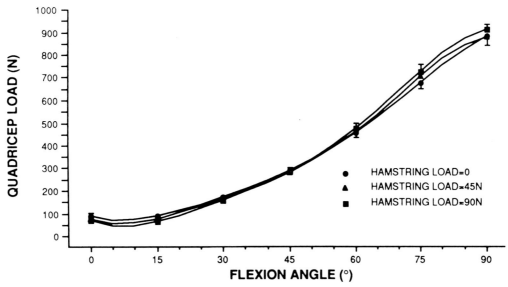

FIG. 18. The effect of hamstring force on quadriceps load with the ACL intact and a 45 N hip load. (From ref. 34, with permission.)

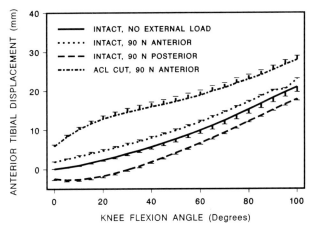

FIG. 19. Anterior tibial translation versus knee flexion in the quadriceps load absent state. Anterior and posterior limits at ±90 N force before and after sectioning the anterior cruciate ligament are shown. (From ref. 48, with permission.)

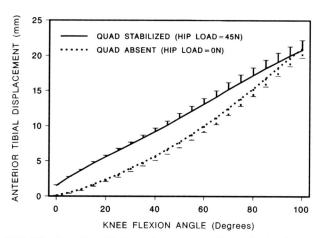

FIG. 20. Anterior tibial translation versus knee flexion for the intact knee in the quadriceps-absent and quadriceps-stabilized states. Note that the curves intersect between 100° and 95° flexion. (From ref. 48, with permission.)

In the quadriceps-stabilized knee, sectioning of the anterior cruciate ligament results in increased anterior displacement of the tibia. The amount of this displacement varies with the hip load and the knee flexion angle (Fig. 22). As the knee is extended from 100° to 70° flexion, the change in anterior tibial displacement is less than 1 mm. The displacement increases to a maximum of 5.0 mm at 20° flexion and then decreases to 2.5 mm at full extension. This displacement is reduced when a hamstring load is added to the ACL sectioned knee (Fig. 23) (34).

The relationship between anterior tibial displacement and knee flexion angle in the quadriceps-stabilized knee has been predicted by several studies that have looked at the orientation of the patellar tendon relative to the tibia (39,49). Smidt (49) reported that the quadriceps exerted an anterior shear force on the tibia between 0° and 70° flexion. Nisell (39) found that the patellar tendon was angled anteriorly in relation to the perpendicular of the tibial plateau from 0° to 100° flexion. The maximum tendon angle was at full extension. As shown in Fig. 22, the maximum anterior tibial displacement after sectioning the ACL occurs at 30° flexion and not at full extension. However, the quadriceps load increases with knee flexion to balance the increasing flexion moment (Fig. 17). Thus, anterior tibial displacement in the quadriceps-stabilized knee is dependent on the force exerted by

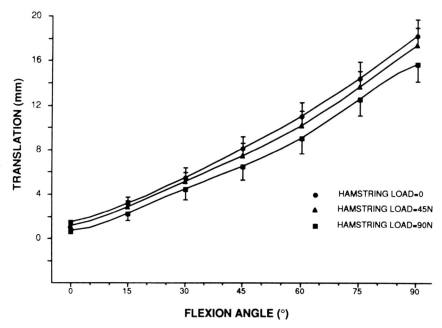

FIG. 21. The effect of hamstring force on anterior tibial translation with the ACL intact and a 45 N hip load. (From ref. 34, with permission.)

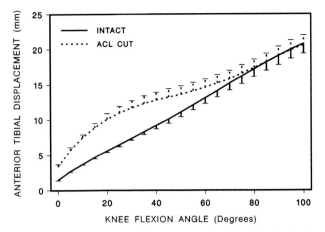

FIG. 22. Anterior tibial translation versus knee flexion in the quadriceps-stabilized state before and after anterior cruciate ligament sectioning. A 45 N hip load was used. (From ref. 48, with permission.)

the quadriceps and the patellar tendon angle. The patellar tendon angle is dependent on the knee flexion angle. In the supine patient, the flexion angle at which the resultant patellar tendon force is perpendicular to the tibial plateau, and no anterior-posterior component is generated due to quadriceps force has been termed the *quadriceps neutral angle* (13,14). Utilizing an instrumented clinical measuring device, the KT-2000, Daniel (13,14) reported that the mean quadriceps neutral angle for 92 normal knees was 71° flexion with a range from 60° to 90° flexion. Interpolating from *in vivo* data presented by Smidt (49), the resultant patellar tendon force during isometric knee extension exercise created no anterior-

posterior shear forces at approximately 70° flexion. Grood et al. (21) demonstrated an abrupt increase in anterior tibial translation beginning at 75°.

Several authors have reported that the hamstrings work synergistically with the ACL to limit anterior tibial displacement. Hamstring-ACL synergy has been reported during walking (24,29,58), squatting (40), knee extension exercise (16), and knee isokinetic exercise (3,50). Based on the available *in vitro* and *in vivo* evidence, it can be postulated that the hamstrings function with the ACL to provide anterior knee stability in either the intact or sectioned state (Fig. 23).

Tibial Rotation

The "screw home" mechanism of the tibia that occurs during the terminal 30° of extension has been described (37). Using the Oxford Rig, it can be demonstrated that quadriceps force has a significant effect on tibial rotation (Fig. 24) (48). In the quadriceps absent state, the maximum internal rotation was 10°. In the quadriceps-stabilized state, internal rotation reached a maximum of 14° throughout the midrange of flexion. The internal rotation was 1.2° to 4.2° greater than in the quadriceps-absent state. One possible explanation for this occurrence is that the patellar tendon probably creates a torsional moment as it leaves the patella captured in the femoral trochlea and travels laterally to insert in the tibial tubercle. Further, addition of a hamstring load will cause a significant decrease in tibial rotation for both the intact and ACL-deficient knee (Fig. 25) (34).

Controversy exists as to whether the anterior cruciate

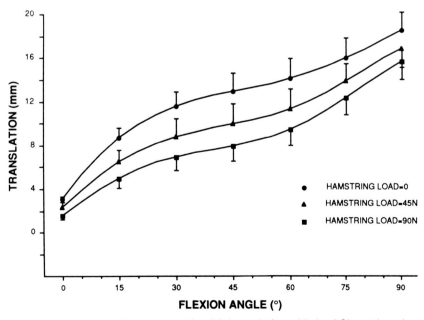

FIG. 23. The effect of hamstring force on anterior tibial translation with the ACL sectioned and a 45 N hip load. (From ref. 34, with permission.)

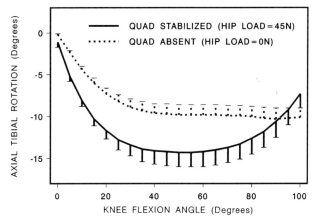

FIG. 24. Axial tibial rotation versus knee flexion for intact knees in the quadriceps-absent and quadriceps-stabilized states. Negative rotation denotes internal rotation of the tibia. (From ref. 48, with permission.)

ligament is an important restraint in limiting axial rotation. Many authors have noted that the presence of anterior-lateral and/or anterior-medial instability in patients with anterior cruciate ligament disruption. Various clinical tests are thought to demonstrate anterior-lateral and anterior-medial rotational instability in the ACL-deficient knee. Lane et al. (28) quantified the total tibial rotation in the quadriceps-stabilized knee. The knees were mounted in an Oxford rig. A 5 N-m rotational torque was applied to the tibial platform of the rig without restricting the freedom of the system. Internal and external torques and hip loads of 0 and 89 N were applied to the intact and ACL-sectioned knee. No significant change in axial rotation occurred between the intact and ACL-sectioned knee for external rotation ($p = 0.24$) or internal rotation ($p = 0.12$) for either the quadriceps-absent or quadriceps-stabilized state (Fig. 26).

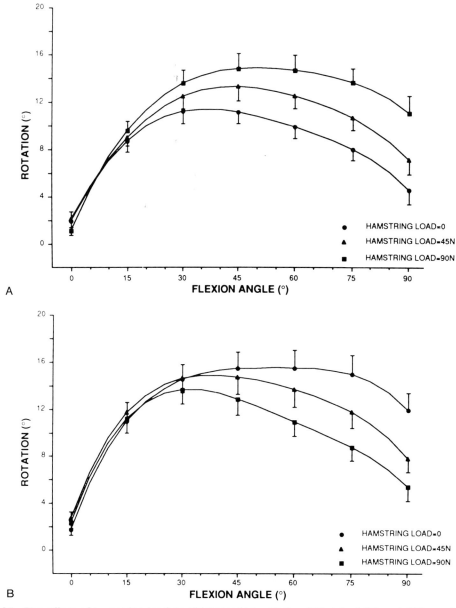

FIG. 25. The effect of hamstring load on tibial rotation with the ACL intact (**A**) and ACL sectioned (**B**) while using a 45 N hip load. (From ref. 34, with permission.

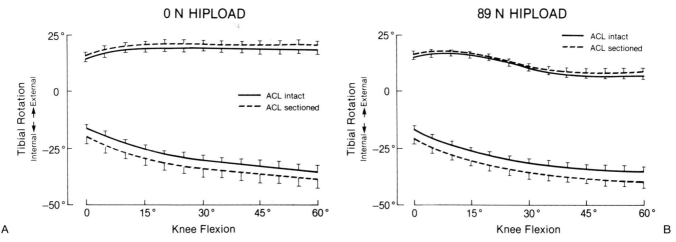

FIG. 26. Axial tibial rotation versus knee flexion in the quadriceps-absent (**A**) and quadriceps-stabilized (**B**) state, before and after anterior cruciate ligament sectioning. A 5 N-m internal and external rotational torque was used to establish the limits of rotational motion. Positive rotation denotes external rotation of the tibia. (From ref. 28, with permission.)

SUMMARY

Many aspects of synovial joint mechanics can only be investigated by *in vitro* experimentation. However, *in vitro* experimentation requires an apparatus for the application of physiological forces acting at the joint without artificially constraining the motion. Peculiar demands, which cannot be met by conventional materials testing machines, are placed on such an apparatus. These demands arise due to the interconnections of intricate capsular, ligamentous, and muscular soft tissues interacting with complex, nonuniform articular surfaces. This chapter has described the relative merits of various loading devices for the knee. It is recommended that muscle-stabilized testing that allows complete 6 *df* motion be utilized. The kinematics of the intact and ACL-sectioned knee have been measured using this type of apparatus. The results provide guidelines for establishing ACL rehabilitation protocols.

REFERENCES

1. Ahmed AM, Hyder A, Burke DL, Chan KH. (1987): *In vitro* ligament tension pattern in the flexed knee in passive loading. *J Orthop Res,* 5:217–230.
1a. Andriacchi TP, Andersson GBJ, Fermier RW, Stern D, Galante JO. (1980): A study of lower-limb mechanics during stair-climbing. *J Bone Joint Surg [Am],* 62A:749–757.
2. Andriacchi T, Stanwyck S, Galante JO. (1986): Knee biomechanics and total knee replacement. *J Arthroplasty,* 1:211–219.
3. Baratta R, Solomonow M, Zhou BH, et al. (1988): Muscular coactivation: the role of the antagonist musculature in maintaining knee stability. *Am J Sports Med,* 16:113–122.
4. Biden E. (1981): *The mechanics of synovial joints* [Thesis]. Oxford, England: University of Oxford.
5. Biden E, O'Connor J. (1990): Experimental methods used to evaluate knee ligament function. In: Daniel D, Akeson W, O'Connor JJ, eds. *Knee ligaments: structure, function, injury and repair.* New York: Raven Press, pp 135–151.
6. Biden E, O'Connor JJ, Goodfellow JW. (1984): Tibial rotations in the cadaver knee. *Trans Orthop Res Soc,* 30:30.
7. Blankevoort L, Huiskes R, deLange A. (1988): The envelope of passive knee joint motion. *J Biomech,* 21:705–720.
8. Boccardi S, Pedotti A, Rodano R, Santambrogio CG. (1981): Evaluation of muscular moments at the lower limb joints by an on-line processing of kinematic data and ground reaction. *J Biomech,* 14:35–45.
9. Bourne R, Goodfellow JW, O'Connor JJ. (1978): A functional analysis of various knee arthroplasties. *Trans Orthop Res Soc,* 24:160.
10. Brantigan OC, Voshell AF. (1941): The mechanics of the ligaments and menisci of the knee joint. *J Bone Joint Surg [Am],* 23A:44–66.
11. Bresler B, Frankel JP. (1950): The forces and moments in the leg during level walking. *Trans ASME,* 72:27–36.
12. Cavanagh PR, Gregor RJ. (1975): Knee joint torque during the swing phase of normal treadmill walking. *J Biomech,* 8:337–344.
13. Daniel DM, Stone ML, Barnett P, Sachs R. (1988): Use of the quadriceps active test to diagnose posterior cruciate ligament disruption and measure posterior laxity of the knee. *J Bone Joint Surg [Am],* 70A:386–391.
14. Daniel D, Lawler J, Malcom L, Biden E, O'Connor J, Goodfellow J. (1982): The quadriceps anterior cruciate interaction. *Orthop Trans,* 6:199–200.
15. Dempster WT. (1955): *Space requirements of the seated operator.* WADC Technical Report, Wright-Patterson Air Force Base, Ohio, pp 123–133.
16. Draganich LF, Jaeger RJ, Kralj AR. (1989): Coactivation of the hamstrings and the quadriceps during extension of the knee. *J Bone Joint Surg [Am],* 71A:1075–1081.
17. Ericson MO, Nisell R. (1987): Patellofemoral joint forces during ergometric cycling. *Phys Ther,* 67:1365–1369.
18. Ericson MO, Nisell R. (1986): Tibiofemoral joint forces during ergometer cycling. *Am J Sports Med,* 14:285–290.
19. Fukubayashi T, Torzilli P, Sherman M, Warren R. (1982): An *in-vitro* biomechanical evaluation of anterior posterior motion of the knee. *J Bone Joint Surg [Am],* 64A:258–264.
20. Goodfellow JW, Hungerford D, Zindal M. (1976): Patellofemoral joint mechanics of pathology: 1. Functional anatomy. *J Bone Joint Surg [Br],* 58B:283–287.
21. Grood E, Suntay W, Noyes F, Butler D. (1984): Biomechanics of the knee extension exercise. *J Bone Joint Surg [Am],* 66A:725–734.
22. Harding ML, Harding L, Goodfellow JW. (1977): A preliminary report of a simple rig to aid the study of the functional anatomy of the cadaver knee joint. *J Biomech,* 10:517–523.
23. Hsieh HH, Walker PS. (1976): Stabilizing mechanisms of the loaded and unloaded knee joint. *J Bone Joint Surg [Am],* 58A:87–93.
24. Kalund S, Sinkjaer T, Arendt-Nielsen L, et al. (1990): Altered timing of hamstring muscle action in anterior cruciate ligament deficient patients. *Am J Sports Med,* 18:245–248.
25. Kaufman KR, An KN, Litchy WJ, Chao EYS. (1991): Physiologi-

cal prediction of muscle forces: Part 2—application to isokinetic exercise. *Neuroscience,* 40:793–804.

26. Kaufman KR, An KN, Chao EYS. (1988): A dynamic mathematical model of the knee joint applied to isokinetic exercise. In: Spilker RL, Simon BR, eds. *Computational methods in engineering.* New York: American Society of Mechanical Engineers, BED-vol 9, pp 157–167.

27. Kelley DL, Dainis A, Wood GK. (1978): Mechanics and muscular dynamics of rising from a seated position. *Biomechanics,* 5:127–134.

28. Lane J, Rangger C, Kaufman K, Irby S, Daniel D. (1991): Evaluation of the ACL in controlling axial rotation. *Trans Orthop Res Soc,* 16:236.

29. Limbird TJ, Shiavi R, Frazer M, et al. (1988): EMG profiles of knee joint musculature during walking: changes inducted by anterior cruciate ligament deficiency. *J Orthop Res,* 6:630–638.

30. Lindahl O, Movin A. (1967): The mechanics of extension of the knee joint. *Acta Orthop Scand,* 38:226–234.

31. Malcom L, Daniel D. (1980): A mechanical substitution technique for cruciate ligament force determinations. *Trans Orthop Res Soc,* 26:303.

32. Markolf K, Mensch J, Amstutz H. (1976): Stiffness and laxity of the knee: the contributions of the supporting structures. *J Bone Joint Surg [Am],* 58A:583–594.

33. Markolf K, Barger W, Shoemaker S, Amstutz H. (1981): The role of joint load in knee stability. *J Bone Joint Surg [Am],* 63A:570–585.

34. More RC, Karras BT, Neiman R, Fritschy D, Woo S-LY, Daniel DM. (1993): Hamstrings—an anterior cruciate ligament protagonist: an *in-vitro* study. *Am J Sports Med* 21(2):231–237.

35. Morrison JB. (1968): Bioengineering analysis of force actions transmitted by the knee joint. *Biomed Eng,* 3:164–170.

36. Morrison JB. (1969): Function of the knee joint in various activities. *Biomed Eng,* 4:573–580.

37. Müller W. (1983): *The knee: form, function and ligament reconstruction.* New York: Springer-Verlag.

38. Neilsen S, Kromann-Andersen C, Rasmussen O, Anderson K. (1984): Instability of cadaver knees after transection of capsule and ligaments. *Acta Orthop Scand,* 55:30–34.

39. Nisell R. (1985): Mechanics of the knee: a study of joint and muscle load with clinical applications. *Acta Orthop Scand,* 56[Suppl 216].

40. Ohkoshi Y, Yasuda K. (1989): Biomechanical analysis of shear force exerted on anterior cruciate ligament during half squat exercise. *Trans Orthop Res Soc,* 35:193.

41. Perry J, Antonelli D, Ford W. (1975): Analysis of knee joint forces during flexed knee stance. *J Bone Joint Surg [Am],* 57A:961–967.

42. Radcliffe CW. (1962): The biomechanics of below knee prostheses in normal level bipedal walking. *Artif Limbs,* 6:16.

43. Reilly DT, Martens M. (1972): Experimental analysis of the quadri-

ceps muscle force and patello-femoral joint reaction force for various activities. *Acta Orthop Scand,* 43:126–137.

44. Schüldt KJ, Ekholm J, Németh B, Arborelius UP, Harms-Ringdahl K. (1983): Knee load and muscle activity during exercises in rising. *Scand J Rehabil Med Suppl,* 9:174–188.

45. Shaw JA, Murray DG. (1973): Knee joint simulator. *Clin Orthop Rel Res,* 94:15–23.

46. Shoemaker SC, Markolf KL. (1985): Effects of joint load on the stiffness and laxity of ligament-deficient knees: an *in-vitro* study of the anterior cruciate and medial collateral ligaments. *J Bone Joint Surg [Am],* 67A:136–146.

47. Shoemaker S, Markolf K. (1986): The role of the meniscus in the anterior-posterior stability of the loaded anterior cruciate-deficient knee. *J Bone Joint Surg [Am],* 68A:71–79.

48. Shoemaker SC, Adams DJ, Daniel DM, Woo S-LY: The quadriceps-anterior cruciate ligament interaction: An *in-vitro* kinematic study of the quadriceps stabilized knee. *Clin Ortho [in press].*

49. Smidt GL. (1973): Biomechanical analysis of knee flexion and extension. *J Biomech,* 6:79–92.

50. Solomonow M, Baratta R, Zhou BH, et al. (1987): The synergistic action of the anterior cruciate ligament and thigh muscles in maintaining joint stability. *Am J Sports Med,* 15:207–213.

51. Sullivan D, Levy M, Sheskier S, Torzilli P, Warren R. (1984): Medial restraints to anterior-posterior motion of the knee. *J Bone Joint Surg [Am],* 66A:930–936.

52. Szklar O, Ahmed AM. (1987): A simple unconstrained dynamic knee simulator. *J Biomech Eng,* 109:247–251.

53. Wahrenberg H, Lindbeck L, Ekholm J. (1978): Knee muscular moment, tendon tension force, and EMG during a vigorous movement in man. *Scand J Rehabil Med,* 10:99–106.

54. Wang CJ, Walker PS. (1974): Rotary laxity in the human knee joint. *J Bone Joint Surg [Am],* 56A:161–170.

55. Winter D. (1980): Overall principle of lower limb support during stance phase of gait. *J Biomech,* 13:923–927.

56. Winter DA. (1983): Moments of force and mechanical power in jogging. *J Biomech,* 16:91–97.

57. Woo SL-Y, Hollis JM, Roux RD, Gomez, MA, Inoue M, Kleiner JB, Akeson WH. (1987): Effects of knee flexion on the structural properties of the rabbit femur-anterior cruciate ligament-tibia complex (FATC). *J Biomech,* 20:557–563.

58. Yasuda K, Sasaki T. (1987): Muscle exercise after anterior cruciate ligament reconstruction: biomechanics of the simultaneous isometric contraction method of the quadriceps and the hamstrings. *Clin Orthop,* 220:266–274.

59. Zachman NJ, Hillberry BM, Kettelkamp DB. (1978): Design of a load simulator for the dynamic evaluation of prosthetic knee joints. *ASME Paper No. 78-DET-59.*

60. Zernicke RF, Garhammer J, Jobe FW. (1977): Human patellar-tendon rupture: a kinetic analysis. *J Bone Joint Surg [Am],* 59A:179–183.

The Anterior Cruciate Ligament: Current and Future Concepts, edited by D.W. Jackson, et al. Raven Press, Ltd., New York © 1993.

CHAPTER 11

Anterior Cruciate Ligament Forces in Activity

John J. O'Connor and Amy Zavatsky

Ligament forces are important when the knee is stabilized dynamically by muscle forces. In this chapter, we will use simple models to show that both the magnitudes of the ligament forces and the flexion ranges over which individual ligaments act depend on the directions and magnitudes of the muscle forces transmitted across the joint. Determining the ligament forces in activity first requires a geometric model of the muscles spanning the joint and a study of the changing directions of the tendons and ligaments with knee flexion.

Many studies have examined ligament strains or ligament forces when the knee is stabilized by muscle forces. However, most such studies have been limited to relatively simple situations such as isometric quadriceps exercises when the configuration of the limb is easily defined. In the *in vitro* studies, tension force was applied to the muscle tendons in a variety of ways (1,7,10,11,14,21, 22,27,33,34,36–38). Similarly, ligament strains or forces were measured or deduced in a variety of ways: by measuring tibiofemoral movements before and after load application and ligament transection (10,37), by direct measurement of ligament strain (1,7,36), or by simulated ligament force (21,27,29,34).

Pope et al. (35) attached a Hall-effect strain transducer to the anteromedial band of the ACL in one subject and measured strain while the subject performed deep squats. Other *in vivo* studies involved the measurement of tibiofemoral translation (15,18,22) or restraining force (39,43) during isometric muscle contractions or the quantification of moments about the knee using a Cybex II isokinetic dynamometer (19,26,42). In most cases (26,39,42,43), a simple mathematical model then was used to calculate the net shear force at the knee, and the ligament forces were not calculated. Kaufman et al. (19) used a more complex optimization model involving

the minimization of muscle activity to deduce the shear force.

The direct measurement of muscle, ligament, and contact forces at the knee *in vivo* is impracticable. Therefore, calculation of these forces, using theoretical models for interpreting experimental data, is likely to remain the principal tool. A recent review (13) cites nearly 100 theoretical models of the knee, increasing in complexity as computing power increased. Nonetheless, few analyses of ligament forces in activity have been performed despite the frequency of ligament damage. Morrison's calculations of ligament forces during walking (25) and its further development by Harrington (12) have stood alone for 20 years.

The main difficulty in such calculation is the number of separate muscle groups that span the knee and can act synergistically or antagonistically. The values of the forces transmitted by the structures of the joint are dynamically indeterminate because the number of unknown forces far exceeds the number of equations available from theoretical dynamics. For this reason, in the large body of literature on gait analysis, the calculations generally are limited to the resultant force and moment transmitted by the joint (9,40). Various optimization techniques have been proposed for predicting muscle activity in walking; using the model to be described below, Collins and O'Connor (6) found that no one criterion appears to be valid throughout the gait cycle.

Electromyographic measurements during normal walking (17) have shown that only one of the main flexor or extensor muscle groups spanning the knee—quadriceps, hamstrings, or gastrocnemius—is active over most of the normal walking cycle. The moment of the muscle force must be balanced with the combined moments of the external and inertial loads about the flexion axis of the joint. Consequently, it is unlikely that the component of the muscle force parallel to the tibial plateau in the sagittal plane also served to balance exactly the corresponding component of the loads. The main structures

---

J. J. O'Connor and A. Zavatsky: Department of Engineering Science, University of Oxford, Oxford OX1 3PJ, England.

available to balance the remainder of the loads are the ligaments. Malcolm and Daniel (21) and O'Connor et al. (29,30,33) have shown that the changing directions of the tendons relative to the bones determine which of the cruciate ligaments is loaded during active extension and flexion. Even in the presence of antagonistic muscle action, precise relationship must exist between extensor and flexor forces to avoid loading the ligaments. The ligaments therefore play an essential role in controlling the stability of the joint during activity.

In this chapter, the sagittal plane model of Chapter 3 is extended to include muscle action, and the interactions between muscle forces and ligament forces are considered. The chapter begins by considering the ligaments to be inextensible straight lines coinciding with the ligament links of the four-bar cruciate linkage in Fig. 1 of Chapter 3. The articular surfaces of the bones are assumed to be rigid, making contact at a point. After a discussion of the factors that govern the relationships between ligament and muscle forces, we will show how these relationships are modified when account is taken of ligament elasticity and recruitment of ligament fibers under load. Further research is necessary to simultaneously examine ligament elasticity, cartilage deformation, and the roles of the menisci and then to study these factors in three dimensions. The chapter concludes with a brief discussion of anterior cruciate ligament forces during normal walking.

NONTURNING LOADS

Using the model developed in Chapter 3, we showed that the flexion axis of the knee during passive movements lies at the point where the neutral fibers of the cruciate ligaments cross. We also showed that the common normal to the articular surfaces at their point of contact passes through the flexion axis. Initially, we will consider that the lines of action of the cruciate ligament forces coincide with the neutral fibers of the four-bar linkage. The ligament forces therefore intersect at the flexion axis. We will consider that the articular surfaces of the tibiofemoral joint are frictionless so that the resultant contact force transmitted between them passes along the common normal at their point of contact. Therefore, this contact force also passes through the flexion axis, where it intersects the lines of action of the two cruciate ligament forces.

Because tibiofemoral contact force and the cruciate ligament forces all intersect at the flexion axis, they can have no turning moment about that axis and cannot by themselves induce or resist flexion or extension. However, these forces are sufficient to balance a "nonturning" load, that is, a load applied to the leg in the sagittal plane whose line of action also passes through the flexion axis. Muscle action is necessary only if the line of action of the load does not pass through the flexion axis.

The Mechanical Center of the Knee

The intersection of the cruciate ligaments, through which the flexion axis of the knee passes, defines the mechanical center of the joint in the sagittal plane. This center is the fulcrum about which external loads and muscle forces exert their leverage. If the line of action of the foot/ground reaction passes anterior to the flexion axis, the knee tends to extend and action is needed from the flexors (either the hamstrings or the gastrocnemius muscles) to stabilize the limb. If this line of action passes posterior to the flexion axis, however, the knee tends to flex, and extensor action (from the quadriceps muscles) is necessary for equilibrium. Ligament geometry is therefore a factor in determining which muscle groups are needed for equilibrium.

Lever-Arms

The perpendicular distance of the line of action of the load from the flexion axis is a direct measure of its tendency to extend or flex the joint and defines the length of the lever-arm of the load. The lever-arm of the load is zero when the load passes through the flexion axis; the load then has neither a flexing nor an extending effect. Likewise, the lever-arms available to the muscles are the perpendicular distances from the flexion axis to their tendons. Calculating the lengths of the muscle lever-arms requires a geometric model of the muscles and their tendons.

THE GEOMETRY OF THE MUSCLE TENDONS

For the mechanical analysis of the joint, we need to describe the way in which the lines of action of the extensor and flexor muscles at the knee move during flexion and extension. The three muscle groups—the quadriceps, gastrocnemius, and hamstrings—will each be represented by a single line, the line of action of the resultant force which that muscle transmits across the knee.

Figure 1 shows the model bones of Fig. 5 of Chapter 3 in three positions, with the addition of these lines.

The Hamstrings Tendon

The hamstrings tendon inserts into the model tibia at a point H posteriorly and distally from the plateau. Point H was taken as a compromise between the attachments of the semimembranosus and the biceps. The tendon is assumed to lie parallel to the femur over the range of flexion. The direction of the tendon and, therefore, of the hamstrings force applied to the tibia, changes over the flexion arc, as indicated by the three diagrams of Fig. 1. Near full extension, the model tendon makes contact with the back of the femoral condyle, as the semimembranosus does, rather than running forward along the

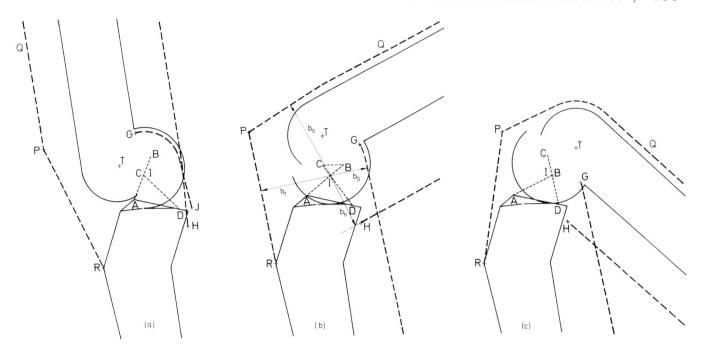

FIG. 1. Models of the bones, the cruciate ligaments, and the muscle tendons at the knee near full extension (**A**), at 70° of flexion (**B**), and a 140° flexion angle (**C**).

outer edge of the femoral condyle as the biceps do. In Fig. 1A, the tendon therefore changes its direction slightly as it passes over the back of the condyle.

The Gastrocnemius Tendon

The gastrocnemius tendon is shown as a single line connecting its point of origin G at the back of the femoral condyle to a point (out of the diagram) representing the insertion of the Achilles tendon on the back of the foot. Within the outline of the model femoral condyle in Figs. 1A and B, the tendon represents a line of action of the resultant gastrocnemius force passing between the two femoral condyles of the human knee. Near extension the line of action of the tendon passes through the point J, where it wraps around the back of the tibial plateau. At higher flexion angles (Figs. 1B and C), the tendon loses contact with the back of plateau. In figure 1C, it loses contact with the back of the femoral condyle and passes directly from its point of origin on the femur to its point of insertion on the heel.

Although the gastrocnemius muscles lie more or less parallel to the back of the tibia, Fig. 1 suggests a small but significant change in direction during flexion and extension, in part caused by the rolling movement of the femur on the tibia (Fig. 5 of Chapter 3).

The Quadriceps Mechanism and the Patellofemoral Joint

The sulcus of the trochlear groove, which guides the patella over the femur in the sagittal plane, is assumed to be circular for this model. In our simplest model of the

quadriceps mechanism (Fig. 1), the patella is represented as a single point P at which the patellar tendon RP intersects the quadriceps tendon QP. It moves on a circular arc about the center T of the circle representing the trochlea. P is the intersection point of the forces applied to the patella by the quadriceps and patellar tendons. The only other significant force applied to the patella in the sagittal plane is the patellofemoral contact force. For equilibrium of the patella, this force must pass through the point where the two tendon forces intersect. The radial line PT is taken to be the line of action of the patellofemoral contact force, always perpendicular to the trochlea.

The point P in the model should be interpreted as the "center of force" of the patella. It is connected to the tibia through the patellar tendon which inserts into the tibial tubercle R. Near extension, the quadriceps tendon QP exits the patella parallel to the femur. At about 70° to 80° of flexion its line of action begins to intersect the femur, and at higher flexion angles the tendon wraps around the surface of the trochlea to form the "tendofemoral" joint.

This model of the quadriceps mechanism is not intended to describe the details of patellar mechanics. A planar model of patellar kinematics and mechanics was described by Yamaguchi and Zajak (41). It accounted for, but did not explain, the rolling movements of the femur on the tibia. The model described in Fig. 1 has been further developed to include a patella (31). Lengsfeld described a similar model that relates the geometry of the extensor mechanism to that of the cruciate ligaments and the tibiofemoral joint (20).

In terms of knee mechanics, the model discussed here reproduces two important features of the natural joint. Because the angle *QPT* between the quadriceps tendon and the line of action of the patellofemoral force is not equal to the angle *RPT* between the patellar tendon and the patellofemoral force, the two tendon forces cannot be equal, and thus the patellofemoral joint does not behave like a simple, frictionless pulley. Maquet (23) came to this conclusion after noting that the lever-arms available to the quadriceps and patellar tendon forces are not equal. The deduction was confirmed experimentally by Bishop and Denham (3), Ellis et al. (8), Huberti et al. (16), and Buff et al. (5). The ratio of the tendon forces at different flexion angles calculated from the model compares reasonably well with measurements made by these authors.

A second feature of quadriceps mechanism geometry that has important mechanical implications is that the model patellar tendon rotates about the tibial tubercle during flexion and extension. This rotation results in part from the rolling of the femur on the tibia and in part, from the cam-like action of the trochlea as it rotates about the flexion axis. The rotation of the natural tendon about the tubercle was described by Matthews et al. (24). Blick et al. (4) measured the backward movement of the patella relative to the tibia over 90° of flexion in specimens stabilized by tension in the quadriceps tendon. They reported a movement of 40 mm, whereas 35 mm was calculated from the computer model of Fig. 1. The theoretical model calculations suggest that about two-thirds of this movement is caused by the cam effect, that is the changing distance from the tendon to the flexion axis, and that one-third is caused by the backward movement of the flexion axis, manifested in the rolling of the femur on the tibia. Buff et al. (5) measured the "patellar mechanism angle"—the angle between the patellar and quadriceps tendons—at different degrees of flexion, and their measurements correspond with our calculations from the model (28). The angle decreases from about 160° at extension to about 110° at approximately 70° of flexion, when trochlear wrap begins, and thereafter increases slowly to about 120° at 140° of flexion. (28)

In short, some of the geometric and mechanical features of the simplest model quadriceps mechanism have been validated by comparison with the results of independent experiments reported in the literature.

The Lever-Arms of the Tendons

The lever-arms of the tendons are their perpendicular distances from the instant center *I* (Fig. 1B). Their lengths were calculated from the geometric model of the knee and are shown plotted against flexion angle in Fig. 2. The lever-arm of the patellar tendon is longer than that of the hamstrings, which, in turn, is longer than that

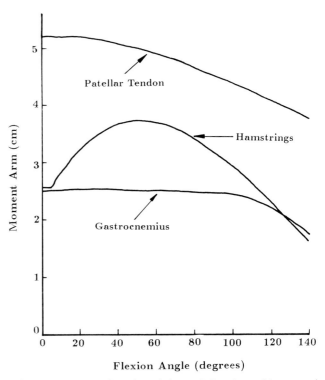

FIG. 2. Lever-arm lengths of the patellar, hamstrings, and gastrocnemius tendons plotted against flexion angle. (From ref. 32, with permission.)

of the gastrocnemius tendons over the whole range of movement. The length of each varies with flexion because the directions of the tendons change and because the flexion axis moves. The lengths of the lever-arms therefore reflect the kinematics of both the tibiofemoral joint and the individual muscle groups. The general calculated pattern of lever-arm length varying with flexion agrees with deductions based on EMG signals by Baratta et al. (2).

A sensitive test of the accuracy of the calculated lever-arm lengths in Fig. 2 is to measure the tensile forces that must be applied to the tendons to stabilize the knee under load. Both Grood et al. (10) and we (28) obtained such measurements *in vitro* for several experimental configurations. In both cases, the results reasonably agreed with our calculations.

LIGAMENT FORCES DURING ISOMETRIC QUADRICEPS EXERCISES

Isometric exercises are frequently used as part of a rehabilitative program after an injury or operation. In the case of ligament injury, exercise can be designed either to load or protect the particular ligament. This isometric quadriceps exercise provides a good illustration of muscle/ligament interactions.

During isometric quadriceps contractions, the knee is held fixed at a constant flexion angle. Figure 3 shows the forces acting on the tibia during this exercise, ignoring

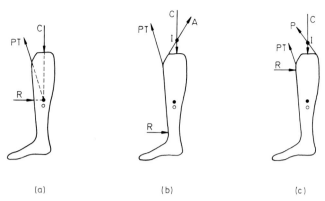

(a)   (b)   (c)

FIG. 3. Isometric quadriceps test. **A:** The tibia in equilibrium under the action of a force *PT* in the patellar tendon, a restraining force *R,* and the tibiofemoral contact force *C*. The lines of action of the three forces meet at *O*. **B:** Load placement distal to *O*; a force *A* is required in the anterior cruciate ligament. **C:** Load placement proximal to *O*; a force *P* is required in the posterior cruciate ligament. (From ref. 6, with permission.)

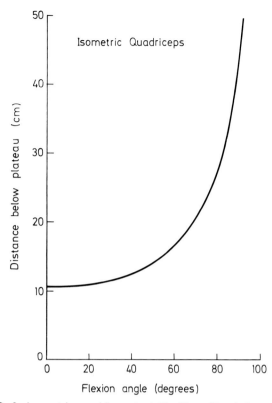

FIG. 4. Isometric quadriceps test. Position of load placement for zero ligament force plotted against flexion angle. If the conditions of the test lie above and to the left of the curve, the ACL is loaded. If they lie below and to the right, the PCL is loaded.

for simplicity the weight of the lower leg. A restraining force *R* is applied to the tibia to prevent extension during quadriceps contraction. The three diagrams show the restraining force applied at different distances from the tibial plateau. As the point of restraint is moved further distal, its lever-arm from the flexion axis of the joint is increased, and the relative value of the patellar tendon force must also increase.

The forces that must be considered to achieve equilibrium of the tibia are the patellar tendon force, *PT,* the tibiofemoral contact force, *C,* the cruciate ligament forces (*A* or *P*), and the restraining force. For each flexion angle, there is a proximal/distal position for the restraint at which no ligament forces are required for equilibrium. This position occurs when the lines of action of the patellar tendon force, the contact force and the restraining force all intersect at a point (*O*) (Fig. 3A). The force *PT* thus simultaneously balances both the flexing effect of *R* and the horizontal component of *R* parallel to the plateau. The component of *PT* perpendicular to the plateau is balanced by the contact force *C*. Because the direction of the patellar tendon force rotates about the tibial tubercle during flexion and the line of action of the contact force moves backward on the tibial plateau, as illustrated in Fig. 1, the point of intersection *O* moves distally with an increasing flexion angle. The calculated distance of *R* below the tibial plateau for zero ligament force is plotted against flexion angle in Fig. 4. Greater than about 90° of flexion, the required position lies more than 40 cm from the tibial plateau and may not be physically achievable.

Figure 4 implies that for a fixed position and direction of the external load *R*, there is a *critical flexion angle* (29,30,32) at which no ligament forces are needed for equilibrium of the tibia. Alternatively, when the flexion angle and the direction of the restraining force are fixed, there is a *critical position* for the external load at which mechanical equilibrium is achieved without ligamentous action.

If the position of *R* is not given by a point on the curve in Fig. 4, the components of *R* and *PT* parallel to the plateau are not equal, and the passive soft tissues must balance the resultant shear force. For simplicity, we will assume that the shear force is balanced by the horizontal component of the force in either the ACL or posterior cruciate ligament. For positions of *R* distal to point *O* (Fig. 3B), a relatively large magnitude of *PT* is needed to balance the greater flexing moment of *R* about the flexion axis of the knee. In this case, the component of *PT* parallel to the tibial plateau is larger than *R*; their resultant force is directed anteriorly, and equilibrium requires a posteriorly directed ligament force, provided by the ACL in the simplest model and by the force *A* in Fig. 3B. The sum of the components of *PT* and *A* perpendicular to the plateau is balanced by *C*.

When *R* is positioned proximal to point *O* (Fig. 3C) and has a shorter lever-arm about the flexion axis of the knee, the corresponding tendon force *PT* is relatively smaller. The resultant of *PT* and *R* is now directed posteriorly, and an anteriorly directed ligament force is needed. In the simplest model, this force is provided entirely by the PCL—the force *P* in Fig. 3C.

As an example, Fig. 5 shows the calculated values of the cruciate ligament forces, expressed as a proportion of the restraining force, plotted against flexion angle for a restraint placement 22 cm below the tibial plateau. The ligament forces are zero at 75° of flexion, the critical flexion angle for the chosen restraint position. Nearer extension, ACL force is required; at flexion angles greater than 75°, PCL force is required. Families of such curves can be drawn for different choices of load placement. The figure also includes the calculated value of the quadriceps force, expressed as a proportion of restraining load. Corresponding families of quadriceps force also can be drawn for different choices of load placement.

The model in Figs. 4 and 5 could form the basis of a physiotherapy program following ligament injury. For instance, if protection of the ACL is desired, load placement and the flexion angle should be chosen so that the conditions of the exercise lie below the curve in Fig. 4. If more proximal load placement is chosen (the region directly below the curve), the ACL will not be loaded at any flexion angle, but the muscle forces involved will be relatively small. More distal load placements involve higher muscle forces but should be attempted only at high flexion angles (to the right of the curve) if the ACL is to be protected.

O'Connor (32) used similar arguments in showing the relationships between antagonistic extensor/flexor forces and cruciate ligament forces; and in defining the circumstances in which quadriceps, hamstrings, and gastrocnemius muscles can act together to completely unload the cruciate ligaments. The latter circumstances also may be of interest in the design of rehabilitation regimens after ligament injury or surgery.

The Effects of Ligament Elasticity

The calculations of ligament forces in Fig. 5 are based on inextensible-line ligament theory. Modeling of the ligaments as arrays of extensible fibers and using geometric compatibility conditions, as in Chapter 3, the mechanisms by which the ligaments of the knee share transmission of shear forces across the joint can be investigated.

We have extended the analysis just described to account for ligament elasticity and fiber recruitment under load, using the model described in Chapter 3 (44). Our calculations show how the ligament forces increase nonlinearly with increasing quadriceps and restraining forces (Fig. 6). As noted earlier, the quadriceps force at the critical flexion angle balances not only the flexing effect of the restraining force about the flexion axis, but also its component parallel to the tibial plateau. At smaller flexion angles, an ACL force is necessary (Fig. 5). However, when the ACL is loaded, it stretches, allowing the tibia to move forward, increasing the inclination of the patellar tendon to the plateau, and *reducing* the horizontal component of its force parallel to the plateau (Fig. 7). The forward movement simultaneously reduces the inclination of the ACL to the plateau and *increases* the horizontal component of its force. With sufficient forward movement, a point can be reached where conditions approach those at the critical flexion angle, that is, an increase in quadriceps force balances the increase in both the flexing effect of the restraining force and its horizontal component. A corresponding increase in the ACL force then is unnecessary; the ACL force has

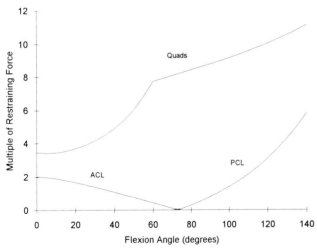

FIG. 5. Isometric quadriceps test. Forces in the ACL, PCL, and quadriceps muscle plotted against flexion angle for restraint placement 22 cm below tibial plateau, on the basis of inextensible ligament theory. (Forces are expressed as multiples of the value of the restraining force.)

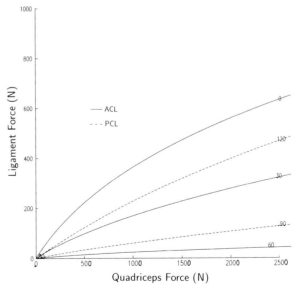

FIG. 6. Isometric quadriceps test. Forces in the ACL and PCL plotted against quadriceps force for restraint placement 22 cm distal to tibial plateau, on the basis of elastic ligament theory with fiber recruitment. Ligament forces are zero at the critical flexion angle of 75°.

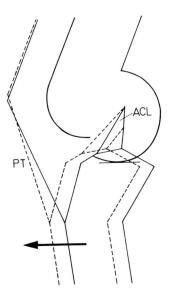

FIG. 7. Changes in direction of the patellar tendon and ACL during anterior displacement of the tibia. (From ref. 6, with permission.)

reached a limiting or asymptotic value and will not change as muscle force is further increased.

Figure 6 shows the calculated values of the ACL and PCL forces plotted against quadriceps force for a number of flexion angles and a load placement 22 cm distal to the tibial plateau. Near the critical flexion angle of 75°, the ligament forces remain relatively small and rapidly approach their asymptotic values. Further from the critical angle, the ligament forces, although growing nonlinearly with increasing quadriceps force, fall short of their asymptotic values for quadriceps forces less than 2500 N. The calculated value of the ACL force was always much less than the reported ultimate strength of young human ACLs (26), even for quadriceps forces of about three times body weight. The potential for these asymptotic values of ligament force may explain why, at certain flexion angles, the muscles at the knee can develop large forces without ligament rupture.

Comparisons with Reported Experimental Results

The results of three experimental studies closely approximate the loading situations shown in Fig. 3. In living human subjects, Jurist and Otis (18) measured tibiofemoral displacements resulting from isometric quadriceps contractions against a quantified restraining load. The directions of anteroposterior tibial translation that they measured are consistent with the patterns of ACL and PCL loading suggested by Fig. 5. Mandt et al. (22) measured quadriceps force and tibial translation in cadaveric knee specimens. The directions of movement found in their experiments for restraining load placements of 20 cm and 30 cm below the plateau are consis-

tent with Fig. 4. The results for the 10 cm load location agree only at 90° flexion. However, the discrepancy can be explained: at lower flexion angles, a restraining load located 10 cm below the tibial plateau is very close to the boundary dividing the regions where anterior and posterior displacements are expected, as shown in Fig. 3.

Using an arthrometer in normal knees, Howell (15) measured the *in vivo* tibial translation produced by an 89-N drawer test, a manual maximum drawer test (MMT), and a maximum isometric quadriceps contraction (QAD) at flexion angles of 15°, 30°, 45°, 60°, and 75°. The distal end of an extension-resistance pad was 29 cm distal to the joint line. During the QAD test, the tibia translated anteriorly at the four lower flexion angles, and it became slightly displaced posteriorly at 75° of flexion. These results are consistent with those presented in Figs. 4 and 5. Howell also found that the anterior tibial translation resulting from QAD was equal to or less than that produced during the 89 N test. The MMT caused twice the anterior tibial translation that accompanied QAD. The limited forward displacement in the QAD test is consistent with our theoretical deduction of asymptotic values of ligament forces in activity, but further experimental evidence is needed.

CRUCIATE LIGAMENT FORCES DURING WALKING

Morrison (25) studied muscle, ligament and contact forces at the human knee joint during walking. Kinematic data from three subjects were acquired using cinematography; the images were digitized manually and used for computer generation of a three-dimensional model of the lower limb during gait. With the knee modeled as a fixed hinge, the relative movements of ligament origins and insertions were determined, and the lines of action of the ligament forces were calculated for each data frame over the gait cycle. The lines of action of the muscle forces were calculated similarly. Kinetic data were acquired simultaneously using a force plate to monitor the magnitude, direction, and line of action of the foot-ground reaction force relative to the leg. Both kinematic and kinetic data were used to calculate the resultant force and moment transmitted by the knee joint for each data frame.

Simplifications were needed to calculate muscle, ligament and contact forces using the equations of dynamics, because the number of unknown forces far exceeds the number of available dynamics equations; the system is dynamically indeterminate. However, EMG data (17) show that not all the muscles are active all the time. After heel-strike, the quadriceps is the only group spanning the knee that is active during early stance. The gastrocnemius muscles resist extension of the knee and the tensor fasciae latae resist adduction during much of midstance; in late stance, the rectus femoris alone resists adduction. Morrison further simplified the calculations by ignoring the brief instants during normal gait when flexor or extensor muscle groups fire simultaneously in antagonism, for instance peri-heel-strike, when the quadriceps and hamstrings act together.

As suggested by Fig. 5, the ligaments act in complementary ways to balance shear forces parallel to the plateau. By assuming that only some of the ligaments bear load at any time, Morrison was able to reduce the number of unknown forces to that of the available dynamics equations and thus to calculate their values. He found that the ACL was loaded during about 65% of the gait cycle, with maximum forces of about 150 N.

Collins and O'Connor (6) used the sagittal plane model of Fig. 1 to consider muscle and ligament forces during normal walking. Their model took account of the rolling movements of the femur on the tibia during flexion and extension. Moreover, they considered all possible dynamically determinate systems of forces at the knee, including those involving antagonistic or agonistic muscle action. Their model was therefore simpler than Morrison's, being two-dimensional, but accounted for factors Morrison omitted. They showed that, over most of the gait cycle and especially during the stance phase, when the joint forces are largest, antagonistic muscle ac-

tion without ligament force is not mechanically possible and that action by a single muscle group at the knee (quadriceps, hamstrings, or gastrocnemius) is more likely. In such circumstances, ligament forces are necessary to balance the resultant of the load and muscle force parallel to the tibial plateau. This principle was described in detail in the earlier discussion of Fig. 3.

Figure 8 shows the force in the ACL for one of their subjects during a single stride, expressed as a proportion of body weight. The figure includes three estimates of the ligament force for three sets of parameters of the four-bar linkage model, with all other conditions the same. The curves demonstrate the extreme parameter sensitivity of the calculated ACL-force values. The calculations of Collins and O'Connor were based on the assumption that the neutral fibers of the ligament links of the four-bar cruciate linkage are located near the centers of the cruciate ligaments. The first set of parameters (Set 1) were chosen based on roentgenographic assessments of the subject's knee (6); the second set (Set 2), based on magnetic resonance imaging, which showed the soft tissues more clearly. The third set (Set 3), located the neutral fibers at the front of the ACL and near the back of the PCL, as described in Chapter 3, and these gave the lowest estimates of ACL forces.

In each case the peak value of the ACL force occurred in early stance, when the quadriceps were active and the

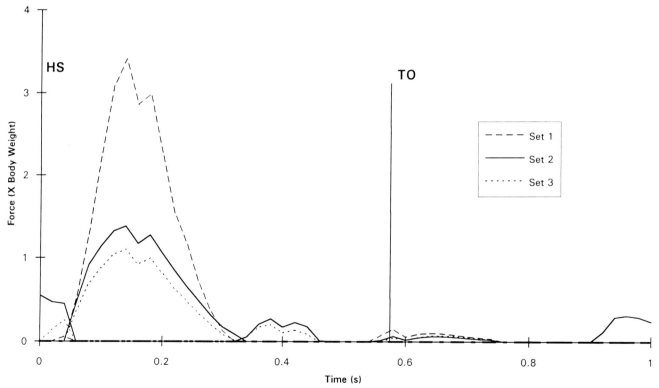

FIG. 8. Level walking. ACL forces during a single step for one subject, based on inextensible ligament theory. Results are presented for three sets of parameters of the four-bar cruciate linkage. *Solid lines,* quadriceps active; *dashed lines,* gastrocnemius active.

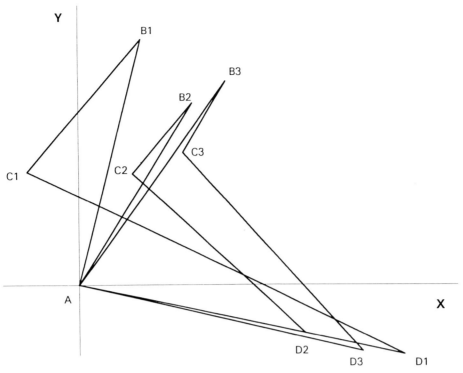

FIG. 9. The four-bar cruciate linkage at 15° flexion for three sets of linkage parameters. The ACL link is most steeply inclined to the tibial plateau for parameter set 1.

flexors quiet (as confirmed by EMG), with the knee bent to about 15°. The estimates for the three sets of parameters differed by a factor of about 3.5, using the same value for the calculated shear force parallel to the plateau. The four-bar linkages in this position for the three sets of parameters are shown superimposed in Fig. 9. At the moment of peak ACL force in gait, the knee is nearly straight, and the ligament is most steeply inclined to the plateau (cf. Figs. 2, 3. and 5 of Chapter 3). As the angle of inclination increases, so does the ligament force required to produce a given shear force parallel to the plateau.[1]

Figure 9 shows that parameter set 1, corresponding to the highest ligament force, gives the highest ligament inclination, and parameter set 3 gives the lowest ligament inclination and lowest ligament force.

This parameter sensitivity has important consequences for the orthopaedic surgeon. If an ACL graft or prosthesis is implanted so that it is positioned "too" vertically when the knee is near extension, it may be subjected not only to unnaturally high forces during passive movement of the joint, but also excessive forces during activity, particularly near extension. Such large forces would be further increased if notch impingement were to occur.

SUMMARY AND CONCLUSION

During some activities, only one main muscle group spanning the knee is exerting force. In such instances, the knee ligaments must be loaded. The ligament forces can be calculated since they must balance the resultant component parallel to the tibial plateau of the muscle forces and external loads. In these circumstances, the ligament forces can be quite large, especially when the ligament is positioned at a steep incline relative to the tibial plateau.

ACKNOWLEDGMENTS

The work described in this chapter was supported by grants from the Arthritis and Rheumatism Council. Amy Zavatsky was supported by a Thouron Award and a Wellcome Trust Prize Studentship. William Davidson's contributions to Figures 8 and 9 were greatly appreciated.

REFERENCES

1. Arms SW, Pope MH, Johnson RJ, Fischer RA, Arvidsson I, Eriksson E. (1984): The biomechanics of anterior cruciate ligament rehabilitation and reconstruction. *Am J Sports Med,* 12:8–18.
2. Baratta R, Solomonow M, Zhou BH, Letson EED, Chuinard R,

---

[1] The shear force S is equal to $L \cdot \cos(\theta)$, where L is the ligament force and θ is its angle of inclination to the plateau. When θ is nearly 90°, small changes in θ produce large changes in $\cos(\theta)$. For instance, cos (89°) = 0.0175, cos (85°) = 0.0872. A change of 4° in the estimate of the ligament angle makes a difference of a factor of five in the estimate of the ligament force necessary to balance a given shear force.

D'Ambrosia R. (1988): The role of the antagonist musculature in maintaining knee stability. *Am J Sports Med*, 16:113–122.

3. Bishop RED, Denham RA. (1977): A note on the ratio between tensions in the quadriceps tendon and infra-patellar ligament. *Eng Med*, 6:53–54.

4. Blick SS, Daniel DM, Foreman K, Davis JL, Focht L. (1990): Kinematics of the quadriceps stabilized anterior cruciate ligament sectioned knee. Unpublished manuscript.

5. Buff H-U, Jones LC, Hungerford DS. (1988): Experimental determination of forces transmitted through the patello-femoral joint. *J Biomech*, 21:17–23.

6. Collins JJ, O'Connor JJ. (1991): Muscle-ligament interactions at the knee during walking. *Proc Inst Mech Eng [H]*, 205:11–18.

7. Draganich LF, Vahey JW. (1990): An *in vitro* study of anterior cruciate ligament strain induced by quadriceps and hamstrings forces. *J Orthop Res*, 8:57–63.

8. Ellis MI, Seedhom BB, Wright V, Dowson D. (1980): An evaluation of the ratio between the tensions along the quadriceps tendon and the patellar ligament. *Eng Med*, 9:189–194.

9. Gilbert JA, Maxwell GM, McElhaney JH, Clippinger FW. (1984): A system to measure the forces and moments at the knee and hip during level walking. *J Orthop Res*, 2:281–288.

10. Grood ES, Suntay WJ, Noyes FR, Butler DL. (1984): Biomechanics of the knee-extension exercise—effect of cutting the anterior cruciate ligament. *J Bone Joint Surg [Am]*, 66A:725–733.

11. Harding ML, Harding L, Goodfellow JW. (1977): A preliminary report of a simple rig to aid study of the functional anatomy of the cadaver human knee joint. *J Biomech*, 10:517–523.

12. Harrington IJ (1976): A bioengineering analysis of force actions at the knee in normal and pathological gait. *Biomed Eng*, 11:167–172.

13. Hefzy MS, Grood ES. (1988): Review of knee models. *Appl Mech Rev*, 41:1–13.

14. Hirokawa S, Solomonow M, Luo Z, Lu Y, D'Ambrosia R. (1991): Muscular co-contraction and control of knee stability. *J Elect Kinesiol*, 1:199–208.

15. Howell SM. (1990): Anterior tibial translation during a maximum quadriceps contraction: is it clinically significant? *Am J Sports Med*, 18:573–578.

16. Huberti HH, Hayes WC, Stone JL, Shybut GT. (1984): Force ratios in the quadriceps tendon and ligamentum patellae. *J Orthop Res*, 2:49–54.

17. Inman VT, Ralston HT, Todd F. (1981): *Human walking*. Baltimore: Williams & Wilkins.

18. Jurist KA, Otis JC. (1985): Anteroposterior tibiofemoral displacements during isometric extension efforts. *Am J Sports Med*, 13:254–258.

19. Kaufman KR, An K-N, Litchy WJ, Morrey BF, Chao EYS. (1991): Dynamic joint forces during knee isokinetic exercise. *Am J Sports Med*, 19:305–316.

20. Lengsfeld M. (1990): Biomechanical model calculations on the influence exerted by the sagittal sliding profile on patello-femoral load. *Unfallchirurgie*, 93:412–417.

21. Malcolm L, Daniel D. (1980): A mechanical substitution technique for cruciate ligament force determinations. *Trans Orthop Res Soc*, 26:303.

22. Mandt PR, Daniel DM, Biden E, Stone ML. (1987): Tibial translation with quadriceps force: an *in vitro* study of the effect of load placement, flexion angle, and ACL sectioning. *Trans Orthop Res Soc*, 33:243.

23. Maquet PGJ. (1976): *Biomechanics of the knee*. Berlin: Springer-Verlag, p 61.

24. Matthews LS, Sonstegard DA, Henke JA. (1977): Load bearing characteristics of the patello-femoral joint. *Acta Orthop Scand*, 48:511–516.

25. Morrison JB. (1968): Bioengineering analysis of force actions transmitted by the knee joint. *Biomed Eng*, 90:164–170.

26. Nisell R, Ericson MO, Nemeth G, Ekholm J. (1989): Tibiofemoral joint forces during isometric knee extension. *Am J Sports Med*, 17:49–54.

27. O'Connor J, Biden E, Bradley J, FitzPatrick D, Young S, Kershaw C, Daniel D, Goodfellow J. (1990): The muscle stabilized knee. In: Daniel DM, Akeson WH, O'Connor JJ, eds. *Knee ligaments: structure, function, injury, and repair*. New York: Raven Press, pp 239–278.

28. O'Connor J, Shercliff T, FitzPatrick D, Biden E, Goodfellow J. (1990): Geometry of the knee. In: Daniel DM, Akeson WH, O'Connor JJ, eds. *Knee ligaments: structure, function, and repair*. New York: Raven Press, pp 163–199.

29. O'Connor J, Shercliff T, FitzPatrick D, Biden E, Goodfellow J. (1990): Mechanics of the knee. In: Daniel DM, Akeson WH, O'Connor JJ, eds. *Knee ligaments: structure, function, injury, and repair*. New York: Raven Press, pp 201–238.

30. O'Connor J, Shercliff T, Goodfellow J. (1988): The mechanics of the knee in the sagittal plane. In: Muller W, Hackenbruch W, eds. *Surgery and arthroscopy of the knee, 2nd Congress of the European Society*. Berlin: Springer-Verlag, pp 12–30.

31. O'Connor J, Zavatsky A. (1990): Kinematics and mechanics of the cruciate ligaments of the knee. In: Mow VC, Ratcliffe A, Woo SL-Y, eds. *The biomechanics of diarthrodial joints*. New York: Springer-Verlag, vol 2, pp 197–242.

32. O'Connor JJ. (1993): Can muscle cocontractions protect ligaments after injury or repair? *J Bone Joint Surg [Br]*, 75B:1:141–148.

33. O'Connor JJ, Goodfellow JW, Young SK, Biden E, Daniel D. (1985): Mechanical interactions between the muscles and cruciate ligaments in the knee. *Trans Orthop Res Soc*, 31:140.

34. Paulos L, Noyes FR, Grood E, Butler DL. (1981): Knee rehabilitation after anterior cruciate ligament reconstruction and repair. *Am J Sports Med*, 9:140–149.

35. Pope MH, Stankewich CJ, Beynnon BD, Fleming BC. (1991): Effect of knee musculature on anterior cruciate ligament strain *in vivo*. *J Elect Kinesiol*, 3:191–198.

36. Renstrom P, Arms SW, Stanwyck TS, Johnson RJ, Pope MH. (1986): Strain within the anterior cruciate ligament during hamstring and quadriceps activity. *Am J Sports Med*, 14:83–87.

37. Reuben JD, Rovick JS, Schrager RJ, Walker PS, Boland AL. (1989): Three-dimensional dynamic motion analysis of the anterior cruciate ligament deficient knee joint. *Am J Sports Med*, 17:463–471.

38. Rovick JS, Reuben JD, Schrager RJ, Walker PS. (1991): Relation between knee motion and ligament length patterns. *Clin Biomech*, 6:213–220.

39. Smidt GL. (1973): Biomechanical analysis of knee flexion and extension. *J Biomech*, 6:79–92.

40. Winter DA. (1979): *Biomechanics of human movement*. New York: John Wiley.

41. Yamaguchi GT, Zajac FJ. (1989): A planar model of the knee joint to characterize the knee extensor mechanism. *J Biomech*, 22:1–10.

42. Yasuda K, Sasaki T. (1987): Muscle exercise after anterior cruciate ligament reconstruction: biomechanics of the simultaneous isometric contraction method of the quadriceps and hamstrings. *Clin Orthop*, 220:266–274, 1987.

43. Yasuda K, Sasaki T. (1987): Exercise after anterior cruciate ligament reconstruction: the force exerted on the tibia by separate isometric contractions of the quadriceps or the hamstrings. *Clin Orthop*, 220:275–283.

44. Zavatsky AB, O'Connor JJ. (1992): Muscle-ligament interaction at the knee during isometric quadriceps contractions. Presented at the meeting of the European Society of Biomechanics, Rome, Abstract 84.

The Anterior Cruciate Ligament: Current and Future Concepts, edited by D.W. Jackson, et al. Raven Press, Ltd., New York © 1993.

CHAPTER 12

Ligament Restraints in Anterior Cruciate Ligament-Deficient Knees

Mohamed Samir Hefzy and Edward S. Grood

Several controversial studies have been published in the literature related to the treatment of the ACL-deficient knee (1,2,7,20). While some investigators report success with nonoperative protocols, others report that patients do poorly without surgical intervention. Recently, Wroble et al. (20) indicated that this difference of opinion may be caused by the heterogeneity of injury in those patients studied. Patients with isolated ACL injuries were evaluated along with patients with injuries to the medial and/or lateral extraarticular structures or both.

Specific knowledge of changes in the three-dimensional knee motions occurring in ACL-deficient knees with and without injuries to the extraarticular structures and menisci seem to be essential when selecting appropriate treatment protocols. The anterior displacement component of the three-dimensional motion of the tibia with respect to the femur in ACL-deficient knees can be considered the sum of two motions: anterior translation of the tibia and tibial axial rotation. These two motions vary depending on the particular ligamentous structures injured in combination with the ACL.

An increase in these two motions has been commonly described by using terms such as anteromedial instability. According to Noyes et al. (16), there is confusion about the meaning of this term. For instance, the descriptive term anteromedial instability does not provide an answer for the following questions: (a) What abnormal motions are described: anterior translation of the tibia, external rotation of the tibia, or both? (b) Is there associated anterior subluxation of the medial tibial con-

dyle? (c) Where is the axis for internal-external rotation of the tibia?

Noyes et al. (16) suggested that rather than using terms such anteromedial instability, clinicians should note the specific motions of anterior translation and external rotation of the tibia that occur with combined injury to the ACL.

Several studies have intended to determine the changes in knee motions that follow isolated or combined cutting of medial and lateral extraarticular structures and menisci in ACL-deficient knees. The following chapter reviews results obtained from these studies, focusing on the contributions of these structures in controlling anterior translations, axial tibial rotations, and varus-valgus angulations in ACL-deficient knees.

THE LIGAMENTOUS RESTRAINTS IN ACL-DEFICIENT KNEES

The Medial Extraarticular Structures

The Anterior Translations

Sullivan et al. (19), Nielsen and Helmig (14), and Shoemaker and Markolf (17) found that the structures of the medial side of the knee joint work to prevent increased anterior translation in ACL-deficient knees. The medial structures include the posterior medial capsule (PMC), the superficial medial collateral ligament, deep medial collateral ligament, and oblique fibers of the medial collateral ligament.

The results reported by Sullivan et al. (19) were obtained by using an *in vitro* knee-testing apparatus with 5 *df* that measured anterior-posterior, medial-lateral, and axial displacement as well as internal-external and valgus-varus rotation (Fig. 1). Sullivan et al. (19) re-

M. S. Hefzy: Biomechanics Laboratories, Department of Mechanical Engineering, University of Toledo, Toledo, Ohio 43606; and Department of Orthopaedic Surgery, Medical College of Ohio, Toledo, Ohio 43606.

E. S. Grood: Noyes-Giannestras Biomechanics Lab, University of Cincinnati, Cincinnati, Ohio 45221.

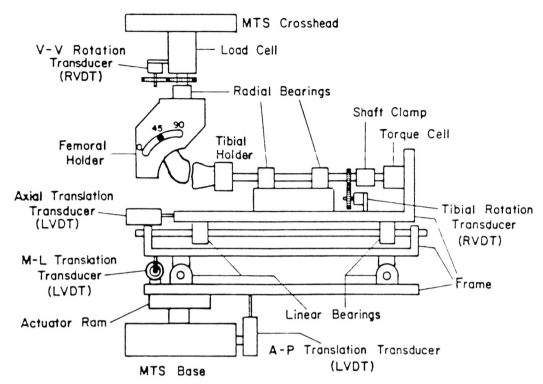

FIG. 1. The knee-testing apparatus with 5 *df* developed at the Hospital for Special Surgery. This apparatus is used to investigate cadaveric knee motions before and after the sectioning of various ligamentous structures. (From ref. 19, with permission.)

ported that, once the ACL was cut, they found no additional increase in anterior displacement following the subsequent sectioning of either the medial part of the capsule or the oblique fibers of the superficial medial collateral ligament, or both. As shown in Fig. 2, when the superficial and deep medial ligaments were sectioned together (the entire medial side), anterior displacement increased at all flexion angles. That is, sectioning the medial structures after cutting the ACL resulted in

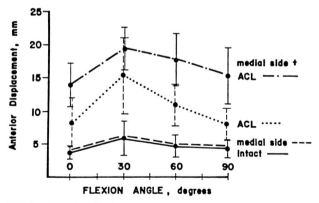

FIG. 2. Anterior displacement resulting from a 100-N anterior force as a function of the angle of flexion. A section of the medial structures increased anterior tibial displacement only after a section of the ACL. The greatest amount of anterior tibial displacement always occurred at 30° of knee flexion. (From ref. 19, with permission.)

displacements that were larger than those found in knees with just the ACL cut. Larger displacements occurred even when the medial meniscus was intact.

Nielsen and Helmig (14) found that lesions to the medial structures did not cause forward tibial displacement when they applied an anterior force. Anterior-posterior displacement was measured for a point located centrally on the posterior side of the tibia, just distal to the insertion of the PCL. Resection of the ACL caused an anterior instability throughout the whole range of motion. As expected, isolated injury to the ACL caused an increase in anterior displacement, making the movement purely translatory. With further transection of the PMC with the MCL intact, Nielsen and Helmig (14) noted no additional increase. After finally resecting the MCL, the anterior displacement increased markedly throughout the whole range of motion.

Recently, Haimes et al. (6) found similar results. They reported that cutting the superficial MCL in an ACL-deficient knee further increased anterior translation at 60° and 90° of flexion, thereby eliminating the difference in anterior translation between 15° and 90° flexion, known to occur in the ACL-deficient knee. Furthermore, cutting the PMC caused an increase in the anterior translation (6).

Shoemaker and Markolf (17) also conducted a ligament sectioning study to determine the effects of sequentially sectioning the ACL and the medial collateral ligament on the primary anterior-posterior translations. A 200 N anterior-posterior load was applied to cadaveric specimens at full extension and at 20° of flexion with and without compressive loads of 320 and 925 N. Tibial rotations were constrained during the application of the force.

Sectioning the ACL produced large increases in anterior laxity; the effects at 20° were somewhat greater than those seen at full extension. Subsequent sectioning of the medial collateral ligament produced an additional increase in the anterior laxity at both flexion angles.

Shoemaker and Markolf (17) also reported that joint compressive loads reduced the increased anterior laxity in ACL-deficient knees at low levels of applied anterior force. Furthermore, once the MCL was cut, at full extension joint loads eliminated the increased laxity. This was not the case at 20° of flexion. These data indicate that joint load plays an important role in limiting tibial displacements in ACL-deficient knees. Shoemaker and Markolf (17) indicate that these results are attributed to the high degree of tibiofemoral congruency and the compression of the menisci, which would tend to prevent tibial anterior excursions.

In summary, the data reported by Sullivan et al. (19), Nielsen and Helmig (14), Haimes et al. (6), and Shoemaker and Markolf (17) indicate that a combined injury to the medial structures and the ACL will produce an increase in anterior displacements at all flexion angles. These data suggest that the MCL provides significant resistance to anterior drawer in ACL-deficient knees and acts as a secondary stabilizer for anterior-posterior displacement.

Axial Tibial Rotations

In 1971 Kennedy and Fowler (8) used x-rays to evaluate the anterior displacements of both tibial condyles in patients having a combined injury to the tibial collateral ligament, medial capsule and the ACL. They found that the displacement of the lateral tibial condyle was equal to that of the medial tibial condyle. Consequently, they concluded that rotatory instability did not exist.

Recently, Kennedy and Fowler's results have been disputed by many investigators (6,11,17). In one of their cadaveric studies, Nielsen et al. (11) measured the knee movements resulting from the application of internal-external rotation torques of 3 N-m at different flexion angles. They reported that cutting the entire ACL caused slight increases in internal rotation in the first 30° of knee flexion. They found no changes in external rotations. As shown in Fig. 3, Nielsen et al. (11) found that further cutting the MCL produced large increases in external tibial rotations of the anteromedial type when they applied external torques to the tibia; these changes in external rotations increased with knee flexion. Nielsen et al. (11) indicate that the anteromedial rotatory instabil-

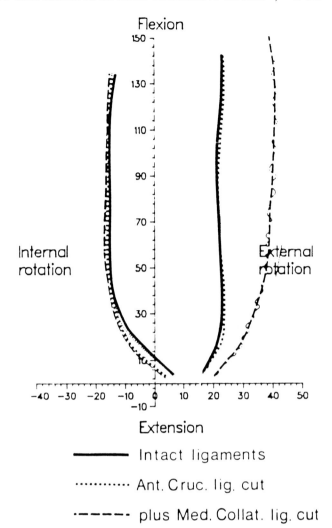

FIG. 3. A mobility pattern showing axial rotation instability. Internal and external rotation correspond to posteromedial and anteromedial rotation, respectively. (From ref. 11, with permission.)

ity caused by the combined resection of the ACL and MCL was about twice that found in one of their previous studies (13) after an isolated cutting of the MCL. These data suggest that an injury to the MCL in ACL-deficient knees causes large increases in external rotations of the anteromedial type.

Recently, Haimes et al. (6) obtained results similar to those obtained by Nielsen et al. (11). They found that significant increases in external rotation occurred when the MCL, the PMC, and the posterior oblique ligament were further cut in ACL-deficient knees. These increases were largest in the flexed knee. However, Haimes et al. (6) reported that increases in external rotation were accompanied by either anterior subluxation of the medial tibial plateau, posterior subluxation of the lateral tibial plateau, or both.

Nielsen and Helmig (14) found that lesions to the MCL and the PMC caused coupled external rotations when they applied an anterior force. Also, Nielsen and Helmig (14) reported that the isolated cutting of the MCL, PMC, or ACL caused no changes in coupled tibial rotations that occur with knee flexion. Combined transection of the MCL and the ACL resulted in an increased coupled external rotation in the flexed position. However, changes in coupled tibial rotation in the extended position were not recorded until the PMC was resected where coupled external tibial rotation increased at all flexion angles, with the largest increase at 90° of flexion.

Shoemaker and Markolf (17) also described the effects of first sectioning the ACL and then the MCL on the primary tibial rotations due to 10 N-m torques. The cadaveric specimens were tested at full extension and at 20° of flexion with and without compressive loads of 320 and 925 N. Results were reported in terms of increase in total laxity as opposed to separating the internal and external components of tibial rotation.

Figure 4 illustrates the paired increases in torsional laxity at both flexion angles, as reported by Shoemaker and Markolf (17). This figure shows that cutting the ACL caused a significant increase in the total torsional laxity only at full extension; results were not affected by application of joint load. Figure 4 also shows that further cutting the MCL produced significant increases in torsional laxity. These increases were larger than those obtained after an isolated cut of the MCL. Also, Shoemaker and Markolf (17) reported that the increases in torsional laxity after sectioning the MCL in ACL-deficient knees were approximately 20% less in the presence of joint load.

Contradictory to the findings of Kennedy and Fowler, Nielsen and Helmig (14), Nielsen et al. (11), and Haimes et al. (6) showed that a combined injury to the medial structures and the ACL will produce an increase in anterior displacement and external rotation in the flexed position. These data suggest that clinical detections of such lesions would require performing the anterior drawer test at 60° or more flexion, with the tibia in an externally rotated position.

Varus-Valgus Angulations

The data reported by Nielsen et al. (11) and Haimes et al. (6) suggest that an injury to the MCL in ACL-deficient knees causes valgus instability which increases with flexion.

Nielsen et al. (11) measured the knee movements caused by the application of varus-valgus torques of 3 N-m in cadaveric specimens at various flexion angles. As shown in Fig. 5, Nielsen et al. reported that cutting the entire ACL caused small valgus instability, maximal at 30° of flexion. They found no changes in varus rotations. Resecting the MCL caused substantially larger valgus rotations when valgus torques were applied to the tibia. These increases in valgus rotations became larger with flexion, but were not present at extension.

Using ab/adduction moments of 20 N-m, Haimes et al. (6) reported that cutting the MCL in ACL-deficient knees caused a significantly increased abduction at all flexion angles except at full extension.

The Lateral Extraarticular Structures

Clinically, the lateral structures are most often involved in complex knee injuries. While several studies have focused on the importance of the lateral compart-

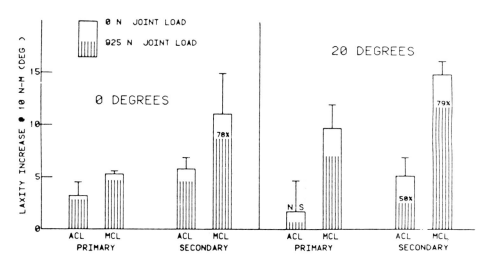

FIG. 4. Mean increases in torsional laxity after the primary and secondary section of the ACL and MCL ligaments. Increases for unloaded specimens are represented by *open bars* (with 1 SD shown); those for loaded specimens are represented by *shaded bars*. The percentage values shown represent significant (*p* < 0.05) proportions of an increase in laxity under load; the larger the percentage shown, the smaller the effect of joint load in limiting laxity. Bars without percentage values indicate that the paired increases in laxity with and without joint load were not significantly different. *NS* above a bar indicates that the increase in laxity under no load was not statistically significant. (From ref. 17, with permission.)

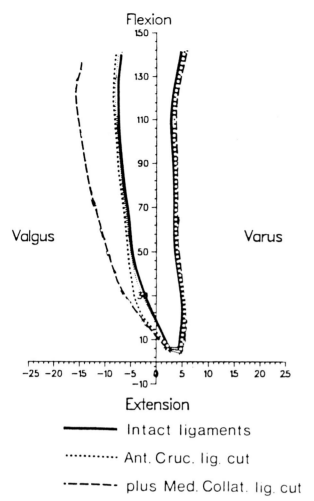

Valgus

Varus

Extension

———— Intact ligaments

·········· Ant. Cruc. lig. cut

– – – – plus Med. Collat. lig. cut

FIG. 5. A mobility pattern showing valgus-varus instability after the successive cutting of the ACL and MCL. (From ref. 11, with permission.)

ment, few studies have reported changes in knee motions of ACL-deficient knees with and without lateral extraarticular injuries.

The lateral structures include the lateral collateral ligament, iliotibial band, and midlateral capsule (anterolateral structures—ALS) and the posterolateral structures (PLS), consisting of the popliteus tendon and posterolateral capsule. It is hard to compare the data reported by various researchers on the evaluation of the ACL-deficient knee with extraarticular injuries since, to our knowledge, no two identically systematic and related studies have been reported in the literature.

Anterior Translations

The data reported by Wroble et al. (21) have shown the importance of the ALS in controlling anterior translation in ACL-deficient knees at 90° flexion. Tibiofemoral motions were determined after application of 100 N of anterior and posterior force when lateral structures were sectioned in ACL-deficient knees. Wroble et

al. (21) reported that cutting the ALS in ACL-deficient knees increased anterior translation in flexion, as shown in Fig. 6. However, increases in motion were highly variable, reflecting the variation in LCL and PLS function.

Wroble et al. (21) also reported that cutting either the LCL or PLS in ACL-deficient knees produced small, statistically significant increases in the anterior translation which were not clinically significant. These data suggest that the LCL acts as a secondary restraint to anterior translation in flexion when the ALS is injured. Wroble et al. (21) also found that cutting the LCL/PLS in an ACL-deficient knee increased anterior translation primarily in extension (Fig. 7), which increased the difference in anterior translation between 20° and 90° flexion. In contrast, cutting the LCL/ALS in an ACL-deficient knee produced larger increases in flexion, thereby decreasing the difference in anterior translation between 20° and 90°. A combined cut of the LCL/ALS/PLS in ACL-deficient knees also produced larger increases in anterior translation in flexion.

A significant finding in the Wroble et al. (21) data is the increased anterior translation of similar magnitude at all flexion angles from 15° to 90°, which is associated with an injury to the ALS in an ACL-deficient knee. This increased anterior laxity is differentiated from the laxity associated with an isolated injury to the ACL because the latter is characterized by an increased anterior translation that reaches a maximum at 30° and decreases substantially at higher flexion angles.

Axial Tibial Rotations

The data obtained from various studies (10,13,21) indicate that greater rotatory instability occurs after combined injury to the lateral structures and the ACL than after injury of the ACL alone. Wroble et al. (21), Lipke et al. (10), and Nielsen et al. (13) have shown that anterolateral (anterior translation of the lateral tibial plateau that occurs with internal rotation) and anteromedial (anterior translation of the medial tibial plateau that occurs with external rotation) rotational instabilities increase in an ACL-deficient knee after the cutting of the extraarticular lateral structures.

The Lipke et al. (10) study was one of several that applied compressive forces to the joint simulating body weight or muscle forces. This study and others prevented ab/aduction and flexion-extension motions while applying rotatory forces. In their study, Lipke et al. (10) designed an apparatus that does not restrict motion in either the sagittal or coronal plane, while applying tibial rotations. In the experiment, flexion changed from zero to 40° of flexion by varying the quadriceps force. Internal-external torques of 15 N-m were applied through a tibial axial rotation mechanism. Ligament sectioning included the ACL, the LCL, and the posterolateral complex.

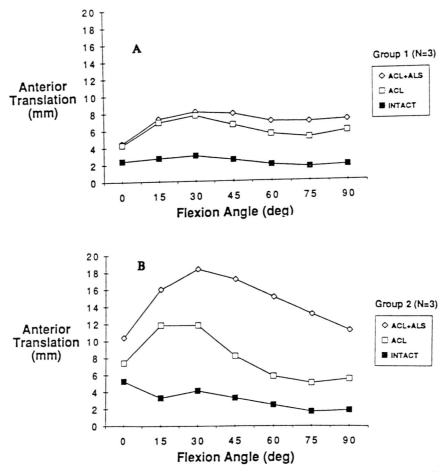

FIG. 6. Limits of anterior translation of 100 N of anterior force for intact specimens, with ACL cut, and with ACL-ALS cut. **A:** In these specimens, anterior translation in the intact state was low and, with the sectioning of the ACL, moderate increases were found throughout the range of motion. Further sectioning of the ALS produced less than 3 mm of increase in anterior translation, predominantly in the flexed knee. **B:** In this group of specimens, anterior translation in the intact state was higher than in Group 1 at low flexion angles. After the cutting of the ACL, anterior translation was markedly increased in the 15° to 30° flexion angle. After the ALS was further sectioned, large anterior translation increases were found at all flexion angles. (From ref. 21, with permission.)

Lipke et al. (10) reported that resecting the ACL caused statistically significant increases in internal rotations, which increased further after they cut the LCL and the posterolateral complex. This would indicate that increased internal rotation of the tibia is detected in ACL-deficient knees. Lipke et al. concluded that the ACL must be insufficient for anterolateral rotational instability to occur (anterior translation of the lateral tibial plateau that occurs with internal rotation). They also concluded that this instability is increased by cutting the LCL and the posterolateral complex. Additionally, Lipke et al. found that external rotations were not statistically affected until the posterolateral complex was injured. As a result, they concluded that anteromedial instability is present only when the posterolateral complex is sectioned.

Wroble et al. (21) measured the changes in limits of tibial axial rotation motion of the ACL-deficient knees

by applying 5 N-m of internal and external moments to the tibia. Wroble et al. (21), consistent with Lipke et al. (10), reported that, for external rotation, significant increases occurred only after a combined resection of the ACL, LCL, and the posterolateral complex. These data, shown in Fig. 8, suggest that the LCL and the posterolateral complex act in concert as a secondary restraint to external rotation.

The results reported by Wroble et al. (21), shown in Fig. 9, indicate that the ALS was important in controlling internal rotation in the flexed knee because there was a consistent increase in the motion when only the ALS was cut in the ACL-deficient knee. The ALS appeared to be less important in controlling anterior translation and internal rotation in extension. This may be explained by the anatomy of the iliotibial band, the main component of the ALS. In extension, fibers of the iliotibial band are poorly oriented to resist anterior transla-

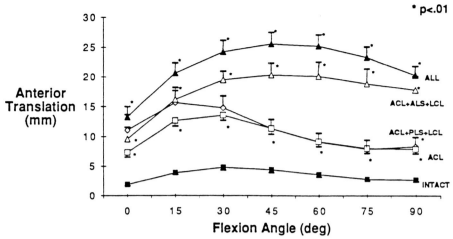

FIG. 7. Limits of anterior translation with 100 N of anterior force for intact specimens and with the ACL, ACL/PLS/LCL, ACL/ALS/LCL, and ALL structures (ACL/ALS/LCL/PLS) cut. Increases in anterior translation with the sectioning of the ACL are statistically significant at all flexion angles. For the ACL/PLS/LCL cut state, the only statistically significant increase was at 0° flexion. For the ACL/ALS/LCL cut state, increases were statistically significant at 15° flexion and above. Increases for the ALL cut state were statistically significant at all flexion angles. Anterior translation for a posterolateral injury is greater at 30° than 90° flexion, but for an anterolateral injury, anterior translation at 30° and 90° flexion is approximately equal. The large effect of the ALS on anterior translation in the flexed knee is seen when the ALS is sectioned in the ACL/PLS/LCL-deficient specimens at 90° (the ALL cut state). (From ref. 21, with permission.)

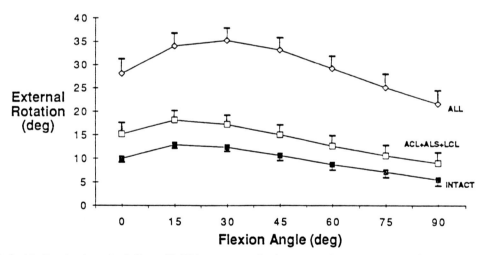

FIG. 8. Limits of external rotation with 5 N-m moment for intact specimens and with ACL/ALS/LCL and ALL structures (ACL/ALS/LCL/PLS) cut. Statistically significant increases were found at all flexion angles for both cut states. The difference between the ACL/ALS/LCL and ACL/ALS/LCL/PLS curves represents the restraining function of the PLS toward external rotation. Note that increases occur at all flexion angles. (From ref. 21, with permission.)

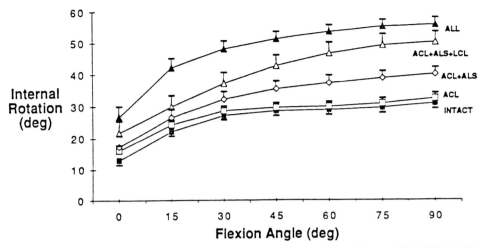

FIG. 9. Limits of internal rotation with 5 N-m for intact specimens and with the ACL, ACL/ALS, ACL/ALS/LCL, and ALL structures (ACL/ALS/LCL/PLS) cut. Increases in internal rotation with a cut ACL are statistically significant, but the magnitude of these increases are small. With ACL/ALS sectioning, increases in internal rotation are statistically significant at 30° flexion and above. Statistically significant increases are found at 15° flexion and above with the ACL/ALS/LCL and at all flexion angles for the ALL cut case. The effect of the PLS on restraining internal rotation in the extended knee can be seen by comparing the ACL/ALS/LCL curve and the ALL cut curve. The difference between these curves reflects sectioning the PLS. The largest differences are found at 15° and 30° flexion. (From ref. 21, with permission.)

tion and internal rotation since they are perpendicular to the anterior-posterior translation axis and parallel to the axis of tibial rotation. In flexion, fibers of the iliotibial band are situated in an ideal position to resist anterior translation and internal rotation since they become oriented parallel to the anterior/posterior translation axis and perpendicular to the internal rotation axis.

Contrary to the Wroble et al. data, Lipke et al. (10) found an increase in internal rotation after injury of the ACL, further increasing when the LCL was also damaged. The Wroble et al. data are generally consistent with the results of Nielsen et al. (11,12) and Gollehon et al. (4), who reported no change in tibial rotation with ACL sectioning. Figure 10 shows the results reported by Nielsen et al. (11) in the study they conducted to determine the rotatory instability after the cutting of the ACL, alone or together with the collateral ligaments. Figure 10 shows that no increases in tibial rotations were found after the cutting of the ACL. Figure 10 also shows that the further cutting of the LCL produced an increase in internal rotation of the anterolateral type in the 50 to 90° range of knee flexion; and an increase in the external rotation of the posterolateral type, which increased with the amount of flexion, but decreased (localized) at about 80° of flexion.

In summary, injury to the ALS in ACL-deficient knee was found to increase internal rotation at 90° flexion, while a combined injury to the LCL and PLS in ACL-deficient knees was found to increase external rotation at all flexion angles. Grood et al. (5) noted similar increases in external rotation at 90° flexion after a combined in-

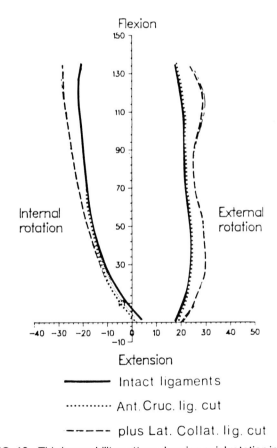

FIG. 10. This is a mobility pattern showing axial rotation instability after the successive cutting of the ACL and LCL. Internal and external rotation correspond to anterolateral and posterolateral rotation, respectively. (From ref. 11, with permission.)

jury to the LCL and PLS in PCL-deficient knees. Grood et al. (5) found that significantly more external rotation can be identified at 0° flexion in knees with an ACL/ PLS/LCL injury than in knees with PCL/PLS/LCL or PLS/LCL injuries.

Combining the results describing the changes in anterior translation and tibial axial rotation that occur after an injury to the lateral extraarticular structures in ACL-deficient knee can be used in the diagnosis of combined injuries to the ACL. In isolated ACL injuries, there is a significant increase in the anterior translation at 30° of flexion. Findings of increased anterior translation in flexion and extension and increased internal rotation at 90° flexion are consistent with an injury to the ALS in an ACL-deficient knee. With a combined injury to the ACL, LCL, and ALS, the increased anterior translation occurs at all flexion angles, along with an associated increase in internal rotation at 90° flexion. A combined injury to the ACL, LCL, and PLS is characterized by large increases in external rotation at all flexion angles. These findings demonstrate the potential usefulness of clinical tests of internal and external rotation. Internal rotation tests performed at 90° of flexion can be used to test the intactness of the iliotibial band in ACL-deficient knees; external rotation tests performed at 30 or 90° can be used to test the intactness of the LCL and PLS.

Varus-Valgus Angulations

Nielsen et al. (11) and Wroble et al. (21) have reported that an injury to the lateral extraarticular structures in ACL-deficient knee produces varus instability, thereby indicating that the primary function of these structures is to restrain adduction.

The results reported by Nielsen et al. (11) are shown in Fig. 11. These results indicate that cutting the LCL in ACL-deficient knees caused a 5° to 10° increase in varus rotations, maximal at about 60° of flexion, when varus torques were applied to the tibia. Furthermore, Fig. 11 indicates that a pivot shift (i.e., anterolateral subluxation of the tibia) was always produced when torques were applied to force the tibia into valgus. Wroble et al. (21) also reported that cutting the LCL in ACL-deficient knees produced large increases in adduction. Additional cuts beyond the LCL caused these increases to become larger at all flexion angles. Wroble et al. (21) found that combined ACL/LCL/ALS cuts resulted in smaller increases in extension than combined ACL/LCL/PLS cuts, apparently due to the tautness of the posterolateral structures in full extension.

The Nielsen et al. data (11) suggest that an injury to the LCL in ACL-deficient knees causes an increase in external rotations of the posterolateral type, as well as a varus instability and a consistent pivot shift when valgus torques are applied in flexion. The Wroble et al. (21)

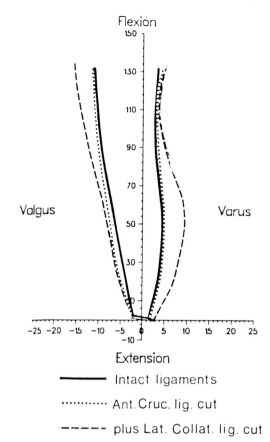

FIG. 11. This is a mobility pattern showing valgus-varus instability after the successive cutting of the ACL and LCL. The apparent valgus instability results from pivot shift. (From ref. 11, with permission.)

data suggest that a combined injury of the PLS and LCL in an ACL-deficient knee is characterized by anterior translation larger in extension than in flexion, increased adduction, and increased external rotation in both flexion and extension.

The Menisci

Noyes et al. (15) reported that meniscal injuries comprise about 60% of the injuries associated with ACL-deficient knees. The results obtained from other studies (9,18) have also supported the clinical observations that the removal of a meniscus from a knee that lacks a functioning ACL has led to a poor surgical result. Levy et al. (9) and Shoemaker and Markolf (18) concluded that in ACL-deficient knees, medial meniscectomy compromises knee stability by allowing additional anterior displacement (9,18).

Levy et al. (9) used the knee testing apparatus developed by Fukubayashi et al. (3) to apply anterior-posterior forces to cadaveric knees. Table 1 lists the results obtained by Levy et al. (9), describing the effects of medial meniscectomy on anterior-posterior tibial dis-

TABLE 1. *Means and standard deviations of the anterior tibial displacement resulting from a force of 100 Newtons in intact knees*

Flexion angle (degrees)	Anterior displacement (mm)		
	Intact (n = 18)	ACL[a] sectioned (n = 10)	ACL sectioned and MM[a] excised (n = 8)
0	4.3 ± 1.6	11.4 ± 4.3	10.4 ± 4.4
30	5.9 ± 2.0	17.4 ± 4.1	21.8 ± 3.9
60	5.4 ± 1.7	16.6 ± 6.8	22.3 ± 3.7
90	4.8 ± 1.4	13.8 ± 5.3	19.7 ± 3.6

These measurements occurred after the resection of the anterior cruciate ligament (ACL) and after a combined cut of the ACL and the medial meniscus. Extracted from *J Bone Joint Surg [Am]*, 64-A: 883–888, 1982.

[a] ACL, anterior cruciate ligament; MM, medial meniscus.

placements before and after the section of the ACL. Anterior displacements were greatest at 30° of knee flexion in intact knees. No statistically significant differences were found in anterior or posterior displacements after the resection of the medial meniscus. As expected, large increases in anterior displacements were found to occur after the cutting of the ACL.

Table 1 shows that further resection of the medial meniscus caused further increases in the anterior tibial displacement at all flexion angles. The greatest and smallest increases occurred at 90° and zero° of flexion, respectively.

Shoemaker and Markolf (18) conducted a study to determine the effects of meniscal injuries on the anterior-

posterior laxity of ACL-deficient cadaveric specimens at 20° of flexion with and without tibial-femoral compressive contact forces. The experimental apparatus utilized by Shoemaker and Markolf (18) did not permit tibial rotation, anterior-posterior forces of 200, 100 and 50 N were applied to the tibia. Compressive load levels were set at 320 and 925 N. The testing sequence included the sectioning of the ACL, creating a bucket-handle tear in the medial meniscus, removing the bucket-handle fragment without damaging the attachments of the horns, removing the rest of the medial meniscus, and performing a complete lateral meniscectomy.

The results obtained by Shoemaker and Markolf (18) are summarized in Table 2. As expected, cutting the ACL caused large, statistically significant increases in anterior translation at all three levels of anterior force, and at all three levels of joint compressions. Shoemaker and Markolf's data (18) (listed in Table 2) indicate that the role of the menisci in controlling anterior translation of the tibia in ACL-deficient knees depends on the amount of both the applied anterior force and the joint load.

Shoemaker and Markolf (18) found that at 200 N of applied tibial force, removal of the bucket-handle fragment did not significantly affect the anterior translation at all levels of joint compression. However, small (10%) but statistically significant increases in the translation were observed after medial meniscectomy; comparable increases were noted after subsequent lateral meniscectomy. For an unloaded ACL-deficient knee, anterior displacement increased by 4 mm after bilateral meniscectomy. These values are comparable with the Levy et al.

TABLE 2. *Means and standard deviations of the anterior tibial displacement for three levels of applied anterior force without joint load and at two levels of compression force in the intact state*

Condition of the specimen	±200 N AP[a] force			±100 N AP force			±50 N AP force		
	0 N[b]	320 N	925 N	0 N	320 N	925 N	0 N	320 N	925 N
Intact	11.3 (±0.6)	11.0 (±1.0)	10.7 (±1.0)	8.7 (±0.8)	8.3 (±0.8)	7.2 (±0.8)	7.2 (±0.8)	6.0 (±0.6)	3.3 (±0.6)[c]
Anterior cruciate ligament sectioned	23.1 (±3.2)[c]	22.9 (±3.2)[c]	21.3 (±4.1)[c]	19.7 (±3.3)[c]	18.6 (±4.0)[c]	11.3 (±3.8)	17.0 (±3.5)[c]	10.7 (±3.5)	4.3 (±1.7)[c]
Bucket-handle tear of medial meniscus removed	23.5 (±3.3)[c]	23.5 (±3.3)[c]	22.7 (±3.7)[c]	20.2 (±3.5)[c]	19.9 (±3.8)[c]	17.3 (±5.1)	17.8 (±3.8)[c]	15.1 (±4.9)	8.1 (±3.3)
Total medial meniscectomy	24.8 (±3.2)	24.8 (±3.2)	24.3 (±3.3)	21.6 (±3.5)	21.5 (±3.5)	19.4 (±4.6)	19.1 (±3.7)	18.1 (±4.9)[c]	13.0 (±4.0)[c]
Bilateral meniscectomy	26.7 (±3.7)	26.9 (±3.5)	26.2 (±3.5)	23.3 (±3.7)	23.2 (±3.5)	21.5 (±3.8)	20.8 (±3.7)	19.4 (±2.3)[c]	12.7 (±6.5)[c]

These measurements occurred after removal of the anterior cruciate ligament, after removal of a bucket-handle tear of the medial meniscus, after total medial meniscectomy, and after bilateral meniscectomy. Mean for six specimens plus or minus one standard deviation. Extracted from *J Bone Joint Surg [Am]*, 68-A: 71–79, 1986.

[a] AP, anteroposterior.

[b] Joint load.

[c] Except where indicated (NS = not significant), all differences are significant.

data (9) (listed in Table 1), showing an increase of 4 mm in anterior displacement at 100 N after medial meniscectomy in ACL-deficient knees at 30° of flexion. Shoemaker and Markolf's translations are smaller since tibial rotations were constrained during the application of the anterior forces. As shown in Table 2, Shoemaker and Markolf (18) also reported that at 50 N of applied tibial force, the translations of the loaded specimens were always significantly smaller than those for unloaded specimens at comparable stages of meniscal sectioning. Furthermore, at 50 N of applied load, significant increases in anterior translations were noted after the removal of the bucket-handle tear and completion of the medial meniscectomy. Further removal of the lateral meniscus did not cause a significant increase in the translation at this low level of applied force.

The Levy et al. (9) and Shoemaker and Markolf (18) data suggest that, in ACL-deficient knees, anterior displacement of the tibia causes the posterior horn of the medial meniscus to move anteriorly until it becomes wedged between the tibial plateau and the femoral condyle. When this occurs, the medial meniscus acts as a stop, thereby preventing further anterior tibial displacements. This indicates that the medial meniscus serves as a secondary restraint to anterior displacement of the tibia. Removing the medial meniscus in the ACL-deficient knee produces additional anterior displacement that lessens its stability.

SUMMARY

1. In ACL-deficient knees, the medial extraarticular structures resist anterior translation and valgus rotation at all flexion angles and resist external rotation in flexion.
2. In ACL-deficient knees, the lateral collateral ligament and the posterolateral structures (popliteus tendon and posterolateral capsule) resist anterior translation in extension, while the iliotibial band and the midlateral capsule resist anterior translation from 15° to 90° of knee flexion.
3. In ACL-deficient knees, the lateral collateral ligament and the posterolateral structures resist external rotation and varus rotation at all flexion angles, while the iliotibial band and the midlateral capsule resist internal rotation in flexion.
4. In ACL-deficient knees, the medial meniscus resists anterior translation at all flexion angles.

REFERENCES

1. Bray RC, Flanagan JP, Dandy DJ. (1988): Reconstruction for chronic anterior cruciate instability: a comparison of two methods after six years. *J Bone Joint Surg [Br]*, 70B:100–105.
2. Clancy WG, Ray JM, Zoltan DJ. (1988): Acute tears of the anterior cruciate ligament: surgical versus conservative treatment. *J Bone Joint Surg [Am]*, 70A:1483–1488.
3. Fukubayashi T, Torzilli PA, Sherman MF, Warren RF. (1982): An *in-vitro* biomechanical evaluation of anterior-posterior motion of the knee: tibial displacement, rotation and torque. *J Bone Joint Surg [Am]*, 64A:258–264.
4. Gollehon DL, Torzilli PA, Warren RF. (1987): The role of the posterolateral and cruciate ligaments in the stability of the human knee: a biomechanical study. *J Bone Joint Surg [Am]*, 69A:233–242.
5. Grood ES, Stowers SF, Noyes FR. (1988): Limits of movement in the human knee: effects of sectioning the posterior cruciate ligament and posterolateral structures. *J Bone Joint Surg [Am]*, 78A:88–97.
6. Haimes JL, Grood ES, Wroble RR, Noyes FR. Limits of motion in the human knee: role of the medial structures in the intact and anterior cruciate ligament deficient knee. Unpublished manuscript.
7. Johnson RJ, Beynnon BD, Nichols CE, Renstrom AFH. (1992): Current concepts review: the treatment of injuries of the anterior cruciate ligament. *J Bone Joint Surg [Am]*, 74A:140–151.
8. Kennedy JC, Fowler PJ. (1971): Medial and anterior instability of the knee: an anatomical and clinical study using stress machines. *J Bone Joint Surg [Am]*, 53A:1257–1270.
9. Levy IM, Torzilli PA, Warren RF. (1982): The effect of medial meniscectomy on anterior-posterior motion of the knee. *J Bone Joint Surg [Am]*, 64A:883–888.
10. Lipke JM, Janecki CJ, Nelson CL, McLeod P, Thompson C, Thompson J, Haynes DW. (1981): The role of incompetence of the anterior cruciate and lateral ligaments in anterolateral and anteromedial instability. *J Bone Joint Surg [Am]*, 63A:954–960.
11. Nielsen S, Ovesen J, Rasmussen O. (1984): The anterior cruciate ligament on the knee: an experimental study of its importance in rotatory knee instability. *Arch Orthop Trauma Surg*, 103:170–174.
12. Nielsen S, Kromann-Andersen C, Rasmussen O, Andersen K. (1984): Instability of cadaver knees after transection of capsule and ligaments. *Acta Orthop Scand*, 55:30–34.
13. Nielsen S, Rasmussen O, Ovesen J, Andersen K. (1984): Rotatory instability of cadaver knees after transection of collateral ligaments and capsule. *Arch Orthop Trauma Surg*, 103:165–169.
14. Nielsen S, Helmig P. (1985): Instability of knees with ligament lesions: cadaver studies of the anterior cruciate ligament. *Acta Orthop Scand*, 56:426–429.
15. Noyes FR, Bassett RW, Grood ES, Butler DL. (1980): Arthroscopy in acute traumatic hemarthrosis of the knee: incidence of anterior cruciate tears and other injuries. *J Bone Joint Surg [Am]*, 62A:687–695.
16. Noyes FR, Grood ES, Torzilli PA. (1989): Current concepts review: the definitions of terms for motion and position of the knee and injuries of the ligaments. *J Bone Joint Surg [Am]*, 71A:465–472.
17. Shoemaker SC, Markolf KL. (1985): Effects of joint load on the stiffness and laxity of ligament-deficient knees: an *in vitro* study of the anterior cruciate and medial collateral ligament. *J Bone Joint Surg [Am]*, 67A:136–146.
18. Shoemaker SC, Markolf KL. (1986): The role of the meniscus in the anterior-posterior stability of the loaded anterior cruciate-deficient knee: effects of partial versus total excision. *J Bone Joint Surg [Am]*, 68A:71–79.
19. Sullivan D, Levy IM, Sheskier S, Torzilli PA, Warren RF. (1984): Medial restraints to anterior-posterior motion of the knee. *J Bone Joint Surg [Am]*, 66A:930–936.
20. Wroble RR, Brand RA. (1990): Paradoxes in the history of the anterior cruciate ligament. *Clin Orthop Rel Res*, No. 259, 183–191.
21. Wroble RR, Grood ES, Cummings JS, Henderson JM, Noyes FR. (1993): The role of the lateral extra-articular restraints in the anterior cruciate ligament deficient knee. *Am J Sports Medicine* 21(2):257–263.

The Anterior Cruciate Ligament: Current and
Future Concepts, edited by D.W. Jackson, et al.
Raven Press, Ltd., New York © 1993.

CHAPTER 13

Functional Evaluation of Normal and ACL-Deficient Knee Using Gait Analysis Techniques

Thomas P. Andriacchi

It has been well documented that the anterior cruciate ligament provides stability and influences the overall kinematics of the knee (13,16,20). There is increasing evidence that there is an interaction between the load or strain in the ACL and patterns of muscle activation (11,16,25). Thus, it is not surprising that loss of the ACL can cause changes in ambulatory function. The variable natural history of the unrepaired ACL is consistent with reported changes in ambulatory function associated with loss of the anterior cruciate ligament. For example, it has been reported that approximately one-third of the patients who had an anterior cruciate deficient knee compensated enough to pursue recreational activities, another third compensated but had to discontinue many activities, and one-third had poorer function (21,22). Perhaps, even the long-term degenerative changes following loss of the ACL can be related to the type of functional changes that are seen in some patients following loss of the ACL.

Treatment of the ruptured anterior cruciate ligament is often complicated by the difficulty in predicting from passive physical examination of the knee which patients will be functionally impaired by the loss of this ligament and which patients will have minimum symptoms. In addition to the initial functional losses which occur primarily during more stressful activities such as running and cutting, long-term degenerative changes to the knee have been demonstrated in subjects following loss of the ACL (1,15–19) in spite of the fact that active athletic participation had been avoided or abandoned. Several studies evaluating both surgical and nonsurgical treatment modalities (7,10,14) have demonstrated immediate improvement in stability to the knee joint following a

number of different types of ACL reconstruction. The long-term efficacy of the various procedures for ACL reconstruction is still unclear. However, it is clear that restoration of function in the short term and prevention of long-term pathological changes to the knee are among the primary goals in the treatment of an ACL rupture. Current methods of clinical examination do not provide an adequate objective assessment of either of these primary treatment goals. The ability to assess the probability of future degenerative changes associated with loss of the anterior cruciate ligament would be extremely valuable in treatment planning and evaluation of the ACL-deficient patients.

Future improvements in methods of treatment should be built upon an ability to objectively assess new procedures. Wroble and Brand (28) have indicated that there is a lack of natural history of long-term follow-up in much of the literature related to the anterior cruciate ligament. They emphasize the need for objective scientific data about the mechanics and function of the ACL on which sound scientific principles can be established for the functional assessment and treatment of patients with ACL loss. It is obviously important to understand the biomechanics associated with functional changes following loss of the ACL. A number of studies have demonstrated that joint loading and muscle loading are directly related and substantially influenced by the way in which an individual ambulates (4,23,25,26). The purpose of this chapter is to examine the way in which gait analysis can be used to improve our understanding of the functional role of the anterior cruciate ligament.

METHODS OF GAIT ANALYSIS

Appropriate technology and instrumentation to conduct functional testing is available from a number of

T. P. Andriacchi: Department of Orthopedic Surgery, Rush-Presbyterian-St. Luke's Medical Center, Chicago, Illinois 60612.

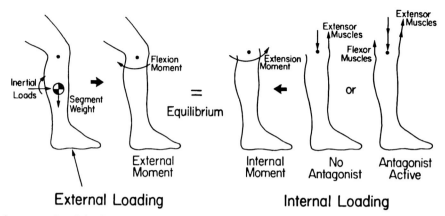

FIG. 1. An example of the balance between external loading producing a moment tending to flex the knee in an equal magnitude (opposite direction) internal moment tending to extend the knee. The internal extension moment is produced by quadriceps contraction (no antagonist) or the net moment produced by the difference between quadriceps contraction and antagonist hamstring contraction.

sources. The availability of this automated instrumentation, however, is not sufficient to provide relevant tests without appropriate protocols and the ability to interpret the complex measurement generated by these tests.

The methodological approach taken for the examples (8,9) in this presentation has been previously described (3–5). Briefly, the lower extremity is idealized as a collection of rigid links with fixed axes of rotation at the joints (12). The ground reaction forces, limb segment masses and inertia are used to calculate joint moments and forces. The basic components of the measurement system include a force platform, optoelectronic system for motion measurement and a computer. The primary limitation of the system was marker movement artifact due to skin movement, a problem common to all systems that require placement of external devices on the skin to measure internal movement of bony segments. Skin motion and joint center approximations will limit the ultimate resolution of measurements of limb kinematics and kinetics. Thus, care must be taken in the appropriate interpretation of these measurements to avoid artifactual effects due to system approximations.

The functional analysis presented here will focus on the moments acting at the knee joint. Previous studies (2–5,8) have demonstrated that these measurements can be interpreted in terms of the loads on muscles, passive soft tissue and joint surfaces. In addition, the joint moments have been shown (4,23,26) to be sensitive indicators of differences between normal and abnormal function.

It is useful to examine the assumptions used as the basis for the interpretation of the joint moments during function. The reader should note that the measurements used to calculate the joint moments are external to the limb and include the ground reaction force, limb segment weight and limb segment inertia (12). Mechanical equilibrium dictates that external forces and moments

must be balanced by internal forces and moments. Forces generated by muscle, passive soft tissue, and joint contact force create these internal moments. If muscles act only synergistically to balance external moments, then one could directly infer internal muscle force in synergistic muscle groupings such as total quadriceps force to balance an external moment tending to flex the knee joint (4). However, if antagonistic muscle activity is present, the external moment reflects the net balance between agonist and antagonist (Fig. 1). The flexion-extension moment at the knee will be described in terms of the net muscular moment which is the differential between antagonist and agonist muscles when inferred from external moment measurements. Thus, if the external moment measured in the laboratory tends to flex the knee, this is described as a "net" demand on the quadriceps to maintain equilibrium. Similarly, a moment that tends to extend the knee is described as a "net" hamstrings moment.

FUNCTIONAL CHANGES AND THE ACL-DEFICIENT KNEE

Functional abnormalities have been reported in patients with arthroscopically documented isolated deficiency of the anterior cruciate ligament when tested (8,9) during level walking, jogging, ascending and descending stairs. The patients were compared with normal subjects tested with identical protocols. Data were collected for the affected and normal limbs of the patients and both extremities for the control subjects. A biomechanical analysis of the functional differences between patients and normal subjects provides important insight into the biomechanics and clinical importance of the ACL.

The measure that demonstrated the greatest change from normal was the flexion-extension moment at the knee. The typical pattern of flexion-extension moment at the knee during normal gait has a number of key features which are highly reproducible during normal gait. The key features include an external moment tending to extend the knee joint (knee flexor muscle demand), as the knee moves into midstance, the external moment reverses its direction (demanding net quadriceps force), as the knee passes midstance the moment again reverses its direction demanding net flexor muscle contraction, and finally, in the preswing phase, the moment tends to flex the knee (demanding net quadriceps muscle contraction) (Fig. 2). Changes from this normal pattern are indicative of changes in the activation patterns of the quadriceps and hamstrings during normal gait.

The patients with the ACL-deficient knee had a significantly lower than normal net quadriceps moment during the middle portion of the stance phase of walking. This type gait has been interpreted as a tendency to avoid or reduce the demand on the quadriceps muscle and has been called a "quadriceps avoidance" (4,8). This "quadriceps avoidance" in ACL-deficient patients may seem surprising since the demands on the quadriceps muscle are relatively low during walking. However, despite the relatively low loads on the knee that occurred during level walking, 75% of the patients studied had the "quadriceps avoidance" gait while 25% had a normal biphasic flexion-extension moment. It is important to note that the magnitude of the moment change during walking between normal subjects and patients was more than 100%.

Patients also had changes in the magnitude of the net quadriceps moment during jogging. However, the greatest percentage of changes from normal was during walking. Thus, the adaptations did not appear to be related to the magnitude of the net quadriceps moment. The net quadriceps moment was approximately 4.5 times greater (in normal subjects) during jogging and when compared to level walking. Patients had approximately a 25% reduction in the net quadriceps moment during jogging and more than a 100% reduction during level walking (Fig. 3). Interestingly, during both the walking and jogging activities the adaptation in the cruciate deficient limb was also evident in the contralateral limb of the patients who developed the functional adaptations. As a result, the magnitude of the moments about the knee in the affected and unaffected limb did not significantly differ during walking or jogging (8). During stair climbing, where the net quadriceps moment was still substantially larger than level walking, the patients and normal subjects had essentially the same pattern and magnitude of quadriceps moment.

The observation that the quadriceps moment had its greatest reduction during level walking when compared to other more stressful activities such as jogging or stair climbing can be explained by examining the relationship between the patellar mechanism and anterior cruciate ligament strain. It has been shown that quadriceps contraction when the knee is near full extension will place strain on the anterior cruciate ligament (6). The strain on the anterior cruciate ligament is caused by the anterior pull of the patellar tendon when the knee is near full extension. Thus, in an ACL-deficient knee, quadriceps

Knee Flexion Moments

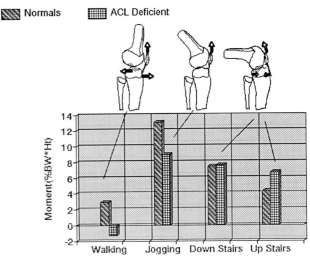

FIG. 3. A comparison of the peak magnitudes of the quadriceps moment during walking, jogging, and stair climbing demonstrates the greatest percentage change in the quadriceps moment during walking. There is a slight reduction during jogging and no significant change during stair climbing. The angle of knee flexion where the maximum quadriceps moment occurs during each activity is shown to illustrate the pull of the patellar tendon where maximum quadriceps contraction occurs for each of these activities.

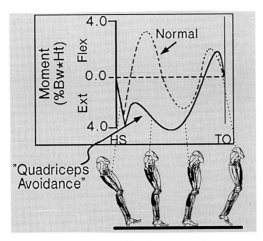

FIG. 2. The normal pattern of flexion-extension moment during the stance phase of walking. Normal subjects walked in a way that produces an oscillating pattern between flexion and extension during stance phase. The majority of the patients with ACL-deficient knees developed a pattern of gait where the flexion-extension moment tends to reduce or avoid the net quadriceps moment. This pattern has been described as a "quadriceps avoidance" gait.

contraction will produce an anteriorly directed force on the tibia when the knee is near full extension. The anterior pull of the patellar mechanism is reduced as the knee approaches 45° of flexion and reverses beyond 45°. Thus, activities such as level walking where quadriceps activation is required when the knee is near full extension for normal function produced an adaptation in patients with ACL-deficient knees. Whereas, activities such as stair climbing, where there is maximum quadriceps contractions, do not require any adaptation for the ACL-deficient knee since the patellar tendon pulls posteriorly on the tibia at these angles of knee flexion. The adaptations in the ACL-deficient knee were greatest during level walking and produced a pattern of walking that reduced or avoided quadriceps contraction and, thus, eliminated the strain on the secondary restraints that would be necessary to balance the anterior pull of the patellar tendon during quadriceps contraction. These results demonstrated that some patients with ACL-deficient knees adapt their ambulatory function while some do not. The physical characteristics of the adaptations appear consistent with the hypothesis that patients avoid or reduce quadriceps contraction during angles of knee flexion where the quadriceps will produce an anteriorly directed force to the tibia (4,6,8). It has been suggested that this adaptation is associated with a reprogramming of the locomotor process since it is not likely that patients adapt to instability movement of the tibia during each step. It is more likely that the adaptation occurs prior to the instability generated from the muscle contraction so the abnormal anterior drawer or strain on secondary restraints to anterior drawer does not occur during these activities of daily living. Perhaps, in patients who do not develop this adaptation, there is a continual strain on the secondary restraints to anterior drawer (menisci and collaterals) causing continuing stretching of these structures and the eventual degenerative problems reported in some ACL-deficient knees.

THE ANTERIOR CRUCIATE LIGAMENT-DEFICIENT KNEE AND STRESSFUL ACTIVITIES

It is possible that patients who tolerate ACL deficiency during high-demand activities compensate with higher than normal hamstring contraction (Fig. 4) during activities where many patients with ACL deficiency report difficulties. Typically, these activities include twisting, pivoting, and running to a stop. It is difficult, from a practical viewpoint, to quantify muscle contraction dynamically using EMG's. However, as previously discussed, net moment magnitudes can be used to interpret changes in the level of muscle contraction when compared to normal controls. The following example illustrates the use of the joint flexion extension moment to identify the presence of net muscular substitution during

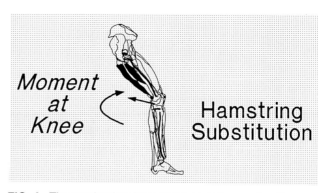

FIG. 4. The mechanism by which hamstring contraction can substitute dynamically for the functional loss of the anterior cruciate ligament.

more stressful activities such as running to a cut and running to a stop.

Patients with ACL deficiency and normal subjects were studied during running to a side-step cut and running to a stop in the gait laboratory (2). The patients were selected on the basis of the history of a trauma of the type associated with an ACL injury and episodes of giving way. The complete rupture of the ACL was confirmed by arthroscopic surgery or at later reconstruction in all subjects. Patients with PCL injury, posterolateral instability, functionally limiting pain, and/or the inability to perform simple activities, running, cutting, or running and stopping maneuvers were excluded from the study.

The patients and control subjects were tested with identical protocols. The cutting maneuver called for each subject running to a specified location (on the force plate) at approximately 2.5 m/sec pace and then cutting at 90° to the direction of progression laterally away from the supporting leg. This maneuver can be described as a lateral side-step cut. The run-to-stop maneuver called for each subject running to a specified location (on the force plate) at approximately a 2.5 m/sec pace and stopping on one limb as if preparing to jump vertically. The external moments were calculated along the axes of flexion-extension, abduction-adduction and internal-external rotation. In addition, knee motion and temporal measurements were quantified. All moments were normalized to the product of body weight times height (bw × ht) to allow comparison among subjects of different sizes.

The typical pattern of flexion-extension moment for both the run-to-stop and run-to-lateral side-step cut activities shows a predominant moment tending to flex the knee (demanding quadriceps muscle balance) during the major portion of since phase. However, the moment tending to extend the knee at the early portion of stance phase was larger in patients with ACL-deficient knees than in normal subjects. This higher extension moment suggests a higher net hamstrings moment and a potential mechanism used in the ACL-deficient knee to compensate for ACL deficiency (Fig. 5). The increased net ham-

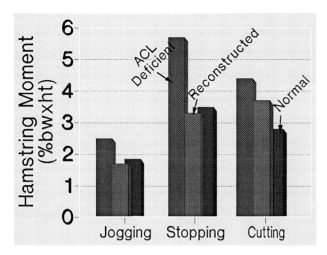

FIG. 5. A comparison of moment magnitudes during running to a cut and running to a stop activity. Patients with ACL-deficient knees tend to compensate by substantially increasing the net hamstring moment during these activities. Following ACL reconstruction, the moments are comparable to normal.

string moment during the early portion of stance phase would dynamically stabilize the knee for the high twisting and adduction moments that occur during these activities. The magnitude of the twisting and adduction moment components during cutting and stopping are substantially higher than those that occur during activities such as level walking. These higher twisting moments may cause the buckling of the knee often reported by the ACL-deficient subject during these activities. Thus, the higher net hamstring moment may be a desirable compensation for the ACL-deficient knee.

Typically, patients with ACL deficiency also tend to reduce the magnitude of the flexion moment and, thus, reduce the net quadriceps moment. The magnitude of the net quadriceps during running is normally five times greater than level walking. This suggests a relatively high demand on the quadriceps muscle when compared to level walking. The reduction of this moment in patients suggests reduced quadriceps strength in the ACL-deficient patients or the presence of antagonistic hamstring activity tending to reduce the net quadriceps moment.

This example suggests that, in the early portion of heel-strike in both the running and cutting and running-to-a-stop activities, the patients develop a higher than normal net hamstring moment in the early portions of the activities. It is possible that the patients activate the hamstring muscles to a greater extent in the early portion of this activity as a preparation for higher rotation in abduction-adduction forces that will occur during the middle portion of that activity. This is likely a method of adaptation that has been developed prior to the particular activity since it requires anticipation of the high loads that will occur later in the activity. It is not likely that the muscles can adapt sufficiently in response to instability generated due to the higher loads which is also due to the rapid onset of the higher loads.

MEDIAL COMPARTMENT LOADING DURING GAIT

The pattern of gait will influence the loading on the knee joint and loading can be related to long-term degenerative changes (23,24,27). Gait abnormalities can be related to loading on the medial compartment of the knee as well as lateral soft tissue structure. It has been shown (23) that a subset of patients with anterior cruciate deficient knees have a higher than normal loading of the medial compartment of the knee based on an analysis of the intrinsic loads acting at the knee during gait. It is useful to look at the mechanics of the knee joint in terms of the factors that influence medial compartment loading during gait.

The external loading (moments and forces) during gait have been used to calculate internal muscle loading and joint loading (25). The sagittal (flexion-extension) and frontal plane (adduction) moments are the primary components contributing to the magnitude of the joint compressive forces, muscle forces and soft tissue stress around the knee joint.

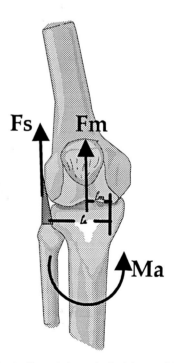

FIG. 6. An illustration of the principal internal forces in the lateral soft tissue structures (Fs) and internal muscle forces (Fm) necessary to balance the external adduction moment (Ma). The force (Fs) acts through the lever arm (L^s), and the muscle force acts through the lever arm (L^m) about the medial compartment. Both of these forces act to prevent lateral compartment lift-off.

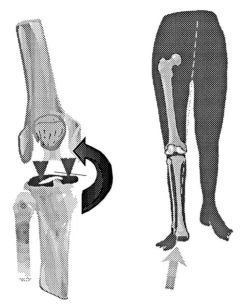

FIG. 7. The adduction moment during walking and its tendency to produce an increased force on the medial compartment of the knee joint. These internal forces are the result of the balance of the muscle and soft tissue forces illustrated in Fig. 6.

It has been shown (23,25) that a critical interaction exists between dynamic muscle forces required to balance the flexion-extension moments and forces in the soft tissue forces needed to stabilize the knee during walking. In particular, the external adducting moment must be balanced by both muscle force and lateral soft tissue pretension in order to maintain contact of both the lateral and medial compartments of the knee (Fig. 6). In the presence of a loss of lateral stability, it is possible for the knee to open up laterally and sustain the entire joint reaction across the medial compartment of the knee joint. Patients with ACL-deficient knees have been examined in the Gait Laboratory and further analyzed using the model to predict the presence of lateral joint opening when lateral instability exists. Patients with combined anterior cruciate ligament deficiency in varus aligned knees can walk in a way where the lateral compartment will open and cause excessively high medial compartment loads (Fig. 7). Lateral lift-off may be associated with the deterioration of the medial compartment in some patients with ACL deficiency and not in others. The condition leading, to lateral lift-off can be identified using quantitative biomechanical testing.

CLOSING COMMENTS

Functional testing can provide unique and important information that is relevant to the treatment and evaluation of the ACL-deficient knee. Quantitative functional testing can supplement clinical examination since it provides information that cannot be obtained from passive physical examination. Further, the information is relevant to the long-term outcome of patients with ACL deficiency and potential pathological changes associated with the ACL-deficient knee. The changes in function associated with the ACL-deficient knee described in this chapter (11,25) are presumably adaptations produced by a subconscious protective mechanism to avoid the excessive anterior displacement of the tibia that can occur in the absence of the anterior cruciate ligament. However, it is not likely that these adaptations are the result of a stimulus that occurs during each cycle of walking for other activities. It is more likely that these adaptations are the result of earlier experiences following the loss of the anterior cruciate ligament. It has been suggested (4) that there is reprogramming of the locomotor process such that the adaptations occur before excessive anterior displacement results. Thus, the adaptations anticipate the instability and, thus, avoid through muscular substitution or avoidance of the external forces producing instability, the actual abnormal displacement.

Testing of ambulatory function or gait analysis is particularly relevant to the ACL-deficient population. The appropriate selection of treatment modalities, rehabilitation and evaluation of patients following treatment can be greatly enhanced through appropriate use of functional testing. These results suggest that all patients do not adapt in the same manner to the loss of the anterior cruciate ligament. It has been shown in other studies (24,27) that the nature of the functional adaptation quantified during gait analysis can be extremely useful in the treatment planning and selection of patients for particular procedures. It is likely that clinical testing of ambulatory function will improve the outcome of treatment or rehabilitation.

REFERENCES

1. Andersson C, Odensten LR, Grood L, GIllquist J. (1989): Surgical or non-surgical treatment of fracture rupture of the ACL: a randomized study with long-term followup. *J Bone Joint Surg,* 71:965–974.
2. Andriacchi TP, Kramer GM, Landon GC. (1985): The biomechanics of running and knee injuries. In: Finerman G, ed. *American Academy of Orthopaedic Surgeons Symposium on Sport Medicine: The Knee.* St. Louis, MO: CV Mosby, pp 23–32.
3. Andriacchi TP, Andersson GBJ, Fermier R, Stern D, Galante JO. (1980): A study of lower limb mechanics during stairclimbing. *J Bone Joint Surg [Am],* 62A:749–757.
4. Andriacchi TP. (1990): Dynamics of pathological motion: applied to the anterior cruciate deficient knee. *J Biomech,* 23[Suppl]: 99–105.
5. Andriacchi TP. (1986): Biomechanics and orthopedic problems: a quantitative approach. In: Skinner JS, Corbin CB, Landers DM, Martin PE, Wells CL, eds. *Future directions in exercise and sport science research.* Champaign, IL: Human Kinetics Books, pp 45–56.
6. Arms SW, Pope MH, Johnson RJ, Fischer RA, Arvidsson I, Eriksson E. (1984): The biomechanics of anterior cruciate ligament rehabilitation and reconstruction. *Am J Sports Med,* 12:8–15.
7. Barrack RL, Bruckner JD, Kneisl J, Inman WS, Alexander AH. (1990): The outcome of nonoperatively treated completed tears of the ACL in active young patients. *Clin Orthop,* 258:192–199.

8. Berchuck M, Andriacchi TP, Bach BR, Reider BR. (1990): Gait adaptations by patients who have a deficient ACL. *J Bone Joint Surg [Am]*, 72A:871–877.

9. Birac D, Andriacchi TP, Bach BR Jr. (1991): Time related changes following ACL rupture. In: *Transactions of the 37th Annual Meeting of the Orthopaedics Research Society,* Anaheim, CA, Section 1, p 231.

10. Bray RC, Dandy DJ. (1989): Meniscal lesions and chronic ACL deficiency: meniscal tears occurring before and after reconstruction. *J Bone Joint Surg [Br]*, 71B:128–130.

11. Branch TP, Hunter R, Donath M. (1989): Dynamic EMG analysis of anterior cruciate deficient legs with and without bracing during cutting. *Am J Sports Med*, 17:35–41.

12. Bresler B, Frankel JP. (1953): The forces and moments in the leg during level walking. *Trans Am Soc Mech Eng*, 48A:62.

13. Butler DL, Noyes FR, Grood ES. (1980): Ligamentous restraints to anterior-posterior drawer in the human knee. *J Bone Joint Surg [Am]*, 62A:259–270.

14. Clancy WG, Ray JM, Zolton DJ. (1988): Acute tears of the ACL: surgical versus conservative treatment. *J Bone Joint Surg [Am]*, 70A:1483–1488.

15. Finsterbush A, Frankl U, Matan Y, Mann G. (1990): Secondary damage to the knee after isolated injury of the ACL. *Am J Sports Med*, 18:475–479.

16. Grood ES, Suntay WJ, Noyes FR, Butler DL. (1984): Biomechanics of the knee extension exercise: effect of cutting the anterior cruciate ligament. *J Bone Joint Surg [Am]*, 66A:725–734.

17. Jacobsen K: Osteoarthritis following insufficiency of the cruciate ligament in man: A clinical study. *Acta Orthop Scand,* 48:520–526.

18. Johnson RJ. (1982): The anterior cruciate ligament: A dilemma in sports medicine. *Int J Sports Med,* 3:71–79.

19. Kannus P, Jarvinen M. (1989): Post-traumatic ACL insufficiency as a cause of osteoarthritis in a knee joint. *Clin Rheumatol,* 8:251–260.

20. Markolf KL, Kochan A, Amstutz HD. (1984): Measurement of knee stiffness and laxity in patients with documented absence of the anterior cruciate ligament. *J Bone Joint Surg [Am]*, 66A:242–253.

21. Noyes FR, Matthews DS, Mooar PA, Grood ES. (1983): The symptomatic anterior cruciate-deficient knee: Part 2. The results of rehabilitation, activity modification and counseling on functional disability. *J Bone Joint Surg [Am]*, 65A:163–174.

22. Noyes FR, Mooar PA, Matthews DS, Butler DL. (1983): The symptomatic anterior cruciate-deficient knee: Part 1. The long-term functional disability in athletically active patients. *J Bone Joint Surg [Am]*, 65A:154–162.

23. Noyes FR, Schipplein OD, Andriacchi TP, Saddemi SR, Weise M. (1992): The anterior cruciate deficient knee with varus alignment: an analysis of gait adaptations and dynamic joint loadings. *Am J Sports Med* 20(6):707–716.

24. Prodromos CC, Andriacchi TP, Galante JO. (1985): A relationship between knee joint loads and clinical changes following high tibial osteotomy. *J Bone Joint Surg [Am]*, 67A:1188–1194.

25. Schipplein OD, Andriacchi TP. (1991): Interaction between active and passive knee stabilizers during level walking. *J Orthop Res,* 9:113–119.

26. Tibone JE, Antich TJ, Fanton GS, Moynes DR, Perry J. (1986): Functional analysis of anterior cruciate ligament instability. *Am J Sports Med,* 14:276–284.

27. Wang J-W, Kuo KN, Andriacchi TP, Galante JO. (1990): The influence of walking mechanics and time on the results of proximal tibial osteotomy. *J Bone Joint Surg [Am]*, 72A:905–913.

28. Wroble RR, Brand RA. (1990): Paradoxes in the history of the ACL. *Clin Orthop,* 259:183–191.

Injury, Healing, Repair, Reconstruction

Our intent in this subsection is to introduce the reader to some of the current research on ligament injury and repair as it relates to the anterior cruciate ligament. The reader will find some new information along with appropriate references to several aspects of ligament healing and ligament grafting, including their cell biology, matrix biochemistry, molecular biochemistry, ultrastructure, and biomechanics. As will become apparent in subsequent sections, basic science work on the ACL is still at a very preliminary stage. Authors are therefore forced to extrapolate, to a large extent, from model systems of other ligaments in which healing is better defined. However, the reader will gain some insights into why the ACL does not appear to heal as well as some other structures and some appreciation for the complexity of the biological processes involved.

Cyril B. Frank

The Anterior Cruciate Ligament: Current and Future Concepts, edited by D.W. Jackson, et al. Raven Press, Ltd., New York © 1993.

CHAPTER **14**

The Cell Biology of Ligaments and Ligament Healing

Patricia G. Murphy, Cyril B. Frank, and David A. Hart

The focus of this chapter is the cell biology of normal, healing, and grafted ligaments, particularly the anterior cruciate ligament (ACL). As is well documented, the healing potential of a complete transection of the anterior cruciate ligament is limited in comparison to other ligaments such as the medial collateral ligament (MCL) (32,34,52,55,87,88). As well, patients with transected ACLs are at a risk to develop degenerative changes within their joints (15,55,67,77,86,101). There are a number of dissimilarities between these two ligaments which may account for the observed differences in healing properties, some of which include gross morphology and anatomical position (18,19,26,30), superficial layers that cover the ligaments (16,18,28), vascularity (16,18, 28), innervation (17,18), cellularity (1,4,18), slight differences in amounts of collagen types (1,4,18), and likely differences in biomechanical loading (18,26,32,83,85, 104,109,113). Many of these variables and others have been studied experimentally; however, it is still uncertain why the ACL heals much less effectively than the MCL. In fact, the general perception is that the injured human ACL does not elicit a functional healing response.

The ultimate goal in all wound healing, including ligament biology, is to regenerate the injured tissue into its original uninjured form (23,24). Wound healing in fetal tissue is capable of forming regenerated tissue without the formation of scar tissue (71,91,93,100,106). In adult ligaments however, healing occurs by the formation of scar tissue which is biomechanically inferior to normal ligament (8,18,22,32,34). Further, while it appears that collateral ligaments are capable of healing by an, albeit inferior, but semifunctional process, (8,18,22,32,34) the ACL appears to be incapable of forming functional scar tissue (50,55,77). Therefore, what may be required is a two step process. First to promote formation of scar tissue in the ACL and secondly to promote conversion of that scar tissue into normal ligament (Fig. 1). To achieve this goal of regeneration, more information regarding the cell biology of the ACL and other ligaments in both the homeostatic state and also during the healing response is required.

This chapter will present the current state of knowledge regarding the cell biology of both normal and healing collateral and cruciate ligaments and their grafts.

NORMAL LIGAMENT CELL BIOLOGY AND PHYSIOLOGY

As discussed in earlier chapters in this monograph, ligaments contain fibroblast-like cells, endothelial cells (microvasculature) and cells of the peripheral nervous system. In addition, a small number of tissue mast cells are also present. The distribution of the cells within each ligament (ACL, MCL, etc.) is not identical, therefore it is likely that the spatial arrangement of cells serves some structure-function relationship within a specific ligament. At the present time, the implications of such fine structure with regard to nutrition, cell-cell communication, neuroendocrine modulation and maintenance of functional homeostasis remains unknown. As most ap-

P. G. Murphy: Joint Injury and Arthritis Research Group, University of Calgary, Calgary, Alberta, Canada T2N 4N1.

C. B. Frank: McCaig Centre for Joint Injury and Arthritis Research, Department of Surgery, The University of Calgary, Calgary, Alberta, Canada T2N 4N1.

D. A. Hart: University of Calgary Health Science Centre, McCaig Centre for Joint Injury and Arthritis Research, Department of Microbiology and Infectious Diseases, Calgary, Alberta, Canada T2N 4N1.

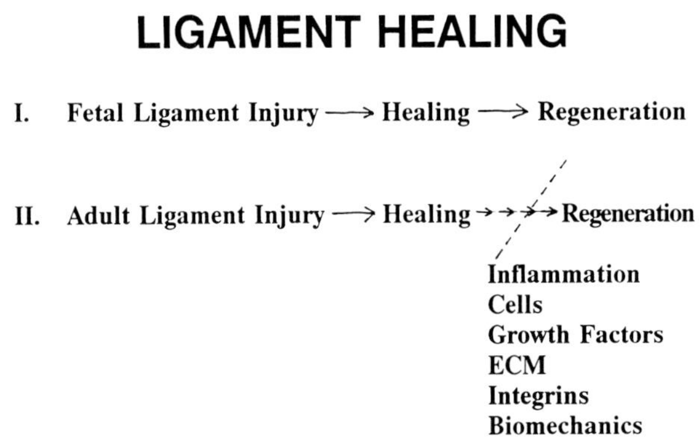

LIGAMENT HEALING

I. Fetal Ligament Injury $\longrightarrow$ Healing $\longrightarrow$ Regeneration

II. Adult Ligament Injury $\longrightarrow$ Healing $\rightarrow \rightarrow \not\rightarrow \rightarrow$ Regeneration

                                         Inflammation
                                         Cells
                                         Growth Factors
                                         ECM
                                         Integrins
                                         Biomechanics

FIG. 1. Factors influencing ligament healing and regeneration.

proaches to investigating grafts, healing injuries, or the cell biology of ligaments leads to the disruption of these spatial arrangements, the analyses discussed below have as a limitation an inability to assess the contribution of such factors to the success or failure of biological grafts and/or scars to regain or maintain function.

Another important aspect of normal ligament cell biology is that it is a dynamic system that changes in cell physiology, cell density, and the availability of exogenous factors which could influence ligament cell activity as an individual progresses from skeletal immaturity to skeletal maturity and finally to "senescence." In addition, within each phase the cells within a ligament must be maintaining the function of the tissue by balancing matrix secretion (anabolic activity) with secretion of proteinases capable of degrading or remodeling matrix components (catabolic activity). At the present time, we do not know if this dynamic state is controlled by a single homogeneous cell population or by separate subsets of cells responsible for either catabolic functions or anabolic functions.

GRAFTS

As mentioned in other chapters, many different types of grafts have been used to replace the torn ACL (20,27,38,61,75,79,84,90,97,99,103). While some are synthetic, the majority are what have become known as "biological." More specifically, some of the biological grafts used in the past have consisted of the patellar tendon, iliotibial band, or semitendinosis. Most are autografts (from the host), but there is some evidence to suggest that allografts may be almost equally effective (84). For both autografts and allografts, a wide range of variability exists in terms of their healing, probably due to variations in the rates of healing processes but also possibly due to variations in the mechanisms themselves. In order to define these mechanisms more clearly, the current understanding of the cell biology of these biological grafts will be discussed below.

The Origin of Cells in Biological Grafts

The healing profile of autografts (PT, MCL, and others) and allografts share basically the same pattern of healing and will be discussed together, although it is conceivable that subtle differences between these tissues exist in either the mechanism or kinetics of healing. Following graft placement there is a fairly rapid loss of cellularity within the graft resulting in a period of graft acellularity (1,6,68–70) (Fig. 2). The basis for this acellularity is unknown but may relate to loss of vascularity and/or innervation since areas of acellularity may be also avascular (9,69). It has been hypothesized that the allograft acellularity was due to an immunological reaction, however, fresh autografts also demonstrate this hypocellularity (1,6,68–70). One explanation for the phe-

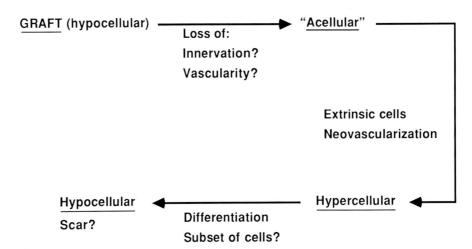

FIG. 2. Cell biology of ligament grafts. The indicated stages of cellular changes during the engraftment process have been demonstrated to occur with both auto- and allografts in a number of animal models and with both patellar tendon and MCL grafts.

nomenon is that an autoimmunological reaction is occurring in frozen-thawed autografts, since others have observed similar responses with frozen-thawed bone (102). However, this seems unlikely since similar patterns are observed in fresh autografts (1,6,68–70). This period of cellular necrosis is followed by repopulation of the graft with cells that are either extrinsic to the graft, cells that are derived from a surviving subset from within the graft (intrinsic), or possibly a combination of both (1,6,68–70). This repopulation results in a period of hypercellularity which persists for a variable amount of time depending upon the type of graft. Eventually, the graft becomes less cellular and histologically more like normal tissue (6,9,69,70). Whether this is due to selection of a subset of extrinsic cells or other factors is not known. Evidence to date, with the patellar tendon, ACL allograft, and MCL autografts would support the theory that these types of grafts, in general, are repopulated by extrinsic cells. This is supported by several observations: a fresh PT or MCL autograft becomes acellular and later is repopulated (6,9,68,69); a frozen PT, MCL, or ACL autograft in which the intrinsic cells are primarily removed (but not entirely) also becomes repopulated (63,68,70); freeze-dried tissue (tendon or fascia lata) is acellular initially and later is repopulated with fibroblasts (62); and a frozen graft that is impermeable to extrinsic cells from the synovial fluid (by the use of dialysis tubing) does not become repopulated (70). These data suggest that the cells which repopulate the graft are extrinsic in origin. This is also observed in ACL allografts where Jackson et al. demonstrated, by molecular methods, that fresh goat ACL allografts are repopulated by host cells (i.e., extrinsic cells) (64). This may not be the result of a presensitized immunological response causing early removal of intrinsic cells since these researchers have demonstrated that no immediate detectable immunological reaction was occurring in the skin from the transplanted animals (64). Also, our research group has demonstrated that presensitization of an animal does not result in an obvious detectable immunological response (C. Frank and D. Hart, unpublished observations). While these data do suggest that these grafts are repopulated by cells extrinsic to the graft, it is possible that some intrinsic cells do contribute (likely as a small minority) to the repopulation of the graft. This is a possibility since it may be difficult, in some models, to verify removal of all of the intrinsic cells (29,68).

Several interesting questions arise with the consensus that the cells that repopulate the graft are extrinsic to the graft. What type of cells are they, from where did they originate, and are they heterogeneous? There are a number of distinct possibilities. These cells may be so-called "mesenchymal stem cells" or other cell types which could have originated within the bone marrow and found their way to the graft either through the vascula-

ture or via the synovial fluid. They could also be a type of "generic fibroblast" precursor that may arise from either the bone marrow or other surrounding connective tissues (for example the periosteum) and when exposed to the proper stimulus, differentiates into the appropriate cell type. There are conflicting reports with respect to the origin of these cells repopulating grafts, but this may simply be a reflection of different mechanisms being operative for different types of grafts or that multiple possibilities exist.

A study performed with patellar tendon autografts demonstrated that extrinsic cells may originate from the synovial fluid (70). Other studies with bone-MCL-bone autografts would suggest that these extrinsic cells may be migrating from some surrounding tissue to form a very thick, cellular epiligament (68) causing progressive repopulation of the ligament from its periphery to its deeper substance. This phenomenon has also been observed in other grafts (6,69). Such observations would suggest that either extrinsic cells are attaching freely to the surface of the ligament and then invading it or that they are migrating through some sort of surface channels. Obviously more research is required to elucidate the answers to these questions if we are to learn how to potentiate the healing process.

Cellular Phenotype

Do these extrinsic cells which repopulate the biological grafts behave like ACL fibroblasts? Are these cells, regardless of their origin, able to arrange the synthesis and secretion of the appropriate proteins and respond to the signals required to enable the graft to "function"? Biochemical data (collagen cross-linking, ratio of type I/type III collagen, and glycosaminoglycan content) and histological data suggest that after becoming exposed to the environment of the ACL, cells within a PT graft may behave more like ACL cells than PT cells. This process has been referred to as "ligamentization" (7). However, such grafts are not normal biomechanically (10,98) and thus are not "ligamentized" in a functional sense. The conflicts in these data could indicate that these grafts are still remodeling and may resemble a form of scar tissue (3,4,31,32,34). This could be a function of their synovial or epiligament/periosteal origin which may yield a biomechanically inferior structure. The concept that the PT graft may evolve into scar tissue may explain the discrepancies observed between the biomechanists and the biochemists with respect to the PT graft replacement approach.

If there is a general consensus that these grafts have not truly replaced the ACL in terms of functionality, regardless of their biochemical or histological appearance, then what stimuli are required to enable these cells and tissues to behave more like an ACL? Recent research has started to address these questions at the cellular level, in an attempt to obtain information regarding the biomechanical and biochemical signals which may enable both better ACL and graft healing. Research has utilized both organ and cell culture to gain more insight into normal ACL behavior and also to compare ACL with the MCL to attempt to explain the variabilities in healing that are observed between these two ligaments. It is also a possibility that these systems may themselves be utilized to promote healing. That is, the use of autologous/nonautologous matrix or cells to replace the injured ligament with or without exogenous stimuli may promote or augment repair in ligaments and may be viable alternatives (see New Directions Chapter). Therefore, characterization of their biochemical behavior is necessary if these alternatives are to be utilized.

ORGAN CULTURE

Many investigators have utilized an organ culture system to analyze several biochemical parameters in ACL, MCL and MCL-scar tissue. The latter has been utilized as a model since there are few good models available to assess the healing potential of the ACL. This usually entails some form of manipulation *in vivo*, subsequent incubation of the tissue *in vitro* for a short period of time, and biochemical analysis of either the tissue or its secreted products. A majority of the studies to date have centered upon the remodeling events that occur during wound healing with particular emphasis upon the regulation between the synthesis of matrix components (anabolic) and the different classes of proteinases that are responsible for the removal or remodeling of these matrix molecules (catabolic). It is obvious that these two must be regulated tightly to maintain homeostasis and also to promote proper healing and remodeling.

Anabolic Regulation

The research surrounding the synthesis of matrix molecules within the ligament has primarily focused upon the production of collagen, since type I collagen is thought to be an important protein both biologically and biomechanically (1,18). The general hypothesis is that increased production of the proper type of collagen or better organization of the collagen (orientation and fibril diameter) produced may enhance the healing response. As reported previously, the relative types and amounts of collagen differ slightly between the MCL and ACL (1,4). The ACL has slightly less type I collagen and more type III collagen than does the MCL (1,34). It has been demonstrated that normal ACL from mature rabbits contains less mRNA for alpha$_1$ procollagen than the normal MCL and that level of message in each cell from

both the ACL and MCL was heterogeneous in that not every cell was expressing detectable levels of this mRNA (107). It was also shown in this study that more alpha$_1$ procollagen mRNA was present at the injury site of the MCL than at the ACL injury site in which no apparent healing was observed (107). Whether such a difference leads to variations in collagen produced is uncertain but if differences in collagen were present, then such results may contribute to the variability in healing that is observed between these two ligaments.

Other matrix components such as fibronectin may also play a role in the healing response. Fibronectin is thought to function as a cell adhesion molecule (78). Therefore, differences in fibronectin between normal ligaments and injured ligaments during repair may influence either recruitment of cells required for healing or may affect the inflammatory process that occurs during healing (23,24,78). It has been documented that the ACL and PCL have approximately twice as much fibronectin as does the MCL (2). This is presumably the result of the synovial layer which surrounds the ACL and PCL, but which is absent in the MCL (2,18). It has also been demonstrated that immobilization of a rabbit stifle joint dramatically decreases the amount of fibronectin detected in both the ACL and MCL (2). The decreases observed in the ACL were more significant than the MCL (2). These changes in fibronectin may be the result of changes in collagen or other matrix components since fibronectin is able to bind these matrix components or these observations may also be related to the expression of proteinases capable of degrading fibronectin (47,59,94). Recently, it has been shown that application of plasma fibronectin to a healing rabbit MCL results in an increase in amount of tissue but this tissue is more disorganized and biomechanically inferior to contralateral MCLs. However, the biomechanics of the tissue did improve with time (13). Additional research is obviously required in order to better determine the role of fibronectin in the healing process.

Recently, attention has focused upon a family of proteins known as integrins which function as cellular receptors and cell adhesion molecules and enable a cell to bind to extracellular matrix components such as collagen, laminin, hyaluronic acid, and fibronectin (59,94). For a more detailed discussion of these and other matrix components see the chapter by McDevitt and Marcelino. With these functions, integrins may play an important role in many cellular processes including wound healing, cellular migration and proliferation, and differentiation of certain tissues (59,94). Variations either in the expression or structure of the integrins has been implicated in pathological disorders such as cancer and inflammatory disorders (59,94). It has also been hypothesized that integrins are involved in the communication that occurs between the matrix and the cell, possibly serving as a biomechanical transducer (60). For the reasons presented above, integrins may be involved both in homeostasis within ligaments and may also function during wound healing. These proteins have been demonstrated to be present both in ligaments and also in ligament cell cultures (37,89). This area has been reviewed more extensively in this monograph by Amiel et al.

Catabolic Regulation

Another important area of the regulation of matrix components involves removal and remodeling by proteinases. One of the systems that is believed to be involved in such tissue remodeling is the plasminogen activator (PA) and inhibitor (PAI) system (47–49). Activation of this system results in the generation of the proteinase plasmin (47–49). Plasmin has a broad substrate specificity and is capable of degrading proteins of the extracellular matrix such as laminin and fibronectin as well as activating other pro-enzymes such as collagenase and stromelysin (47–49). Therefore, activation of this system may result in an amplification of extracellular matrix remodeling (47–49). These systems could be especially important in ligament tissue since type I collagen is a major protein component of the extracellular matrix of ligaments and activation of collagenase by plasmin may result in extensive remodeling events. As one may suspect, uncontrolled or inappropriate expression of either of these enzymes (and/or others) or of their inhibitors may result in abnormal remodeling during healing.

Investigations have demonstrated that both rabbit and human ligaments are capable of producing PAs in vitro and therefore, these tissues could be capable of producing these enzymes in vivo which may contribute to remodeling during wound healing (33,51). It has been demonstrated that ligaments isolated from both immature and mature rabbits express PAs and that heterogeneity in expression exists between and within different ligaments (33,51,80). That is, expression of PA differs between different ligaments and also differs along the length of a ligament (33,51,80). The PA profile of the ACL was shown to be different from the MCL (33,51,80). More specifically, the PA activity in the ACL femoral insertional area was higher than in the tibial insertional area (33,51). This polarity in expression in the ACL was opposite to the MCL (33,51). The PA expression in the MCL was higher in the tibial insertional area than in the femoral area (33,51). This was apparently not the result of overt differences in cellularity and was intrinsic to the ligament substance since removal of the epiligament resulted in the same results (51). Other studies have indicated that different ligaments also display differences in basal PA activity (80). For instance, the ACL produces the least amount of PA while the MCL and LCL seem to produce similar amounts of PA, al-

though both secrete more PA than the ACL (80) (D. Hart, C. Clary, and P. Murphy, manuscript in preparation). Therefore, ligaments are not simply heterogeneous along the length of the ligament but also between different ligaments. This same heterogeneity and polarity was also observed in human ligaments (ACL and MCL) that were analyzed (33). Recent investigations have revealed similar patterns of expression with MCL, LCL, and ACL tissue from porcine, canine, ovine, and equine sources, therefore, the findings appear to represent a general biological observation and are not species specific (D. Hart, P. Murphy, S. Lenz, and C. Clary, manuscript in preparation). Identification of the PA by biochemical techniques indicated that the PA expressed by these ligaments is of the urokinase family (UK-like) (51,80,81). These findings have recently been confirmed in rabbit ligament cell cultures using molecular techniques (81). t-PA (vascular PA) was not detected in any of these samples (51,80,81). These findings are consistent with the hypothesis that PAs may be involved within the remodeling in ligaments in both homeostasis and also during healing, since UK is known to be involved in matrix remodeling in other systems (47–49) and t-PA is more involved in vascular fibrinolysis (47). Further analysis has indicated that the inhibitor of PAs (PAI) are also expressed in the same polarity by these ligaments (51,80). The PAI expressed by these tissues is thought to be PAI-1, which was demonstrated using cell culture and molecular techniques (81).

These enzymes are also of interest since it has been demonstrated that their expression can be influenced by biomechanical and biological stimuli in vivo (105). For example, immobilization of an immature rabbit stifle joint influences the secretion of PA and the expression of PA varies depending upon the duration of immobilization (105). Immobilization of a joint and analysis of the PA secreted in the rabbit MCL 2 to 4 weeks postimmobilization resulted in a decrease in PA activity (and also in collagen synthesis) (105). However, more prolonged immobilization resulted in an increase in PA secretion while collagen synthesis remained suppressed (105). These findings correlate well with both loss of biomechanical function and loss of matrix material and therefore, PAs may be one of the factors contributing to these changes. This data also indicates that an immature rabbit MCL alters its biochemical behavior with altered biomechanical stimulation. This is also observed in the mature rabbit stifle joint where it was demonstrated that immobilization led to reduced collagenase secretion with prolonged immobilization (44,45). Although immobilization appears to be affecting the expression of these proteinases in an opposite manner, these data indicate that immobilization (or an altered biomechanical environment) is able to alter biochemical or metabolic functions. Other investigators have demonstrated in vitro that connective tissues isolated from rabbit joints produce collagenase and also an inhibitor to collagenase (43). These studies have shown that the level of collagenase was similar in the ACL and MCL but higher in the patellar tendon (43). While no apparent differences are evident between different ligaments in a homeostatic state, further studies have indicated that a transected ACL produces more collagenase than its contralateral ACL (5). The production of this collagenase may contribute to the loss of matrix continuity, to the acellularity, and also to the possible retraction of the ACL (5). It could also contribute to any remodelling that may be attempted by the ACL. Further experiments are necessary to determine whether these speculations are accurate, but these data do suggest that an alteration in proteolytic activity may be involved in these processes. These data also indicate that ligaments are capable of producing proteinases in response to biomechanical or biochemical stimuli and that proper control over the expression of proteinases is required during both homeostasis and repair. It is known that the expression of proteinases and inhibitors is influenced by a variety of mediators some which include inflammatory agents, neuropeptides, and growth factors (47–49).

Inflammatory Regulation

Inflammation is an early event that is observed in adult but not fetal wound healing (71,91,93,100,106) (Fig. 3). Inflammation is initially characterized by an increase in vascular permeability in which the integrity of the vascular wall is altered, resulting in extravasation of both the fluid and the cells within the vasculature (23,24). These cells include inflammatory cells such as macrophages and polymorphonuclear leukocytes (PMNs). Such cells are able to perform several functions includ-

ing: possible recruitment of other inflammatory cells as well as potential stem cells, removal of damaged tissue, and the production and release of factors such as growth factors that may aid the healing process (23,24). Inflammatory cells and their mediators are also able to produce substances such as oxygen radicals and cytokines that may be detrimental to healing (23,24). It has been demonstrated that prolonged inflammation has a negative effect on wound healing (23,24). It has also been shown that fetal wound healing does not exhibit a response that resembles inflammation in nonfetal tissue, suggesting that, at least in the fetus, inflammation is either unnecessary or may be detrimental to wound healing. It is possible that because of other differences, wound healing in the fetus does not require inflammation to occur. Nonetheless, consideration of the inflammatory response is necessary in both immature and mature tissue.

It has been speculated that differences between ACL and MCL healing may be due to exposure to different environments since the ACL is intraarticular and the MCL is extraarticular (18,19,26,30). This is especially valid when the ACL is ruptured, thus exposing it to the synovial fluid which may contain inflammatory cells and their mediators (18,24). Interestingly, synovial fluid, but not purified hyaluronic acid, can also influence the activity of both ACL and MCL ligament cells in culture (82). Thus it was of interest to determine the influence of mediators such as IL-1 upon the expression of PAs in ligament tissue. It was determined that the levels of PA in ligament tissue increased with the addition of IL-1 (33,51). It was also demonstrated that incubation of ligament tissue with aspirin, indomethacin, and corticosteroids resulted in reduction of basal PA activity in both human and rabbit ligaments (33,51). These are interesting observations since these enzymes and mediators are present in these tissues and they may disrupt healing if overexpression is present. Furthermore, the antiinflam-

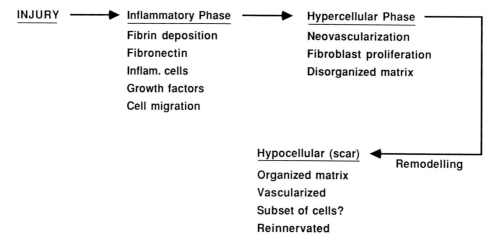

FIG. 3. Cell biology of wound healing. The indicated sequence of events has been demonstrated for a number of model systems. Whether or not ACL injuries initiate and follow the same sequence is still controversial.

matory drugs tested are used in the treatment of joint injuries and some of the efficacy at the cellular level may relate to the expression of such enzymes.

Neurogenic Regulation

As is well documented, ligaments function to guide and direct motion (18,113). They also serve to restrict and protect the joint from certain movements (18,113). Ligaments may also function in a neurosensory capacity including proprioception (sense of joint position), which may have an influence on motion (11,14,66) (see also the chapter by Brand). It has been shown in a number of animal models that joint components including synovium and ligaments are innervated and may potentially function as proprioceptors (17,25,40,53,95). The ACL (human and cat), for example, is innervated and contains nerve endings which could function as mechanoreceptors, proprioceptors, and nociceptors (pain perception) (40,53,66,95,114). Specifically, the ACL mechanoreceptors resemble Golgi-like, Ruffini-like, and Pacinian-like corpuscular nerve endings (66,114). These are nerve endings which transmit mechanical stimuli into electric potentials. It has also been shown that separate regions within a ligament may be innervated differently (17,18,28). This has been observed in the MCL where the epiligament may be more heavily innervated than the ligament substance (17,18,28). The MCL epiligament may also contain more myelinated nerve fibers than does the deep ligament substance, although both may contain unmyelinated fibers (17,18,28). There are a few nerve fibers deep within the ligament which may function as proprioceptive fibers (17,18,28). These differences may result in altered functions within different regions of a ligament.

It has been reported that many nerves mediate their responses through the actions of neurotransmitters as well as neuropeptides such as Substance P and calcitonin gene-related product (CGRP) (56,74,76). These neuropeptides are multifunctional in that they are capable of causing vasodilation, plasma extravasation, and angiogenesis (56,74,76). Substance P is capable of functioning as a chemoattractant to neutrophils and is mitogenic to certain cell types (56,74,76). These peptides mediate their effect through receptors and are functional at very low concentrations (56,74,76). It has been demonstrated that collateral ligament nerves contain both Substance P and CGRP (39,96). This has been shown in both the MCL substance as well as the MCL epiligament (96). Innervation may also influence healing since neuropeptides increase during healing of the MCL (39). It is possible that these neuropeptides may contribute to the transmission of information to the fibroblasts within the ligament since the nerves within ligaments may be sensory neurons (17,18,28,39). This information may be

biomechanical or biological in nature. Therefore, it was of interest to determine the effects of such neuromediators upon the fibroblasts within ligaments.

Recent studies have utilized an organ culture system to determine the effects of Substance P on the expression of plasminogen activator and inhibitor in rabbit joint connective tissues. It has been determined that different connective tissues respond in a unique manner to Substance P, which may reflect the extent of their innervation (80). That is, MCL epiligament and synovium increase PA secretion in response to Substance P while the midsubstance of the MCL and ACL were either not responsive to this neuropeptide or yielded a very modest change in PA expression (80). Similar observations have been obtained using connective tissues obtained from domestic dogs. Such findings indicate that certain areas and types of ligaments are responsive to the neuropeptide Substance P. The observed variability in responsiveness may be a result of differential receptor expression by the different connective tissues, however the data also correlate well with the degree of innervation within these structures (17,18,28,96). These data, as well as other methodological approaches (histology), lend confidence to using this type of system to measure the responsiveness of these structures to other mediators. That is, the use of an organ culture system to analyze ligament behavior, albeit *in vitro*, may be useful since the ligaments seem to maintain their phenotype and therefore enable additional studies to be conducted.

Growth Factor Regulation

An exciting area of investigation that is currently very popular focuses on the possible influence of polypeptides known as growth factors upon the repair process (23,24). A large number of growth factors or growth modulators are known. Some of these are very cell specific while others are more multispecific (23,24). In that regard, multispecific growth factors may elicit different effects on different cells (proliferation, secretion of proteins, differentiation) (23,24). Cells respond to peptide growth factors via specific cell surface receptors (23,24). Responsiveness to growth factors can be accomplished in an autocrine, paracrine, or endocrine fashion (Fig. 4). Other growth regulators, such as estrogens or corticosteroids exert their effects on cells via intracellular binding proteins.

In the context of injury, the hypothesis is that lack of, or inappropriate expression of specific growth factors leads to scar formation and thus inhibits regeneration of the injured tissue. Therefore, application of these missing factors or regulation of endogenous factors may encourage more effective healing and possibly promote regeneration. Much of this research stems from the localization of these factors in the tissues and also in the

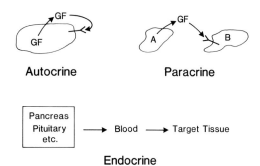

FIG. 4. Diagrammatic representation of autocrine, paracrine, and endocrine regulation by growth factors and cytokines.

inflammatory cells that infiltrate the site of injury (23,24). Such inflammatory cells include platelets, macrophages/monocytes, neutrophils, and possibly multipotent cells (23,24). Platelets produce and secrete platelet-derived growth factor (PDGF), transforming growth factor beta (TGF-B), and epidermal growth factor (EGF) (23,24). Macrophages that are activated produce PDGF, TGF-B, basic fibroblast growth factor (bFGF), and transforming growth factor alpha (TGF-a) (23,24). Acidic fibroblast growth factor (aFGF) and insulin-like growth factors I and II (IGF) are other growth factors that may also be involved in wound healing (23,24). Initially thought of as primarily mitogenic for certain cells, growth factors are also able to function in other capacities (23,24). Some growth factors are able to act as chemoattractants, are able to induce cell migration, and in some instances are able to promote angiogenesis (23,24). It has also been shown that growth factors display high specificity with respect to both the cell type that they influence and also the response of that particular cell to the growth factor (23,24). This specificity may be the result of the expression of unique receptors for the various growth factors on the different cell types (23,24). It may also be due to the use of different intracellular signaling mechanisms for different cell types (signal transduction) (23,24).

Growth factors are also of interest because of their acceleration of wound healing in a variety of models (23,24). There are many variables in studies using growth factors, some of which include: the optimal growth factor or factors, the optimal dose, the type of application, the duration of application, and the assessment of "better healing" are all important criteria to assess. The use of different growth factors with different models involved in a different treatment regimen makes it difficult to interpret results, but in a general sense these growth factors are capable of accelerating wound healing, but this is a very specific response.

One of the rationales for using growth factors in healing, at least in orthopaedics, likely originated from the observation that mineralized bone contains a considerable quantity of growth factors (FGF, PDGF, and TGF-

B) and also that fractured bone heals quite well (12,54). Whether the application of exogenous growth factors to fractured bone results in increased healing is controversial. The application of growth hormone to fractured bone, in some studies, results in increased bone formation (46) while other studies indicate that growth hormone does not cause bone formation and does not influence the biomechanics of fractured bone (21). Other studies indicate that the addition of aFGF to fractured bone results in an increase in the size of the fracture callus, however, it did not alter the mechanical strength of the callus (65). It is likely that these factors are promoting the synthesis of cell and matrix components while not necessarily organizing the matrix which may influence the mechanical strength of a structure. It is also possible that premature biomechanical testing may bias the results seen in these studies. Other studies, in tendon, have demonstrated that exercise increases the detection of IGF-1 in rat Achilles and tibialis anterior tendon (41,42). It was also shown that the IGF-1 concentration was highest in the area with the highest amount of mechanical stress (41,42). These results suggest that biomechanical loading may influence the expression of growth factors and may be an important consideration during stress as well as healing.

To our knowledge, no *in vivo* growth factor studies have yet been performed in ligament tissues. However, an *in vitro* study to assess the effects of growth factors upon both normal and healing rabbit ligaments has recently been completed (P. Murphy and D. Hart, manuscript in preparation). It was of interest to determine the influence of growth factors upon PA and PAI expression. An organ culture system was utilized in which the ligaments (ACL, MCL, MCL-scar, and LCL) examined were first removed of all overlying tissue, divided longitudinally and then divided into three or four equal pieces. The pieces of ligament were then incubated with and without the growth factor overnight. The samples then were analyzed for PA/PAI activity. Of the growth factors tested (acidic and basic FGF and IGF-1), none of them produced any detectable change in PA/PAI activity of any of these tissues (P. Murphy and D. Hart, manuscript in preparation). This may be the result of a number of variables some of which include: inability of the growth factor to reach the cells, lack of a receptor for the growth factor, a dosage problem (too little or saturation with endogenous growth factor), changes not detected, alterations in other molecules that were not measured, or no change with the addition of these growth factors. Despite these limitations, it would be of interest to determine if other growth factors have an influence in this system.

Other Regulation

Other factors may also be involved in regulating healing. These include possible age and gender (hormonal) influences upon ligament healing. It has been demonstrated that aging results in a decreased ability to remodel or repair bone (35). It has also been shown that certain immunological diseases which influence joint integrity also show a preponderance toward one gender or another. For instance, it is known that there is a prevalence toward the female gender in diseases such as rheumatoid arthritis and systemic lupus erytheymatosus and the severity of these diseases is altered during pregnancy and post menopause, therefore, suggesting that sex hormones may have an effect on the disease process (50,57,58). It is also quite possible that either age and/or gender may influence ligament homeostasis and healing (108,110–112). With these thoughts in mind, an organ culture system was utilized to determine if any differences existed in PA/PAI expression of connective tissues between male and female rabbits. It was also of interest to determine if these tissues would respond in a different manner to estrogen. Using this system, it was determined that the synovium from both male and female rabbits and the MCL epiligament from female, but not male rabbits, decreased PA expression with the addition of estrogen while there was no detectable response in either the MCL substance or the ACL from both male and female rabbits (L. Roux, P. Murphy, and D. Hart, manuscript in preparation). Such observations indicate that gender could contribute to the responsiveness of a tissue to exogenous stimuli which may result in differences in healing responses.

CELL CULTURE

In addition to the research performed on connective tissues utilizing an organ culture system, recently researchers have also adopted a cell culture system to determine if differences exist, at the cellular level, between the cells of the ACL and other joint components. There are some primary concerns when utilizing a cell culture system such as this one, the first of which is to determine what type of cells are being cultured and whether selection for a subpopulation of cells is occurring. That is, is the population of cells obtained *in vitro* representative of cells within the ligament? Another concern is what influence matrix has upon cellular phenotype and does removal of this matrix alter this phenotype? Finally, are the cells maintaining their phenotype *in vitro* and can this system be utilized to increase our understanding how ligament cells function and how we may influence them to promote healing/regeneration? These concepts will be addressed below.

Several laboratories have now begun to use such cell culture systems to answer some of these important questions. Our laboratory has focused on characterizing cells derived from ligaments in an attempt to address some of the issues presented above. The first priority was to determine what types of cells were present within the ligament cell preparations so in the future these cells may be used *in vivo*. The problem was addressed using biochemical and histological approaches. Cells were analyzed biochemically (cellular proliferation, collagen typing, PA/PAI expression, and rate of hyaluronic acid secretion) and it was determined that cells isolated from rabbit ligaments are biochemically distinct from those isolated from rabbit synovium. More specifically, it was demonstrated that synovial fibroblasts have a higher proliferation rate, produce more type III collagen, secrete a unique PA activity, and have a fourfold higher rate of secretion of hyaluronic acid than do ligament fibroblasts (ACL and MCL) (81). It has also been determined that ACL fibroblasts proliferate more slowly than MCL fibroblasts and secrete slightly different ratios of collagen subtypes (92). The types of collagen secreted are relatively consistent with what is observed within these tissues, which suggests that these cells are ligament fibroblasts (4,92). This phenomenon of different rates of proliferation is also observed with similar cells isolated from other species (D. Hart, C. Clary, P. Murphy, manuscript in preparation). To determine the relative contribution of inflammatory cells within the ligament and synovial cell populations, histochemical differential staining techniques were employed. Stains specific for macrophage/monocytes and mast cell stains were also utilized. It was determined that less than 1% of the ligament cell fibroblast population were inflammatory cells, with some macrophage and mast cells detected (P. Murphy and D. Hart, unpublished observations). Other possible cell types within the ligament cell preparation include cells of the endothelial lineage which have very defined growth requirements (60,72) and also have a distinct morphological appearance (72). It is unlikely that the ligament cultures contain a significant contribution of endothelial cells since ligament fibroblasts have a high rate of proliferation and are easily cultured, ligament cells have a different morphology than do endothelial cells, and t-PA (vascular PA) has not been detected with the ligament cell cultures under any conditions, although endothelial cells express t-PA (47). Further studies are currently being conducted to substantiate these findings.

CELLULAR DIFFERENCES BETWEEN THE ACL AND THE MCL

Anabolic Regulation

Investigations have proceeded at the cellular level in an attempt to determine whether differences exist between the ACL and the MCL which may account for the differences observed in their healing responses. Some of these differences may be biochemical in nature and could involve the matrix proteins or adhesion proteins which the cells use to bind to the matrix. As mentioned above, ongoing investigations have determined that differences exist between ACL and MCL fibroblasts in the ratios of the types of collagen produced. That is, cells isolated from both rabbit ACL and MCL secreted mainly type I collagen but ACL fibroblasts secreted slightly more type I and less type III collagen than MCL cells (92). Although these ratios are slightly different than what has been reported for their respective tissues, they are very similar to the tissue data and may reflect differences in methodology (4,92). It has also been demonstrated that ACL and MCL fibroblasts, when grown in culture, produce a protein containing extracellular matrix. It was of interest to determine whether there was something different (a deficiency or an inhibitory substance) between the ACL and MCL matrices which may have resulted in their different proliferation rates. That is, could the proliferation rate of cells isolated from ACL increase when cultured upon the MCL matrix or could MCL cell conditioned medium stimulate their proliferation? Such experiments resulted in no detectable differences in the proliferation rate of ACL fibroblasts. Therefore, the results indicated that the MCL fibroblasts were not producing anything which may stimulate the growth of the ACL cells (P. Murphy, M. Dobson, and D. Hart, unpublished observations).

Other investigators have determined that there are differences between the cells from human ACL and MCL with respect to adhesion characteristics. Akeson et al. (73) have shown that both cell types increase their adhesion when cultured onto fibronectin-coated surfaces as compared to a plastic surface. They have also demonstrated that, in general, MCL fibroblasts are more adherent to fibronectin than cells from the ACL (73). This may be important since adhesion may reflect both migration and localization of cells during healing (23,24,59,94). Other studies indicate that rabbit ACL cells may be more adherent based upon integrin expression since ACL fibroblasts produce more VLA B5 than MCL (89). In addition it has also been shown that there is a difference between cells isolated from rabbit ACL and MCL with respect to migration (36). That is, MCL fibroblasts are able to migrate out of the tissue at a faster rate than ACL fibroblasts (36). Although these two investigations suggest different findings, they may be related to one another since adhesion and migration are important components of the healing response.

Catabolic Regulation

In an attempt to determine whether the cells used in these cell culture experiments were maintaining their phenotype in the absence of a normal extracellular matrix, experiments similar to the organ culture investigations were performed. That is, were cells derived from ACL, MCL, MCL-epiligament, MCL-scar, and synovium responding to mediators in a fashion similar to what was observed when they were in an organ culture environment. Similar experiments using the neuropeptide Substance P, as well as the growth factors described earlier were performed. It was demonstrated that the addition of Substance P evoked a similar pattern of responsiveness in the cell cultures as it had in the organ cultures (80). That is, the cells isolated from rabbit synovium as well as from the epiligament of the MCL were more responsive (increased PA/PAI secretion) than were cells derived from the deep ligament substance of the MCL or ACL (the MCL fibroblasts were slightly more responsive than were the ACL fibroblasts) (80). The same pattern of expression was also observed with the growth factors FGF and IGF-1 (P. Murphy and D. Hart, manuscript in preparation). No detectable change in expression of PA/PAI was observed in any of the cell types tested, although other growth factors may elicit a response. These results correspond to what was observed in the organ culture system. It was determined that these cells maintain their responsiveness toward estrogen in culture with a pattern similar to what was observed in the organ culture. However, only cells from female rabbits have been utilized to date. These data, as well as other, suggest that these cells are maintaining a similar phenotype with what is seen in the organ culture and possibly may be responding in a similar fashion to their pattern of responsiveness *in vivo*. These studies have also demonstrated that the cells isolated from the different ligaments and different parts of a ligament are biochemically and phenotypically distinct from one another. Such studies indicate that cells derived from different ligaments maintain unique phenotypes when cultured *in vitro*. Such findings have implications for future investigations of ligament healing.

CONCLUSIONS

This chapter has presented the current state of information regarding the cell biology of ligaments with particular emphasis upon the factors which may be involved in ACL healing. As one may appreciate, wound repair is an extremely complex event and our current understanding of wound healing in ligaments is limited. There may be a number of different reasons why the ACL heals much less effectively than other ligaments. In addition, the inability of this ligament to repair may be the result of combinations of these factors. Therefore, accumulation of biological and biomechanical information pertaining to normal ACL behavior is critical for determining the variables required for a proper healing response. Comparison of the biological and biomechanical behavior of scar tissue with uninjured tissue may provide some indication of what is important in the healing of ligaments. It may also provide some information as to how we may increase the healing/regeneration response of the ACL so that a functional replacement or a regenerated tissue might occur.

ACKNOWLEDGMENTS

The authors wish to acknowledge Judy Crawford and Linda Marchuk for assistance in preparation of this manuscript. They also wish to recognize Carol Clary, Larissa Roux, and Mark Dobson for their research contributions to this manuscript. The authors apologize to those researchers whose work was not cited due to the space limitations of this manuscript. These studies were supported by the Canadian Arthritis Society, the Alberta Heritage Foundation for Medical Research, and the Medical Research Council of Canada. P.G.M. was supported by AHFMR and the Canadian Arthritis Society Studentships, C.B.F. and D.A.H. are AHFMR Scholars.

REFERENCES

1. Amiel D, Billings E Jr, Akeson WH. (1990): Ligament structure, chemistry, and physiology. In: Daniel D, Akeson WH, O'Connor J, eds. *Knee ligaments: structure, function, injury, and repair.* New York: Raven Press, pp 77–91.
2. Amiel D, Foulk RA, Harwood FL, Akeson WH. (1990): Quantitative assessment by competitive ELISA of fibronectin (Fn) in tendons and ligaments. *Matrix,* 9:421–427.
3. Amiel D, Frank CB, Harwood FL, Akeson WH, Kleiner JB. (1987): Collagen alteration in medial collateral ligament healing in a rabbit model. *Connect Tissue Res,* 16:357–366.
4. Amiel D, Frank CB, Harwood FL, Fronek J, Akeson WH. (1983): Tendons and ligaments—a morphological and biochemical comparison. *J Orthop Res,* 1:257–265.
5. Amiel D, Ishizue KK, Harwood FL, Kitabayashi L, Akeson WH. (1989): Injury of the anterior cruciate ligament: the role of collagenase in ligament degeneration. *J Orthop Res,* 7:486–493.
6. Amiel D, Kleiner JB, Akeson WH. (1986): The natural history of the anterior cruciate ligament autograft of patellar tendon origin. *Am J Sports Med,* 14:449–462.
7. Arniel D, Kleiner JB, Roux RD, Harwood FL, Akeson WH. (1986): The phenomenon of "ligamentization": anterior cruciate ligament reconstruction with autogenous patellar tendon. *J Orthop Res,* 4:162–172.
8. Andriacchi T, Sabiston P, DeHaven K, Dahners L, Woo SL-Y, Frank C, Oakes B, Brand R, Lewis J. (1988): Ligament: injury and repair. In: Woo SL-Y, Buckwalter JA, eds. *Injury and repair of the musculoskeletal soft tissues.* Park Ridge, Illinois: American Academy of Orthopaedic Surgeons, pp 103–132.
9. Arnoczky SP, Tarvin GB, Marshall JL. (1982): Anterior cruciate ligament replacement using patellar tendon: an evaluation of graft revascularization in the dog. *J Bone Joint Surg [Am],* 64:217–224.
10. Ballock RT, Woo SL, Lyon RM, Hollis JM, Akeson WH. (1989): Use of patellar tendon autograft for anterior cruciate ligament reconstruction in the rabbit: a long-term histologic and biomechanical study. *J Orthop Res,* 7:474–485.
11. Barrack RL, Skinner HB. (1990): The sensory function of knee ligaments. In: Daniel D, Akeson WH, O'Connor J, eds. *Knee ligaments: structure, function, injury, and repair.* New York: Raven Press, pp 95–114.
12. Bonewald LF, Mundy GR. (1990): Role of transforming growth factor-beta in bone remodelling. *Clin Orthop Rel Res,* 250:261–276.
13. Boynton MD, Cannistra LM, Walsh WR, Sasken HF, Russell MS, Akelman E. (1992): Early effects of local fibronectin application on ligament healing. *Orthop Trans,* 17:77(abst).
14. Brand RA. (1989): A neurosensory hypothesis of ligament function. *Med Hypotheses,* 29:245–250.
15. Brandt KD, Braunstein EM, Visco DM, O'Connor B, Heck D, Albrecht M. (1991): Anterior (cranial) cruciate ligament transection in the dog: a bona fide model of osteoarthritis, not merely of cartilage injury and repair. *J Rheumatol,* 18:436–446.
16. Bray RC, Fisher AW, Frank CB. (1990): Fine vascular anatomy of adult rabbit knee ligaments. *J Anat,* 172:69–79.
17. Bray RC, Fisher AW, Salo P, Hennenfent BW, Rossler R, Frank CB. (1989): Neurovascular anatomy of collateral knee ligaments as revealed by vascular injection and metallic impregnation techniques. *Orthop Trans,* 13:670(abst).
18. Bray RC, Frank CB, Miniaci A. (1991): Structure and function of diathrodial joints. In: McGinty JB, ed. *Operative arthroscopy.* New York: Raven Press, pp 79–123.
19. Burks, RT. (1990): Gross anatomy. In: Daniel D, Akeson WH, O'Connor J, eds. *Knee ligaments: structure, function, injury, and repair.* New York: Raven Press, pp 59–76.
20. Campbell TDJ. (1990): Anterior cruciate ligament reconstruction: using patellar tendon grafts. *AORN J,* 51:944–954,956.
21. Carpenter JE, Hipp JA, Gerhart TM, Rudman CG, Hayes WC, Trippel SB. (1992): Failure of growth hormone to alter the biomechanics of fracture healing in a rabbit model. *J Bone Joint Surg [Am],* 74A:359–366.
22. Chimich D, Frank C, Shrive N, Dougall H, Bray R. (1991): The effects of initial end contact on medial collateral ligament healing: a morphological and biomechanical study in a rabbit model. *J Orthop Res,* 9:37–47.
23. Clark RAF, Henson PM. (1988): *The molecular and cellular biology of wound repair.* New York: Plenum Press.
24. Cohen IK, Diegelman RF, Linblad WJ. (1992): *Wound healing: biochemical and clinical aspects.* Philadelphia: Saunders.
25. De Avila GA, O'Connor BL, Visco DM, Sisk TD. (1989): The mechanoreceptor innervation of the human fibular collateral ligament. *J Anat,* 162:1–7.
26. Dye SF, Cannon WDJ. (1988): Anatomy and biomechanics of the anterior cruciate ligament. *Clin Sports Med,* 7:715–725.
27. Ekstrand J. (1989): Reconstruction of the anterior cruciate ligament in athletes, using a fascia lata graft: a review with preliminary results of a new concept. *Int J Sports Med,* 10:225–232.
28. Eng K, Rangayyan RM, Bray RC, Frank CB, Anscomb L, Veale P. (1992): Quantitative analysis of fine vascular anatomy of articular ligaments. *IEEE Trans Biomed Eng,* 39:296–306.
29. Frank C, Edwards P, McDonald D, Bodie D, Sabiston P. (1988): Viability of ligaments after freezing: an experimental study in a rabbit model. *J Orthop Res,* 6:95–102.
30. Frank C, Woo S, Andriacchi T, Brand R, Oakes B, Dahners L, DeHaven K, Lewis J, Sabiston P. (1988): Normal ligament: structure, function, and composition. In: Woo SL-Y, Buckwalter JA, eds. *Injury and repair of the musculoskeletal soft tissues.* Park Ridge, Illinois: American Academy of Orthopaedic Surgeons, pp 45–101.
31. Frank CB, Amiel D, Akeson WH. (1983): Healing of the medial collateral ligament of the knee—a morphological and biochemical assessment in rabbits. *Acta Orthop Scand,* 54:917–923.
32. Frank CB, Amiel D, Woo SL-Y, Akeson WH. (1985): Normal ligament properties and ligament healing. *Clin Orthop Rel Res,* 196:15–25.
33. Frank CB, Hart DA. (1990): The biology of tendons and ligaments. In: Mow VC, Ratcliffe A, Woo SL-Y, eds. *Biomechanics of diathrodial joints.* New York: Springer-Verlag, pp 39–62.
34. Frank CB, Woo SL-Y, Amiel D, Gomez MA, Harwood FL, Akeson WH. (1983): Medial collateral ligament healing: a multidisciplinary assessment in rabbits. *Am J Sports Med,* 11:379–389.
35. Frost HM. (1992): The role of changes in the mechanics usage set points in the pathogenesis of osteoporosis. *J Bone Miner Res,* 7:253–261.
36. Geiger MH, Amiel D, Green MH, Most D, Berchuck M, Akeson WH. (1992): Rates of migration of ACL and MCL derived fibroblasts. *Orthop Trans,* 17:75(abst).
37. Gesink DS, Pacheco HO, Kuiper SD, Schreck PJ, Amiel D, Akeson WH, Woods VL. (1992): Immunohistochemical localization of B1-integrins in anterior cruciate and medial collateral ligaments of human and rabbit. *J Orthop Res,* 17:667(abst).

38. Gomez T, Ratzlaff C, McConkey JP, Dean E, Thompson JP. (1990): Semitendinosus repair augmentation of acute anterior cruciate ligament rupture. *Can J Sport Sci,* 15:137–142.

39. Gronblad M, Korkala O, Konttinen YT, Kuokkanen H, Liesi P. (1991): Immunoreactive neuropeptides in nerves in ligamentous tissue: an experimental neuroimmunohistochemical study. *Clin Orthop,* 265:291–296.

40. Halata Z, Haus J. (1989): The ultrastructure of sensory nerve endings in human anterior cruciate ligament. *Anat Embryol Berl,* 179:415–421.

41. Hansson HA, Dahlin LB, Lundborg G, Lowenadler B, Paleus S, Skottner A. (1988): Transiently increased insulin-like growth factor 1 immunoreactivity in tendons after vibration trauma. *Scand J Plast Reconstr Surg Hand Surg,* 22:1–6.

42. Hansson HA, Engstrom AMC, Holm S, Rosenquist AL. (1988): Somatomedin C immunoreactivity in the Achilles tendon varies in a dynamic manner with the mechanical load. *Acta Physiol Scand,* 134:119–208.

43. Harper J, Amiel D, Harper E. (1988): Collagenase production by rabbit ligaments and tendon. *Connect Tissue Res,* 17:253–259.

44. Harper J, Amiel D, Harper E. (1989): Collagenases from periarticular ligaments and tendon: enzyme levels during the development of joint contracture. *Matrix,* 9:200–205.

45. Harper J, Amiel D, Harper E. (1990): Immunochemical characterization and determination of collagenase activity in periarticular tendon and ligaments during the early development of stress deprivation. *Orthop Trans* (abst), 15:535.

46. Harris WH, Heaney RP. (1969): Effect of growth hormone on skeletal mass in adult dogs. *Nature,* 223:403–404.

47. Hart D, Rehemtulla A. (1988): Plasminogen activators and their inhibitors: regulators of extracellular proteolysis and cell function. *Comp Biochem Physiol,* 90B:691–708.

48. Hart DA. (1992): Regulation of plasminogen activators in connective tissues: potential for thrombolytic therapy in collagen-vascular diseases. *Fibrinology (Suppl),* 6:43–48.

49. Hart DA. (1992): Dysregulation of plasminogen activators in cancer—potential role in invasion, metastasis, and as a prognostic indicator. *Fibrinology (Suppl),* 6: 11–15.

50. Hart DA, Fritzler MJ. (1989): Regulation of plasminogen activators and their inhibitors in rheumatic diseases: new understanding and the potential for new directions. *J Rheumatol,* 16:1184–1191.

51. Hart DA, O'Brien MD, Walsh SL, Frank CB. (1988): Plasminogen activators and inhibitors in rabbit connective tissues. *Fibrinology,* 2:171(abst).

52. Hastings DE. (1980): The non-operative treatment of collateral ligament injuries of the knee joint. *Clin Orthop,* 147:22–28.

53. Haus J, Halata Z. (1990): Innervation of the anterior cruciate ligament. *Int Orthop,* 14:293–296.

54. Hauschka PV, Mavrakos AE, Iafrati MD, Doleman SE, Klagsbrun M. (1986): Growth factors in bone matrix. *J Biol Chem,* 261:12665–12674.

55. Hefti FL, Kress I, Fasel J, Morscher EW. (1991): Healing of the transected anterior cruciate ligament in the rabbit. *J Bone Joint Surg [Am],* 73:373–383.

56. Hokfelt T. (1991): Neuropeptides in perspective: the last ten years. *Neuron,* 7:867–879.

57. Holmdahl R, Jansson L. (1988): Estrogen-induced suppression of collagen induced arthritis. *Brain Behav Immun,* 2:123–132.

58. Holmdahl R, Jansson L, Anderson M. (1986): Female sex hormones suppress development of collagen induced arthritis in mice. *Arthritis Rheum,* 29:1501–1508.

59. Hynes RO. (1992): Integrins: versatility, modulation, signalling in cell adhesion. *Cell,* 69:11–25.

60. Ingebar D. (1991): Integrins as mechanochemical transducers. *Curr Opin Cell Biol,* 3:841–848.

61. Jackson DW, Grood ES, Arnoczky SP, Butler DL, Simon TM. (1987): Cruciate reconstruction using freeze dried anterior cruciate ligament allograft and a ligament augmentation device (LAD): an experimental study in a goat model. *Am J Sports Med,* 15:528–538.

62. Jackson DW, Grood ES, Arnoczky SP, Butler DL, Simon TM. (1987): Freeze dried anterior cruciate ligament allografts: preliminary studies in a goat model. *Am J Sports Med,* 15:295–303.

63. Jackson DW, Grood ES, Cohn BT, Arnoczky SP, Simon TM, Cummings JF. (1991): The effects of *in situ* freezing on the anterior cruciate ligament: an experimental study in goats. *J Bone Joint Surg [Am],* 73A:201–213.

64. Jackson DW, Simon TM, Kurzweil PR, Rosen MA. (1992): Survival of cells after intra-articular transplantation of fresh allografts of the patellar and anterior cruciate ligaments. *J Bone Joint Surg [Am],* 74A:112–118.

65. Jingushi S, Heydemann A, Kana SK, Macey LR, Bolander ME. (1990): Acidic fibroblast growth factor injection stimulates cartilage enlargement and inhibits cartilage gene expression in rat fracture healing. *J Orthop Res,* 8:364–371.

66. Johansson H, Sjolander P, Sojka P. (1991): A sensory role for the cruciate ligaments. *Clin Orthop,* 265:161–178.

67. Kannus P, Jarvinen M. (1989): Posttraumatic anterior cruciate ligament insufficiency as a cause of osteoarthritis in a knee joint. *Clin Rheumatol,* 8:251–260.

68. King GJW. (1991): *A biomechanical evaluation of orthotopic ligament transplantation in a rabbit model* [Thesis]. Calgary, Alberta: University of Calgary.

69. Kleiner JB, Arniel D, Harwood FL, Akeson WH. (1989): Early histologic, metabolic, and vascular assessment of anterior cruciate ligament autografts. *J Orthop Res,* 7:235–242.

70. Kleiner JB, Arniel D, Roux RD, Akeson WH. (1986): Origin of replacement cells for the anterior cruciate ligament autograft. *J Orthop Res,* 4:466–474.

71. Krummel TM, Nelson JM, Diegelman RF, Lindlad WJ, Salzberg AM, Greenfield LJ, Cohen IK. (1987): Fetal response to injury in the rabbit. *J Pediatr Surg,* 22:640–645.

72. Kubota Y, Kleinman HK, Martin GR, Lawley TJ. (1988): Role of laminin and basement membrane in the morphological differentiation of human endothelial cells into capillary-like structures. *J Cell Biol,* 107:1589–1598.

73. Kwan MK, Sung PKL, Akeson WH. (1992): Adhesion characteristics of human ligament fibroblasts. *Orthop Trans,* 17:76(abst).

74. Macaulay VM, Carney DN. (1991): Neuropeptide growth factors. *Cancer Invest,* 9:659–673.

75. Makisalo SE, Paavolainen PP, Lehto M, Skutnabb K, Slatis P. (1989): Collagen Types I and III and fibronectin in healing anterior cruciate ligament after reconstruction with carbon fibre. *Injury,* 20:72–76.

76. Mantyh PW. (1991): Substance P and the inflammatory and immune response. *Ann NY Acad Sci,* 632:263–271.

77. McDaniel WJ Jr, Dameron TB Jr. (1983): The untreated anterior cruciate ligament rupture. *Clin Orthop,* 172:90–92.

78. McDonald JA. (1988): Fibronectin: a primitive matrix. In: Clark RAF, Henson PM, eds. *The molecular and cellular biology of wound repair.* New York: Plenum Press, pp 405–435.

79. Meyers JF. (1991): Allograft reconstruction of the anterior cruciate ligament. *Clin Sports Med,* 10:487–498.

80. Murphy PG, Frank CB, Hart DA. (1991): Regulation of plasminogen activator and plasminogen activator inhibitor expression by connective tissues and connective tissue cells. In: *Combined Meeting of the ORS of USA, Japan, and Canada.* Calgary: The Organizing Committee of the Orthopaedic Research Societies, vol 1, p 10(abst).

81. Murphy PG, Frank CB, Hart DA. (1991): Rabbit MCL and ACL fibroblasts express plasminogen activator and inhibitor in culture: evidence for differences from synovial fibroblasts. *Orthop Trans,* 16:110(abst).

82. Nickerson DA, Joshi R, Williams S, Ross SM, Frank CB. (1992): Synovial fluid stimulates the proliferation of rabbit ligament fibroblasts *in vitro. Clin Orthop Rel Res,* 274:294–299.

83. Noyes FR. (1977): Functional properties of knee ligaments and alterations induced by immobilization: a correlative biomechanical and histological study in primates. *Clin Orthop Rel Res,* 123:210–242.

84. Noyes FR, Barber SD, Mangine RE. (1990): Bone-patellar ligament-bone and fascia lata allografts for reconstruction of the anterior cruciate ligament. *J Bone Joint Surg [Am],* 72:1125–1136.

85. Noyes FR, DeLucas JL, Torvik PJ. (1974): Biomechanics of anterior cruciate ligament failure: an analysis of strain-rate sensitivity and mechanisms of failure in primates. *J Bone Joint Surg [Am],* 56A:236–253.

86. Noyes FR, Matthews DS, Mooar PA, Grood ES. (1983): The symptomatic anterior cruciate-deficient knee. *J Bone Joint Surg* [*Am*], 65A:163–174.

87. O'Donoghue DH. (1955): An analysis of end results of surgical treatment of major injuries to the ligaments of the knee. *J Bone Joint Surg* [*Am*], 37A:1–13.

88. O'Donoghue DH, Frank GR, Jeter GL, Johnson W, Zeiders JW, Kenyon R. (1971): Repair and reconstruction of the anterior cruciate ligament in dogs: factors influencing long term results. *J Bone Joint Surg* [*Am*], 53A:710–718.

89. Pacheco HO, Gesink DS, Woods VL, Nagineni CN, Amiel D, Akeson WH. (1992): Integrin and fibronectin isoform expression in cultured rabbit anterior cruciate and medial collateral ligament fibroblasts. In: *Combined Meeting of the ORS of USA, Japan, and Canada.* Calgary: The Organizing Committee of the Orthopaedic Research Societies, vol 1, p 102(abst).

90. Paulos LE, Cherf J, Rosenberg TD, Beck CL. (1991): Anterior cruciate ligament reconstruction with autografts. *Clin Sports Med,* 10:469–485.

91. Robinson BW, Goss AN. (1981): Intrauterine healing of fetal rat cheek wounds. *Cleft Palate,* 18:251–255.

92. Ross SM, Joshi R, Frank CB. (1990): Establishment and comparison of fibroblast cell lines from the medial collateral and anterior cruciate ligaments of the rabbit. *In Vitro Cell Dev Biol,* 26:579–584.

93. Rowsell AR. (1984): The intra-uterine healing of fetal muscle wounds: experimental study in the rat. *Br J Plast Surg,* 37:635–642.

94. Ruoslahti E. (1991): Integrins. *J Clin Invest,* 87:1–5.

95. Schutte MJ, Dabezies EJ, Zimny ML, Happel LT. (1987): Neural anatomy of the human anterior cruciate ligament. *J Bone Joint Surg* [*Am*], 69:243–247.

96. Sharkey K, Bray RC. (1990): Innervation patterns of the collateral knee ligaments as revealed by silver staining and immunohistochemistry. *Soc Neurosci,* 16:882(abst).

97. Shino K, Inoue M, Horibe S, Hamada M, Ono K. (1990): Reconstruction of the anterior cruciate ligament using allogeneic tendon: long-term followup. *Am J Sports Med,* 18:457–465.

98. Shino K, Kawasaki T, Hirose I, Gotoh I, Inoue M, Ono K. (1984): Replacement of the anterior cruciate ligament by an allogenic tendon graft: an experimental study in the dog. *J Bone Joint Surg* [*Am*], 66:672–681.

99. Shino K, Kimura T, Hirose H, Inoue M, Ono K. (1986): Reconstruction of the anterior cruciate ligament by allogeneic tendon graft: an operation for chronic ligamentous insufficiency. *J Bone Joint Surg* [*Br*], 68B:739–746.

100. Siebert JW, Burd AR, McCarthy JG, Weinzweig J, Ehrlich HP. (1990): Fetal wound healing: a biochemical study of scarless healing. *Plast Reconstr Surg,* 85:495–504.

101. Sommerlath K, Lysholm J, Gillquist J. (1991): The long-term course after treatment of acute anterior cruciate ligament ruptures: a 9 to 16 year followup. *Am J Sports Med,* 19:156–162.

102. Stevenson S, Fredricks RW, Zart DJ, Li XQ, Bensusan J, Davy D, Klein L, Goldberg VM. (1989): The interaction and effects of freezing and histocompatibility on the incorporation of allogenic cortical grafts in rats. *Orthop Trans,* 14:269(abst).

103. Turner IG, Thomas NP. (1990): Comparative analysis of four types of synthetic anterior cruciate ligament replacement in the goat: *in vivo* histological and mechanical findings. *Biomaterials,* 11:321–329.

104. Viidik A. (1990): Structure and function of normal and healing tendons and ligaments. In: Mow VC, Ratcliffe A, Woo SL-Y, eds. *Biomechanics of diathrodial joints.* New York: Springer-Verlag, pp 3–38.

105. Walsh S, Frank CB, Hart DA. (1992): Immobilization alters cell metabolism in an immature ligament. *Clin Orthop Rel Res,* 277:277–288.

106. Whitby DJ, Ferguson MWJ. (1991): The extracellular matrix of lip wounds in fetal, neonatal, and adult mice. *Development,* 112:651–668.

107. Wiig ME, Amiel D, Ivarsson M, Nagineni CN, Wallace CD, Arfors KE. (1991): Type I procollagen gene expression in normal and early healing of the medial collateral and anterior cruciate ligaments in rabbits: an *in situ* hybridization study. *J Orthop Res,* ·9:374–382.

108. Woo SL-Y, Hollis JM, Adams DJ, Lyon RM, Takai S. (1991): Tensile properties of the human femur-anterior cruciate ligament-tibia complex: the effects of specimen age and orientation. *Am J Sports Med,* 19:217–225.

109. Woo SL-Y, Young EP. (1991): Structure and function of tendons and ligaments. In: Mow VC, Hayes WC, eds. *Basic orthopaedic biomechanics.* New York: Raven Press, pp 199–243.

110. Woo SL, Orlando CA, Gomez MA, Frank CB, Akeson WH. (1986): Tensile properties of the medial collateral ligament as a function of age. *J Orthop Res,* 4:133–141.

111. Woo SL-Y, Ohland KJ, Weiss JA. (1990): Aging and sex-related changes in the biomechanical properties of the rabbit medial collateral ligament. *Mech Ageing Dev,* 56:129–142.

112. Woo SL-Y, Peterson RH, Ohland KJ, Sites TJ, Danto MI. (1990): The effects of strain rate on the properties of the medial collateral ligament in skeletally immature and mature rabbits: a biomechanical and histological study. *J Orthop Res,* 8:712–721.

113. Woo SL-Y, Young EP, Kwan MK. (1990): Fundamental studies in knee ligament mechanics. In: Daniel D, Akeson WH, O'Connor J, eds. *Knee ligaments: structure, function, injury, and repair.* New York: Raven Press, pp 115–134.

114. Zimny ML, Schutte M, Dabezies E. (1986): Mechanoreceptors in the human anterior cruciate ligament. *Anat Rec,* 214:204–209.

The Anterior Cruciate Ligament: Current and Future Concepts, edited by D.W. Jackson, et al. Raven Press, Ltd., New York © 1993.

CHAPTER 15

Adhesion Macromolecules of the Ligament: The Molecular Glues in Wound Healing

Cahir A. McDevitt and Jose Marcelino

Wound healing necessarily involves the migration of inflammatory and connective tissue cells from the surrounding tissue or circulation into the area of the wound. The healing process also involves remodeling of the tissue with, finally, the deposition of a new extracellular matrix. Adhesion proteins are specialized proteins that play pivotal roles in both the migratory and remodeling processes (76). Fetal development and the metastasis of a tumor are two other processes in which cell motility, and therefore adhesion proteins, play a key role. Adhesion proteins bind cells to macromolecules of the extracellular matrix (see the previous chapter by Murphy, Frank and Hart for description of graft healing process). Some also can bind one macromolecule to another macromolecule in the extracellular matrix, thus organizing those molecules into higher ordered structures. The manner in which adhesion proteins endows tissues with different levels of organization has been referred to as "tissue engineering" by the Keystone Conference organizers. The role of adhesion proteins in cell motility and tissue engineering constitutes one of the most active and exciting research frontiers in medical research today.

The adhesion proteins of ligaments have only begun to be investigated. Certain general principles, however, appear to apply to a wound healing process generally, and we shall extrapolate from data obtained from other tissues in this review.

THE MOLECULAR BASIS OF CELL ADHESION

Cell adhesion may be viewed as a multistep process *in vitro* involving, initially, attachment to the adhesion pro-

tein or polysaccharide such as hyaluronan (formerly called hyaluronic acid), followed by spreading of the cells and organization of the membrane and cytoskeleton into mature adhesion contacts called "focal adhesion plaques"(67). Stationary, anchorage dependent, nontransformed cells are generally enriched in adhesion plaques. In contrast, highly migratory cells, including transformed cells, generally have fewer adhesion plaques (for references, see 2).

Cells must bind to adhesion proteins to move. However, as McCarthy et al. have pointed out, "cells must adhere sufficiently to the substrata to generate the traction force required for motility, yet not be so adherent that they are incapable of breaking adhesions and translocation" (51). There are a range of adhesion proteins available in ligament for cells, as there are cell surface receptors for interacting with these proteins. Clearly, cell-matrix interaction is a complex phenomenon and the different adhesion proteins very probably have different roles to play. We shall confine our discussion to five adhesion proteins: fibronectin, Type VI collagen, thrombospondin, tenascin, and laminin.

FIBRONECTIN

Fibronectin (from the Latin, *nectere,* to bind; *fibra,* a fiber) was the first adhesion protein to be identified and studied in detail. It should be noted, however, that the concentration of fibronectin in ligaments has not been established. Quantitatively, it may be a minor adhesion protein in the tissue.

The fibronectin molecule is composed of two elongated subunits that are bound near one extremity by a disulfide bond to form a V-shaped structure (Fig. 1). Each subunit is composed of distinct structural domains that interact with specific receptors on the surface of cells

C. A. McDevitt and J. Marcelino: Section of Musculoskeletal Biology, Department of Biomedical Engineering, The Cleveland Clinic Foundation Research Institute, Cleveland, Ohio 44106.

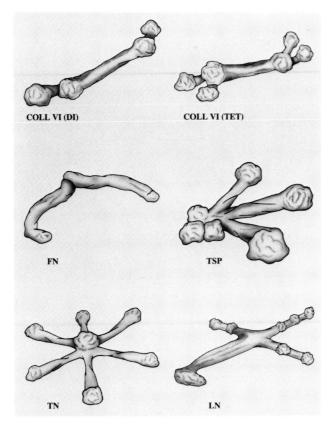

FIG. 1. Space-filling models showing shapes of adhesion proteins. These models were drawn from electron micrographs in which the protein was rotary shadowed. *COLL VI (DI)*, two dumbbell-shaped molecules (i.e., monomers of Type VI collagen) associate laterally to form the dimer (*DI*) shown here. The globular extremity of one molecule interacts with the triple helix between the globular domains of the second molecule. *COLL VI (TET)*, tetramer of Type VI collagen formed by two dimers associating in a scissors-like configuration. The two larger inner globes represent two globular domains of the monomeric molecule that are unresolved in the electron microscope. Tetramers are considered to associate longitudinally to form the fibrils of Type VI collagen (microfilaments) that are seen in Figs. 2 and 3. *FN*, fibronectin, with its two arms joined by disulfide linkages at one extremity. *TSP*, thrombospondin. The protein is composed of three polypeptides, each composed of a small globular domain and then a thin strand connected to a large globular domain at the carboxyl extremity. *TN*, tenascin. Sometimes referred to as hexabrachion in the literature, with its characteristic stellate appearance. *LN*, laminin, showing the cross-like structure.

or with other matrix macromolecules that include collagen, fibrin and heparin (93). These domains are formed by segments of repeating polypeptides that share similarities in their respective amino acid sequences and repeat themselves. The repeats have been called Type I, Type II and Type III repeats (83). Type I and II are characterized by intramolecular disulfide bonded repeats; Type III is composed of conserved aromatic residues. Fibronectin interacts with cells, collagen and heparin by noncovalent bonds. The interaction with fibrin (or fibrinogen) and collagen can be covalently cross-linked by factor IIIa

transglutaminase (64). This interaction anchors fibronectin in the fibrin clot, thus permitting cells to migrate into the wound.

Along with its fibrin binding domain, fibronectin also has a domain that binds both native and denatured collagens (22,78). The importance of this interaction allows the reconstruction of the disrupted matrix, although the possibility of fibronectin interfering with collagen fibrillogenesis should be noted (41).

In addition to its binding capacity toward collagen, proteoglycan, integrins, and fibrin, fibronectin is also capable of binding to hyaluronan (37), tenascin (16), entactin (seelaminin) (91), thrombospondin (21), and Type VI collagen (53).

The interaction between cells and fibronectin is mediated by a distinct family of cell surface receptors called integrins (36). Such integrins, specifically the $\alpha 5\beta 1$, have been shown to bind to the cell binding domain through the tripeptide sequence, arginine-glycine-aspartic acid (RGD in the more recent, single letter nomenclature for amino acids) (79). Cell surface proteoglycans, such as syndecan (25), also bind to fibronectin. The sulfate groups of the heparan sulfate proteoglycans interact with the arginine residues within the heparin binding domain of fibronectin (38).

Alternative splicing of the pre-mRNA gives rise to multiple forms of fibronectin. Variation in the relative proportion of these isoforms can modulate cell behavior (83). With the three alternately spliced segments of fibronectin (EIIIA, EIIIB, and V), the V region plays an important role in plasma and cellular fibronectin structure and function. The presence (V+) or absence (V_0) of the V region within the molecule determines its solubility. Plasma fibronectin is predominantly $V+V_0$ (one subunit has the V region while the other does not) and the remainder being V+ homodimers (83). This $V+V_0$ heterodimeric structure allows the molecule to remain soluble in the blood but also allows the molecule to be incorporated into the extracellular matrix (83). Although plasma and cellular fibronectin share similar (but not identical) primary structure and glycosylation, the two types of fibronectin can be distinguished through its quaternary structure. In the rat, cellular fibronectin is composed mainly of V+ homodimers while plasma fibronectin is mainly $V+V_0$ heterodimers (83).

Fibronectin in Wound Healing

Fibronectin plays many roles in wound healing, including chemattraction of fibroblasts, cell adhesion, wound contraction and deposition of the new matrix. As noted above, fibronectin is cross-linked to fibrin by plasma transglutaminase in the plasma clot that initially forms in the wound. Fibroblasts, stimulated by growth factors, are attracted into the wound by chemotactic fragments of fibronectin. Once within the fibrin clot, the fibroblasts attach to the fibronectin. Deposition by the fibroblasts of matrix macromolecules then occurs, including Type I and III collagen, hyaluronan, fibronectin, proteoglycans, and thrombospondin (57).

Fibronectin is an active player in the inflammatory phase of wound healing, particularly in the activation and aggregation of platelets (86). The RGD sequence in fibronectin binds to the GpIIb-IIIa receptor in platelets (73). Peptides containing the RGD sequence (32) and monoclonal antibodies against the GpIIIb-IIIa complex (74) inhibit adhesion of platelets to fibronectin. Fibronectin can also mediate platelet adhesion to nonfibrillar Type I and III collagens, but not their fibrillar forms (69). Activated platelets then release a collection of adhesion proteins that include thrombospondin and von Willebrand factor, as well as proteinases and growth factors (89).

Fibronectin promotes wound contraction by linking cellular stress fiber (i.e., actin filaments) with collagen. As wound healing progresses, the concentration of fibronectin decreases and the remodeled matrix is then predominantly Type I collagen and proteoglycans (47).

Fibronectin also acts as an opsonin by binding to bacteria and cellular/tissue debris that are then subsequently phagocytized by macrophages (50).

Along with its chemotactic activity toward endothelial cells required for vascular formation and subsequent delivery of nutritional goods (10) and fibroblasts, fibronectin has also been shown to be chemotactic toward monocytes (20). This activity then supports the molecule's opsonic function in tissue remodeling, an important phase in wound healing.

TYPE VI COLLAGEN

When ligaments are ground in liquid nitrogen and extracted with a solution of 4M guanidine hydrochloride, an effective solvent for proteins, Type VI is one of the major proteins mobilized from the tissue. It is thus one of the major proteins in the tissue apart from Type I/III collagen. Its classification as a collagen is misleading: it does not form cross-links to form an insoluble fibrillar meshwork and its properties are those of an adhesion glycoprotein.

Type VI collagen is a ubiquitous component of all connective tissues, including ligaments. Its macromolecular form is that of thin fibrils, made up of a building block that is a tetramer of the dumbbell shaped Type VI molecules. It is first necessary to describe the molecular form of Type VI collagen before discussing its function and the fibrils it forms.

The Structure of Type VI Collagen

Type VI collagen is a truly distinctive protein. It has a dumbbell-shaped structure, comprised of three genetically distinct α chains that form a relatively short triple helix with large globular domains at each extremity (Reviewed in 18). Two molecules of Type VI collagen associate to form dimers (Fig. 1). This is accomplished by disulfide bridging between the globular domain of one molecule and the triple helix of the other. Two dimers associate scissors-fashion to form a tetramer (Fig. 1). The tetramer is considered the functional form of Type VI collagen in tissues. The α chains migrate on electrophoresis under reduced conditions as a ladder of three to four bands between 185 kDa and 260 kDa ($\alpha3$ chain) and a broad band (or two bands) at 140 kDa ($\alpha1$ and $\alpha2$ chains) (54,92). Digestion of the globular domains of the intact Type VI collagen molecule with pepsin gives rise to three fragments of apparent MR 70 kDa ($\alpha1$), 55 kDa ($\alpha2$), and 40 kDa ($\alpha3$) that represent the Gly-X-Y repeat segment of the triple helix, collagenous domain with some attached, nonhelical peptide (92). Sequencing of chicken (8), and human (19) Type VI collagen cDNA has revealed at least 9 RGD sequences in the triple helix. The nonhelical portions contain 15 repeat segments, each 200 residues, nine of which are located in the $\alpha3$ chain (4,80) and three each in the $\alpha1$ and $\alpha2$ (18) chains. The repeating segment bears homology with the collagen binding motif of von Willebrand factor and cartilage matrix protein (8,18,19). The $\alpha3$ chain also contains segments that bear homology with the Type III repeat of fibronectin and the Kunitz inhibitors of serine proteinases (8,19), respectively.

Type VI Collagen in Ligaments

Early work by Gibson and Clearly (31) demonstrated that Type VI collagen was a constituent of ligamentum nuchae. Using cationic dyes (35) in an electron microscopic study of rabbit medial collateral ligament, Bray and colleagues discovered that the extracellular matrix was subdivided by electron dense "seams" that interconnected cells (11). These seams consisted mainly of thread-like, beaded microfilaments whose dimensions and appearance were similar to those of Type VI collagen (40,87). This is illustrated in the electron micrograph of rabbit medial collateral ligament shown in Fig. 2, which shows the meshwork of the alternating thin and thick microfilaments. Immunoelectron microscopy with gold labeled anti-Type VI collagen antibodies confirmed the identity of these microfilaments as Type VI collagen (12). Similar microfilaments have been observed in skin and cartilage (40). The alternating thin and thick segments of one (or maybe two) Type VI collagen microfilaments are shown in the high power electron micrograph in Fig. 3. The periodicity in these filaments is close to 100 nm, corresponding to the approximate length of the tetramer of Type VI collagen shown in Fig. 1. Bray (12), from the appearance of stereo pairs in sequential slices,

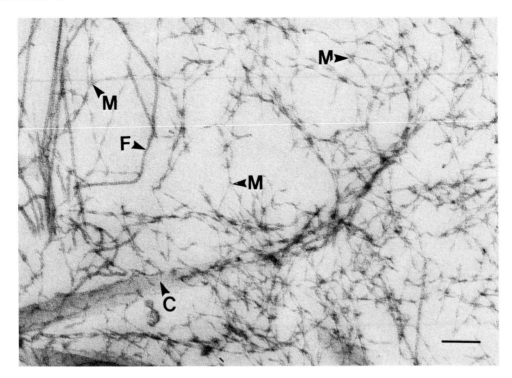

FIG. 2. Electron micrograph of midsubstance of 4-month-old rabbit medial collateral ligament that has been digested with testicular hyaluronidase. The tissue was fixed in glutaraldehyde containing ruthenium hexamine trichloride (RHT) followed by a postfixation in osmium tetroxide containing RHT (see ref. 11 for details). The micrograph shows a well-dispersed network of Type VI collagen microfilaments. The microfilaments appear as thin strands with alternating thick and thin segments. Association between different microfilaments is always at a thick segment (*M*). Banded fibrils, mainly of Type I/III collagen, are also evident (*C*). A 10-nm-diameter microfibril (*F*), clearly distinguishable from the Type VI collagen microfilaments, is also evident and probably represents a fibrillin-elastin microfibril. (×70,000, bar: 200 nm) (Courtesy of Dr. Doug Bray.)

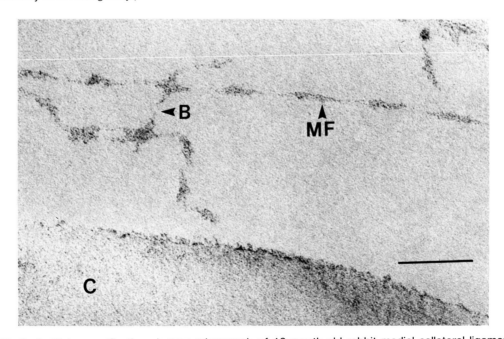

FIG. 3. A: High-magnification electron micrograph of 10-month-old rabbit medial collateral ligament, fixed as described in Fig. 2. The strand (*MF*) represents one, or maybe two, Type VI collagen microfilaments. The periodicity of this microfilament is about 100 nm, approximating the length of a Type VI collagen tetramer. (×250,000) Microfilaments crossing over and making contact at their thick segments are also evident (**B**). A single Type I/III collagen fibril (**C**) is evident at the bottom of the picture.

has proposed that these thin and thick segments represent a spiral.

The role, if any, of hyaluronan in the microfilaments has yet to be established. Type VI collagen binds to hyaluronan (54) *in vitro*. It is as yet unclear whether the Type VI collagen decorates strands of hyaluronan in the microfilaments in Figs. 2 and 3. Figure 3 shows an interconnection between the thick regions of two microfilaments, involving, perhaps, some other matrix protein. These fibrils make contact with the Type I/III collagen fibrils in ligaments, as well as the fibroblasts in the tissue. The Type VI collagen molecule, with its domains for interacting with itself to form tetramers and fibrils, as well as those domains for interacting with other matrix molecules such as hyaluronan and the surface of cells, is thus elegantly tailored to function as an adhesion protein in ligaments.

Type VI Collagen and Cell Attachment

Electron microscopic studies of ligament (12) and cartilage (40) demonstrate that Type VI collagen fibrils are often in contact with cell surfaces. Purified pepsinized Type VI collagen (that lacks, therefore, its globular domains) attached a range of fibroblast and tumor cell lines as well as embryo arterial smooth muscle cells (2). The unfolded α2 (VI) and α3 (VI) chains also showed attachment that were, not surprisingly, sensitive to RGD containing peptides (2).

We addressed the issue of chondrocyte and fibrochondrocyte attachment to Type VI collagen by the more difficult, but more physiologically meaningful approach of purifying the highly insoluble, intact, nonpepsinized Type VI collagen (54). We found that intact Type VI collagen did indeed attach and spread chondrocytes and fibrochondrocytes, but by an RGD-independent mechanism (56).

Type VI Collagen in Wound Healing

Rupture of the anterior cruciate ligament elicits osteoarthritic changes in the articular cartilage of dogs (52). Type VI collagen is enriched in this experimental osteoarthritic cartilage, presumably as a "wound healing" or repair response (55).

Type VI collagen is confined to the periphery of full thickness wounds in rabbit corneas at one week after initiation of the defect (66). Thereafter, however, the level of Type VI collagen increased substantially in the healing wound. Immunoelectron microscopy demonstrated Type VI collagen pericellularly, suggesting that its cell adhesion capacity was a key property in the healing process.

Thickening of the ligamentum flavum has been implicated in low-back pain (39). In these ligaments the normal elastic meshwork was ruptured, and the resultant fibrosis appeared hyaline and was rich in Type VI collagen. This was interpreted by the authors as a reparative process.

THROMBOSPONDIN

Thrombospondin is a protein that binds to cell surfaces and is present in ligaments (61). It was first identified by Baenziger et al. (4) in 1971 as the major protein released by the α granules of platelets after challenge with thrombin. Our laboratory identified thrombospondin as a constituent of hyaline cartilage and demonstrated that it is synthesized by chondrocytes in culture (63). We then demonstrated that it is also present in ligaments, meniscus and the intervertebral disc and is synthesized by ligament fibroblasts and meniscal fibrochondrocytes in culture (61). It would appear that thrombospondin is a secreted product of most mesenchymal and epithelial cells (80).

Thrombospondin is composed of three identical polypeptide chains, each of absolute molecular weight 146 kDa, but that migrate in electrophoretic gels under reduced conditions with an apparent molecular weight of 180 kDa. Each polypeptide appears in the electron microscope as a thin strand that bears globular domains at each extremity (Fig. 1) The strands are joined at a hinge region by disulfide bonds. Like fibronectin, thrombospondin contains discrete functional domains that bind to other matrix molecules, including fibronectin, fibrinogen, plasminogen, sulfated glycolipid, Type V collagen, and calcium (28,46).

Thrombospondin and Wound Healing

Thrombospondin is released from stimulated platelets and becomes incorporated, presumably by binding to fibrinogen, into the fibrin clot (75). As early wounds are filled with a fibrin clot, it is not surprising that thrombospondin has been implicated in wound healing in human skin (75), rat skeletal muscle (88), and bovine corneal endothelium (65).

Thrombospondin is concentrated in the dermis along the lateral and deep margins of the wounds at 2, 3, 5 and 7 days after induction of the incision in human volunteers (75). The protein is then apparently cleared from the extracellular matrices as it is no longer detectable in these sites in most 14-day-old wounds. Thrombospondin is enriched, however, around the vascular channels of day 7 and day 14 wounds (75). Raugi et al. (75) suggested a role for thrombospondin in the early organization of the extracellular matrix in the wound healing process.

An elegant study by Watkins et al. (88) explored the role of thrombospondin in rat soleus muscle which had been crushed with a hemostat and then allowed to heal *in vivo.* Care was taken in these experiments not to injure the muscle tendons. Fibrin networks appeared immediately after crushing, followed within a few hours by an ordered accumulation of thrombospondin in the connective tissue surrounding the muscle fiber and the blood vessel. Thrombospondin levels appeared maximal at 3 to 6 days postinjury, and decreased thereafter to near normal levels after 7 days, coincident with the appearance of regenerating muscle fibers (88). Fibrin, in contrast, was only present in trace quantities at 5 days after injury. Electrophoresis suggests that the thrombospondin incorporated into the injured site was in a polymerized state (88). The thrombospondin may have been associated with some other matrix component, such as a collagen.

The results of Watkins et al. (88) on the regenerating muscle that was crushed and of Raugi et al. (75) on wound healing in human skin are in striking agreement. Their data suggest that thrombospondin is a key, but transient, factor in the elaboration of a new extracellular matrix.

The Molecular Mechanisms of Thrombospondin in Wound Healing

The data reviewed above suggest that the role of thrombospondin may be twofold: (a) as a constituent, presumably adhesion protein, in the organization of the new extracellular matrix; (b) as a possible participant in angiogenesis. The capacity of thrombospondin to bind other matrix macromolecules is probably operative in the organization of the new matrix. In its role as a cell binding protein, however, thrombospondin may function also as a "detachment factor" for some cells in which migration (e.g., into the healing wound) may be facilitated. As noted below, the interaction of thrombospondin with endothelial cells seems particularly complex.

Thrombospondin as an Adhesive Protein

While thrombospondin binds to the surface of many cells, it does not seem to be a classical adhesion protein, like fibronectin, laminin and Type VI collagen, that attach and spread cells. The nature and consequences of the interaction of thrombospondin with cells appears to be much more complex, as Sage and Bornstein (80) have noted. Thrombospondin attaches chondrocytes (62), some fibroblasts, keratinocytes, neurons, and a variety of transformed cells (80) as well as *Staphylococcus aureus* (80). Fragmentation of the molecule with proteinases and evaluation of the isolated fragments has implicated a range of cell-attachment sites in thrombospondin. Among these are: (a) the NH_2-terminal globular domain

that binds heparin; (b) the RGDA sequence, located in the calcium binding domain, that attaches to $\beta 3$ integrin receptors on the cell surface (44,80); (c) the COOH-terminal globe that contains a non-RGD attachment site (44). This latter binding site was identified by expressing the COOH-terminal 212 amino acids in a bacterium and demonstrating that the resultant fusion protein was effective in supporting cell attachment, even though it lacks an RGD sequence (44).

Angiogenesis is a multistep process involving migration, attachment and proliferation of endothelial cells (5). Thrombospondin appears to influence this series of events by mechanisms whose complexity is not understood. While thrombospondin promotes attachment of bovine aortic endothelial cells, it inhibits formation of focal adhesion plaques and spreading of the cells (67). Thrombospondin also inhibits the proliferation of endothelial cells from a variety of different sources. The effect seems to be specific for endothelial cells, as thrombospondin actually increases proliferation of vascular smooth muscle cells and human foreskin fibroblasts (5). These observations, collectively, support a role for thrombospondin as an inhibitor of angiogenesis, a property of the molecule that may have a therapeutic application.

LAMININ

The classical laminin, which has a molecular weight of about 900 kDa, is a multidomain glycoprotein found as a major constituent of basement membranes (6). Rotary shadow electron microscopy reveals the characteristic cross-like structure of the molecule (13). The molecule is composed of three distinct polypeptide chains (A, B 1, and B2) cross-linked by disulfide bonds (72). Each chain has six domains (I to VI) and an extra EGF-like and globular domain (IIIa and IVa, respectively) in the A chain (72). Laminin has been observed to self-aggregate in a calcium-dependent manner and its interaction with other laminin molecules is mediated by the globular domain, VI (14). Extraction of laminin was first accomplished from EHS murine tumor by using 0.5M NaCl and chelating agents where laminin couples with another basement membrane protein called nidogen/entactin in a 1:1 complex (1). The characterization of laminin's biological functions is accomplished by fragmenting the molecule with limited enzyme digestion. Fragments such as the Pl, El, and E8 have been shown to have mitogenic or cell attachment properties or both (64,65,70). In the proteolytic fragmentation of the molecule, a cryptic cell attachment site with the pentapeptide sequence TRY-ILE-GLY-SER-ARG (YIGSR) has been localized in the inner part of the cross-like structure of the molecule (66). Interaction with other basement membrane molecules is another important aspect of laminin. The molecule's interaction with nidogen/entactin has been localized in the inner part (Pl fragment) of laminin and has significance as a mediator for laminin-coll IV interaction, although direct laminin-coll IV interaction has been observed (71). In addition to its interactions with other laminin molecules, Type IV collagen and entactin/nidogen, laminin also binds to heparan sulfate proteoglycan (29) and binds more avidly to heparin (81).

Laminin fragments also have some growth factor-like activity in terms of promoting neurite outgrowth and mitogenicity on several types of cells (23,42,70). This biological property of the molecule has been localized both in the Pl and E8 fragments (3). Receptors for laminin have been shown to be several members of the integrin family and also some nonintegrin types (58,60). Of the nonintegrin binding proteins, most of the focus has been on the 67 kDa receptor that has been found in many cell types and has been observed to have a high affinity for laminin (58,60). The 67 kDa receptor has been shown to bind the pentapeptide sequence YIGSR (33) and other sites in the molecule (see 59 for an extensive review of laminin receptors).

The Role of Laminin in Wound Repair

Laminin shares several similarities with fibronectin in terms of its role in wound healing. Like fibronectin, platelets adhere to laminin at considerable shear rates (34). This adhesion is possibly mediated mainly by the $\alpha6\beta1$ integrin and the presence of calcium at physiological concentrations (34). This calcium requirement is possibly necessary for laminin aggregation which is then preferred by platelets. Laminin is also chemotactic for neutrophils, which are mainly responsible for preventing bacterial infection (42) and mast cells (85). During neovascularization, laminin possibly helps in mediating vessel formation. In an *in vitro* angiogenesis model, human umbilical endothelial cells were revealed to be capable of forming "endotubes" (capillary-like structures) when plated on Matrigel (reconstituted basement membrane matrix enriched with laminin) and influenced by interferon α but inhibited by IFNΓ (49). Madri and Pratt (48) have shown previously that plating of microvascular endothelial cells on selected basement membrane components such as laminin results in the formation of tubelike structures. If the same cells were plated on Type I or III collagen, there was no formation of tube-like structure. Laminin seems to appear more prominently during or after tissue remodeling as revealed by the molecule being present only after reepithelialization and wound closure (30). The Pl fragment of laminin has also been detected in human serum during wound healing, showing maximum levels within 7 postoperative days (7). This obser-

vation supports laminin's role as an important marker for wound repair.

TENASCIN

Another important extracellular matrix protein is tenascin, a name coined by Chiquet-Ehrismann (15) that pertains to the same molecule isolated independently by several laboratories. Tenascin's unique spider-like structure is observed under rotary shadow electron microscopy (27). Tenascin has a large molecular weight of about 1.9×10^6 Da and is composed of six long arms: three arms are disulfide linked to each other at the T junction to form a trimer and two trimers are then disulfide bonded to each other at the central globule to form the whole molecule (26). Under reducing conditions, human tenascin runs as three major bands in SDS-PAGE with the apparent molecular weights of 320K, 230K, and 220K (17). Within each arm, different domains exist: a heptad, EGF-like and fibronectin Type III repeats plus a terminal segment that bears similarity to fibrinogen (26). Tenascin expression is predominantly confined to organogenesis (within the mesenchyme around the developing organs), wound healing and tumors (82). Despite tenascin's temporal and spatial expression during embryogenesis and pathology, immunohistochemical studies reveal the expression of the molecule in several normal adult tissues (45), suggesting a more ubiquitous type of expression.

Some of the proposed biological functions of tenascin include: inhibition of cell attachment on fibronectin, inhibition of epithelial cell-cell adhesion, hemagglutination, immunosuppression of T lymphocytes, and as a cell adhesion protein that does not promote cell spreading (15,77). The contrary functions of tenascin in terms of cell adhesion have been investigated and the adhesive and antiadhesive properties have been localized in two independent sites within each subunit of the molecule (84).

Tenascin in Wound Healing

The role of tenascin in wound healing has just been recently investigated. Although it has been proposed that tenascin has a limited spatiotemporal distribution, with its restriction to embryonic tissues, tumors and wounds, the molecule's expression in normal adult tissues (24) possibly reflects the continuation of the similar role(s) that tenascin played during embryogenesis, i.e., maintenance of epithelial-stromal interaction that is required for organogenesis (24) and cell migration (90). Furthermore, the prominence of tenascin in several types of tumor may implicate roles as a marker for undifferentiated tumor and a possible aid in the diagnosis of tumors by means of monoclonal antibodies for the molecule (9).

Tenascin, like the other adhesion molecules that have been discussed, is also prominent in wounds (82). Its role in inducing cell migration counterbalances the effects of fibronectin. Mechanically, this is accomplished by the reduction of focal adhesions in spread cells by tenascin, as has been observed in bovine aortic endothelial cells (68). In addition, tenascin has been shown to inhibit T-cell activation in a fashion similar to the reduction of focal adhesions (93). This activity would be advantageous in regulating T-cell activity (77), such as cytotoxicity, that in turn may be damaging if left unchecked.

SUMMARY

As noted above, the adhesion proteins play important roles in the mobility and attachment of cells, and in the assembly of the new extracellular matrix within the wound area. Clearly, the different adhesion proteins play different roles in this process. Knowing more about these interactions should aid in developing biological prostheses for the ligament.

ACKNOWLEDGMENTS

We wish to thank Dr. Doug Bray, University of Lethbridge, Alberta, Canada, for generously supplying the electron micrographs of Figs. 2 and 3 and for providing us with access to data prior to publication. We also thank Ms. Judy Christopher for editorial and typing assistance. Support from the National Institutes of Health (ROLI-AR39569) and the Edison BioTechnology Center of Ohio is acknowledged.

REFERENCES

1. Aeschlimann D, Paulsson M. (1991): Cross-linking of laminin-nidogen complexes by tissue transglutaminase. *J Biol Chem,* 266:15308–15317.
2. Aumailley M, Mann K, von der Mark M, Timpl M. (1989): Cell attachment of collagen Type VI and Arg-Gly-Asp dependent binding to its alpha 2(VI) and alpha 3(VI) chains. *Exp Cell Res,* 181:463–474.
3. Aumailley M, Nurcombe V, Edgar D, Paulsson M, Timpl R. (1987): The cellular interactions of laminin fragments: cell adhesion correlates with two fragment-specific high affinity binding sites. *J Biol Chem,* 262:11532–11538.
4. Baenziger NL, Brodie GN, Majerus PW. (1971): A thrombin-sensitive protein of human platelet membranes. *Proc Natl Acad Sci USA,* 68:240–243.
5. Bagavandoss P, Wilks JW. (1990): Specific inhibition of endothelial cell proliferation by thrombospondin. *Biochem Biophys Res Commun,* 170:867–872.
6. Beck K, Hunter I, Engel J. (1990): Structure and function of laminin: anatomy of a multidomain glycoprotein. *FASEB J,* 4:148–160.
7. Bentsen KD, Lanng C, Hirslev-Petersen K, Risteli J. (1988): The amino terminal propeptide of Type III procollagen and basement membrane components in serum during wound healing in man. *Acta Chir Scand,* 154:97–101.
8. Bonaldo P, Colombatti A. (1989): The carboxyl terminus of the chicken α3 chain of collagen VI is a unique mosaic structure with glycoprotein Ib-like, fibronectin Type III, and Kunitz modules. *J Biol Chem,* 264:20235–20239.
9. Bourdon MA, Wikstrand CJ, Furthmayer H, Mathews TJ, Bigner DD. (1983): Human glioma mesenchymal extracellular matrix antigen defined by monoclonal antibody. *Cancer Res,* 43: 2796–2805.
10. Bowersox JC, Sorgente N. (1982): Chemotaxis of aortic endothelial cells in response to fibronectin. *Cancer Res,* 42:2547–2551.
11. Bray DF, Frank CB, Bray RC. (1990): Cytochemical evidence for a proteoglycan-associated network in ligament extracellular matrix. *J Orthop Res,* 8:1–12.
12. Bray DF, Bray RC, Frank CB. (1993): Ultrastructural immunolocalization of Type VI collagen and chondroitin sulfate in ligament. *J Orthop Res, (in press).*
13. Bruch M, Landwehr R, Engel J. (1989): Dissection of laminin by cathepsin C into its long arm and short arm structures and localization of regions involved in calcium dependent stabilization and self association. *Eur J Biochem,* 185:271–279.
14. Charonis AS, Tsilibary EC, Yurchenco PD, Furthrnay R, Coritz A. (1985): Binding of laminin to Type IV collagen: a morphological study. *J Cell Biol,* 100:1848–1853.
15. Chiquet-Ehrismann R. (1990): What distinguishes tenascin from fibronectin? *FASEB J,* 4:2598–2604.
16. Chiquet Ehrismann R, Kalla P, Pearson CA, Beck K, Chiquet M. (1988): Tenascin interferes with fibronectin action. *Cell,* 53:383–390.
17. Chiquet M, Fambrough DM. (1984): Chick myotendinous antigen: II. A novel extracellular glycoprotein complex consisting of large disulfide-linked subunits. *J Cell Biol,* 98:1937–1946.
18. Chu M-L, Pan T-C, Conway D, et al. (1990): The structure of Type VI collagen. In: Fleischmajer R, Olsen BR, Kuhn K, eds. *Structure, molecular biology, and pathology of collagen,* vol 580. New York: New York Academy of Sciences, pp 55–63.
19. Chu M-L, Zhang R-Z, Pan T-C, et al. (1990): Mosaic structure of globular domains in the human Type VI collagen α3 chain: similarity to von Willebrand factor, fibronectin, actin, salivary proteins and aprotinin type protease inhibitors. *EMBO J,* 9:385–393.
20. Clark RAF, Wikner NE, Doherty DE, Norris DA. (1988): Cryptic chemotactic activity of fibronectin for human monocytes resides at the 120-kDa fibroblastic cell-binding fragment. *J Biol Chem,* 263:12115–12123.
21. Dardik R, Lahav J. (1989): Multiple domains are involved in the interaction of endothelial cell thrombospondin with fibronectin. *Eur J Biochem,* 185:581–588.
22. Dessau W, Adelmann BC, Timpl R, Martin GR. (1978): Identification of the sites in collagen α chains that bind serum anti-gelatin factor (cold-insoluble globulin). *Biochem J,* 169:55–59.
23. Edgar D, Timpl R, Thoenen H. (1984): The heparin-binding domain of laminin is responsible for its effects on neurite outgrowth and neuronal survival. *EMBO J,* 3:1463–1468.
24. Ekblom P, Aufderheide E. (1989): Stimulation of tenascin expression in mesenchyme by epithelial-mesenchymal interactions. *Int J Dev Biol,* 33:71–79.
25. Elenius K, Salmivirta M, Inki P, Mali M, Jalkanen M. (1990): Binding of human syndecan to extracellular matrix proteins. *J Biol Chem,* 265:17837–17843.
26. Erickson HP, Bourdon MA. (1989): Tenascin: an extracellular matrix protein prominent in specialized embryonic tissues and tumors. *Annu Rev Cell Biol,* 5:71–92.
27. Erickson HP, Inglesias JL. (1984): A six-armed oligomer isolated from cell surface fibronectin preparations. *Nature,* 311:267–269.
28. Frazier WA. (1987): Mini-review: thrombospondin. A modular adhesive glycoprotein of platelets and nucleated cells. *J Cell Biol,* 105:625–632.
29. Frenette GP, Ruddon RW, Krzesicki RF, Naser JA. (1989): Biosynthesis and deposition of a noncovalent laminin-heparan sulfate proteoglycan complex and other basal lamina components by a human malignant cell line. *J Biol Chem,* 264:3078–3088.
30. Fujikawa LS, Foster CS, Gipson IK, Colvin RB. (1984): Basement membrane components in healing rabbit corneal epithelial wounds: immunofluorescence and ultrastructural studies. *J Cell Biol,* 98:128–138.
31. Gibson MA, Clearly EG. (1982): A collagen like glycoprotein from elastic rich tissues. *Biochem Biophys Res Commun,* 105: 1288–1295.

32. Ginsburg M, Pierschbacher MD, Ruoslahti E, Marguerie G, Plow E. (1985): Inhibition of fibronectin binding to platelets by proteolytic fragments and synthetic peptides which support fibroblast adhesion. *J Biol Chem,* 260:3931–3936.

33. Graf J, Iwamoto Y, Sasaki M, Martin GR, Kleinman HK, Robey FA, Yamada Y. (1987): Identification of an amino acid sequence in laminin mediating cell attachment, chemotaxis, and receptor binding. *Cell,* 48:989–996.

34. Hindriks G, Jsseldijk MJ, Sonnenberg A, Sixma JJ, de Groot PG. (1992): Platelet adhesion to laminin: Role of Ca2+ and Mg2+ ions, shear rate, and platelet membrane glycoproteins. *Blood,* 79:928–935.

35. Hunziker EB, Herrmann W, Schenk RK. (1982): Improved cartilage fixation by ruthenium hexamine trichloride (RHT). *J Ultrastruct Res,* 81:1–12.

36. Hynes RO. (1992): Integrins: versatility, modulation, and signaling in cell adhesion. *Cell,* 69:11–25.

37. Isemura M, Yosizawa Z, Koide T, Ono T. (1982): Interaction of fibronectin and its proteolytic fragments with hyaluronic acid. *J Biochem,* 92:731–734.

38. Jaikaria NS, Rosenfeld L, Khan MY, Danishefsky I, Newman SA. (1991): Interaction of fibronectin with heparin in model extracellular matrices: role of arginine residues and sulfate groups. *Biochemistry,* 30:1538–1544.

39. Kawahara E, Oda Y, Katsuda S, Nakanishi I, Aoyama K, Tomita K. (1991): Microfilamentous Type VI collagen in the hyalinized stroma of the hypertrophied ligamentum flavum. *Virchows Arch A Pathol Anat Histopathol,* 419:373–380.

40. Keene DR, Engvall E, Glanville RW. (1988): Ultrastructure of Type VI collagen in human skin and cartilage suggests an anchoring function for this filamentous network. *J Cell Biol,* 107:1995–2006.

41. Kleinman FK, Wilkes CM, Martin GR. (1981): Interaction of fibronectin with collagen fibrils. *Biochemistry,* 20:2325–2330.

42. Kleinman HK, Cannon FB, Laurie GW, Hassell JR, Aumailley M, Terranova VP, Martin GR, DuBois-Dalcq M. (1985): Biological activities of laminin. *J Cell Biochem,* 27:317–325.

43. Kleinman HK, Graf J, Iwamoto Y, Sasaki M, Schasteen CS, Yamada Y, Martin GR, Robey FA. (1989): Identification of a second active site in laminin for promotion of cell adhesion and migration and inhibition of *in vivo* melanoma lung colonization. *Arch Biochem Biophys,* 272:39–45.

44. Kosfeld MD, Pavlopoulos TV, Frazier WA. (1991): Cell attachment activity of the carboxyl-terminal domain of human thrombospondin expressed in *Escherichia coli. J Biol Chem,* 266:24257–24259.

45. Koukoulis GK, Gould VE, Bhattacharyya A, Gould JE, Howeedy AA, Virtanen I. (1991): Tenascin in normal, reactive, hyperplastic, and neoplastic tissues: biologic and pathologic implications. *Hum Pathol,* 22:636–643.

46. Lawler J. (1986): Review: the structural and functional properties of thrombospondin. *Blood,* 67:1197–1209.

47. Lynch SE. (1991): Interactions of growth factors in tissue repair. In: *Clinical and experimental approaches to dermal and epidermal repair: normal and chronic wounds,* New York, Wiley-Liss, pp 341–357.

48. Madri JA, Pratt BM. (1986): Endothelial cell-matrix interactions: *in vitro* models of angiogenesis. *J Histochem Cytochem,* 34:85–91.

49. Maheshwari RK, Srikantan V, Bhartiya D, Kleinman HK, Grant DS. (1991): Differential effects of interferon gamma and alpha on *in vitro* model of angiogenesis. *J Cell Physiol,* 146:164–169.

50. Martin DE, Reece MC, Maher JE, Reese AC. (1988): Tissue debris at the injury site is coated by plasma fibronectin and subsequently removed by tissue macrophages. *Arch Dermatol,* 124:226–229.

51. McCarthy JB, Sas DF, Furcht LT. (1988): Mechanisms of parenchymal cell migration into wounds. In: Clark RAF, Henson PM, eds. *The molecular and cellular biology of wound repair.* New York: Plenum Press, pp 281–319.

52. McDevitt CA, Gilbertson EMM, Muir H. (1977): An experimental model of osteoarthritis: early morphological and biological changes. *J Bone Joint Surg [Br],* 59B:24–35.

53. McDevitt CA, Marcelino J. (1993): Inact Type VI collagen binds to fibronectin. *Trans Orthop Res Soc,* Park Ridge, Ill, 18:72.

54. McDevitt CA, Marcelino J, Tucker L. (1991): Interaction of intact Type VI collagen with hyaluronan. *FEBS Lett,* 294:167–170.

55. McDevitt CA, Pahl JA, Ayad S, Miller RR, Uratsuji M, Andrish JT. (1988): Experimental osteoarthritic articular cartilage is enriched in guanidine-soluble Type VI collagen. *Biochem Biophys Res Commun,* 157:250–255.

56. McDevitt CA, Sarrimanolis NI, Miller RR. (1991): Type VI collagen is a potent cell adhesion protein for cartilage chondrocytes and meniscal fibrochondrocytes. *Trans Orthop Res Soc,* 16:346.

57. McDonald JA. (1988): Fibronectin: a primitive matrix. In: Clark RAF, Henson PM, eds. *The molecular and cellular biology of wound repair.* New York: Plenum Press, pp 405–435.

58. Mecham, RP. (1991): Laminin receptors. *Annu Rev Cell Biol,* 7:71–91.

59. Mecham RP. (1991): Receptors for laminin on mammalian cells. *FASEB J,* 5:2538–2546.

60. Mercurio AM, Shaw LM. (1991) Laminin binding proteins. *Bioessays,* 13:469–473.

61. Miller RR, McDevitt CA. (1991): Thrombospondin in ligament, meniscus and intervertebral disc. *Biochim Biophys Acta,* 1115:85–88.

62. Miller RR, McDevitt CA. (1989): Thrombospondin promotes articular chondrocyte attachment but not spreading. *Glycoconjugate J,* 6:429.

63. Miller RR, McDevitt CA. (1988): Thrombospondin is present in articular cartilage and is synthesized by articular chondrocytes. *Biochem Biophys Res Commun,* 153:708–714.

64. Mosher DF, Schad PE. (1979): Cross-linking of fibronectin to collagen by blood coagulation factor XIIIa. *J Clin Invest,* 64:781–787.

65. Munjal ID, Blake DA, Sabet MD, Gordon SR. (1990): Thrombospondin: biosynthesis, distribution, and changes associated with wound repair in corneal endothelium. *Eur J Cell Biol,* 52:252–263.

66. Murata Y, Yoshioka H, Kitaoka M, Iyama K-I, Okamura R, Usuku G. (1990): Type VI collagen in healing rabbit corneal wounds. *Ophthalmic Res,* 11:144–151.

67. Murphy-Ullrich JE, Hook M. (1989): Thrombospondin modulates focal adhesions in endothelial cells. *J Cell Biol,* 109:1309–1319.

68. Murphy-Ullrich JE, Lightner VA, Aukhil I, Yan YZ, Erickson HP, Hook M. (1991): Focal adhesion integrity is down regulated by the alternatively spliced domain of human tenascin. *J Cell Biol,* 115:1127–1136.

69. Nievelstein PF, D'Alessio PA, Sixma JJ. (1988): Fibronectin in platelet adhesion to human collagen Types I and III. *Arteriosclerosis,* 8:200–206.

70. Panayotou G, End P, Aumailley M, Timpl R, Engel J. (1989): Domains of laminin with growth factor activity. *Cell,* 56:93–101.

71. Paulsson M, Aumailley M, Deutzmann R, Timpl R, Beck K, Engel J. (1987): Laminin-nidogen complex: extraction with chelating agents and structural characterization. *Eur J Biochem,* 166:11–19.

72. Paulsson M. (1992): Basement membrane proteins: structure, assembly, and cellular interactions. *Crit Rev Biochem Mol Biol,* 17(1/2):93–127.

73. Phillips DR, Charo IR, Scarborough RM. (1991): GPIIb-IIIa: the responsive integrin. *Cell,* 65:359–363.

74. Plow EF, McEver RP, Coller BS, Woods VL, Marguerie GA, Ginsburg MH. (1985): Related binding mechanisms for fibrinogen, fibronectin, von Willebrand factor, and thrombospondin on thrombin-stimulated human platelets. *Blood,* 66:724–727.

75. Raugi GJ, Olerud JE, Gown AM. (1987): Thrombospondin in early human wound tissue. *J Invest Dermatol,* 89:551–554.

76. Rudolph R, Cheresh D. (1990): Cell adhesion mechanisms and their potential impact on wound healing and tumor control. *Clin Plast Surg,* 17:457–462.

77. Ruegg CR, Chiquet-Ehrismann R, Alkan SS. (1989): Tenascin, an extracellular matrix protein, exerts immunomodulatory activities. *Proc Natl Acad Sci USA,* 86:7437–7441.

78. Ruoslahti E. (1988): Fibronectin and its receptors. *Annu Rev Biochem,* 57:375–413.

79. Ruoslahti E, Pierschbacher MD. (1987): New perspectives in cell adhesion: RGD and integrins. *Science,* 238:491–497.

80. Sage EH, Bornstein P. (1991): Extracellular proteins that modulate cell-matrix interactions. SPARC, tenascin, and thrombospondin. *J Biol Chem,* 266(23):14831–14834.

81. Sakashita S, Engvall E, Ruoslahti E. (1980): Basement membrane glycoprotein laminin binds to heparin. *FEBS Lett,* 116:243–246.

82. Sakakura T, Kusano I. (1991): Tenascin in tissue perturbation repair. *Acta Pathol Jpn,* 41(4):247–258.

83. Schwarzbauer JE. (1991): Alternative splicing of fibronectin: three variants, three functions. *Bioessays,* 13:527–533.

84. Spring J, Beck K, Chiquet-Ehrismann R. (1989): Two contrary functions of tenascin: dissection of the active sites by recombinant tenascin fragments. *Cell,* 59:325–334.

85. Thompson HL, Burbelo PD, Yamada Y, Kleinman HK, Metcalfe DD. (1989): Mast cells chemotax to laminin with enhancement after IgE-mediated activation. *J Immunol,* 143:4188–4192.

86. Thurlow PJ, Kenneally DA, Connellan JM. (1990): The role of fibronectin in platelet aggregation. *Br J Haematol,* 75:549–556.

87. von der Mark H, Aumailley M, Wick G, Fleischmajer R, Timpl R. (1984): Immunochemistry, genuine size and tissue localization of collagen VI. *Eur J Biochem,* 142:493–502.

88. Watkins SC, Lynch GW, Kane LP, Slayter HS. (1990): Thrombospondin expression in traumatized skeletal muscle. *Cell Tissue Res,* 261:73–84.

89. Wencel-Drake JD, Painter RG, Zimmerman TS, Ginsberg MH. (1985): Ultrastructural localization of human platelet thrombospondin, fibrinogen, fibronectin, and von Willebrand factor in frozen thin section. *Blood,* 65:929–938.

90. Whitby DJ, Longaker MT, Harrison MR, Adzick NS, Ferguson MW. (1991): Rapid epithelialization of fetal wounds is associated with the early deposition of tenascin. *J Cell Sci,* 99:583–586.

91. Wu C, Reing J, Chung AE. (1991): Entactin forms a complex with fibronectin and co-localizes in the extracellular matrix of the embryonal carcinoma-derived 4CQ cell line. *Biochem Biophys Res Commun,* 178:1219–1225.

92. Wu J-J, Eyre DR, Slayter HS. (1987): Type VI collagen of the intervertebral disc: biochemical and electron-microscopic characterization of the native protein. *Biochem J,* 248:373–381.

93. Yamada KM. (1983): Cell surface interactions with extracellular materials. *Annu Rev Biochem,* 52:761–799.

The Anterior Cruciate Ligament: Current and Future Concepts, edited by D.W. Jackson, et al. Raven Press, Ltd., New York © 1993.

CHAPTER 16

The Molecular Signals in Ligament Healing

David Amiel, Monica Wiig, and Marcel Nimni

The poor inherent healing capacity of the anterior cruciate ligament is well recognized (4,6,13,19). By contrast, studies on the medial collateral ligament have shown the intrinsic capability of this tissue to heal following injury (5,7,12,20). Ligament healing is a complex process and is affected by multiple factors (i.e., nutrient delivery, biomechanical forces, and the intrinsic capacity of the cells to synthesize extracellular matrix components to support the healing process).

Approximately 70% of the dry weight of the normal ligament is composed of collagen (1). The major component of the collagens present in ligament is collagen Type I, which is a heterotrimer of two $\alpha_1(I)$ chains and one $\alpha_2(I)$ chain. During the repair of interstitial tears of the ligaments, new extracellular matrix has to be synthesized in order to replace and remodel the damaged/injured tissue (2). Since collagen Type I is the major constituent of ligament, it is valuable to examine the nature of collagen synthesis at the site of injury. Evidence from other studies (10,14,15,17,18) suggests that collagen synthesis is predominantly regulated at the pretranslational level. We have used an *in situ* hybridization technique to monitor the levels of pro $\alpha_1(I)$ collagen mRNA in normal and healing MCL and ACL. This method will allow us to clarify the collagen Type I gene expression in normal MCL and ACL, and also during the early stage of their healing.

MATERIALS AND METHODS: ANIMAL MODEL

Male New Zealand white rabbits with closed epiphyses and 10 to 12 months old weighing 3.5 kg + 0.2 kg

were used for the study. Under general anesthesia and with sterile technique, a longitudinal incision was made over the medial aspect of the right knee of each animal. The fascia was divided longitudinally and the MCL exposed at the joint line. The ACL on the same knee was exposed by a medial parapatellar incision. The lacerations of the ACL and MCL were made with a razor-thin, square-edged microsurgical blade in the horizontal direction through the midsubstance of the ligament, leaving fibers on both sides of the laceration intact. The laceration represents approximately 60% of the ligament's width. The repair sites were assessed at 3, 7, 14 and 28 days post-surgery.

RESULTS

Gross Appearances

Representative pictures of the MCL and ACL at 3, 14 and 28 days postlaceration are shown in Fig. 1A–F. In the gross observation we defined healing as complete bridging of the laceration (i.e., Fig. 1A). In the MCL, healing occurred very quickly as the defect became filled with watery granulation tissue by 7 days. At the 3 and 7 day time periods, 5 of the 6 MCLs that were healed as defects were filled with a translucent "membrane." By 14 days all lacerations in the MCLs (3/3) were covered by a more hypertrophic ligamentous-like tissue (i.e. Fig. 1B), which seemed to increase only slightly by 28 days (Fig. 1C).

With the exception of one bridged laceration at 14 days, the lacerations in the ACLs didn't heal (Fig. 1D–F). The sharp edges created at the time of surgery were rounded off.

In Situ Hybridization

We used a cDNA probe corresponding to human pro $\alpha_1(I)$ collagen for detecting the levels of procollagen Type

D. Amiel and M. Wiig: Department of Orthopaedic Surgery, University of California, San Diego, School of Medicine, La Jolla, California 92093.

M. Nimni: University of Southern California–Orthopaedic Hospital, Los Angeles, California 90007.

Medial Collateral Ligament (MCL)

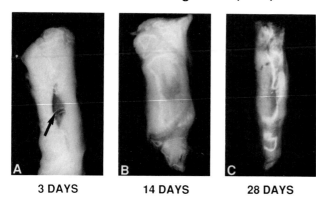

3 DAYS 14 DAYS 28 DAYS

Anterior Cruciate Ligament (ACL)

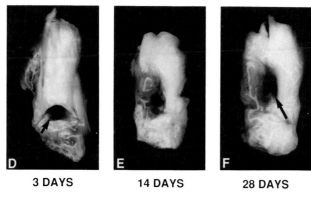

3 DAYS 14 DAYS 28 DAYS

FIG. 1. Gross appearance of the MCL (**A–C**) and ACL (**D–F**) at 3, 14, and 28 days postlaceration. A: MCL. *Arrow* indicates the presence of a thin translucent membrane covering the injury site. D–F: ACL. *Arrows* show the site of laceration (uncovered hole).

relatively small number of cells producing procollagen Type I mRNA in normal MCL and ACL was found to be rather homogeneously distributed throughout the ligament. More grains were observed in the tissue sections of MCL than in ACL (Fig. 3A,B), suggesting higher levels of mRNA in the fibroblastic cells of MCL. Light microscopy observations of grains and the relative number of cells expressing the procollagen gene, i.e. expressed by the qualitative assessment of the [32]p autoradiography, were higher in all MCL tissue sections. There was no difference in the level of procollagen mRNA between the ligaments of the right and left knees in the normal control animals.

An increased expression of the procollagen Type I gene was observed in the healing MCL and ACL when compared to normal ACL and MCL tissues. The strongest signal was detected adjacent to the laceration sites. By 3 days postlaceration, the levels of procollagen Type I mRNA were slightly higher in both MCL and ACL liga-

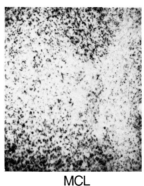 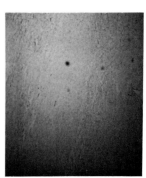

MCL
14 days postsurgery

RNAse treated MCL
14 days postsurgery

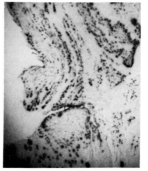 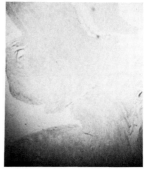

ACL
14 days postsurgery

RNAse treated ACL
14 days postsurgery

FIG. 2. Micrographs illustrating the expression of Type I procollagen mRNA in MCL and ACL. The tissue sections either were subjected to no RNAase treatment (*left*) or were incubated with RNAse A (100 µg/ml) in Tris-EDTA for 30 min at 37°C (*right*). Note the lack of silver grains in the RNAse-treated sections. (×6)

I mRNA in rabbit MCL and ACL tissues. This cDNA fragment has been shown to be specific for procollagen Type I mRNA in *in situ* hybridization studies in human tissue (16). We have conducted initial studies to assess possible nonspecific binding of the labeled probe to the rabbit ligament tissue sections during hybridization and washing. Removal of mRNA from the tissue sections of both MCL and ACL by RNAase treatment prior to hybridizations resulted in no signals (Fig. 2). When labeled bacteriophage DNA fragments were used as probes, no silver grains were observed in the tissue sections. The above two negative controls rule out the possibility of nonspecific binding of the pro α_1(I) collagen probe to the tissue sections during hybridization and subsequent washing steps.

The number of silver grains observed in the tissue sections after hybridization and autoradiography was taken as a measure of the levels of pro collagen mRNA. The

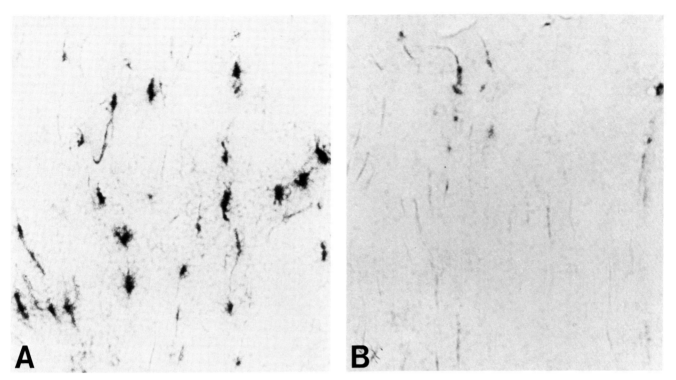

FIG. 3. Photomicrographs from normal MCL (**A**) and ACL (**B**) show the expression of Type I procollagen mRNA. A: The MCL shows a higher level of mRNA due to both more cells expressing the mRNA and a higher intensity per cell. B: In the ACL, the cells that express Type I procollagen mRNA are sparsely distributed within the ligament. (×31)

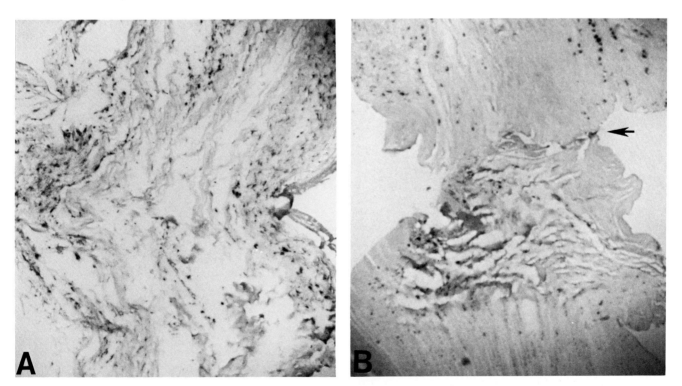

FIG. 4. The levels of Type I procollagen mRNA in MCL (**A**) and ACL (**B**) 3 days postlaceration. The expression is only slightly increased compared with normal. *Arrow* represents injury site. (×6)

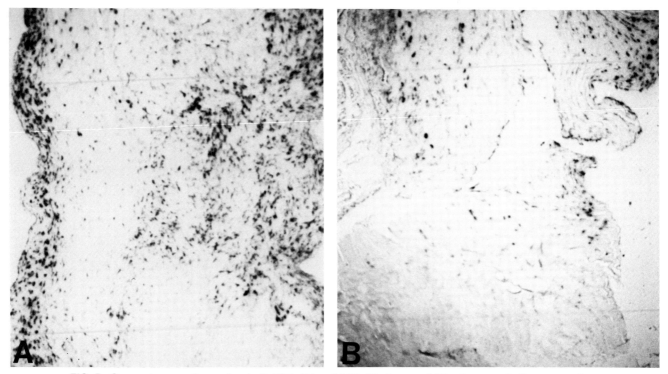

FIG. 5. Seven days postlaceration both MCL (**A**) and ACL (**B**) show a striking increase in the expression of Type I procollagen gene (×6).

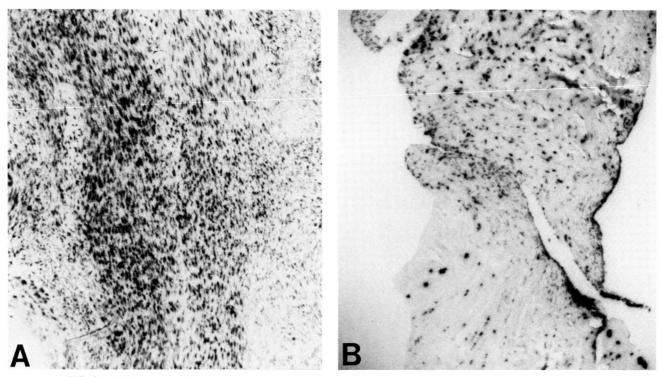

FIG. 6. At 14 days postlaceration, the labeling intensity has reached its maximum in both MCL (**A**) and ACL (**B**). The expression is especially strong in the MCL. (×6)

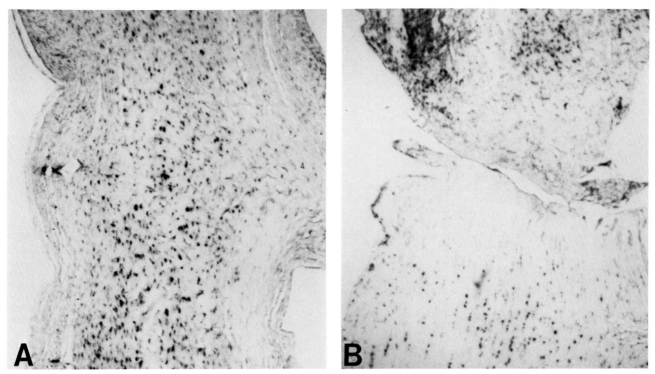

FIG. 7. The expression of Type I procollagen gene at 28 days is still higher than normal in both MCL (**A**) and ACL (**B**) but is less than the amount expressed at 14 days. (×6)

ments (Fig. 4A,B) than in the normal ligaments. At 7 days both MCL and ACL showed a striking increase in the levels of procollagen Type I mRNA (Fig. 5A,B), reaching its highest level at 14 days post laceration (Fig. 6A,B). The expression of the procollagen Type I gene was still higher than normal at 28 days postinjury (Fig. 7A,B), but less than the amount expressed at 14 days. The MCL healing site always expressed a considerably higher level of the procollagen Type I gene than the ACL healing site at all corresponding post laceration intervals studied.

In the healing ACL, the expression of the procollagen Type I gene was more pronounced at the femoral side of the laceration when compared to the tibial side (Figs. 4B,5B,6B,7B,8).

DISCUSSION

A higher level of procollagen mRNA was detected consistently in normal MCL than in normal ACL, suggesting higher collagen synthetic activity in the MCL. The increased level of procollagen Type I mRNA in healing MCL and ACL demonstrates higher collagen synthetic rates of cells in order to remodel the injured tissues for repair. At all corresponding stages of healing, the level of collagen mRNA was observed to be much higher in MCL than ACL, and seemed to reach a peak at 14

days. The pro α_1(I) collagen mRNA, with a relatively short half-life of 5 to 10 hr (8,9) is a precise marker of the synthesis of collagen. Under normal conditions the turnover rate of collagen is very slow, because of the long half-life (300 to 500 days) of this protein (11). Upon injury, new extracellular matrix has to be synthesized to replace the torn and/or degenerating tissue. Cellular components of the ligaments, especially those in the injured areas, had to increase their synthetic activities.

An increased level of procollagen Type I mRNA in healing MCL, and consequent elevation of the collagen synthesis, might be responsible for earlier repair of this tissue. Lower levels of collagen gene expression in ACL causes slower collagen synthesis, thereby delaying the repair process. Another possibility of lack of healing in the ACL rabbit model, as proposed by Amiel et al. in 1990 (3), is that the injury to the synovial sheath exposes ligamentous substance to the degradative effects of synovial proteases. It could as well be due to intrinsic degradative capabilities, e.g. collagenase production by the injured ACL itself. MCL, on the other hand, situated outside the intrasynovial space, is less exposed to the hostile environment of synovial fluids, and therefore may be less subjected to attack by proteolytic enzymes.

In this *in situ* hybridization study we also observed a very low level of the α_1(I) procollagen mRNA at the tibial side of the ACL's laceration site, which could be due

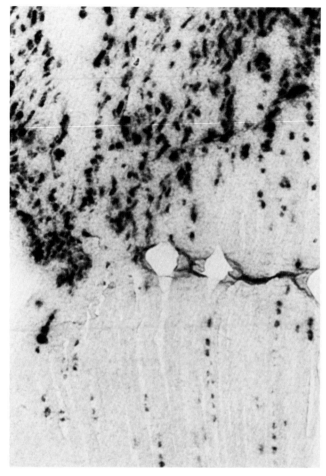

FIG. 8. Photomicrographs of the ACL 14 days postlaceration showing the lack of Type I procollagen gene expression at the tibial side (*lower half*) of the laceration compared to the femoral side (*upper half*). (×18)

to reduced nutrient supply associated with poor vascularity.

ACKNOWLEDGMENT

We wish to acknowledge the support of NIH grants AR07484, AR34264, and the Malcolm and Dorothy Coutts Institute for Joint Reconstruction and Research.

REFERENCES

1. Amiel D, Frank CB, Harwood FL, Fronek J, Akeson WH. (1984): Tendons and ligaments: a morphological and biochemical comparison. *J Orthop Res,* 1:257–265.

2. Amiel D, Frank CB, Harwood FL, Akeson WH, Kleiner JB. (1987): Collagen alteration in medial collateral ligament healing in a rabbit model. *Connect Tissue Res,* 16:357–366.

3. Amiel D, Billings E Jr, Lyon R, Kitabayashi L, Harwood FL, Woo SL-Y, Akeson WH. (1990): Collagenase activity in anterior cruciate ligament (ACL): the protective role of the synovial sheath. *Orthop Res Soc,* 15(1):269.

4. Arnold JA, Coker TP, Heaton LM, Park JP, Harris WD. (1979): Natural history of anterior cruciate tears. *Am J Sports Med,* 7:305–313.

5. Clayton ML, Miles JS, Abdulla M. (1968): Experimental investigations of ligamentous healing. *Clin Orthop,* 61:146–153.

6. Feagin JA Jr, Curl W. (1976): Isolated tear of the anterior cruciate ligament: 5-year followup study. *Am J Sports Med,* 4:95–100.

7. Frank C, Woo SL-Y, Amiel D, Harwood F, Gomez M, Akeson W. (1983): Medial collateral ligament healing: a multidisciplinary assessment in rabbits. *Am J Sports Med,* 11:379–389.

8. Hamalainen L, Oikarinen J, Kivirikko K. (1985): Synthesis and degradation of Type I procollagen mRNAs in cultured human skin fibroblasts and the effect of cortisol. *J Biol Chem,* 260: 720–725.

9. Kahari V-M, Vuorio EI. (1987): Increased half-lives of procollagen mRNAs may contribute to the elevated procollagen mRNA levels in cultured scleroderma fibroblasts. *Med Sci Res,* 15:417–418.

10. Mauch C, Hatamochi A, Scharffetter K, Krieg T. (1988): Regulation of collagen synthesis in fibroblasts within a three-dimensional collagen gel. *Exp Cell Res,* 178:493–503.

11. Neuberger A, Slack HGB. (1953): The metabolism of collagen from liver, bone, skin and tendon in the normal rat. *Biochem J,* 53:47–52.

12. O'Donoghue DH. (1955): An analysis of end results of surgical treatment of major injuries to the ligaments of the knee. *J Bone Joint Surg [Am],* 37A:1–13.

13. O'Donoghue DH, Frank GR, Jeter GL, Johnson W, Zeiders JW, Kenyon R. (1971): Repair and reconstruction of the anterior cruciate ligament in dogs: factors influencing long-term results. *J Bone Joint Surg [Am],* 53A:710–718.

14. Rowe DW, Moen RC, Davidson JM, Byers PH, Bornstein P, Palmiter RD. (1978): Correlation of procollagen mRNA levels in normal and transformed chick embryo fibroblasts with different rates of procollagen synthesis. *Biochemistry,* 17:1581–1590.

15. Rowe LB, Schwartz J. (1983): Role of procollagen mRNA levels in controlling the rate of procollagen synthesis. *Mol Cell Biol,* 3:241–249.

16. Sandberg M, Vuorio E. (1987): Localization of Types I, II, III collagen mRNA's in developing human skeletal tissues by *in situ* hybridization. *J Cell Biol,* 104:1077–1084.

17. Sandmeyer S, Smith R, Kien D, Bornstein P. (1981): Correlation of collagen synthesis and procollagen mRNA levels with transformation in rat embryo fibroblasts. *Cancer Res,* 41:830–838.

18. Uitto J, Perejda AJ, Abergel RP, Chu ML, Ramirez F. (1985): Altered steady state ratio of Type I, III procollagen mRNAs correlates with selectively increased Type I procollagen biosynthesis in cultured keloid fibroblasts. *Proc Natl Acad Sci USA,* 82:5935–5939.

19. Wiig ME, Amiel D, VandeBerg J, Kitabayashi L, Harwood FL, Arfors K-E. (1990): The early effect of high molecular weight hyaluronan (hyaluronic acid) on anterior cruciate ligament healing. *J Orthop Res,* 8:425–434.

20. Woo SL-Y, Gomez MA, Inoue M, Akeson WH. (1987): New experimental procedures to evaluate the biomechanical properties of healing canine medial collateral ligament. *J Orthop Res,* 5:425–432.

The Anterior Cruciate Ligament: Current and Future Concepts, edited by D.W. Jackson, et al. Raven Press, Ltd., New York © 1993.

CHAPTER 17

Collagen Fiber Changes in the Exercised, Immobilized, or Injured Anterior Cruciate Ligament

Pascal S. Christel and Donald F. Gibbons

Collagen is involved in different structures and tissues of the human body (29) and contributes to their biomechanical functions (5,7,8,9,15,30,33). The study of the ultrastructural assembly of collagen may be important in the understanding of the biomechanical performance of ligament and tendon tissue (15,16). Thus, it appears appropriate to collect more information on the ultrastructure of the anterior cruciate ligament after injury and try to bring some insight to its ability to heal.

Careful examination of ultrastructure of ligaments and other connective tissues has led to the conclusion that variation in structure exists and relates to several factors: function, species, and anatomical situation (12). Several investigators have evaluated the ultrastructure of the ACL (6,36). From scanning electron microscopy micrographs, Danylchuk et al. (6) have described the presence of epitenon sheaths surrounding collagenous subfasciculi in human and bovine ACL. Yahia and Drouin (36) have shown that a helical wave pattern occurs in the ACL with a planar waveform found only in the central part of the ligament fascicles. Clark and Sidles (4) have further described increased interfascicular substance near insertion sites for the human, canine, and rabbit ACL.

Morphometric analyses of fibril diameter distributions from Transmission Electron Microscopy (TEM) micrographs have been performed on a variety of collagenous tissues. Parry and Craig have shown broadening and increased bimodality of the collagen fibril distribu-

tion with age from an initially narrow, unimodal distribution at birth in rat-tail tendon, as well as in the superficial flexor tendon and suspensory ligament of the horse (24–26). Moore and De Beaux (17) have reported similar results in the rat extensor digitorum longus and have shown that the volume fraction of organized collagen increased with maturation. Frank et al. (11) have shown increased bimodality of fibril distributions with maturation in rabbit MCL.

There is a paucity of data concerning ultrastructure of injured ligaments. However, the study of ruptured ligament structure may be useful in the understanding of the mechanisms of ligament healing as well as tissue modification of its properties. This chapter will review normal ACL ultrastructure and its modifications following intense exercise, stress protection, or injury.

THE NORMAL HUMAN ACL ULTRASTRUCTURE

In human ACLs, Strocchi et al. (31) have observed two types of collagen fibrils: small with a smooth contour (with a single diameter peak at 45 nm) and large with irregular contour exhibiting a trimodal distribution (three peaks at 35, 50, and 70 nm). Oakes, in a previous chapter by Frank et al. (10), reported studying the collagen fibril population obtained from 4 cadaver ACL specimens, 10 ACL specimens from young (<30 years) patients, and 6 biopsies from older patients (>30 years) who had sustained recent tears. It was found that collagen fibrils less than 100 nm in diameter form 85% of the cross-sectional area in the normal human ACL. Cadaver ACL had more of the larger fibers than did the "normal" ACL.

P. S. Christel: Orthopaedic Research Laboratory and Orthopaedic Surgery Department, Lariboisìere Saint-Louis Medical School, University of Paris, F-75010 Paris, France.

D. F. Gibbons: Biosciences Research Laboratory, 3M Center, St. Paul, Minnesota 55144.

In a recent study, Neurath and Stofft (18,19) have shown that the fibril diameters in injured ACLs exhibited an unimodal distribution (79.3 ± 19.9 nm), and the average macroperiodicity was 63.2 ± 4.2 nm.

THE EFFECTS OF EXERCISE ON ACL STRUCTURE

Following the demonstration that exercise can influence ligament-bone junction strength (3,31,32) and collagen ultrastructure (27,28), Oakes et al. (21–23) have studied the effects of an intensive four-week exercise program on rat knee ligaments and patellar tendon structure in comparison with a control, non exercised, group. Fibril diameters and fibril occupied areas for each diameter group were calculated in order to quantify the relative amount of collagen represented by each fibril class. They found significantly both more smaller diameter (80 to 100 nm) and less larger fibrils in the exercised ACL. This was reflected in the decrease in percentage area occupied by the large-diameter group (125 to 175 nm). The control ACL had more fibrils with diameters in the 125 to 162 nm range. However, this increase in small-diameter fibrils may be responsible for the decreased elastic stiffness in the ligaments of exercised animals (14). Although the number of fibrils in the exercised ACL, compared to control ACL, was increased, the total cross-sectional area of the control ACL was larger than that of the exercised group. This indicates that little change in the tensile strength of the exercised ligaments should be detected (14,34,35). Oakes et al. (22,23) further submitted rats to a program of alternating days of swimming and treadmill running during one month. The TEM study of the removed ACL showed (a) a significant 29% increase in number of collagen fibrils per unit area in ACL from the exercised group compared to controls; (b) a significant fall in mean fibril diameter from 966 ± 115 Å in the controls to 830 ± 30 Å in the loaded ACL; (c) as a consequence of the two previous observations, the major cross-sectional area of collagen fibrils was found in the 1125 Å diameter group in the exercised ACL and in the 1500 Å diameter group in the control ACL. However, total collagen fibril cross-sectional area was approximately the same in both the exercised and nonexercised ACL. The authors concluded that ACL fibroblasts deposit tropocollagen as smaller diameter fibrils when subjected to intensive one month intermittent loading rather than accretion and increase in size of the large collagen fibrils.

THE EFFECTS OF STRESS PROTECTION ON THE ACL

Effects of stress protection on the structural and mechanical properties of ACLs are not well documented.

Noyes (20) has reported that immobilization of the knee reduced the mechanical strength of the ACL in dogs. Binkley and Peat (2) have shown that after 6 weeks of immobilization of the rat MCL, the small fibrils decreased in number. Keira et al. (13) have studied the effects of the release of ACL bone tibial insertion in dogs on cross-sectional area and tensile strength of ACL after 6 and 12 weeks. The cross-sectional area significantly increased in the relaxed group compared to the sham group, while the tensile strength was significantly lower for the relaxed group at 12 weeks only.

THE ULTRASTRUCTURE OF LIGAMENT HEALING

Healing phases of ligaments have been divided into four phases and we will review them mostly from an ultrastructural point of view. Complementary reading on the morphology of ligament healing may be found in Akeson et al. (1).

Phase I (inflammation). TEM of a 1-week ruptured rabbit MCL shows fine random collagen fibrils and abundant ground substance composed of a mixture of newly synthesized matrix materials. Fibroblasts are present with an abundant rough endoplasmic reticulum, suggesting that they are synthesizing collagenous matrix. Macrophages containing phagocytized erythrocytes may be commonly observed.

Phase II (matrix and cellular proliferation). On TEM, the cells appear to actively synthesize matrix. The healing ligament is bigger than the normal ligament and contains significantly more total collagen than at the previous phase. However, the collagen concentration is lower than that in a normal ligament. There is unidentified fibrous material associated with heterogeneous and disorganized collagen fibrils embedded within an amorphous ground substance. Elastin starts to appear in the scar.

Phase III (remodeling). After several weeks, fibroblasts and macrophages are decreasing in number. The density of the scar collagen matrix is increasing. The cells are less active ultrastructurally. Collagen fibrils are slightly increasing in diameter and are more densely packed.

Phase IV (maturation). After several months the ligament scar matrix gradually matures to a tissue that is still slightly disorganized and hypercellular. Activity level, immobilization, and primary surgical repair strongly influence both scar quantity and quality.

THE ULTRASTRUCTURE OF TIBIAL STUMPS FROM TORN ACLS

We had the opportunity to define the long-term, time-dependent ultrastructure of human ACL after traumatic

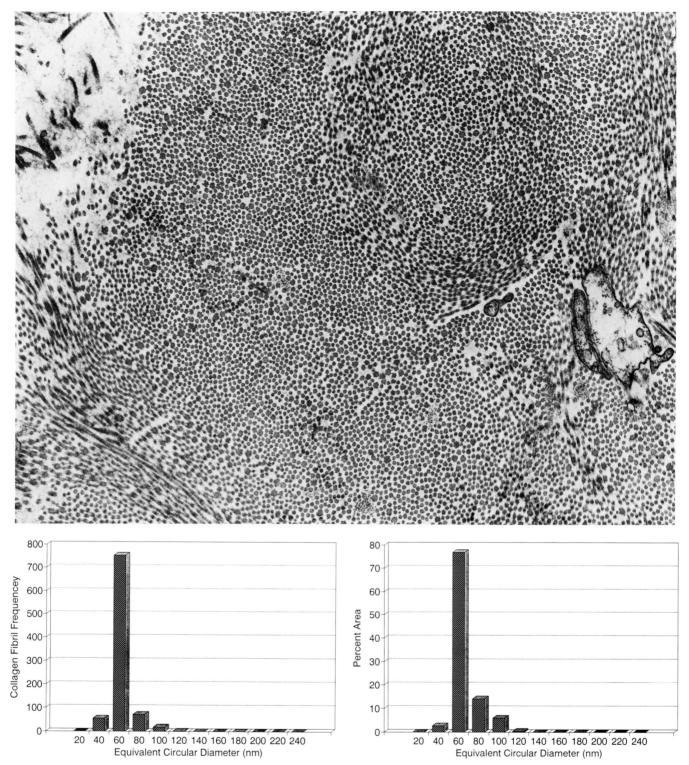

FIG. 1. Transverse section through a 4-day ruptured ACL near the tibial insertion, with corresponding histograms. Almost all fibers are small (<100 nm). (×26,200)

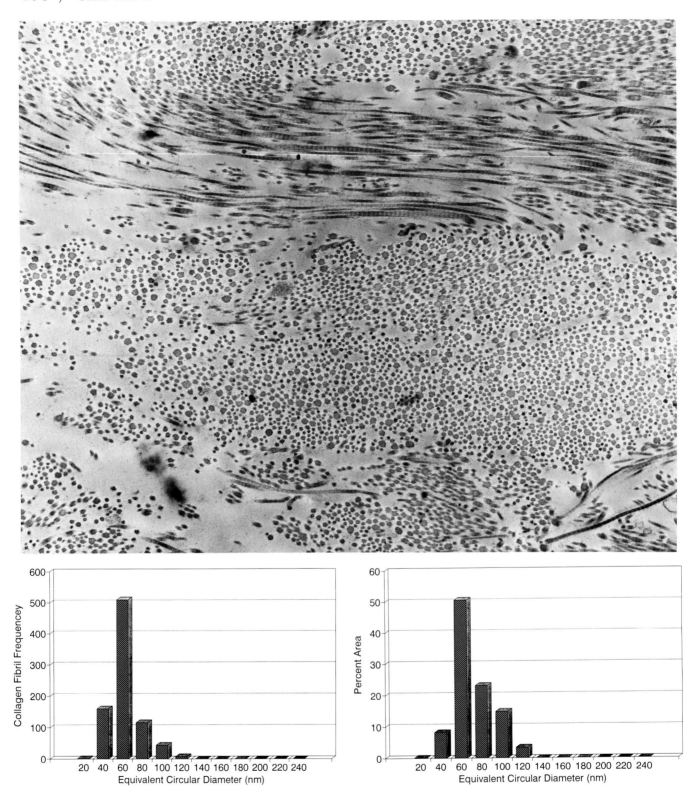

FIG. 2. Transverse section through a 4-day ruptured ACL near the frayed end, with corresponding histograms. Larger fibrils (100 to 120 nm) can be seen. (×26,500)

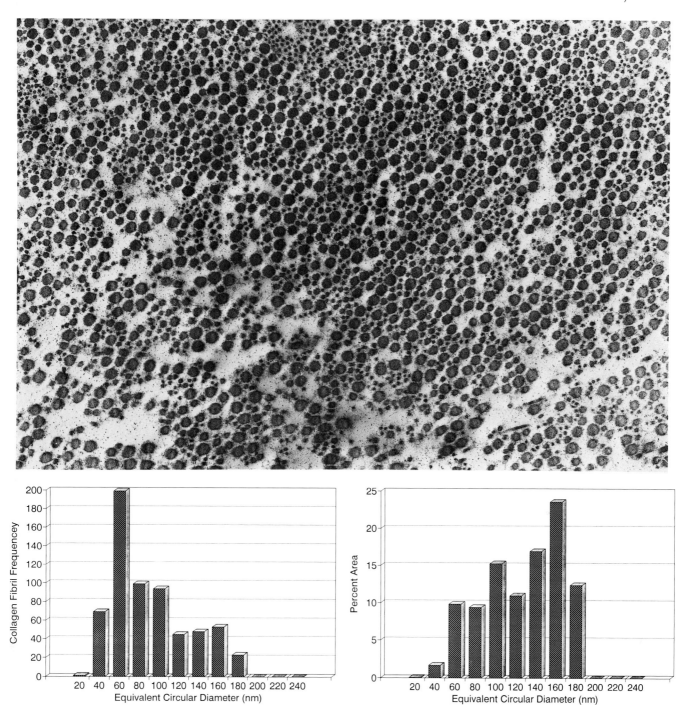

FIG. 3. Transverse section through a 2-month ruptured ACL with corresponding histograms showing a mixture of large and medium fibrils. (×25,000)

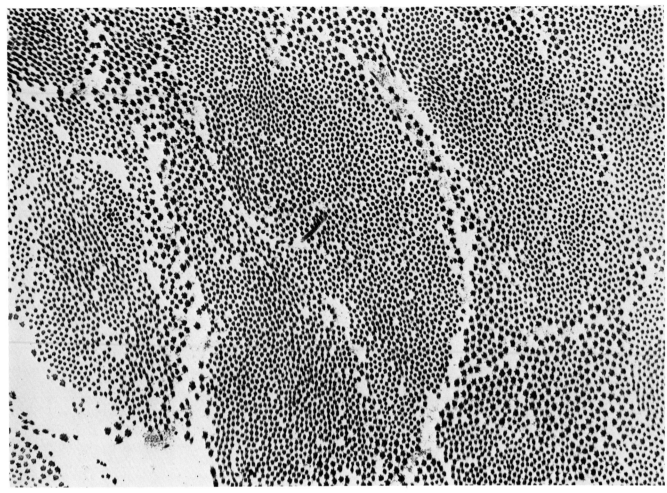

FIG. 4. After 2 months, some regions are still well organized, mostly made of small-diameter fibrils except for interesting patterns of lines or networks of larger diameter fibrils.

rupture. Collagen fibril diameters were quantitatively analyzed in 7 specimens from patients aged 17 to 25 . All had grades II or III pivot shifts and gross anterior drawer preoperatively (2 or 3+). The time of disability, between the initial trauma and surgery, ranged from 4 days to 6 years.

All ACL stumps, still attached on the tibia, were collected during surgery and the specimens immediately fixed in formalin. For TEM processing, a complete slice was taken across the center of the specimen. The whole slice was fixed in 2.5% glutaraldehyde, in 0.1 M sodium phosphate, buffered at pH 7.4, with 0.1 M sucrose for 30 to 60 minutes. After washing, the samples were postfixed in 1% osmium tetroxide (4% aqueous solution in buffer) for 1 hour. They were then washed in distilled water, en bloc stained for 20 minutes with 4% uranyl acetate in 30% acetone, and dehydrated with a graded acetone series, (30, 50, 70, 95, and 100%). After infiltrating in a 50/50 mixture of 100% acetone and Spurr resin for 30 to 90 minutes, the samples were put through four changes of Spurr resin over 20 to 24 hours. The whole tissue slices were then cut into blocks and embedded in flat molds. Polymerization was performed at 60° C for 1 to 3 days.

The cross-section cut from the stump was usually divided into six pieces. Thick sections were cut and stained with toluidine blue stain. The blocks were sectioned on a Sorvall MT2-B ultramicrotome. After trimming, 1 μm sections were made for light microscopy. Selected blocks were then further trimmed and sectioned at 100 nm for TEM using a diamond knife. Sections were collected on copper grids, dried and stained for 10 minutes with 2% aqueous uranyl acetate. After washing they were further stained with Reynold's lead citrate for 3 minutes. All samples were observed under a JEOL 100B transmission electron microscope.

TEM prints were acquired into the Quantimet 570 image analysis system (LEICA) by means of a video camera on a copy stand. In order to identify and separate collagen fibrils, images were first thresholded into "binaries". Then morphological processing using a disk structuring element was applied. Finally, an "open" filter was performed to eliminate noise and to trim fibrils to their

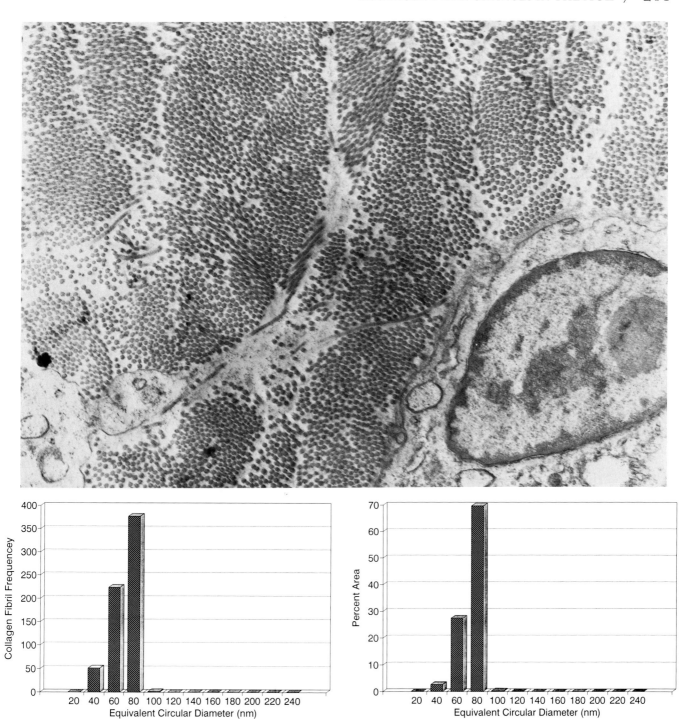

FIG. 5. Transverse section through a 13-month ruptured ACL with corresponding histograms. Cells look healthy and collagen fibrils shows an almost uniform distribution. (×25,000)

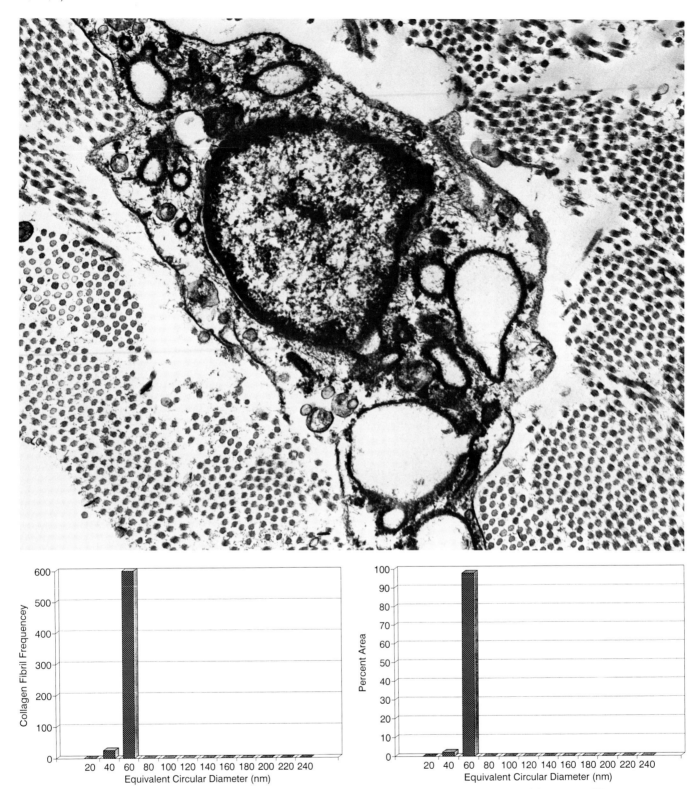

FIG. 6. Transverse section through a 1-year 7-month ruptured ACL with corresponding histograms. The section shows mostly 60-nm fibrils and includes a typical cell still producing collagen. Note large vacuoles in cell. (×42,800)

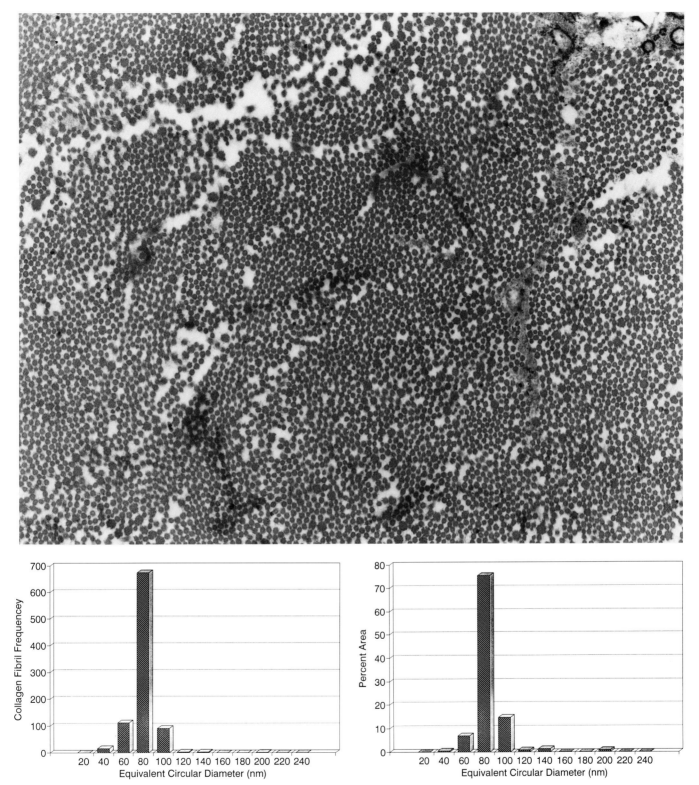

FIG. 7. Transverse section through a 2-year 6-month ruptured ACL with corresponding histograms. Collagen fibrils clearly peak at 80 nm, however, with still a few 140- to 160-nm large fibrils. (×26,500)

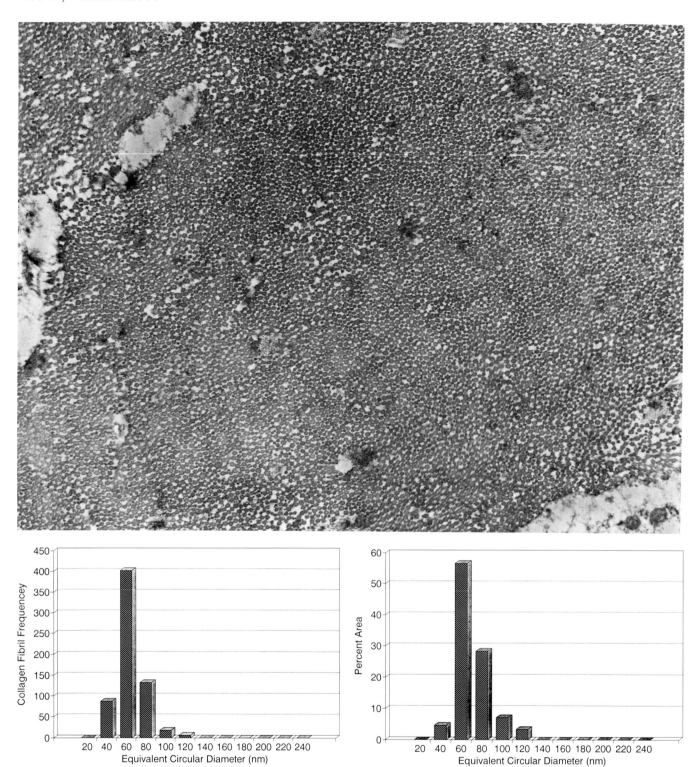

FIG. 8. Transverse section through a 3-year 8-month ruptured ACL near border of a fascicle with corresponding histograms. Significant large fibrils are still present. (×26,500)

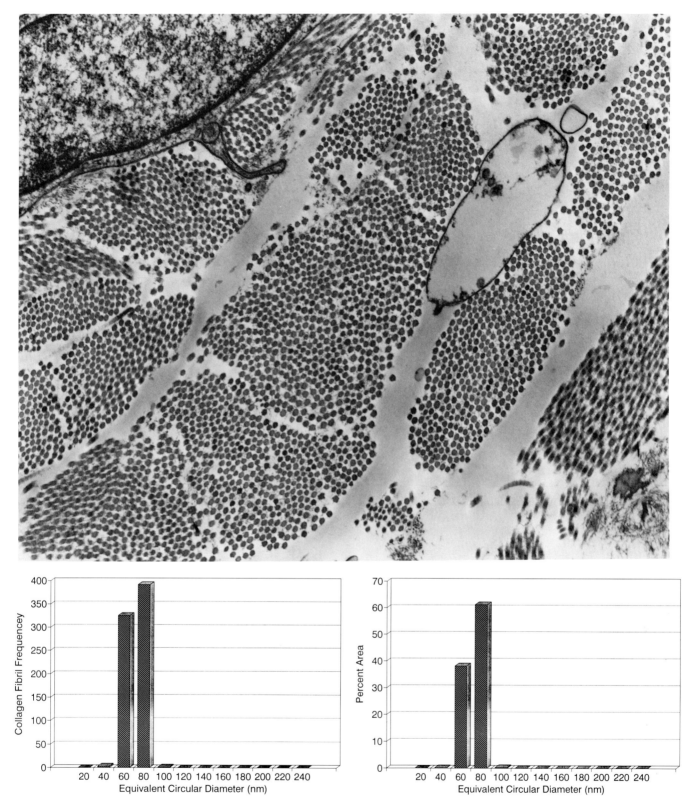

FIG. 9. Transverse section through a 6-year ruptured ACL with corresponding histograms. On this section, collagen fibrils peak at 80 nm, and one area has larger collagen fibrils, up to 100 nm. (×42,800)

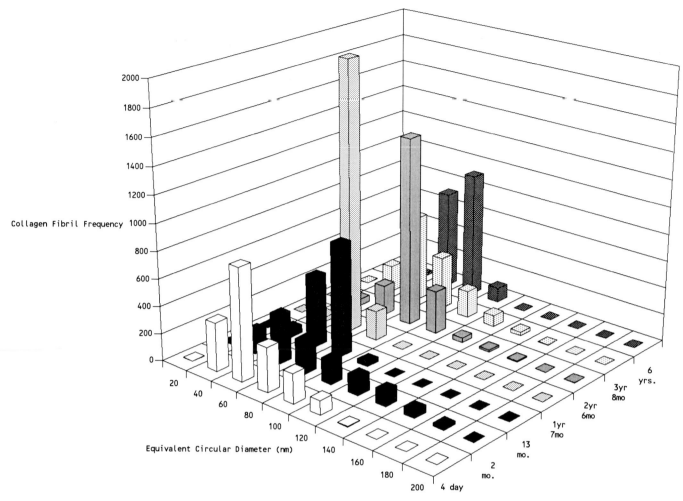

FIG. 10. Time evolution of the histogram profiles of mean data for number of fibrils (*left*) and percentage area occupied for each diameter group (*right*) for all studied ACL stumps.

proper boundaries. The images were analyzed for Area and Aspect Ratio. Equivalent Circular Diameter was calculated from Area. Particles were excluded if Aspect Ratio was over 2.0. These results were then printed to a file.

Files were then imported into Quattro Pro (version 4.0, Borland). The equivalent Circular Diameters were separated into bins and counted using the Frequency function. These results were used to generate a histogram plot. In order to get a plot of the percentage area for each diameter bin, the area column was first summed. Each individual fibril area was then divided by this total to generate a percent area column. An extract function was then performed to list all fibrils where the diameter fallen into a given bin. The percent area column in this extracted list was summed, thus giving the percent area value for that bin. This extraction was repeated for each bin, and the results were plotted versus diameter bins.

Case 1: 4 days postinjury. This specimen was considered as a control. Near the tibial insertion almost all fi-

brils were small (Fig. 1), 75% being in the 60-nm range. Close to the frayed end, 100- to 120-nm fibrils were readily seen (Fig. 2).

Case 2: 2 months postinjury. Several areas exhibited transition from degenerated region, then transition to mixture of large and medium fibrils (Fig. 3) with little or no evidence for degeneration. Sixty percent of the fibrils were over 100 nm. Other regions were still quite organized, consisting of all small-diameter fibrils except for some interesting patterns formed by lines or networks of larger diameter fibrils (Fig. 4).

Case 3: 13 months postinjury. All the blocks showed basically a uniform distribution of collagen fibers diameters, 95% being in the 60- to 80-nm range. The closest section from the stump edge had scar tissue transitional to fascicles. Cells appeared healthy and not compromised (Fig. 5).

Case 4: 1 year 7 months postinjury. Thick sections showed many regions of adipose tissue. Image analysis

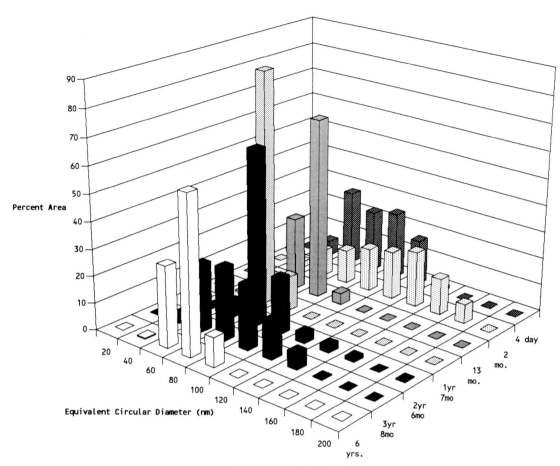

FIG. 10. *Continued.*

demonstrated uniform size of collagen fibers, 60 nm average (Fig. 6). Most of the sections were quite cellular, but did not appear to exhibit degeneration yet. Cells appeared quite healthy, however, with vacuoles in their cytoplasm in most cases.

Case 5: 2 years 6 months postinjury. Thick sections showed significant adipose in one of four. Overall, the tissue was not very cellular. Collagen fiber diameters were quite uniform, 75% at 80 nm (Fig. 7), with a few 140- to 160-nm large fibers.

Case 6: 3 years 8 months postinjury. Thick sections showed rips and holes suggesting that some areas were calcified. Several sections showed that significant larger diameter fibrils, over 100 nm, were still present (Fig. 8). Other areas exhibited some evidence of beginning degeneration.

Case 7: 6 years postinjury. Thick sections showed adipose in all areas. Regions of scar tissue appeared to be mixed with regions of more uniform collagen fibril diameters (Fig. 9). There was slight evidence for degeneration and scar tissue initiating near the synovium. Ninety percent of the fibrils were in the 60- to 80-nm range, and only a small area had larger collagen diameter to any

extent at 100 nm. Cells exhibited cytoplasmic vacuolization and many did not appear healthy.

From the previous data, it is clear that the ruptured ACL ultrastructure strongly depends on the observed region. Large and small fibers may be associated for a long period of time after injury. The time evolution of the histogram profiles of mean data for number of fibrils and percentage area occupied for each diameter group is summarized in Fig. 10. It can be seen that the general trend is a disappearance of the over 100-nm collagen fibril; however, large fibrils may be observed for a long time (Case 6). From this study it is clear that ACL stumps slowly evolved toward degeneration, with disappearance of large collagen fibrils, adipose and cellular degeneration. The disturbance of the blood supply to the ligament following the injury may induce cell hypoxia and may also account in the variation observed in the fibril diameter distribution from zone to zone. Persistence of large collagen fibrils, even after 2 years (Case 5), could be related to a pseudocontinuity made by fibrous attachment between the ACL stump and the PCL synovial sheath. This could provide some degree of functional loading of the remaining ACL stump.

CONCLUSION

The ultrastructural modifications of the ruptured human ACL show a complex evolution that is not as simple as has been suggested by animal experiments. When injured, the ACL is not loaded anymore and its vascular supply is disturbed. This might be responsible for migration of fascicular boundaries and explain some of the fibroblasts and collagen fibrils diameter changes. However, other reasons for fibril changes may be related to the modification of the local concentration in hyaluronate and GAGs.

REFERENCES

1. Akeson WH, Frank CB, Amiel D, et al. (1985): In: Finerman G, ed. *American Academy of Orthopaedic Surgeons Symposium on Sports Medicine: The Knee.* St. Louis, MO, CV Mosby, pp 111–151.
2. Binkley JM, Peat M. (1986): The effects of immobilization on the ultrastructure and mechanical properties of the medial collateral ligament of rats. *Clin Orthop,* 203:301–308.
3. Cabaud HE, Chatty A, Gildengorin V, et al. (1980): Exercise effects on the strength of the rat anterior cruciate ligament. *Am J Sports Med,* 8:79–86.
4. Clark JM, Sidles JA. (1990): The interrelation of fiber bundles in the anterior cruciate ligament. *J Orthop Res,* 8:180–188.
5. Craig AS, Einkenberry EF, Parry DAD. (1987): Ultrastructural organization of skin: classification on the basis of mechanical role. *Connect Tissue Res,* 16:213–223.
6. Danylchuk KD, Finlay JB, Kreek JP. (1978): Microstructural organization of human and bovine cruciate ligaments. *Clin Orthop,* 131:294–298.
7. Fitton-Jackson S. (1968): In: Gould BS, ed. *Treatise on collagen.* London: Academic Press, vol 2, pp 1–66.
8. Flint MH. (1976): In: Longrace JJ, ed. *The ultrastructure of collagen.* Springfield, IL, Charles C Thomas, pp 191–198.
9. Flint MH, Craig AS, Reilly HC, Gillard GC, Parry DAD. (1984): Collagen fibril diameters and glycosaminoglycan content of skins: indices of tissue maturity and function. *Connect Tissue Res,* 13:69–81.
10. Frank C, Woo SL-Y, Andriacchi T, et al. (1988): In: Woo SL-Y, Buckwalter J, eds. *Injury and repair of the musculoskeletal soft tissues.* Park Ridge, Illinois: American Academy of Orthopaedic Surgeons, pp 43–101.
11. Frank C, Bray D, Rademaker A, Chrusch C, Sabiston P, Bodie D, Rangayyan R. (1989): Electron microscopic quantification of collagen diameters in the rabbit medial collateral ligament: a baseline for comparison. *Connect Tissue Res,* 19:11–25.
12. Hart RA, Woo SL-Y, Newton PO. (1992): Ultrastructural morphometry of anterior cruciate and medial collateral ligaments: an experimental study in rabbits. *J Orthop Res,* 10:96–103.
13. Keira M, Yasuda K, Hayashi K, Yamamoto N, Kaneda K. (1992): Mechanical properties of the canine anterior cruciate ligament chronically relaxed by elevation of the tibial insertion. In: *Trans Orthop Res Soc,* Park Ridge, Illinois: American Academy of Orthopaedic Surgeons 17:661.
14. Larsen N, Parker AW. (1982): In: Howell ML, Parker AW, eds. *Sports medicine: medical and scientific aspects of elitism in sports.* Brisbane: Australian Sports Medicine Federation, vol 8, pp 63–73.
15. Matthew C, Moore MJ, Campbell L. (1987): A quantitative ultra-

structural study of collagen fibril formation in the healing extensor digitorum longus tendon of the rat. *J Hand Surg [Br],* 12:313–320.
16. Michna H. (1984): Morphometric analysis of loading-induced changes in collagen-fibril populations in young tendons. *Cell Tissue Res,* 236:465–470.
17. Moore MJ, De Beaux A. (1987): A quantitative ultrastructural study of rat tendon from birth to maturity. *J Anat,* 153:163–169.
18. Neurath MF. (1992): Collagen types (III, IV, VI, VII) pattern and ultrastructure of ruptured cruciate ligaments. In: *Transactions of the 1st World Congress of Sports Trauma, Palma de Mallorca, Spain,* pp 44–45.
19. Neurath MF, Stofft E. (1992): Collagen ultrastructure in ruptured cruciate ligaments. An electron microscopic investigation. *Acta Orthop Scand* 63(5):507–510.
20. Noyes F. (1977): Functional properties of knee ligaments and alterations induced by immobilization: a correlative biomechanical and histological study in primates. *Clin Orthop,* 123:210–242.
21. Oakes BW, Parker AW, Norman J. (1981): In: Russo P, Gass G, eds. *Human adaption.* Williamsberg, KY: Cumberland College of Health Sciences, pp 223–230.
22. Oakes BW, Parker AW, Norman J. (1982): Changes in collagen fiber populations in young rat cruciate ligaments in response to a one month intensive exercise program. *Connect Tissue Res,* 9:212.
23. Oakes BW, Leslie J, Jacobsen J, et al. (1982): In: Howell ML, Parker AW, eds. *Sports medicine: medical and scientific aspects of elitism in sports.* Brisbane: Australian Sports Medicine Federation, vol 8, pp 39–62.
24. Parry DAD, Craig AS. (1977): Quantitative electron microscope observation of collagen fibrils in rat-tail tendon. *Biopolymers,* 16:1015–1031.
25. Parry DAD, Craig AS. (1978): Collagen fibrils and elastic fibers in rat-tail tendon: an electron microscopic investigation. *Biopolymers,* 17:843–855.
26. Parry DAD, Craig SA, Barnes GRG. (1978): Tendon and ligament from the horse: an ultrastructural study of collagen fibrils and elastic fibers as a function of age. *Proc R Soc Lond [Biol],* 203:293–303.
27. Parry DAD, Barnes GRG, Craig AS. (1978): A comparison of the size distribution of collagen fibrils in connective tissues as a function of age and a possible relation between fibril size distribution and mechanical properties. *Proc R Soc Lond [Biol],* 203:305–321.
28. Parry DAD, Craig AS. (1984): In: Ruggeri A, Motta PM, eds. *Ultrastructure of the connective tissue matrix.* Boston: Martinus Nijhoff, pp 34–64.
29. Penttinen R, Frey H, Aalto M, Vuorio E, Marttala T. (1980): In: Viidik A, Vuust J, eds. *Biology of collagen.* New York: Academic Press, pp 87–105.
30. Shore RC, Berkovitz BKB, Moxham BJ. (1988): A quantitative ultrastructural study of the extra cellular matrix of the sheep incisor peridontium. *Res Vet Sci,* 44:190–193.
31. Strocchi R, de Pasquale V, Gubellini P, et al. (1992): The human anterior cruciate ligament: histological and structural observations. *J Anat* 108:515–519.
32. Tipton CM, Matthes RD, Maynard JA, et al. (1975): The influence of physical activity on ligaments and tendons. *Med Sci Sports,* 7:165–175.
33. Viidik A. (1979): In: Akkas N, ed. *Progress in Biomechanics.* Amsterdam: Sijtthoff & Noordhoff, pp 75–113.
34. Woo SL-Y, Amiel D, Akeson WH, et al. (1979): Effects of long term exercise on ligaments, tendons and bone of swines. *Med Sci Sports,* 11:105.
35. Woo SL-Y, Ritter MA, Amiel D, et al. (1980): The biochemical and biomechanical properties of swine tendons—long term effects of exercise on the digital extensors. *Connect Tissue Res,* 7:177–183.
36. Yahia L-H, Drouin G. (1989): Microscopical investigation of canine anterior cruciate ligament and patellar tendon: collagen fascicle morphology and architecture. *J Orthop Res,* 7:243–251.

The Anterior Cruciate Ligament: Current and Future Concepts, edited by D.W. Jackson, et al. Raven Press, Ltd., New York © 1993.

CHAPTER 18

Collagen Ultrastructure in the Normal ACL and in ACL Graft

Barry W. Oakes

NORMAL ACL STRUCTURE

The human anterior cruciate ligament is composed of collagen fibrils, 30 to 175 nm in diameter, which are parallel at high magnification (Fig. 1) (2). These fibrils form fiber bundles 1 to 20 μm in diameter, running almost parallel to the long axis of the ligament. These fiber bundles coalesce to form a subfascicular unit, which varies from 100 to 250 mm in diameter. Three to 20 subfasciculi are collected together to form a collagen fasciculus that can be several millimeters in diameter (1–3,9).

AGE-RELATED CHANGES IN NORMAL HUMAN ACL

Collagen fibril profiles from the ACL of different age specimens were analyzed using transmission electron microscopy (5). ACL specimens with an age range from 16 weeks fetal to 73 years old were divided into four age groups: fetal, adolescent, adult, and late adulthood. In the three fetal specimens, Frogameni and Jackson demonstrated a uniform population of small-diameter collagen fibrils; greater than 90% of the fibrils and 91% of the area quantified were made up of fibrils with diameters in the 25- to 50-nm range. No fibrils greater than 100 nm were seen. The adolescent sample (14 year old boy, n = 1) also demonstrated a uniform population of slightly larger fibrils; again, no large-diameter fibrils were seen. Sixty-six percent of the fibrils and 69% of the area were composed of fibrils in the 50- to 75-nm-diameter range.

B. W. Oakes: Department of Anatomy, Monash University, Clayton, 31 68 Australia.

In the young adult (aged 21, n = 1), the collagen fibril diameters became bimodal in distribution, with 56% of the fibrils and 25% of the area in the 25- to ~50-nm range; 42% of the fibrils and 66% of the cross-sectional area were made up of fibrils in the range of 75 to 125 nm. In later adult life (ages >65 years, n = 2), there was a return to a predominance of small-diameter fibrils. Although only 38% of the cross-sectional area was made up of small-diameter fibrils, 74% of the fibrils were in the 25- to 50-nm range. (Figs. 2 and 3).

COLLAGEN FIBRIL POPULATIONS IN HUMAN ACL AUTOGRAFTS AND ALLOGRAFTS

ACL Patellar Tendon Autografts

In order to gain some biological insight into collagen remodeling mechanisms within human cruciate ligament grafts Oakes (4,6,7) reported quantitative collagen fibril analyses of biopsies obtained from autogenous ACL patellar tendon grafts. These biopsies were obtained from patients subsequently requiring arthroscopic intervention because of stiffness, meniscal and/or articular cartilage problems or removal of prominent staples used for fixation. Most of the ACL grafts were obtained from the central one-third of the patellar tendon as a free graft (n = 33); some were left attached distally (n = 8). These biopsies represented approximately 20% of the total free grafts performed over the 6 years of the study. The clinical ACL stability of the biopsy group differed little from the remainder. All had a Grade II–III pivot shift (jerk) preoperatively [10 to ~15 mm anterior drawer neutral (ADN)], eliminated postoperatively in 87% of patients (0.5 mm ADN). Subsequent clinical re-

FIG. 1. Electron micrograph demonstrating parallel collagen fibrils in the anterior cruciate ligament of a 14-year-old boy. (×52,000)

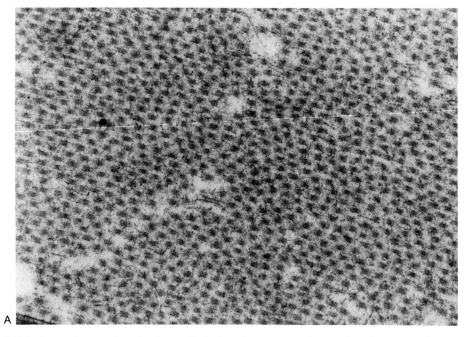

A

FIG. 2. Electron micrographs of collagen fibrils from human anterior cruciate ligaments of various ages. All biopsies were taken from the peripheral region of the middle of the ACL after synovial clearage. (×52,000) **A.** Sixteen-week fetal ACL demonstrating a uniform small-diameter collagen fibril profile. **B:** Fourteen-year-old male ACL demonstrating larger fibrils but a relatively homogeneous pattern. **C:** Forty-six-year-old male ACL. Note the appearance of small- and large-diameter fibrils giving a ''bimodal'' appearance. **D:** Seventy-three-year-old male ACL (from total knee arthroplasty). There is a multimodal distribution of collagen fibril diameters with evidence of peripheral disintegration of some of the fibrils.

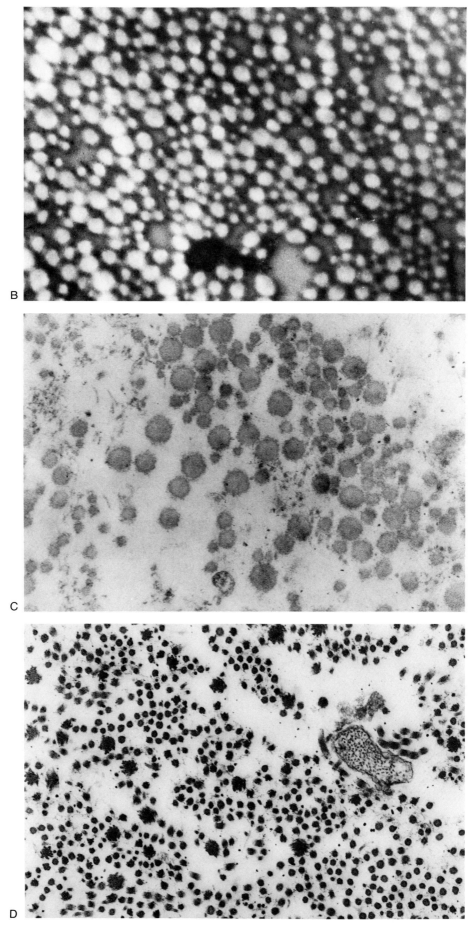

FIG. 2. *Continued.*

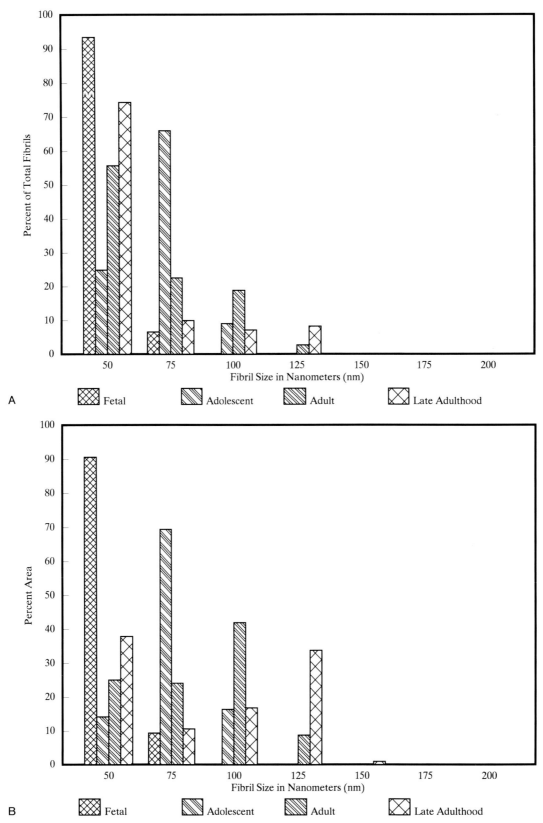

FIG. 3. Histograms demonstrating the populations of collagen fibrils as a function of age in the human anterior cruciate ligament corresponding to Fig. 7. **A:** Distribution of the number of fibrils with various diameters. **B:** Percentage area occupied by each fibril diameter group relative to the total fibril area quantified.

view at 3 years showed an increase in ADN with a return in 20% of a grade I pivot shift.

A total of 39 biopsies have been quantitatively analyzed for collagen fibril diameter populations in patients aged 19 to 42 years with patellar tendon autografts. These data were compared with collagen fibril populations obtained from biopsies of cadaver ACLs (n = 5) and also biopsies of ACLs from young (<30 years, n = 10) and older patients (30 years, n = 6) who had sustained a recent tear. Biopsies were also obtained from normal patellar tendons at operation (n = 7) and also cadavers (n = 3). The results (Fig. 4) from the collagen fibril diameter morphometric analysis in all the ACL patellar tendon autografts clearly indicated a predominance of small-diameter collagen fibrils. Absence of an ordered "regular crimping" of collagen fibrils was observed by both light and electron microscopy, as was a

less parallel arrangement of fibrils. The collagen fibrils were not tightly packed as in normal ligament. In other words, the extrafibril noncellular space was greatly increased compared to the normal adult ACL. In most biopsies capillaries were present and the majority of fibroblast-appearing cells were viable.

Quantitatively (Figs. 4–6), (a) large-diameter collagen fibrils (>100 nm diameter) form a large proportion (approximately 45%) of the percentage cross-sectional area in the normal human patellar tendon. (b) Collagen fibrils <100 nm diameter form a large proportion (approximately 85%) of the percentage cross-sectional area in the normal human ACL. (c) In all the incorporated ACL grafts, collagen fibrils <100 nm in diameter (majority 25 to 75 nm diameter) are the major contributor to the collagen fibril cross-sectional area, be they "young" (9 month) or "old" grafts (5 to 9 years). (See Fig. 4.)

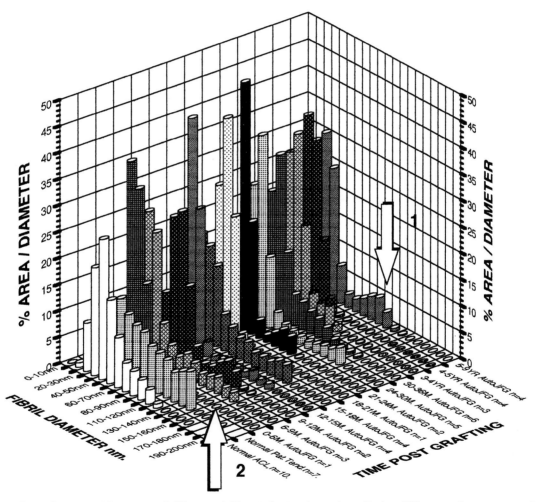

FIG. 4. Summary histogram of all human ACL patellar tendon autografts (n = 39) versus time compared to the normal young ACL (n = 10) and normal young patellar tendon (n = 7) expressed as percentage area per diameter fibril group. Note the presence of large fibrils (>100 nm) in the older 5- to 9-year-old grafts (*Arrow 1*) and the rapid loss of <100-nm fibrils in the 0- to 6-month postgraft group (*Arrow 2*) which are present in the donor patellar tendon (to the *left* of Arrow 2).

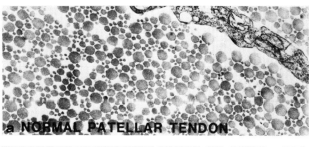

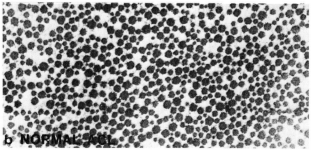

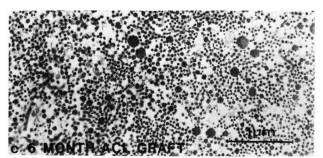

FIG. 5. Transverse section electron micrographs. **A:** Normal young (<30 years old) human patellar tendon. Note the large- and small-diameter fibrils. **B:** Normal human ACL (<30 years old). Note smaller fibrils compared to the patellar tendon. **C:** Six-month human ACL patellar tendon autograft. Note the predominance of small fibrils and the remains of the larger "donor" patellar tendon fibrils. (all ×34,000) See Figs. 2 and 4 for quantitative histograms.

Autogenous ACL patellar tendon grafts (Jones' free grafts) were divided into six monthly age periods post-grafting ($n = 39$) and are shown in Fig. 4 as % area/diameter group versus diameter of fibrils and are compared to the normal ACL and normal patellar tendon. Note in the earliest graft obtained at 6 months the large number of small fibrils and the loss of the large fibrils from the patellar tendon graft (Arrow 2). The large cross-section represented by the small-diameter fibrils persists through all age groups of grafts with a suggestion of a decline in the small fibril representation in percent cross-sectional area at least after 4 years of grafting and an increase in the cross-sectional area of fibrils larger than 100 nm in grafts older than 5 to 9 years (Fig. 4: last column on the graph, Arrow 1). These data were collected from that obtained from the work of two surgeons (O.D.and

L.M.), but the same profile has been obtained from ACL graft biopsies graciously sent by other surgeons both nationally and internationally indicating that this remodeling procedure is independent of the surgical technique and is dependent on the basic mechanisms of collagen remodeling with "foreign" intraarticular collagen (4).

Human ACL Hamstring and Iliotibial Band ACL Autografts

Since the 1988 (6) report we have had an opportunity to collect more ACL autograft biopsies from both patients who have had a strip of iliotibial tract or the medial hamstrings used as an ACL replacement. Fifteen iliotibial ACL autografts (graft age, 10 months to 6 years) and 9 hamstring grafts (graft age, 10 months to ~6 years) have been quantitated for collagen fibril size. Eighteen ACL graft biopsies have been obtained from other surgeons both national and international. The mean %area/%area/diameter for the normally used graft tissues (i.e., normal patellar tendon, normal iliotibial tract, and normal semitendinosus) is compared with the normal ACL and the mean %area/diameter group for 39 Jones' free grafts, 9 hamstring grafts, and 15 iliotibial tract grafts (Fig. 6). Note with all these autogenous grafts that small fibrils <100 nm predominate compared to the normal ACL collagen fibril profile. Some large fibrils are present in the hamstring grafts, which probably reflects remnants of the original large fibrils in the normal hamstring tendons rather than the formation of large fibrils from preexisting medium-sized fibrils. This persisting small number of large fibrils seen in the hamstring grafts is not seen with the iliotibial band or the patellar tendon autografts (4).

The unimodal profile of small-diameter fibrils was observed in most of the ACL autografts whether they were patellar, hamstring tendon, or iliotibial in origin (Fig. 6). This was a constant observation indicating that collagen remodeling occurs with all these tissues within 3 to 4 months postsurgery and is independent of the surgeon. Large fibrils were observed in a few biopsies obtained from autografts older than 12 months but these were the exception.

Human ACL Allografts

Human ACL allograft specimens were studied as above for the autografts with quantitative collagen fibril analyses (8). The allograft specimens were procured at the time of second look arthroscopy from the superficial region of the midzone of ACL grafts after synovial clearage. The grafts used for the ACL reconstruction were usually from fresh-frozen allogeneic Achilles or tibialis

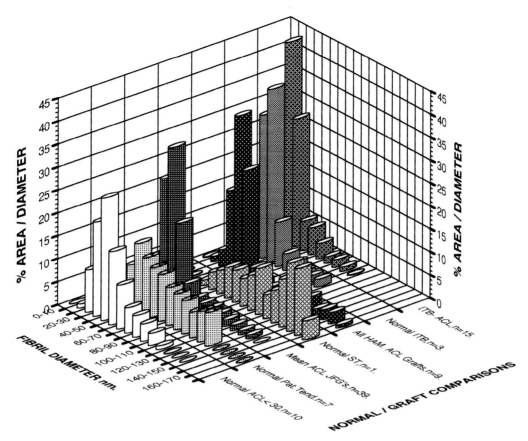

FIG. 6. Grand summary direct comparison of collagen fibril profiles for normal tissues used for ACL grafting [patellar tendon (*n* = 7), iliotibial band (*n* = 3), semitendinosus (*n* = 1)] with ACL autografts derived from the same tissues expressed as % area per diameter group. Note that large-diameter fibrils of >100 nm are found predominantly in the hamstring semitendinosus and to a lesser extent in the normal patellar tendon. The iliotibial band has a profile not unlike that of the normal ACL. Note that all the autografts [patellar tendon Jones' free ACL grafts (*JFG*) (*n* = 39), hamstring ACL grafts (*n* = 9), and iliotibial band ACL grafts (*n* = 15)] have predominantly small-diameter fibrils.

posterior or anterior tendons and were implanted 3 to 96 months prior to biopsy. In the ACL reconstruction technique, a fresh-frozen allograft 8 to 9 mm in diameter consisting of part of the Achilles tendon, the tibialis anterior or posterior, and peroneal or other thick flexor tendons without any bone attached to their ends was used as an ACL substitute. The tendons were fixed into drill holes made into the anatomical ACL attachment sites of the femur and the tibia with sutures, buttons, or staples. Postoperatively, the knee was immobilized for 2 to 5 weeks, and then full weight bearing was allowed at 2 to 3 months, jogging was recommended at 5 to 6 months, and full activity was allowed at 9 to 12 months.

Thirty-eight patients who had undergone allograft ACL reconstruction from 3 to 96 months previously and whose anteroposterior stability had been adequately restored were randomly selected. The restored stability of the involved knees was carefully confirmed with both Lachman and pivot shift signs and an objective quantita-

tive knee instability testing apparatus. All of these patients were subjected to second-look arthroscopy as a part of the procedure to remove hardware installed for graft fixation. Thirty-five graft biopsies were obtained from this patient group. Their age ranged from 15 to 37 years at the time of reconstruction. The biopsy specimens were obtained as shown in Table 1. The normal

TABLE 1. *Number of specimens obtained in relation to graft* in vivo *time*

Anterior cruciate ligament graft age (mo)	Number of biopsies
3	2
6	5
12	12
13–24	7
25–48	5
49–96	5

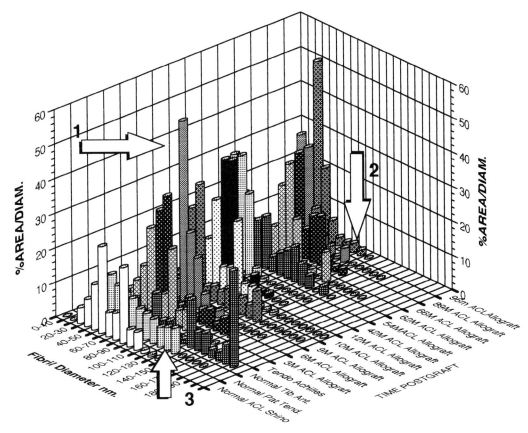

FIG. 7. Summary of all human ACL allografts versus time postgrafting compared to the normal young ACL, normal patellar tendon, and reconstituted tibialis anterior and Achilles tendons expressed as % area per diameter group. Note the early predominance of the small fibrils at 3 months postgraft (*Arrow 1*) and their persistence even at 96 months postgraft in the majority of biopsies examined. Some large fibrils are present (*Arrow 2*) at 96 months, but the majority of the large fibrils present in the donor tissues are removed (*to the right of Arrow 3*).

tissues used were compared with the normal ACL and the ACL allografts and are shown in Figs. 7 and 8.

Allograft Results versus Time

By 3 months postoperatively ($n = 2$) there was a predominance of small-diameter fibrils which accounted for >85% of the total cross-sectional area of these biopsies, with a tail of larger fibrils making the fibril distribution bimodal in shape. At 6 months ($n = 5$) the fibril distribution was now unimodal with most (approximately 90%) of the fibril cross-sectional area in <100-nm-diameter group. Fibrils >100 nm were obviously fewer than in the 3 month specimens. By 12 months ($n = 12$) almost all the cross-sectional area resided in <100-nm-diameter fibrils and there was almost complete absence of the large, 100-nm fibrils in most samples.

These observations suggest at least that most of the original large-diameter fibrils in the ACL allografts are replaced by newly synthesized, smaller diameter colla-

gen fibrils or that large fibrils undergo disaggregation (see Fig. 2D).

These observations parallel those described above for ACL autografts which also demonstrated within 6 months postimplantation the loss of large-diameter collagen fibrils of patellar tendon origin. It could be concluded therefore that the remodeling process has a similar time frame in both ACL tendon allografts and patellar tendon ACL autografts.

CONCLUSION

In reconstructing the ACL, the surgeon attempts to reproduce the morphology, orientation, strength, length, and function of the normal ACL. Despite surgical advances in ACL reconstruction techniques that have led to the substitution of the ACL with numerous biologic replacement tissues, the studies described have shown that reproduction of the normal ACL ultrastructure has not yet been achieved.

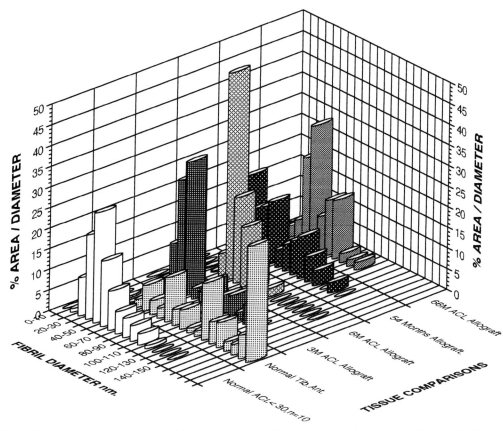

FIG. 8. Summary comparison of "older" and "younger" human ACL allografts. An "atypical" 54-month allograft and a "typical" 66-month-old allograft with the normal ACL and tibialis anterior expressed as % area per diameter group. Note that the "atypical" 54-month allograft has a fibril profile *almost* matching that of the normal ACL, but it is more distinctly bimodal. The 66-month ACL allograft also is bimodal compared to the normal young ACL.

ACKNOWLEDGMENT

The author acknowledges the support and encouragement of two close colleagues without which this work would not have been possible, Owen Deacon and Iain McLean. Also I thank Professor Konei Shino for the privilege of being able to work with him on the ACL allograft study. The author also acknowledges the support of the Australian NH and MRC and the Australian Orthopaedic Association for their support. Also thanks to M. Cross, J. Fox, J. Hart, I. Henderson, G. Keene, N. Thompson, and D. Young for supplying biopsies from their patients and to Michael Knight and Gabriel Ng, R. Bland-Coshall, Joan Clark, and Terry Martin and staff for their excellent technical support.

REFERENCES

1. Amiel D, Frank C, Harwood F, Fronek J, Akeson W. (1984): Tendons and ligaments: a morphological and biochemical comparison. *J Orthop Res,* 1:257–265.
2. Amiel D, Billings E Jr, Akeson WH. (1990): Ligament structure, chemistry, and physiology. In: Daniel D, Akeson W, O'Connor J, eds. *Knee ligaments, structure, injury and repair.* New York: Raven Press, pp 77–91.
3. Clark JM, Sidles JA. (1990): The interrelation of fiber bundles in the anterior cruciate ligament. *J Orthop Res,* 8:180–188.
4. Deacon OW, McLean LD, Oakes BW, Cole WG, Chan D, Knight M. (1991): Ultrastructural and collagen typing analyses of autogenous ACL grafts—an update. Presented at the meeting of the International Knee Society, Toronto, Ontario, May.
5. Frogameni AD, Jackson DW. (1992): Age-related changes in the human anterior cruciate ligament: electron microscopic analysis of collagen fibril diameters. Unpublished study.
6. Frank C, Woo SL-Y, Andriacchi T, et al. (1988): Normal ligament: structure, function, and composition. In: Woo SL-Y, Buckwalter JA, eds. *Injury and Repair of the Musculoskeletal Soft Tissues.* Park Ridge, Illinois: American Academy of Orthopaedic Surgeons, pp 45–101.
7. Oakes BW. (1989): Connective tissue adaptation to loading; fibroblasts, fibres, fibrils and free grafts. In: *Proceedings of the First International Olympic Committee World Congress of Sports Sciences, Colorado Springs, Colorado, October 28–Nov 3.* Park Ridge, Illinois: American Academy of Orthopaedic Surgeons, pp 156–160.
8. Shino K, Oakes BW, lnoue H, Horibe S, Nakata K. (1990): Human ACL allograft: collagen fibril populations studied as a function of age. *Trans Orthop Res Soc,* 15:520.
9. Yahia L-H, Drouin G. (1988): Collagen structure in human anterior cruciate ligament and patellar tendon. *J Materials Sci,* 23:3750–3755.

The Anterior Cruciate Ligament: Current and Future Concepts, edited by D.W. Jackson, et al. Raven Press, Ltd., New York © 1993.

CHAPTER 19

Collagen Remodeling in ACL Reconstruction (Goat Model)

Anthony D. Frogameni, Douglas W. Jackson, and Timothy M. Simon

The reconstructed anterior cruciate ligament in both goats and humans does not reestablish the normal bimodal distribution of collagen fibril diameters that appears to be a structure-specific phenomenon seen in native ACL. The changes in fibril diameter that occur during the "ligamentization" of transplanted tendon is different from that seen in normal collagen maturation (1,2,4,16).

Using data collected from various authors, Parry and Craig (22) attempted to correlate ultimate tensile strength to fibril diameter (Table 1). They noted that collagen fibrils are composed of similarly directed collagen molecules. The collagen fibrils are circular in cross-section. There was no evidence that anastomosing fibrils occur *in vivo* in any connective tissue. The ends of a collagen fibril were rarely, if ever, seen in electron microscopic sections. In fact, Parry and Craig (22) followed the courses of 1,000 fibrils in rat tendon over 14 serial sections without observing either a fibril originating or terminating. From these small numbers they concluded that collagen fibril distributions are a heterogeneous group of "infinitely" long cylindrical fibrils of various diameters. In the canine anterior cruciate ligament, Clark and Sidles (8) followed peripheral fascicles from origin to insertion. They did not observe any evidence of fibril crossing, interweaving or termination. However, Trotter and Wofsy (27) examined 5,639 rat tendon fibrils over a length of 4.26 mm and encountered 4 ends in this group. They concluded that collagen fibrils have intratendinous ends and that the ends are associated with fibril tapering (Fig. 1).

From their extensive studies of collagen, Parry et al. (20–22) have made several conclusions:

1. During fetal development and at birth, the distribution of collagen fibril diameters is primarily unimodal.
2. Mass-average diameter of collagen fibrils increases between birth and maturity.

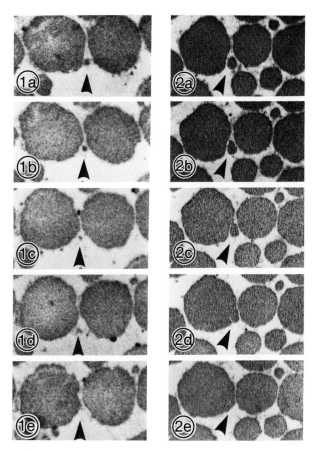

FIG. 1. Serial electron micrographs of collagen fibrils from rat extension digitorum longus tendon demonstrating intratendinous ends (*arrow*). These fibril terminations are associated with fibril tapering. (From ref. *27*, with permission.)

A. D. Fromageni, D. W. Jackson, and T. M. Simon: Southern California Center for Sports Medicine, Long Beach Memorial Medical Center, Long Beach, California 90806.

TABLE 1. *Samples of rat tendon, skin, and cartilage relating tensile strength to the mass-average diameter of collagen fibrils*

Measurement	Mature tendon	Skin	Cartilage
Ultimate tensile strength (MPa)	60	12	1.2
Young's modulus (MPa)	400–1,200	20–100	10
Collagen fibril diameter (nm)	160–240	90–130	70

From Parry et al., ref. 20.

3. Collagen subjected to high tensile stresses has a bimodal distribution of fibril diameters at maturity.
4. As tissues age past maturity, the average diameter of collagen fibrils decreases.
5. The ultimate tensile strength of connective tissue is likely correlated with the mass-average diameter of the collagen fibrils.

ACL ALLOGRAFTS (ACL REPLACING AN ACL) IN A GOAT MODEL

ACL allografts used to reconstruct the ACL in the goat model have failed to duplicate the structural and mechanical properties of the complex collagen scaffolding that comprises the normal ACL (11). In our preliminary studies, mechanical function did not follow the normal appearing cellular and microvascular form seen in the transplants. Grossly and on histological examination, the allograft ACLs at one year appeared similar to the normal ACL. Early unrestricted activity of the goats following transplantation did not have deleterious effects on the revascularization of the ligament, did not alter the ACL fiber transition into the bone plugs, nor did it have a deleterious effect on the incorporation of the bony plugs.

There were no apparent detrimental immunological effects on the incorporation of the allografts and no significant cellular inflammatory response associated with the bony plug incorporation site at the one year observation period. None of the ACL allografts were reabsorbed. The bulk of all the ACL allografts at one year had a cross sectional area similar to that at the time of implant.

In animal models to date, no transplanted biological tissues, allograft or autograft, have been reported to have mechanical properties after remodeling that were equal or better than those in the graft at the time of implantation. The graft replacements following incorporation have approached 30% to 80% of their time zero maximum force to failure values (7,9,12–14,17,28). It is commonly believed that the stronger the biological ACL substitute is at the time of implantation the potential is it will be stronger at follow-up. This has been the contention based on uniaxial loading of ACL reconstructions.

The goat model, as do all animal models, present several problems in studying ACL allografts (5,6,11). All animal models present variations from the human.

There is presently no ideal animal model for direct comparison with the human ACL. The goat ACL and its surgical repair differs from the human ligament: (a) The goat ligament maximum load to failure values are higher than the human ACLs (2,301 ± 155 N versus 1,725 ± 269 N, respectively). (b) There is greater difficulty in protecting the ACL transplants in the goat during the early postoperative phase which potentially places increased demands on the surgical reconstruction. (c) The anterior cruciate ligament tibial attachment in the goat is broader and the anterior limb crosses the meniscal attachment. (d) There is 1 ± 0.1 mm of anterior posterior translation in the goat knee. This constitutes a difficult end point to duplicate in a reconstruction.

The results of our experience with ACL allografts will serve as a baseline for future investigations. Although the desired mechanical and structural properties of the ACL allografts were not reestablished, the fiber orientation, the developed vascular network, and lack of cellular (immune) infiltration following transplantation were all encouraging.

THE EFFECTS OF FREEZE-THAWING ALONE ON THE *IN SITU* GOAT ACL

To demonstrate the effects of biological incorporation on a devitalized collagen graft, Jackson, et al. developed a multiple freeze-thaw technique to kill the cells and interrupt the vascular supply of the anterior cruciate ligament (13). This model simulates a biological (autogenous) graft in which the collagen fibers are anatomically oriented and have physiological tensioning of individual fibers and anatomic fixation to bone. The effects of repopulation of cells and of revascularization on this ideally placed and tensioned graft were then studied in relation to changes in mechanical and structural properties at time zero, six weeks, and six months.

At 6 months, no statistically significant differences were noted between treated and contralateral control ligaments relative to anterior-posterior translation, maximum force to rupture, stiffness in the linear region of the force-length curve, modulus of elasticity in the linear region, strain to maximum stress or maximum stress. The only significant difference observed was an increase in the cross-sectional area of the ligament. This increase was 22% and 42% greater than the control ligaments at 6 weeks and 6 months, respectively. These observations are in contrast to a previous study by Jackson et al. following replacement of the anterior cruciate ligament with an ACL allograft and an ACL allograft supplemented with a 3M ligament augmentation device (LAD; 3M, St. Paul, Minnesota) (12). In those studies, an average reduction in maximum strength of 75% for the allografts and 50% for the allografts that had a ligament augmentation device was found at one year. The authors concluded that devitalized, devascularized anterior cruciate ligaments do not lose their ultimate strength if the anatomical position and the orientation of the collagen fibers are not altered.

The loss in strength that occurs postoperatively in allografts and autografts used to reconstruct the anterior cruciate ligament may not be the natural sequela of the revascularization and healing process, but, rather, the consequence of improper orientation and tensioning of the graft. The specific events that are involved in the loss of strength need to be clarified.

The revascularization of these anterior cruciate ligaments that were subjected to the freeze-thaw procedure was also different from that observed in the previous experience with allografts of the anterior cruciate ligament. The freeze-thaw treated anterior cruciate ligaments had less vascular response at six months and one year. They did have a similar periligamentous hypervascular response present in the fat pad, the periligamentous tissue, and the synovial tissue in the posterior compartment. Another difference from the previous goat model experience was that the freeze-thaw procedure did not have altered anterior-posterior stability of the knee. With either an allograft or an autogenous graft, we have been unable to reestablish the inherent anterior-posterior stability of 1 ± 0.1 millimeter of the knee (stifle joint) of the goat.

The freeze-thaw technique represents the ideal operative placement of a biological graft. The collagen fibers are in the proper anatomical position, with the appropriate length, as well as physiologically tensioned and biologically fixed to bone. If there had been an associated increase in anterior-posterior translation in these studies in the goat model, the potential use of a biological grafts alone to obtain this goal would be questionable.

GOAT EM COLLAGEN FIBRIL ANALYSES

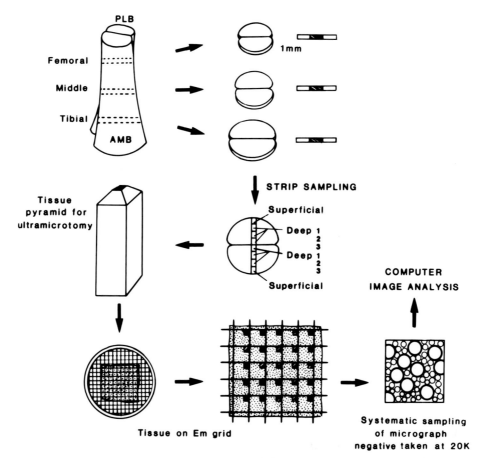

FIG. 2. Preparation of goat ACL for quantitative collagen fibril analyses of the femoral, middle, and tibial regions by strip sampling and also systematic random sampling of thin sections on the EM grids.

The maintenance of normal stability was accompanied by the unexpected finding of an increase in the cross-sectional area of the treated anterior cruciate ligament, which was present at six weeks and six months. The increase in the size of the ligament that was treated with the freeze-thaw technique was associated with a significant change in the size of collagen fibrils. There was an increase in smaller diameter collagen fibrils and of their density. This increase in cross-sectional area was associated with a robust biological response. ACL reconstructions in animal models and the cross-sectional area of the incorporated grafts have been reported to be inversely correlated with the amount of anterior-posterior translation at 6 and 12 months in three different studies of animals (29).

COLLAGEN REMODELING IN GOAT ACL AUTOGRAFTS AND ALLOGRAFTS

The aim of a study by Oakes et al. (19) was to quantify in detail the collagen fibril remodeling process in the adult goat patellar tendon ACL autografts as a function of three defined anatomic sampling sites over a 12-months time frame and to compare these observations with those already described for human ACL auto and allografts which were single "representative" biopsies from the grafted ACL.

Eight mature female adult goats were used in this study. The central one third of the patellar tendon was taken over the top of the lateral femoral condyle after a Gigli saw grooved the ACL graft track for isometry. The graft was stapled under a periosteal flap to the lateral femoral condyle. The ACL grafts were sampled at times, $T = 0, 6, 12, 24,$ and 52 weeks. Two goats were killed at each time interval and the ACL grafts obtained and prepared for quantitative ultrastructural collagen fibril analyses. The normal ACL ($T = 0$, $n = 5$) and ACL patellar tendon grafts ($n = 7$) were divided into thirds and 1-mm-thick sections were cut from the femoral, middle, and tibial thirds. This section was then cut into a strip, and four sections were obtained; two were deemed "superficial" and contained a synovial surface and two were deemed "deep." From each section two ultrastructural thin sections were analyzed systematically on copper 400 mesh grids. Systematic random sampling was done such that about 10% of the grid spaces the sections covered were photographed for later quantitative ultrastructural collagen fibril analyses (See Fig. 2). The patellar tendon was sampled in the central region and two blocks per tendon were analyzed as above, $n = 3$. The collagen fibril profiles were directly quantitated from electron micrograph negatives and the collagen fibril population profile obtained were subjected to Komolgorov-Smirnov statistical analysis. Figure 3 shows representative electron micrographs of goat patellar tendon autografts

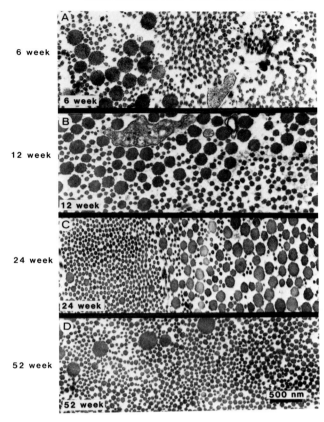

GOAT ACL PATELLAR TENDON AUTOGRAFTS

FIG. 3. Representative transverse electron micrographs of goat patellar tendon autografts versus time postgrafting. **A:** 6 weeks, **B:** 12 weeks, **C:** 24 weeks, **D:** 52 weeks. Note the progressive loss of large fibrils and the increase of the small fibrils with time postgraft.

from 6 to 52 weeks postgrafting reflecting the increasing numbers of small-diameter collagen fibrils with time.

In another study by Jackson et al. using the goat model, transmission electron micrographs of patellar tendon and reconstructed ACL (from both autogenous and allograft patellar tendon) were analyzed six months postoperatively (14). In normal patellar tendon, 80% of the collagen fibril diameters were in the range of 100 to 200 nm. The normal goat ACL had 80% of the collagen fibril diameters in the 100 to 150 nm range, but no 200-nm fibrils were seen. The 6-month autograft group demonstrated large increases in the number of 25- to 50-nm-diameter fibrils; these small-diameter fibrils accounted for 84% of the fibril population. However, in the allograft group, only 54% of the collagen fibrils at six months postoperative were in the 25 to 50 nm range (Fig. 4). These findings correlated with the allograft replacement retaining a greater percentage of large-diameter collagen fibrils and being slower to remodel into small-diameter fibrils. The cross-sectional area of the autografts at six months was 164% of the control ACL as compared to 78% for the allografts. The strengths of the autografts and allografts were 62% and 27% of control ACL strength

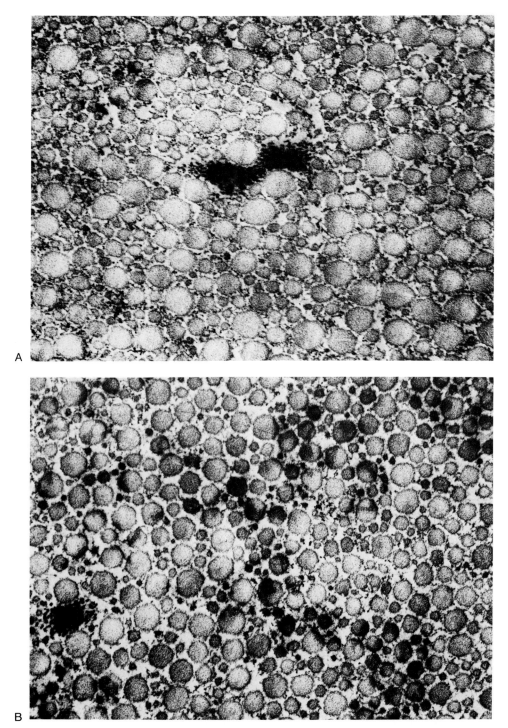

FIG. 4. Transmission electron micrographs from tissue obtained from a skeletally mature Spanish female goat (×52,000) **A:** Normal patellar tendon demonstrating large-diameter collagen fibrils in the range of 100 to 200 nm. **B:** Normal anterior cruciate ligament. Smaller collagen fibrils present; none of the fibrils exceed 150 nm in diameter. **C:** Six-month postoperative specimen following ACL reconstruction using patellar tendon autograft. There is a predominance of small-diameter fibrils in the 25 to 50 nm range. **D:** Six-month postoperative specimen following ACL reconstruction using patellar tendon allograft. Note the persistence of large-diameter fibrils (greater than 100 nm).

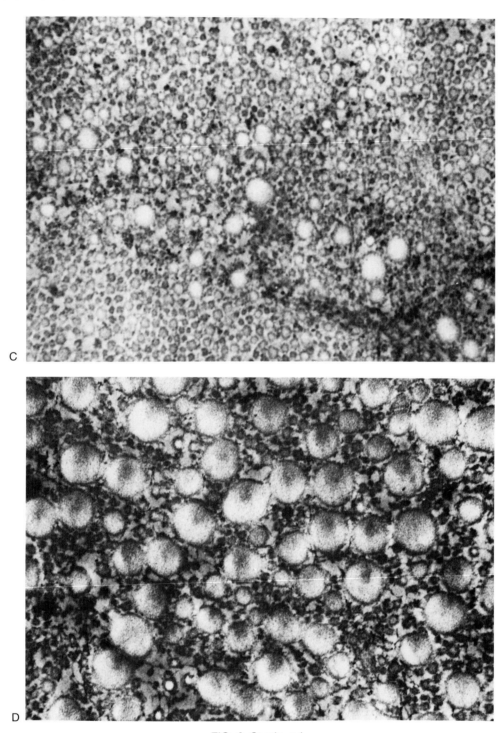

FIG. 4. *Continued.*

respectively. This data is consistent with the work by Parry and Craig (22), indicating that the tensile strength of a tissue is proportional to the diameters of its collagen fibrils. However, the authors noted the fact that since the study concluded at six months, it is possible that the collagen fibrils may continue to enlarge as the cells respond to the environment. However, Oakes' work suggests that large collagen fibrils diameter in allograft sub-

stitution are slow to decrease with time (19,25). Similarly, the predominance of small-diameter collagen fibrils documented in autogenous grafts that have been used to reconstruct the human anterior cruciate ligament have persisted regardless of the origin of the graft, the surgeon, or the time after the operation (10).

The study by Jackson et al. comparing two commonly used patellar tendon grafts (autografts and fresh frozen allografts) demonstrated in the goat model that at the six-month time period the autograft has significantly less inflammatory response, a more robust biological response, and improved mechanical and structural properties in comparison to a similar sized allograft (14). The altered and delayed response in the allograft remains a challenge. However, neither tissue replacement demonstrated the formation of large-diameter collagen fibrils seen in native ACL tissue. Similarly, the tensile strength of normal ACL has not been reproduced with reconstructive surgery in the goat model. The response in the allograft tissue may be missing some stimulus present in the autograft tissue. The cells that repopulate the two grafts seem to be of similar origin (2,15).

These studies suggest that small-diameter collagen fibrils are synthesized at the expense of large-diameter fibrils during the repair process after ACL reconstruction. The fact that allografts retain a higher percentage of large-diameter fibrils may indicate slower replacement of large collagen fibrils during repair. The increase in cross sectional area in the autografts suggests a more robust remodeling. Another mechanism for the observed change to a small-diameter collagen fibril may be related to a change in the type of glycosaminoglycans synthesized by the replacement "fibroblasts" (18,24,26). Amiel et al. (3) have shown that the rabbit cruciate ligaments have more GAGs than the patellar tendon; this may be an important factor in determining collagen fibril populations.

In a preliminary human study, similar sized patellar tendon allografts and autografts have not been reported to have a significantly different failure rate (23). This may be due to several factors: (a) a difference between the human and the goat's biological response to an allograft ACL reconstruction; (b) the differences in strength and stability being too small to be clinically significant; (c) the human clinical data available to make these comparisons is too limited at this time.

SUMMARY

Ideally, surgery to reconstruct the anterior cruciate ligament attempts to reproduce the structural, biochemical and mechanical properties of the native ACL. However, this has not been accomplished by current techniques in the animal model. Biological grafts undergo cellular repopulation after intraarticular substitution. The replacement cells do not appear to synthesize large-diameter collagen fibrils. The graft tissue in the animal model is mechanically weaker than native ACL. Reasons for this may involve factors related to surgical techniques, the surrounding milieu, failure to achieve cell differentiation, or degeneration of the fibril structures. Animal studies have shown that allografts used to reconstruct the ACL undergo a slower and less robust response than au-

tografts. Further studies are necessary to clarify these differences and similarities.

REFERENCES

1. Amiel D, Frank CB, Hardwood FL. (1984): Tendons and ligaments: a morphological and biochemical comparison. *J Orthop Res,* 1:257–265.
2. Amiel D, Kleiner JB, Hardwood FL, Raux R, Akeson WH. (1986): Anterior cruciate ligament (ACL) reconstruction with autogenous patellar tendon (PT): the process of "ligamentization." *Trans Orthop Res Soc,* 11:57.
3. Amiel D, Kleiner JB. (1988): Collagen. In: Nimni ME, Olsen B, eds. *Biochemistry of tendon and ligament, vol 3, Biotechnology.* Cleveland: CRC Press, pp 223–251.
4. Amiel D, Billings E, Akeson WH. (1990): Ligament structure, chemistry and physiology. In: Daniel D, ed. *Knee ligaments: structure, function, injury and repair.* New York: Raven Press, pp 77–91.
5. Arnoczky SP, Rubin RM, Marshall JL. (1979): Microvasculature of the cruciate ligaments and its response to injury: an experimental study in the dog. *J Bone Joint Surg [Am],* 61A:1221–1229.
6. Arnoczky SP, Warren RF, Ashlock MA. (1986): Replacement of the anterior cruciate ligament using a patellar tendon allograft: an experimental study. *J Bone Joint Surg [Am],* 68A:376–385.
7. Clancy WG, Narechania RG, Rosenberg TD. (1981): Anterior and posterior cruciate ligament reconstruction in rhesus monkeys. *J Bone Joint Surg [Am],* 63A:1270–1284.
8. Clark JM, Sidles JA. (1970): The interrelation of fiber bundles in the anterior cruciate ligament. *J Orthop Res,* 8:180–188.
9. Curtis RJ, Delee JC, Drez DJ. (1985): Reconstruction of the anterior cruciate ligament with freeze dried fascia lata allografts in dogs: a preliminary report. *Am J Sports Med,* 13:408–414.
10. Frank C, Woo SL-Y, Andriacchi T, Brand R, Oakes B, Dahners L, DeHaven K, Lewis J, Sabiston P. (1988): Normal ligament: structure, function and composition. In: Woo SL-Y, Buckwalter JA, eds. *Injury and repair of the musculoskeletal soft tissues.* Park Ridge, Illinois: American Academy of Orthopaedic Surgeons, pp 45–101.
11. Jackson DW, Grood ES, Arnozcky SP, Butler DL, Simon TM. (1987): Freeze dried anterior cruciate ligament allografts: a preliminary study in a goat model. *Am J Sports Med,* 15:295–302.
12. Jackson DW, Grood ES, Arnozcky SP, Butler DL, Simon TM. (1987): Cruciate reconstruction using freeze dried anterior cruciate ligament allograft and a ligament augmentation device (LAD): an experimental study in a goat model. *Am J Sports Med,* 15:528–538.
13. Jackson DW, Grood ES, Cohn BT, Arnozcky SP, Simon TM, Cummings JF. (1991): The effects of *in situ* freezing on the anterior cruciate ligament. *J Bone Joint Surg [Am],* 73A:201–213.
14. Jackson DW, Grood ES, Goldstein J, Rosen MA, Kurzweil PR, Cummings JF, Simon TM. (1992): Anterior cruciate ligament reconstruction using patellar tendon autograft and allograft—a comparative study in goats. *Am J Sports Med [in press].*
15. Jackson DW, Simon TM, Kurzweil PR, Rosen MA. (1992): Survival of cells after intra-articular transplantation of fresh allografts of the patellar and anterior cruciate ligaments. *J Bone Joint Surg [Am],* 74A:112–123.
16. Monter GS, Bezerra MSF, Junqueira LCU. (1984): Collagen distribution in tissues. In: Ruggeri A, Motta PM, eds. *Ultrastructure of the connective tissue matrix.* The Hague: Martinus Nijhoff, pp 65–91.
17. Noyes FR, Butler DL, Grood ES. (1984): Biomechanical analysis of the human ligament grafts used in knee ligament repairs and reconstruction. *J Bone Joint Surg [Am],* 66A:344–352.
18. Oakes BW. (1988): Ultrastructure studies on knee joint ligaments: quantitation of collagen fibre population in exercised and control rat cruciate ligaments and in human anterior cruciate grafts. Injury and repair of the musculoskeletal soft tissues. In: Buckwalter J, Woo SL-Y, eds. *Proceedings of the Soft Tissue Repair Conference, Savannah, GA.* Park Ridge, Illinois: American Academy of Orthopaedic Surgeons, vol 2, pp 66–82.

19. Oakes BW, Knight, M, McLean ID, Deacon O. (1992): Goat ACL autograft collagen remodelling—quantitative collagen fibril analyses over one year. *Proceedings of AOSSM, San Diego,* pp 45–46.
20. Parry DAD, Barnes GRG, Craig AS. (1978): A comparison of the size distribution of collagen fibrils in connective tissues as a function of age and a possible relation between fibril size distribution and mechanical properties. *Proc R Soc Lond [Biol],* 203:305–321.
21. Parry DAD, Craig AS, Barnes GRG. (1978): Tendon and ligament from the horse: an ultrastructural study of collagen fibrils and elastic fibers as a function of age. *Proc R Soc Lond [Biol],* 203:293–303.
22. Parry DA, Craig AS. (1984): Growth and development of collagen fibrils in connective tissue. In: Ruggeri A, Motta PM, eds. *Ultrastructure of the connective tissue matrix.* The Hague: Martinus Nijhoff, pp 34–62.
23. Saddemi SR, Frogameni AD, Fenton PJ, Hartman J, Hartman W. (1991): Comparison of perioperative morbidity in ACL reconstruction: autograft vs. allograft. Presented at the 10th Annual Meeting of the Arthroscopy Association of North America, San Diego, CA July 6–9, 1992.
24. Scott JE, Hughes EW. (1986): Proteoglycan-collagen relationships in developing chick and bovine tendons: influence of the physiological environment. *Connect Tissue Res,* 14:267–268.
25. Shino K, Oakes B, Inoue M, Horibe S, Nakata K, Ono K. (1990): Human allografts: collagen fibril populations as a function of age of the graft. *Trans Orthop Res Soc,* 15:520.
26. Toole BP, Lowther DA. (1968): The effect of chondroitin sulphate-protein on the formation of collagen fibrils *in vitro. Biochem J,* 109:857–866.
27. Trotter JA, Wofsy C. (1989): The length of collagen fibrils in tendon. *Trans Orthop Res Soc,* 14:180.
28. Van Rens TJG, van den Berg AF, Huskies R. (1986): Substitution of the anterior cruciate ligament: a long term histologic and biomechanical study with autogenous pedicled grafts of the iliotibial band in dogs. *Arthroscopy,* 2:139–154.
29. Walz KA, Grood ES, Noyes FR, Butler DL, Jackson DW, Drez DJ. (1989): Anterior-posterior translation in reconstructed knees correlates with graft cross-sectional area. *Trans Orthop Res Soc,* 14:511.

The Anterior Cruciate Ligament: Current and Future Concepts, edited by D.W. Jackson, et al.
Raven Press, Ltd., New York © 1993.

CHAPTER 20

The Biomechanical Properties of Normal and Healing Ligaments

Mark A. Gomez

Clinical and basic science investigations over the last 70 years have contributed much to our understanding of the role of the anterior cruciate ligament (ACL) (3,5,12). These studies have demonstrated that the ACL is a complex anatomical structure that plays an intricate role in providing normal knee joint motion. However, the potential of an injured ACL to permit normal joint motion is unclear.

Clinical studies in the literature have shown that the nonoperative treatment of full and partial tears of the ACL produces varying results. For example, Bonamo et al. (2) found in 73 younger patients (average age 26 years) who had undergone conservative treatment of an ACL-deficient knee, that 11% had excellent results, 32% had good results, 22% were considered fair, and 35% were classified poor at an average 1-year follow-up. However, if one looked at the 30 patients followed between 4 and 8.5 years in this same population, 50% had poor results. Giove et al. (7) treated another patient population (age 18 to 40 years) with torn ACLs nonoperatively and found that even though all of the patients returned to some level of sports activity, there was a high incidence of anterior instability. With regard to partial tears of the ACL, Kannus and Jarvinen and Finsterbush et al. (6,13) indicate that nonoperative methods are generally successful, but the latter authors have shown that secondary damage can still occur. Of 42 cases with a partial tear of the ACL, 11 cases went on to a complete tear, 2 acquired a meniscal tear and 3 resulted in a loose or subluxed anterior horn of the medial meniscus. What these clinical findings infer is that an ACL has low tolerance for injury and its potential for healing is questionable.

Normal function of the knee joint depends in part on the biomechanical properties of the ligament structures. Due to the paucity of information regarding the biomechanical behavior of anterior cruciate ligament especially from the standpoint of healing properties (11,17), the remainder of this chapter will provide information on what *is* known about the properties of both normal and injured/healing ligaments obtained from studies of the medial collateral ligament (MCL).

THE BIOMECHANICAL PROPERTIES OF NORMAL LIGAMENT

The literature abounds with descriptions of the structural as well as mechanical properties of ligament tissue. For that matter, the "biomechanical properties" of ligaments are also frequently mentioned. What is not always clear is the distinction between all these engineering terms. The next few sections will address the definitions of these properties and what these properties are for normal ligament tissue.

Structural Properties

If one clamps the two ends of a ligament and then proceeds to stretch it to the point of failure while recording both the amount of stretch and the load simultaneously, then one has essentially obtained the structural properties of that ligament. This load-deformation behavior is nonlinear, and a function of both the cross-sectional area and length of the ligament. Figure 1 demonstrates how the load rises in an exponential fashion as the deformation increases. This figure also shows that if the cross-sectional area is increased while maintaining the same ligament length, the load will go up even faster

M. A. Gomez: University of Colorado Health Sciences Center, Denver, Colorado 80262.

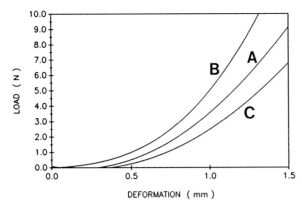

FIG. 1. Load-deformation or structural properties of ligament with particular cross-section and length (**A**), ligament with the same length as A but with a larger cross-section (**B**), and ligament with the same cross-section as A but longer length (**C**).

as the ligament is stretched (Fig. 1B). Conversely, if the cross-sectional area is kept the same and the ligament length is increased, the load does not increase in the same fashion (Fig. 1C). This behavior explains why the term "structural" is used when describing the structural properties of a ligament. A short ligament that has a big cross-section will behave in a stiffer fashion than one that has a small cross-section and is very long. This concept explains why one cannot always compare the load-deformation curves between anatomically similar ligaments. For instance, the biological variability between ACLs may result in varying cross-sections or one sample may be clamped "shorter" than another when performing tensile tests. In order to account for these differences in size and shape and to permit comparisons between tissues, the concept of "mechanical" properties is used.

Mechanical Properties

The mechanical properties of ligaments are sometimes referred to as the material or stress-strain properties of the ligament substance. Thus, the terms *mechanical properties, material properties,* and *stress-strain properties* are all essentially equivalent and are used to describe the intrinsic nature of the ligament substance. These properties are not dependent on the size or shape of the ligament structure. This is because the structural or load-deformation properties are normalized: the measured load is divided by the cross-sectional area and defines the stress. The difference between the new length and the original length of the ligament is divided by ligament's original length to obtain the strain. The technical side of actually obtaining these stress-strain properties is well reviewed in the literature (10,18).

As mentioned above, the load-deformation curve for ligament has a nonlinear shape. This behavior occurs because of the stress-strain or mechanical properties of the ligament. However, the overall shape of the curve is

dictated not only by the stresses or strains applied to the ligament, but also by the history of their application. In layman's terms, the ligament "remembers" what stresses or strains it has undergone and is affected by any subsequent application of stress or strain. For example, Fig. 2 shows what happens if a ligament is first loaded to a certain level and then unloaded. One can see that the load goes up in an exponential fashion and then goes down in a similar, but not exact manner. The reason for this disparity is that the ligament has adapted to the imposed strain condition through a loss of energy. (Note: the loss in energy is defined by the area between the loading and unloading curves and is defined as the hysteresis). Again, in nontechnical jargon, the ligament "remembers" the loading phase during the unloading part of the cycle. Now if this same (low) deformation is applied in a continuous cyclic fashion, then the difference between curves approaches zero and the ligament behaves in a "pseudoelastic" way. That is, the loading and unloading curves are repeatable and considered equivalent. This cyclic adaptation is essentially what happens when one stretches to loosen up before a physical workout. It permits a joint to move or deform with less load than if no cyclic strain history or stretching had been performed. Does the ligament recover from an applied stress or strain history? The answer is affirmative, but the length of time it takes depends on the level of stress or strain applied and even the temperature of the ligament (18).

Knowledge of the time-dependent nature of ligament tissue is important not only for the understanding of how the ligament contributes to joint function, but also how one evaluates the ability of a healing ligament to provide for normal joint motion. For example, given a knee with a partial tear of the ACL, the initial clinical test of anterior drawer may show good stability. However, if a repetitive cyclic load is applied over time, the anterior subluxation of the knee may increase more than that of normal knee because of the inferior time dependent mechanical properties of the injured ligament. This point will be expanded upon in the next section.

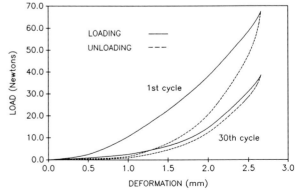

FIG. 2. Graph showing the effect of a cyclic strain history on the load-deformation behavior of a bone-ligament-bone complex.

Finally, it should be mentioned that the term "biomechanical properties" is usually used to describe both the structural and the mechanical properties of the ligament. Some may argue about this definition, so the final recommendation for aspiring biomechanicians is to understand fully the distinction between structural and mechanical properties and you cannot go wrong.

THE BIOMECHANICAL PROPERTIES OF HEALING LIGAMENT

The following sections will describe the biomechanical properties of surgically transected rabbit MCL after 6 and 12 weeks of healing (9).

The Structural Properties of Healing Bone-Ligament-Bone Complexes

Gross Morphology

Healing of the MCL occurs at both 6 and 12 weeks postoperation. The ligament ends become well approximated and no extreme tissue proliferation is in evidence at the site of transection. At 6 weeks, the healing tissue is pink in color with some translucency, but has a normal white, glistening appearance proximal and distal to the healing site. However, the cross-sectional area of the healing substance hypertrophies significantly. An average value of 6.4 ± 0.2 mm^2 is measured compared to 3.7 ± 0.1 mm^2 for the control ligament ($p < 0.05$). At 12 weeks, healing ligaments have similar characteristics as those described above, but the healing region shows a more normal white color. Significant hypertrophy of the midsubstance cross-sectional area can again be observed compared to that of control ligaments (i.e., 6.2 ± 0.5 mm^2 versus 4.1 ± 0.1 mm^2, respectively, $p < 0.05$).

Load-Deformation Behavior

The average load-deformation or structural properties for a healing bone-ligament-bone (BLB) structure are shown in Fig. 3. One can see that after 12 weeks of healing, the structural properties of the BLB structure approach those of normal. Also, this structure is more capable of resisting a particular deformation than one that has undergone only 6 weeks of healing. What these properties imply is that the function of the joint will be compromised, particularly after only 6 weeks of healing.

The Mechanical Properties of Healing Ligament

Stress-Strain Behavior

The mechanical properties of healing collateral ligaments at 6 and 12 weeks posttransection are vastly inferior to those of a normal ligament. This is dramatically

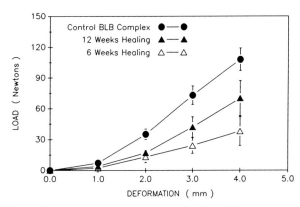

FIG. 3. The structural properties of healing BLB complexes after 6 and 12 weeks of healing compared to those of a control.

displayed in Fig. 4 which shows that stress values for normal tissue are almost an order of magnitude higher than those of healing tissues at a defined level of strain. It is further seen that only slight improvements in the mechanical properties of the healing substance are made between 6 and 12 weeks.

Why is there such an astounding return of the structural properties by 12 weeks if the mechanical properties are so inferior (and similar) at both time periods? To begin with, a poor material can withstand a higher load if there is more of it. There is an increase in the cross-sectional area of the healing ligament, but this increase is similar at both time periods. Thus, if there is going to be a difference in structural properties between 6 and 12 weeks of healing, then it will be due changes in the length of the structure being tested. One has to remember first that the structural properties reported here are for a bone-ligament-bone complex. This means that the load is experienced by the bones, the ligament *and* the insertion sites. An examination of the tibial insertion site after 6 weeks of healing demonstrates atrophy of the substance and/or the bone (Fig. 5). By 12 weeks, however, the insertion site appears improved with no apparent gaps and a parallel fiber orientation of the ligament's collagen fibers (Fig. 6). Thus, considering the similar mechanical properties for the healing ligament tissue, the

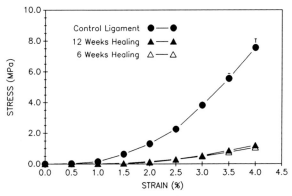

FIG. 4. The mechanical properties of healing ligament after 6 and 12 weeks of healing compared to those of a control.

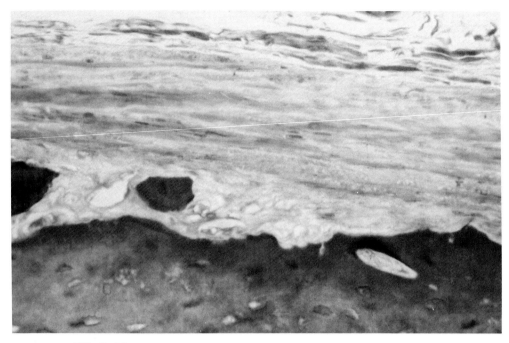

FIG. 5. Micrograph of tibial insertion after 6 weeks of ligament healing.

main reason for the difference in structural properties between BLB complexes at 6 and 12 weeks, is the fact that the insertion site can deform more easily while under load at the earlier time period.

Time-Dependent Behavior

The time-dependent behavior of ligaments is also affected by healing. By applying a cyclic deformation to the healing BLB structures, there is a distinct drop in the cyclic load by the tenth cycle. After 6 weeks of healing, the normalized load value (i.e. the load at the 10th cycle divided by that for the first cycle) is $79 \pm 4\%$ compared to $94 \pm 1\%$ for the control side. After 12 weeks, the normalized load value increases to $85 \pm 2\%$. These changes in the load value after the application of a cyclic strain history show how important the time-dependent properties of the healing structure are in determining the ligament's contribution to knee stability. For example, if a single deformation cycle is applied to a healing BLB structure at 12 weeks, the resistant load will be very similar to that

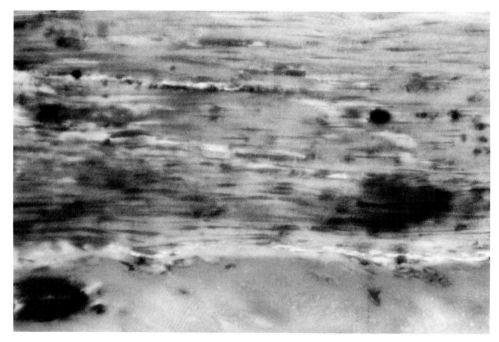

FIG. 6. Tibial insertion site after 12 weeks of ligament healing.

obtained for a normal specimen. However, if this cycle is repeated ten times, the load can drop by as much as 15% compared to 6% for a normal BLB structure and possibly indicate an unstable joint.

THE FUNCTIONAL POTENTIAL OF PARTIALLY TORN ACL

The literature has shown the distinct roles of different anatomical regions of the ACL during various joint loading conditions (1,4,14–16). Considering these intraligamentous functional differences, it may be possible for a particular band of the ACL to be disrupted under particular loading conditions. If there is a complete tear of this particular band, no or limited healing is the prognosis. However, it may be that the remaining tissue has the potential to remodel in order to help provide for more normal joint function.

Experiments have been performed in rabbits to examine how increasing the tension on medial collateral ligaments affects the biomechanical properties of the ligament (8). Tension in the MCL was increased by placing a stainless steel pin, 9.5 mm long and 1.6 mm in diameter, perpendicularly underneath and distal to the joint line. This pin was held to the tibial periosteum by 5-0 nylon sutures sewn through holes drilled in each end of the pin and maintained *in vivo* for 12 weeks. The results of these experiments are summarized below.

The Structural Properties of Ligament Subjected to Increased Tension

Gross Morphology

The surface of MCL which undergoes an increased stress regimen is similar to that of a normal ligament. However, the overall tissue appears slightly swollen. This is supported by the fact that there is hypertrophy of the ligament cross-section albeit insignificant as compared to normal ligaments (4.5 ± 0.1 versus 5.2 ± 0.9 mm^2, $p > 0.05$).

Load-Deformation Behavior

Structurally, ligaments which experience an increased tension regimen behave similarly to that of a normal ligament. Thus, they can potentially provide the same contribution to joint function.

The Mechanical Properties of Ligament Subjected to Increased Tension: Stress-Strain Behavior

Despite similarities in the structural properties of the ligament with increased tension compared to those of a normal ligament, the stress-strain properties are consider-

ably different (Fig. 7). With added tension over 12 weeks, a ligament can withstand a higher stress for a given strain. Given the fact that the cross-sectional area does not change and the structural properties are not changed for the ligament which has undergone increased stresses, it is assumed that the ligament is longer. Thus, even though the ligament as a material is improved, it can have the same load-deformation characteristics as a normal ligament and provide for more normal joint function.

Now given the situation where a partial tear of the ACL has occurred *and* the remaining tissue has substantial injury, is there the potential for adequate healing? The clinical studies referenced in the Introduction indicate the possibility, but it is not proven. Further, if healing is possible, what factors would provide for an ideal clinical result? Again, experiments using a transected rabbit MCL show that the level of stress the ligament experiences during healing may be very important with regard to producing optimum biomechanical properties. The next few sections will characterize the biomechanical properties of transected MCL subjected to increased tension after four weeks of healing (9). Tension was again applied utilizing the stainless steel pin described above. Animals were divided into 6 and 12 week groups: 4 weeks of healing plus 2 weeks tension and 4 weeks healing plus 8 weeks of tension.

The Structural Properties of Healing Ligament: The Effect of Increased Tension

Gross Morphology

In the 6-week group, the cross-sectional area for healing MCL which undergoes the stress regimen increases to an average of 6.1 ± 0.2 mm^2 compared to 3.9 ± 0.1 mm^2 for control MCL ($p < 0.05$). With an additional 6 weeks of applied tension, the cross-sectional area reduces slightly in size with a value of 5.9 ± 0.7 mm^2, but is still significantly higher than the control value.

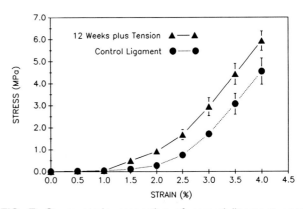

FIG. 7. Stress-strain properties of normal ligament compared to those of one that has undergone an increased tension regimen.

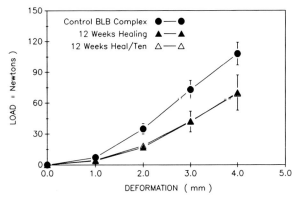

FIG. 8. Structural or load-deformation properties of BLB complexes after 12 weeks of ligament healing with and without tension compared to those of normal.

Load-Deformation Behavior

The average load-deformation or structural properties for a healing bone-ligament-bone structure with added tension from the 12-week group are shown in Fig. 8. One can see that the structural properties of the BLB structure are the *same* as those of the 12-week group without tension and also approach those of normal.

The Mechanical Properties of Healing Ligament: The Effect of Increased Tension: Stress-Strain Behavior

Positive changes are seen with the addition of tension to the healing MCL. Higher stresses for a given strain are achieved compared to ligament allowed to simply heal (Fig. 9). The fact that changes are seen in these mechanical properties with concomitant similarities to the structural properties of ligaments which do not under go an increased stress regimen, one finds support for the concept that the impetus for ligament remodeling is normal

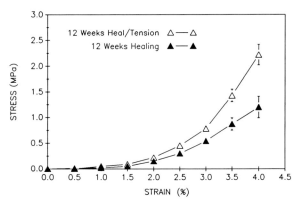

FIG. 9. Mechanical or stress-strain properties of healing ligament at 12 weeks posttransection with and without increased tension.

joint function. The load-deformation properties dictate joint function and in this case are maintained during healing regardless of the mechanical or material properties of the ligament.

FUTURE DIRECTIONS

The biomechanical properties of ACL postinjury are unknown. If the strain levels are too high (i.e., a complete tear of the ACL), then the ligament's healing potential is completely compromised. On the other hand, if injury strain levels are low (i.e., a partial tear of the ACL), then the remaining tissue may have some ability to heal. Future studies should therefore address the questions of whether or not the ACL truly does have the potential to heal and if this ability is a function of the level of strain at injury. A good starting point would be to compare data from ACL studies to that obtained for injured MCL in which healing mechanisms are more readily apparent. Comparative studies such as these could potentially dictate the correct mechanical *and* biological environment necessary for achieving ACL healing and ultimately, normal biomechanical properties.

REFERENCES

1. Arnoczky SP. (1983): Anatomy of the anterior cruciate ligament. *Clin Orthop*, 172:19–25.
2. Bonamo JJ, Fay C, Firestone T. (1990): The conservative treatment of the anterior cruciate deficient knee. *Am J Sports Med*, 18:618–623.
3. Cabaud HE. (1983): Biomechanics of the anterior cruciate ligament. *Clin Orthop*, 172:26–31.
4. Danylchuk KD, Finlay JB, Kreek JP. (1978): Microstructural organization of human and bovine cruciate ligaments. *Clin Orthop*, 131:294.
5. Fick R. (1911): Anatomie und mechanik der gelinke unter berucksichtigung der bewegenden muskelen. In: von Bardeleben K, Fischer G, eds. *Handbuch der anatomie des menschen*, band II, teil III Jena: Fisher.
6. Finsterbush A, Frankl U, Matan Y, Mann G. (1990): Secondary damage to the knee after isolated injury of the anterior cruciate ligament. *Am J Sports Med*, 18:475–479.
7. Giove TP, Miller SJ, Kent BE, Sanford TL, Garrick JG. (1983): Non-operative treatment of the torn anterior cruciate ligament. *J Bone Joint Surg [Am]*, 65A:184–192.
8. Gomez MA. (1988): *The effect of tension on normal and healing medial collateral ligaments* [Dissertation]. La Jolla, CA: University of California, San Diego.
9. Gomez MA, Woo SL-Y, Amiel D, Harwood F, Kitabayashi L, Matyas JR. (1991): The effects of increased tension on healing medial collateral ligaments. *Am J Sports Med*, 19:347–354.
10. Gomez MA, Woo SL-Y, Inoue M, Amiel D, Harwood FL, Kitabayashi L. (1989): Medial collateral ligament healing subsequent to different treatment regimens. *J Appl Physiol*, 66:245–252.
11. Hefti FL, Kress A, Fasel J, Morscher EW. (1991): Healing of the transected anterior cruciate ligament in the rabbit. *J Bone Joint Surg [Am]*, 73A:373–383.
12. Hey Groves EW. (1920): The cruciate ligaments of the knee joint: their function, rupture and the operative treatment of the same. *Br J Surg*, 7:505.

13. Kannus P, Jarvinen M. (1987): Conservatively treated tears of the anterior cruciate ligament. *J Bone Joint Surg [Am]*, 69A:1007–1012.
14. Trent PS, Walker PS, Wolf B. (1976): Ligament length patterns, strength and rotational axes of the knee joint. *Clin Orthop*, 117:263.
15. Wang C, Walker PS, Wolf B. (1973): The effect of flexion and rotation on the length patterns of the ligaments of the knee. *J Biomech*, 6:587.
16. Welsh RP. (1980): Knee joint structure and function. *Clin Orthop*, 147:7.
17. Wiig ME, Amiel D, VandeBerg J, Kitabayashi L, Harwood FL, Arfors KE. (1990): The early effect of high molecular weight hyaluron (hyaluronic acid) on anterior cruciate ligament healing: an experimental study in rabbits. *J Orthop Res*, 8:425–434.
18. Woo SL-Y, Lee TQ, Gomez MA, Sato S, Field FP. (1987): Temperature dependent behavior of the canine medial collateral ligament. *J Biomech Eng*, 109:68–71.

SECTION IV

ACL Reconstruction and Substitutes (Biologic)

The evaluation and treatment of a patient with a deficient anterior cruciate ligament draws upon and combines historical data and objective measurements to formulate a recommendation. The available literature is helpful, but it contains many articles that are contradictive and inconclusive. The questions that must be answered for the patient remain "Who needs ACL surgery" and "What are the benefits of ACL surgery?" In this section the authors review the current information that is available for making decisions on treatment selection.

Once the decision is made to reconstruct the ACL, the surgeon has considerable data available regarding the structural and mechanical properties of potential grafts. What properties exist after the incorporation of these grafts are not as precisely defined. Many different soft tissue ACL reconstructions are proposed in the orthopedic literature. It will require prospective, randomized, well-controlled, and long-term follow-up studies to give the type of information necessary to formulate better criteria for graft selection in the future.

Reconstruction of the ACL requires attention to various principles, surgical techniques, and intraoperative considerations. These include tunnel site selection and preparation, positioning of the graft, tensioning of the graft, and fixation of the graft. Presently, the grafts that substitute for an ACL are composed of parallel collagen fibers and serve as a check rein against abnormal anterior tibial displacement but do not reestablish normal joint kinematics. Duplicating the complex properties of the ACL in the future will probably require individual bundles to be reconstructed and selectively tensioned. Of the surgical options available, the most simplistic approach to a ruptured ACL is an acute repair. Reestablishing the continuity of the fibers by utilizing the residual ruptured ACL collagen and fibroblasts seems ideal. Experimental and clinical research has failed to document reproducible success with ACL repair alone. The technique of augmenting the primary repair continues to be evaluated and explored. Most surgeons are reconstructing, rather than repairing, the ACL. Two autografts have emerged as the most commonly used ACL replacements. These are bone-patellar tendon-bone and semitendinosus tendon. While bone-patellar tendon-bone autograft is considered by many to be the gold standard, other clinicians are obtaining favorable results with the semitendinosus tendon. The placement of these two grafts is quite similar and can be performed using arthroscopically-assisted techniques.

Over the past decade, there has been increased interest in allografts as an alternative graft source for ACL reconstruction. Clinical and laboratory investigations have contributed considerable insight into allograft sterility, immunogenicity, intraarticular considerations, and remodeling. Prosthetic ligament replacement of the ACL to date has had an increasing failure rate with time. The preliminary experience with a prosthetic ACL allows special consideration for future designs, coatings, new materials, altered surgical techniques, and indications. The desirability for a synthetic or biological graft to replace the ACL, other than an autograft, remains high and will stimulate research in this area.

The experience to date demonstrates that reconstruction of the anterior cruciate ligament is not without potential complications. Three specific considerations around the theme of loss of motion include notch fibrosis and impingement, capsular fibrosis, and patellar entrapment. Every surgeon performing this type of surgery should be familiar with prevention and early recognition of these particular complications to minimize potential disability.

The success of the surgical ACL reconstruction is further dependent on the postoperative course. Rehabilitation has the potential to affect the graft's incorporation and ultimate function. Relative immobility, protected healing, muscular atrophy, limitations in motion, various graft loads, bracing, and weight bearing are all considerations that are incorporated into the rehabilitation environment after an ACL reconstruction. Successfully treating an ACL-deficient knee requires individualized patient selection, precise surgical technical considerations, avoidance of complications, and appropriate rehabilitation.

Douglas W. Jackson

The Anterior Cruciate Ligament: Current and Future Concepts, edited by D.W. Jackson, et al. Raven Press, Ltd., New York © 1993.

CHAPTER 21

The Use of Knee Laxity Testers for the Determination of Anterior-Posterior Stability of the Knee

Pitfalls in Practice

Braden C. Fleming, Bruce D. Beynnon, and Robert J. Johnson

The integrity of the ACL has been traditionally diagnosed through the clinical examination. The examination requires the application of forces or moments to the knee joint, an evaluation of the resulting displacement (translation and/or rotation), and the determination of an endpoint (8,25,31–33,44,54,62,66). The tests commonly used to evaluate ACL function in the midsagittal plane are the anterior drawer test (ADT) and Lachman test (66). During the Lachman test, posterior and anterior shear forces are applied to the proximal tibia and the resulting translation of the tibia with respect to the femur is graded with the knee at 15° to 30° flexion. The ADT is performed in a similar fashion with the knee flexed to 90°. The accuracy, sensitivity/specificity, and reproducibility of these examination techniques remain controversial.

It is not possible to determine the accuracy of the clinical ADT and Lachman test since there is no quantitative measurement of the loads applied or the resulting displacements that occur. These tests are qualitative by nature.

The usefulness of the clinical exam is determined by its sensitivity and specificity. Sensitivity is the percentage of patients with an ACL deficiency who demonstrate a positive test result. Specificity is a measure of a test's ability to correctly identify patients who do not have an ACL deficiency. For the isolated acute ACL injury without anesthesia, sensitivities reported for the ADT range from 10% to 93% when performed by experienced examiners (1,14,15,19,37,40). All of these studies except for that of Fetto and Marshall (19) report ADT sensitivities less than 54%, an extremely high rate of false negatives. Torg et al. (66) popularized the Lachman test as a "reliable and reproducible" method for assessing the isolated ACL injury reporting a sensitivity of 95%. Others have reported sensitivities ranging from 75% to 100% (1,9,15,37,40,64). The specificity of the ADT and Lachman test is greater than or equal to 95% (40,64).

Inter- and intraexaminer variations due to differences in clinical testing technique and data interpretation have been reported (9,21,49,58,64). Daniel (9) reported the comprehensive clinical study performed by the "International Knee Documentation Committee" using ten experienced clinical examiners and concluded that "clinical motion tests are clinician specific." Clinical examinations have also been shown to be dependent on examiner experience (49,58). These findings indicate that clinical laxity examination techniques are subjective, emphasizing the need for *objective* diagnostic instrumentation.

The goal of instrumented knee laxity systems is to objectively quantify the clinical term "knee joint stability." Although the clinical Lachman test is capable of detecting an ACL deficiency, an objective measurement of midsagittal plane laxity would be extremely useful. In addition, it would be particularly helpful in patients who

B. C. Fleming, B. D. Beynnon, and R. J. Johnson: McClure Musculoskeletal Research Center, Department of Orthopaedics, University of Vermont Medical School, Burlington, Vermont 05405.

have undergone ACL reconstruction surgery since reconstructed grafts do not necessarily provide a similar endpoint as the normal ACL. In theory, instrumented laxity testers could be an asset in determining the extent of an ACL tear, and would compliment the diagnosis if they proved to have a greater sensitivity and specificity than the Lachman test. The ideal laxity tester should also be accurate, reproducible, versatile, comfortable, easy to use, and inexpensive.

If accurate and reproducible, instrumented laxity testers would enhance clinical research. Long term follow-up studies of ACL reconstruction necessitate an objective measurement system that is safe, accurate, reproducible, and user independent to prevent data biasing. These devices could also prove beneficial in determining the success of brace and prosthesis design.

There is no consensus in the literature regarding the usefulness of instrumented knee laxity testing. The experimental methods and statistical analyses differ. Therefore, comparisons between studies are difficult. This chapter will to review the instrumented laxity testers that are currently used to measure A-P laxity of the knee and will review the accuracy, sensitivity/specificity, and reproducibility of these systems.

KNEE LAXITY INSTRUMENTATION

There are a variety of techniques used to "objectively" measure A-P translation during Lachman and drawer testing. Anterior-posterior laxity has been measured using radiographic templates (16,23,29,34,39,41,43,50,57,67). However, these techniques require multiple x-ray exposures, are expensive, time consuming and cumbersome. The reproducibility of x-ray techniques have not been verified *in vivo* since additional x-ray exposures would be required (68). The usefulness of uniplanar x-ray techniques at documenting ACL ruptures remains questionable (34,35,41,63–65).

Several investigators have developed instrumented systems, utilizing displacement, rotation, and/or load transducers, to quantify tibiofemoral motion in the midsagittal plane (10,16,17,36,46,61). The challenge to knee instrumentation systems is to externally measure bone to bone motion through the soft tissue surrounding the tibia and the femur. Although the tibia has distinct bony prominences on which a device may be mounted, the soft tissue envelope surrounding the femur does not provide rigid points for attachment.

In 1978, Markolf et al. (46) presented the "UCLA device" which consists of a dental chair with a tapered metal thigh clamp and patellar block to stabilize the femur. A spring loaded linear potentiometer which was mounted to the thigh fixation system measured A-P displacement at the tibial tubercle relative to the fixation unit while an instrumented load applicator measured the

A-P forces applied to the tibia immediately below the tibial tubercle during the ADT and Lachman test. A portable version of this device has since been developed (48).

In 1984, Johnson et al. (36) utilized a cable system to measure A-P laxity during the ADT and Lachman test. This was a one degree of freedom system designed to measure A-P displacement. The two cables were attached to the proximal tibia and to the medial femoral condyle by Velcro straps. The cables wrapped around pulleys connected to angular potentiometers calibrated to measure tibial and femoral displacement. The relative tibiofemoral displacement was calculated by subtracting the absolute femoral displacement from the absolute tibial displacement. Using this device, the clinician performs the ADT and Lachman test in the normal "hands on" clinical fashion. The system was designed to measure tibiofemoral displacement up to the end point perceived by the examiner as the ACL becomes taut.

The most popular of the instrumented laxity testing devices was introduced by Daniel et al. (10) in 1985. The device is a one degree of freedom system capable of measuring A-P translation with the knee flexed to 25 ($\pm$5)°. The device is now commercially available as the KT-1000 Knee Ligament Arthrometer (Table 1). This portable tester is strapped to the anterior tibia. A paddle which rests against the anterior aspect of the patella is used to measure patellar displacement relative to the tibia. The accuracy of the KT-1000 is based on the assumption that the patella remains fixed to the distal aspect of the femur. Thigh and foot supports maintain anatomical alignment throughout the test protocol. A dial gauge is used to mechanically measure displacement between the body of the KT-1000 and the patellar paddle. This displacement is interpreted as the relative tibiofemoral displacement. The instrumented handle of the KT-1000 measures the forces applied to the proximal tibia. When the load limits of $\pm$67 and $\pm$89 N have been reached, the device emits an audible "beep." At each load interval the examiner reads the resulting displacement off the dial gauge. There is a variation of the KT-1000 which records the

TABLE 1. *Commercially available laxity testing devices*

Device	Manufacturer	DOF
CA-4000*	Orthopaedic Systems, Inc. Hayward, CA	4
Genucom	Faro Medical Technologies, Inc. Montreal, QUE	6
KT-1000	Medmetric Corp.	1
KT-2000	San Diego, CA	
Stryker	Stryker Corp. Kalamazoo, MI	1

* The CA-4000 and the Knee Signature System (KSS) are equivalent systems. The KSS was originally distributed by Acufex Microsurgical, Inc., Norwood, MA. The KSS is now distributed by OSI (Hayward, CA), the company that originally developed and manufactured the device.

load-displacement curve directly to an X-Y plotter. This device is called the KT-2000. Both devices are based on the same mechanical principles.

The apparatus developed by Shino et al. (61) in 1987 consisted of a chair with a calf support and a thigh clamp. The calf support comprised a hinged foot holder which permitted tibial rotation. The proximal tibia was supported by clamps which allowed displacement to occur in the A-P plane. Anterior-posterior loads were applied to the proximal tibia through this clamp. The distal thigh was secured to a chair by four adjustable metal shells. Two linear "plunger type" transducers measured patellar and tibial displacement. Tibiofemoral displacement was calculated by the difference between the two transducers. Forces of ±250 N were applied mechanically through the tibial clamp.

The device developed by Edixhoven et al. (16,17) in 1987 fixed the thigh and tibia in a fashion similar to the UCLA device and the Shino apparatus, however, the foot was not free to rotate. The differential method of determining tibiofemoral displacement was employed by positioning displacement transducers at the tibial tuberosity and anterior aspect of the patella. Loads through ±180 N were manually applied with a spindle and measured with a load cell at the level of the tibial tuberosity.

COMMERCIAL LAXITY INSTRUMENTATION

Besides the KT-1000 described above, there are several other commercial knee laxity systems available at the time of preparation of this chapter (Table 1). The Stryker ligament tester is the simplest of these devices. The device straps to the lower limb. A spring-loaded displacement gauge measures A-P displacement relative to the patella. A hand-held load applicator has a calibrated spring gage to measure A-P force.

The CA-4000 is manufactured and marketed by Orthopaedic Systems, Inc. This same device was originally marketed as the Knee Signature System (KSS) by Acufex Microsurgical, Inc. The CA-4000 is an electrogoniometer linkage that measures joint motion in four degrees of freedom; A-P translation of the tibia (with respect to the patella), flexion-extension, axial rotation, and varus-valgus angulation. A device that measures motion in multiple degrees of freedom theoretically enables the examiner to monitor and control motions that will influence the A-P laxity measurement (i.e., flexion-extension, axial rotation) providing a more reproducible test. The electrogoniometer attaches to the thigh and lower limb using elastic straps. Anterior-posterior loads are applied to the proximal tibia at the level of the tibial tuberosity with a hand-held load cell.

The Genucom is a complex computerized device consisting of a six degree of freedom electrogoniometer, and

a dynamometer capable of measuring the external forces and moments applied to the knee during laxity testing. Unlike the other devices which measure motion of the tibia relative to the patella, the Genucom attempts to measure tibiofemoral motion directly. The patient is strapped on a test seat and a restraining clamp is situated around the distal thigh. In a digitization procedure, the Genucom establishes a coordinate system within the knee joint on which applied loads and tibiofemoral motion are referenced. A soft tissue compensation protocol determines the amount of motion artifact that is due to the soft tissue compressed between the thigh clamp and the femur. A variety of tests may then be performed to determine the ligamentous integrity of the knee joint, including the Lachman test, ADT, A-P translation of the medial and lateral tibiofemoral compartments, and variations of the pivot shift test.

DATA INTERPRETATION

The terms anterior laxity, A-P laxity, and anterior stiffness are not precisely defined (55). As generalized terms, anterior and A-P laxity are the amount of tibiofemoral displacement occurring in the midsagittal plane between defined load limits. Anterior stiffness is defined as the tangent slope of the anterior load deflection curve at a specified load (Fig. 1). The confusion within these definitions are the load limits employed. Originally, Markolf et al. (46) defined A-P laxity as the displacement occurring between ±100 N. In a subsequent study, they changed their laxity limits to ±200 N to increase test

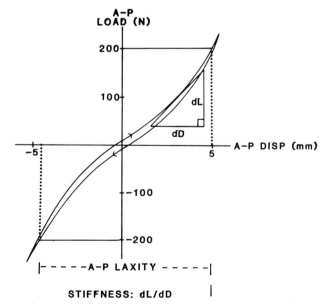

FIG. 1. Typical A-P load displacement curve of the normal knee. Laxity is defined as the displacement occurring between predefined load limits. Stiffness is the tangent slope of the curve at a predefined load level. (From ref. 47, with permission.)

sensitivity (47). Johnson et al. (36) defined "primary laxity" as the amount of displacement that occurred between perceived end points. They did not objectively measure the applied shear loads. Daniel et al. (10) measured anterior laxity between 0 and +89 N. To quantify the clinical end point, they also measured the relative change in displacement occurring between 67 and 89 N of anterior shear force. This measurement was coined the "anterior compliance index." Anterior-posterior laxity has also been defined between −89 and 133 N (13), ±180 N (16,17), and ±200 N (61). Furthermore, Markolf et al. (46,47) and Shino et al. (61) calculated anterior stiffness at 100 N and 50 N of anterior shear force, respectively.

Many investigators have reported laxity measurements of normal "control" subjects and ACL-deficient patients using knee laxity instrumentation (1–3,5, 7,10,11,13,17,18,21,22,27,28,42,46,51,53,56,59–61, 64,68–71). Table 2 summarizes those studies which report the midsagittal plane laxity of a sample normal population. It is obvious from Table 2 that the different devices do not produce equivalent laxity measurements. Furthermore, some of the studies utilizing the same test device are contradictory. Using the KT-1000, Daniel et al. (11) report normal laxity values (3 to 13.5 mm) similar to the laxity values reported by Gurtler et al. (26) (2 to 19 mm) for patients documented as ACL deficient. These findings have led to several recommendations that should help "standardize" results: (a) to routinely perform laxity testing using the same instrumented device, (b) to use each patient as their own control by performing bilateral examinations and making right-left comparisons, (c) to evaluate knee laxity at higher load limits, (d) to perform A-P laxity measurements, and (e) to standardize knee flexion angles and the load limits at which displacements are measured.

Recording systems are not standardized (1,9,18,21, 28,53,59,60,64). Therefore, the numerical results of one device may not be generalized with the results of another device. The data presented in Table 2 support this finding.

There is a wide distribution of anterior laxity, A-P laxity, and anterior stiffness values in both the normal population and ACL-deficient population (5,10,46,47,61). For example, Daniel et al. (11) found that the anterior laxity (+89 N) ranged from 3 to 13.5 mm with a mean of

TABLE 2. *Laxiety values for normal control subjects. Summary of* in vivo *Lachman test studies*

Study	Device used	Flex angle	Load limit	Anterior laxity	A-P laxity
Andersson (2)	Stryker	20°	±90 N	3.0 mm	7.0 mm
			±180 N	5.0 mm	10.0 mm
Boniface (5)	Stryker	20°	+89 N	2.7 mm	—
Daniel (10)	KT-1000	20°	±89 N	5.7 mm	8.4 mm
Daniel (11)	KT-1000	30°	Max	8.5 mm	—
Edixhovan (17)	custom	25°	±90 N	2.6 mm	4.9 mm
			±180 N	3.4 mm	6.4 mm
Emery (18)	Genucom	30°	±90 N	—	12.2 mm
Fleming (21)	Genucom	30°	±90 N	—	10.6 mm
	KSS	30°	±90 N	—	7.6 mm
Forster (22)	KT-1000	25°	+89 N	4.4 mm	—
Highgenboten (28)	Genucom	20°	±93 N	7.8 mm	9.0 mm
	KT-1000	20°	±89 N	4.7 mm	6.6 mm
	Stryker	20°	±89 N	2.4 mm	5.6 mm
Markolf (46)	UCLA	20°	±100 N	2.6 mm	5.5 mm
Markolf (47)	UCLA	20°	±200 N	—	10.0 mm
McQuade (51)	Genucom	20°	±93 N	1.6 mm	5.5 mm
		30°	±93 N	4.3 mm	9.0 mm
Riederman (59)	KSS	30°	±89 N	5.2 mm	7.5 mm
			±178 N	7.5 mm	10.7 mm
Sherman (60)	KT-1000	20°	+89 N	5.5 mm	—
	UCLA	20°	+89 N	3.4 mm	—
Shino (61)	custom	20°	±200 N	6.6 mm	12.4 mm
Steiner (64)	Genucom	20°	±89 N	3.8 mm	5.5 mm
	KSS	20°	±89 N	4.7 mm	7.9 mm
	KT-1000	25°	±89 N	3.9 mm	6.9 mm
	Stryker	20°	±89 N	2.9 mm	6.4 mm
Torzilli (68)	Genucom	30°	±93 N	5.5 mm	7.6 mm
	KT-1000	30°	±69 N	5.1 mm	7.1 mm
White (69)	custom	30°	?	2.4 mm	—
Wroble (70)	Genucom	30°	±90 N	—	9.2 mm
Wroble (71)	KT-1000	25°	±89 N	—	7.1 mm

7.2 (±1.9) mm using the KT-1000 on 240 subjects with no history of knee injuries. In 65 acute ACL disruptions, they determined that anterior laxity ranged from 6 to 19 mm with a mean of 11.4 (±2.9 mm). The laxity of both populations fit a normal distribution, with considerable overlap between the two groups. In an effort to remove the variation between normal subjects, authors have proposed the use of bilateral laxity comparisons (10,11,46–48). One must assume that the uninjured knee is representative of normal laxity for that particular patient. Several studies conclude that the assumption is valid, that each patient serves as their own control (11,59,61,71). In the above example, Daniel et al. (11) found that 88% of the normal population had right-left anterior laxity differences of less than 2 mm. In the acute ACL-deficient patients, only 9% had right-left differences less than 2 mm.

To the contrary, Markolf et al. (46,47) reported a high scatter in the right-left A-P laxity differences in the normal and ACL-deficient populations using the UCLA device (Fig. 2). Individual right-left differences varied 26 to 35% for A-P laxity and 19 to 24% for anterior stiffness in the normal population. Shino et al. (61) reported no significant differences in the normal population for anterior laxity, A-P laxity or anterior stiffness. However, an analysis of the normal female population alone indicated a significant right-left difference in total A-P laxity. Edixhoven et al. (17) determined that 95% of the normal population had right-left A-P laxity within 2.1 mm using their custom testing device.

By evaluating A-P laxity at higher load limits, the overlap between the normal and ACL-deficient population distribution curves is reduced since the mean laxity of the ACL-deficient population is increased relative to the increase demonstrated in the normal knee. In turn, the sensitivity of the instrumented Lachman test is increased (2,11,17,47,61). Markolf and associates (47) compared the stiffness and laxity values in patients with a documented ACL deficiency and found that differences in A-P laxity between normal and chronic ACL-deficient knees were best detected at ±200 N when compared to ±100 N. The A-P laxity for normal knees averaged 9.6 and 7.4 mm at ±200 N for the Lachman and ADT, respectively. The chronic ACL-deficient knees were found to demonstrate a significant increase with mean A-P laxity values of 15.1 and 9.8 mm, respectively. In response, Daniel et al. (11) introduced the manual maximum test while performing a study designed to measure anterior laxity in the acute ACL-deficient patient. The acute ACL-deficient knee demonstrates less laxity in comparison to the knee of the chronic patient (3,7,11,23). The manual maximum test requires the examiner to apply a maximum anterior load after the +89 N load level has been reached to accentuate the anterior displacement difference of the tibia between the normal and ACL-deficient knee. A manual maximum anterior displacement difference (uninjured-injured) of 3 mm or more is indicative of an ACL disruption. The manual maximum test increased the diagnostic accuracy of the KT-1000 from 62% to 92% (11). The commercial version of the KT-1000 has since been upgraded to include a "beep" signifying a 133 N anterior shear load to help standardize the manual maximum load level.

Many investigators have concluded that a measure of total A-P displacement is more reproducible and less variable than anterior displacement alone (2,9,16,52, 59). Shino et al. (61) are the only investigators to recommend anterior laxity over total A-P displacement. The sigmoid shape of the joint load-deflection curve and the posterior directed preload on the tibia due to gravity make the precise definition of the neutral resting position of the tibiofemoral joint difficult to isolate. The typical load-deflection curve of the normal knee has a region where the slope is approximately zero over a range of displacement values at the transition between the posterior push and the anterior pull of the applied shear loads. Therefore, the true zero load-displacement point is difficult to accurately select. By utilizing a specified posterior shear load as the displacement reference, the nondistinct zero load-displacement point becomes irrelevant. When performing total A-P laxity measurements, the examiner

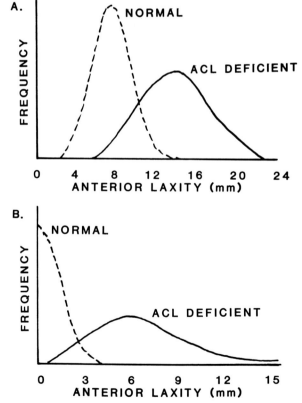

FIG. 2. Frequency distribution for anterior laxity at 89 N for normal and chronic ACL-deficient knees. **A:** Actual displacement. **B:** Side-to-side difference. (From ref. 11, with permission.)

must be aware that a PCL injury will also increase A-P laxity. To diagnose a PCL disruption, Daniel et al. (12) introduced the quadriceps active test on the KT-1000. In 41 out of 42 knees with a documented PCL injury an active quadriceps contraction caused an anterior translation of the tibia relative to the femur with the knee flexed at 90°. There was no anterior translation in the uninjured contralateral knee of the same patient population.

A direct comparison of laxity data across the studies in Table 2 is difficult because the load limits and flexion angles used to measure laxity are not standardized. The load limits vary between 67 and 200 N. As discussed above, laxity differences between the ACL-deficient and normal knees are greatest at higher loads. However, the test becomes difficult to perform and may cause pain to the patient if the loads are too great. When performing laxity tests on a newly reconstructed knee joint, high shear loads may also stretch out the graft or cause fixation slippage during initial graft healing. To the contrary, the anterior stiffness is best calculated at lower load limits before the secondary stabilizers become engaged (11,17,47,61). To make comparisons across studies it is important to standardize load limits and include a reading at a low and high load level. The majority of studies have made anterior displacement measurements at 89 N. This load level is good for stiffness determination. With the addition of a higher load level the sensitivity of the instrumented Lachman test is improved (11,16, 47,61).

The reported flexion angles for the instrumented Lachman test range from 15° to 30°. In the cadaveric model, Fukubayashi et al. (24) evaluated A-P laxity at flexion angles throughout the range of motion. The greatest A-P displacement occurred at 30° flexion. With the Genucom, McQuade (51) found the A-P laxity at 20° to be 61% less than the A-P laxity at 30° (Table 2). Andersson and Gillquist (2) found the anterior laxity at 25° to be significantly greater than the laxity at 15° using the Stryker system. Therefore, standardization of flexion angle is essential.

Axial rotation also influences A-P translation of the knee. Fukubayashi et al. (24) found axial rotation an important consideration in analyzing A-P displacement. Permitting free rotation of the tibia increased A-P laxity up to 30%. Bargar et al. (4) documented the effect of axial rotation on the drawer sign using the UCLA device. They concluded that maximum A-P displacement occurred when the foot was rotated externally by 15°.

ACCURACY

Accuracy is the ability of a device to conform to a known standard. All of the components of an instrumentation system are individually calibrated by the manufacturer and may be assumed to be relatively accurate.

However, it is important to determine the accuracy of the whole system as it measures A-P motion of the knee. Since the objective of knee instrumentation systems is to evaluate internal ligament integrity through an external measure of tibiofemoral displacement, a direct bone to bone displacement measurement is required. There are currently two methods which may be used. First, cadaveric studies which permit direct bone to bone measurement may be utilized. Second, *in vivo* measurement using stereoradiography may be employed. A prerequisite for either method is that the resolution and accuracy of the direct bone to bone measurement system is greater than the resolution and accuracy required by the laxity system with which it is to be compared.

Several cadaveric studies have been performed. Daniel et al. (10) determined the correlation coefficient between skeletal pin motion and the KT-1000 as 0.97 with a standard error of 0.4 mm. Edixhoven et al. (16) used stereoradiography to measure the A-P laxity of cadaveric specimens with tantalum beads embedded in the tibia and femur. Measurements were simultaneously performed on their custom laxity tester. The laxity tester gave errors of approximately 10% at ±180 N. Fleming et al. (21) compared the A-P laxity of cadaveric specimens on the Genucom and KSS systems. The specimens were then mounted on a Materials Test System (MTS) and the "true" tibiofemoral motion was then compared. There was no significant difference between the Genucom and the MTS during the Lachman test, while the KSS system measured significantly less displacement. Shino et al. (61) compared the A-P laxity in cadaveric specimens with *in vivo* data measured with their testing apparatus. They found that the A-P laxity of the cadavers was significantly greater than A-P laxity of patients. The authors attribute these differences to the compliant soft tissue interference. A drawback to these cadaveric models is that femoral motion is altered or eliminated by the fixation of the specimen to the testing platform of the laxity tester. Actual *in vivo* measurements are necessary.

Staubli and Jakob (63) made simultaneous *in vivo* radiographic and KT-1000 laxity measurements. They found no correlation between the two methods on the intact knees, however, both methods correctly identified 13 of the 16 ACL-deficient patients as ACL deficient. Since the x-ray technique did not involve a stereo measurement technique utilizing precise landmarks, one must question the accuracy and reproducibility of the radiographic method employed (34,35,41,65,68). Jonsson et al. (38) used an *in vivo* stereo radiographic technique to determine the accuracy of anterior laxity measurements of the KT-1000 on normal and ACL-deficient patients. Tantalum beads were inserted in the tibia and femur to provide landmarks for motion measurement. Their results suggest that both devices demonstrate a similar measure of anterior laxity in normal knees (KT-1000 at 5.8 mm, x-ray method at 4.9 mm). However, the KT-1000 underestimated the difference between normal and ACL-deficient knees by 2.5 mm. The authors concluded that one must question the value of the KT-1000 in the assessment of reconstructive surgery. Unfortunately, the authors made the comparison between these two measurement techniques at different load limits. Therefore, a fair assessment of the accuracy of knee laxity instrumentation systems remains to be performed.

SENSITIVITY/SPECIFICITY

The studies which directly compare instrumented laxity measurements with a direct measure of bone to bone displacement using cadavers or x-ray techniques indicate that knee laxity instrumentation systems are less accurate then desired. The relative value of these devices may be in determining the status of the ACL with greater precision than the clinical exam. An effective way of determining the clinical usefulness of instrumented laxity testers is to examine the ratio of true positive tests (sensitivity) to the total number of true positive and false negative tests expressed as a percentage. The ratio of true negative tests (specificity) to the combined total of true negative plus false positive tests expressed as a percentage would require arthroscopically examining a normal population to verify whether or not the knee is indeed "normal." Studies that report specificity values should include reliable certification of a normal ACL.

There have been several studies which have determined the sensitivities and/or specificities of the instrumented laxity testers. The sensitivity and specificity of the clinical Lachman test to detect a ruptured anterior cruciate ligament falls between 75 and 100% (Table 3). Three of these six studies report sensitivities of 98% or greater (1,7,15). It should be noted that these measurements were performed on normal and ACL-deficient patients. The clinical result of patients with a reconstructed

TABLE 3. *Sensitivities of knee laxity instrumentation systems. Summary of literature**

Device	Sensitivity	Specificity	References
Clinical lachman	75%–100%	95%	1, 7, 11, 37, 40, 64
Clinical ADT	10%–93%	95%	1, 14, 15, 19, 37, 40
Genucom	45%–70%	65%	1, 64
KSS	85%–95%	81%–95%	52, 64
KT-1000	75%–95%	70%–85%	1, 11, 60, 63, 64
Stryker	75%–92%	70%–85%	1, 2, 6, 64
UCLA	90%–95%	—	60

* Sensitivity and specificity values vary depending on load limits and flexion angles tested. Value chosen to represent a particular study is the highest one reported for any combination of test parameters on the non-anesthetized patient.

ACL may be more difficult to interpret. The reported sensitivities and specificities of instrumented knee laxity testers range from 45% to 95% with the majority of studies falling in the 80% and 90% range (Table 3).

The sensitivity and specificity of a test is dependent on the threshold value chosen to separate a patient into the injured or noninjured group. By increasing the threshold value, the specificity of the test is increased, however, the sensitivity is decreased. By increasing the threshold it is more difficult to prove an ACL-deficient patient to be ACL deficient. In contrast, a decrease in the threshold limit for a particular laxity tester will increase the test's sensitivity and decrease the specificity. Steiner et al. (64) reported the sensitivities and specificities of different instrumented laxity testers and clinical examination techniques on a group of normal and ACL-deficient subjects. They also reported the diagnostic correctness of the sample population. Diagnostic correctness is the percent of all subjects, both normal and ACL deficient, that are correctly identified by the particular test method. The diagnostic correctness for the clinical Lachman test was 85%, whereas the diagnostic correctness of the KSS was 90%, the Stryker was 85%, the KT-1000 was 80% and the Genucom was 60%.

REPRODUCIBILITY

A measurement of reproducibility is an important index in evaluating the usefulness of instrumented laxity testers. An instrumented laxity tester must meet two criteria. First, the device must be reproducible for one examiner over time (test/retest). Second, the device must be reproducible across examiners (Examiner 1/Examiner 2). If the inter- or intraexaminer variability is greater than the threshold limit used to separate normal from ACL-deficient patients, then the device is not a useful clinical tool. Even higher precision is needed if these devices are to be used to diagnose the extent of a partial tear. For plotting the success of an ACL reconstruction, both the inter- and intraexaminer variability must be minimal to detect any laxity changes that may occur over time.

The reproducibility of the different instrumented laxity systems currently in use have been performed by many investigators (2,16,18,21,22,27,28,42,45,51,59, 61,64,68,70,71). Using a variety of statistical methods, interexaminer variability and intraobserver variables such as trial-trial, installation-installation, and day-day effects have been analyzed. Reproducibility has been statistically addressed using correlation coefficients, analysis of variance, coefficients of variation, and 95% confidence limits. Correlation coefficients are not a precise method for evaluating reproducibility. A correlation is a qualitative measure indicating that two methods demonstrate a similar increase in laxity. More quantitative measures result from analysis of variance which may be designed to isolate the sources of variability. The coefficients of variation, which is the standard deviation divided by the mean, is a useful indicator of the degree of variability. However, this value is dependent on the size of the mean and is not useful in determining differences between normal and ACL patient populations. Ninety-five percent confidence limits provide a range of values about the mean in which 95% of the laxity values of a sample population will fall. If the 95% confidence limits are greater than the threshold set to determine an ACL deficiency, the device should not be considered a useful clinical tool.

Daniel and Stone (13) report the intraexaminer (test/retest) variation of the KT-1000 to be less than 2.5 mm in 87% of normal knees tested. The intraexaminer correlation coefficients for the KT-1000 are approximately 0.85 (27,28). Torzilli et al. (68) report coefficients of variation ranging from 8 to 33% across normal subjects. Ninety percent and 95% confidence limits are reported at 1.6 and 2.4 mm, respectively (64,71). Furthermore, Wroble et al. (71) determined significant day to day variations using the KT-1000. Using the Stryker device, Andersson and Gillquist (2) determined the intraexaminer correlation coefficients for A-P laxity to be 0.8 and 0.9 for ACL-deficient and normal knees, respectively, while King and Kumar (42) determined that 22% of normal subjects had R-L differences greater than 2 mm for one or more of the trials. For the Genucom, several authors report correlation coefficients ranging from .84 to .96 (18,27,28), coefficients of variation ranging from 13 to 87% (18,53,68), and 95% confidence limits ranging 1.6 to 5.4 mm (21,51,64,70). For the KSS, 95% confidence limits ranging from 2.6 to 3.6 mm have been reported (21,59,64). Riederman et al. (59) report that smaller 90% confidence limits are present at lower shear loads and recommends that forces of ±89 N over ±180 N for A-P laxity testing. In contrast, the device developed by Edixhoven et al. (16) was most reproducible in measuring total A-P translation between ±180 N reporting coefficients of variation ranging from 2 to 8% across the normal population. Edixhoven found trial to trial variations to be negligible, however, day to day variations were substantial. Ideally, several installation to installation trials should be performed to evaluate an instrument laxity tester.

The interexaminer (Ex1/Ex2) A-P laxity variability of instrumented testers have also been reported. Malcom et al. (45) compared the variability between two examiners using the KT-1000 and determined that both examiners agreed with one another 93% of time using 2 mm as the threshold limit. However, Forster et al. (22) found that 28% of a population of normal control subjects displayed a side to side anterior laxity difference between 2 and 4 mm using five different KT-1000 examiners. Hanten et al. (27) reported the KT-1000 interexaminer reli-

ability coefficient as .85. Using the Stryker device, Andersson and Gillquist (2) report the correlation coefficient between two examiners to be 0.9 and 0.6 for the injured and contralateral normal limb, respectively, while King and Kumar (42) determined that 20% of the normal knees tested by two independent examiners demonstrated greater than 2 mm variation. Fleming et al. report interexaminer correlation coefficients of .88 for the KSS and .67 for the Genucom (21). Several authors (18,21,71) have reported significant interexaminer differences between the mean A-P laxity of normal knees as measured by the Genucom. Edixhoven et al. (16) determined the interexaminer variability of their laxity testing device to be significant but not as great as the day to day intraexaminer variability.

The reproducibility of the instrumented laxity testing devices is ambiguous. There are several factors that influence the reliability of these devices: the device, examiner experience, the diagnostic threshold limit and the patient population tested. One may eliminate the interexaminer variability problem by evaluating knee laxity using one examiner. This is practical in the clinic on a daily basis, however, following patient success over time requires the same examiner to be present throughout the study. Examiner experience has been shown to influence reproducibility results. All of the investigators reporting reproducibility studies claim to use highly trained examiners. In the study of Steiner et al. (64), the manufacturers of the devices designated the examiner to perform the laxity tests. The findings of Steiner et al., raises questions related to the reproducibility of instrumented laxity testers.

CLINICAL VERSUS LAXITY INSTRUMENTATION TESTERS

There are several studies which have directly compared instrumented laxity testing to the clinical exam. Anderson and Lipscomb (1) compared the clinical exam versus the Genucom, KT-1000 and Stryker laxity testers and found significant correlations with all three devices. The sensitivity of the clinical exam was greater than any of the three instrumented devices tested. In another study, Fleming et al. (21) found significant correlations between the KSS, Genucom, and clinical Lachman test. The clinical Lachman test proved to be more reliable. Gurtler et al. (26) found a significant correlation between the clinical exam and KT-1000 measurements and that the clinical laxity grades were represented by specific ranges of A-P displacement values as measured by the KT-1000. However, Howe et al. (30) were not able to correlate a specific grade of clinical laxity with actual A-P displacement measurements using the Genucom. The most complete comparison between instrumented laxity testers and the clinical exam was performed by Steiner et al. (65). They found significant correlations between the clinical exam and the KSS, KT-1000, and Stryker instrumented testers. They reported no significant correlation between the clinical exam and the Genucom. This is contrary to Oliver and Coughlin (56). Steiner et al. (64) reported the reproducibility of the clinical exam to be equivalent to that of the instrumented devices.

SPECIFIC PROBLEMS: THE PITFALLS OF INSTRUMENTATION SYSTEMS

In reviewing the literature, it is obvious that there are several problems inherent to laxity measurement techniques. These errors are dependent on the device-examiner unit.

Device-dependant factors include the method of soft tissue fixation and the reference position of the load and displacement measurement. Device fixation to the soft tissue structures surrounding the lower limb, particularly around the femur, poses quite a challenge. In a study evaluating device fixation, Edixhoven et al. (16) concluded that complete fixation of an instrumented device is impossible. Within the soft tissue envelope, the femur moved and the flexion angle of the knee changed with applied load. In another study, Fleming et al. (21) observed that an increase in the soft tissue bulk about the femur results in a decrease in reproducibility. One possible solution to improve fixation is to increase the pressure about the thigh, however, patient discomfort and therefore, patient apprehension is increased. The instrumented laxity testers utilize different methods of fixation. Some of the devices are mounted to the soft tissues surrounding the femur and tibia, while others bypass the femoral soft tissues by attaching directly to the anterior portion of the tibia measuring displacement of the tibia relative to the patella. This placement is chosen because the soft tissue bulk is minimal over the patella.

The displacement reference is another possible factor accounting for device dependent error. Some of the devices measure displacement of the tibia relative to the patella whereas others measure displacement of the tibia with respect to the femur. Edixhoven (16) compared stereoradiographic measurements of knee laxity with their device and concluded that the error due to patellar motion was negligible, ranging between 1 to 3% of the total A-P displacement, and thus the assumption that the patella remains fixed to the femur is valid. The Genucom utilizes an elaborate digitization method to establish a coordinate system at the center of the knee joint in which loads and displacements are referenced. Wroble et al. (70) determined that digitization errors had a significant impact on A-P laxity measurements using the Genucom.

Instrumented laxity testers utilize different references for applied load. The Genucom references loads at the center of the knee joint, whereas devices such as the CA-4000 and the Stryker measure loads at the point of application (at the tibial tuberosity). Anterior-posterior laxity measurements decreased as the point of load application on the tibia is moved distally (2,21). The load resisted at the knee joint is decreased as the applied load to the tibia is shifted distally. This was proven in a free body analysis and verified experimentally (21). The shear load must also be applied in the midsagittal plane perpendicular to the longitudinal axis of the tibia. Loads out of plane will not produce the same amount of anterior motion. The different knee laxity testers apply the shear loads at different sites, which may account for some of the discrepancies between devices. Variability within a device may be related to deviations in load applicator placement.

Another source of potential error is examiner dependent. Examiners must be experienced and instrumented laxity testing requires strict attention to detail (1,13,28,59,60,64). Daniel states that the most significant examiner problem when using the KT-1000 is the examiners ability to apply constant pressure to the patellar pad (13). The study executed by Emery et al. (18) determined significant differences between examiners using the Genucom. The manufacturers attributed these differences due to inconsistent testing technique. Faro Medical Technologies gives a certification course to train potential Genucom examiners with a yearly update for recertification. However, Fleming et al. (21) repeated the study using certified Genucom technicians and found similar results. Patient position has an effect on A-P laxity measurements (16,64). Edixhoven et al. (16) concluded that patient positioning is the major factor influencing reproducibility. Shifting the patient within the restraints will alter reference positions of the applied load and displacement as well as altering the soft tissue fixation. The examiner must pay attention to the direction and magnitude of the loads applied (2,21,64).

It is also up to the examiner to be aware of patient comfort and apprehension. Laxity testing requires the patient to be completely relaxed throughout the test cycle. Patient guarding has been shown to significantly decrease A-P laxity (up to 76%) and increase anterior stiffness (up to four times) (1,16,21,47,61,70). Many investigators have shown that instrumented laxity test results become more reproducible in subsequent testing sessions (16,60,68,71). The patient learns to relax and not to fight the test. Furthermore, shear forces greater than 200 N cause the patient to contract the thigh muscles due to discomfort (61). When performing a clinical Lachman test, the clinician supports the limb with his/her hands. Thus the clinician may sense patient apprehension and has the ability to encourage the patient to relax. Using instrumented laxity testers, except for the Genucom, the examiner is further removed from the patient since the hands are placed on the device. The loss of contact between examiner and patient may be one reason that the clinical exam proves more reliable than the instrumented testers. If the examiner is not attentive to patient comfort and apprehension, the output of any instrumented laxity tester will not be valid.

PRACTICALITY IN CLINIC/RESEARCH

It is obvious that there is substantial controversy in the literature on the accuracy, efficacy and reproducibility of instrumented laxity testers. It should be noted that most of these investigations report data averaged over a sample population. With large sample sizes, errors due to testing technique and patient apprehension may not be as apparent. In determining the usefulness of a clinical diagnostic tool, the device should be evaluated on a patient to patient basis. An example is shown in the works of Markolf et al. (46,48). No side to side differences were found in the sample normal population tested, however, a considerable amount of variability in the laxity measurement for any individual patient (26 to 35%) was reported. Therefore, an evaluation of knee laxity testers should key in on both the variability within a patient (reproducibility) and a sensitivity/specificity/diagnostic correctness analysis.

The studies which have evaluated reproducibility of the clinical Lachman test indicate significant differences between examiners (9,21). However, these studies have made the task of identifying the ACL injury very stringent. Instead of asking the simple question of whether or not the ACL is intact, these studies have required the clinicians to estimate the millimeters of translation (9) or to grade laxity on an eight point scale (21,58). The lack of reproducibility of the clinical Lachman test in the literature may therefore be artificially low. With the clinical Lachman test, Steiner et al. (64) used a five point clinical scale (0, 1+, 2+, 3+, and 4+) and found its reproducibility to be equivalent to the commercially available laxity testers. With a complete clinical knee exam, including the pivot shift test, the sensitivity of the ACL diagnosis is 98% (1).

The sensitivity, specificity, diagnostic correctness and reproducibility indices of the clinical exam are equivalent to, if not better than the various instrumented laxity testers. Instrumented testers do not replace the standard clinical evaluation techniques. However, instrumented laxity testers may augment a clinical diagnosis by increasing confidence in the clinical examination. From a clinical standpoint, one must weigh the cost of purchasing the system, training a technician or examiner to perform the tests, and the time commitment, as well as technician costs.

The clinician and investigator desire an objective measurement system for A-P laxity for initial examinations and postreconstruction ACL evaluations. As a research tool, knee laxity instrumentation systems require several installation-to-installation trials to help reduce intra-examiner variability. The current instrument laxity testers are less accurate, reproducible, and sensitive than many investigators and clinicians find acceptable (16,20, 64,70).

In a survey designed to analyze current trends in repair and rehabilitation of knee ligament injuries, Campbell et al. (6) contacted 125 orthopaedic surgeons. Of the 101 surgeons that responded, 61% use the KT-1000 for the preoperative evaluation. Of those that do not use the KT-1000, 36% use the manual exam, 26% use the Stryker, 8% use the Genucom, 8% use the Telos, a stress x-ray technique, and 5% use a personal system. Despite the ambiguity present in the literature, instrumented laxity testers are used in many settings. Objective measurements are a necessary part of evaluating ACL-deficient patients and reconstructions. Improvements in design and application of these devices will continue to be part of future advances in this field.

ACKNOWLEDGMENTS

This work was supported by National Institutes of Health Grants AR40174 and AR39213.

REFERENCES

1. Anderson A, Lipscomb A. (1989): Preoperative instrumented testing of anterior and posterior knee laxity. *Am J Sports Med,* 17:387–392.
2. Andersson C, Gillquist J. (1990): Instrumented testing for evaluation of sagittal knee laxity. *Clin Orthop,* 256:178–184.
3. Bach B, Flynn W, Warren R, Kroll M, Wickiewicz T. (1987): KT-1000 evaluation of normal, acute and chronic anterior cruciate ligament knees. *Trans Orthop Res Soc,* 12:194.
4. Bargar W, Moreland J, Markolf K, Shoemaker S. (1983): The effect of tibial-foot rotatory position on the anterior drawer test. *Clin Orthop,* 173:200–203.
5. Boniface R, Fu F, Ilkhanipour K. (1986): Objective anterior cruciate ligament testing. *Orthopedics,* 9:391–393.
6. Campbell J, Wills R, Arstone K, Feagin J. (1992): Current trends in repair and rehabilitation of anterior cruciate ligament injuries, medial collateral ligament injuries, and meniscal injuries. ACL Study Group, Aspen, Colorado, January 1992.
7. Dahlstedt L, Dalen N. (1989): Knee laxity in cruciate ligament injury: value of examination under anesthesia. *Acta Orthop Scand,* 60:181–184.
8. Daniel D. (1990): Diagnosis of a ligament injury. In: Daniel D, Akeson W, O'Connor J, eds. *Knee ligaments: structure, function, injury, and repair.* New York: Raven Press, pp 3–10.
9. Daniel D. (1991): Assessing the limits of knee motion. *Am J Sports Med,* 19:139–147.
10. Daniel D, Malcom L, Losse G, Stone M, Sachs R, Burks R. (1985): Instrumented measurement of anterior laxity of the knee. *J Bone Joint Surg [Am],* 67A:720–726.
11. Daniel D, Stone M, Sachs R, Malcom L. (1985): Instrumented measurement of anterior cruciate ligament disruption. *Am J Sports Med,* 13:401–407.
12. Daniel D, Stone M, Barnett P, Sachs R. (1988): Use of the quadriceps active test to diagnose posterior cruciate ligament disruption and measure posterior laxity of the knee. *J Bone Joint Surg [Am],* 70A:386–391.
13. Daniel D, Stone M. (1990): KT-1000 anterior-posterior displacement measurements. In: Daniel D, Akeson W, O'Connor J, eds.

Knee ligaments: structure, function, injury, and repair. New York: Raven Press, pp 427–447.

14. DeHaven K. (1983): Arthroscopy in the diagnosis and management of the anterior cruciate ligament deficient knee. *Clin Orthop,* 172:52–56.

15. Donaldson W, Warren R, Wickiewicz T. (1985): A comparison of acute anterior cruciate ligament examinations: initial versus examination under anesthesia. *Am J Sports Med,* 13:5–10.

16. Edixhoven PH, Huiskes R, DeGraaf R, Von Rens TH, Slooff T. (1987): Accuracy and reproducibility of instrumented knee drawer tests. *J Orthop Res,* 5:378–487.

17. Edixhoven PH, Huiskes R, DeGraaf R. (1989): Anteroposterior drawer measurements in the knee using an instrumented test device. *Clin Orthop,* 247:233–242.

18. Emery M, Moffroid M, Boerman J, Fleming B, Howe J, Pope M. (1989): Reliability of force/displacement measures in a clinical device designed to measure ligamentous laxity at the knee. *J Orthop Sports Phys Ther,* 10:441–447.

19. Fetto J, Marshall J. (1980): The natural history and diagnosis of anterior cruciate ligament insufficiency. *Clin Orthop,* 147:29–38.

20. Fleming B, Beynnon B, Nichols C, Johnson R, Pope M. 1993: An *in vivo* comparison of anterior tibial translation and strain in the anteromedial band of the anterior cruciate ligament. *J Biomech* 26:51–58.

21. Fleming B, Johnson R, Shapiro E, Fenwick J, Howe J, Pope M. (1992): Clinical versus instrumented knee testing on autopsy specimens. *Clin Orthop* 282:196–207.

22. Forster J, Warren-Smith C. (1989): Is the KT-1000 knee ligament arthrometer reliable? *J Bone Joint Surg [Br],* 71B:841–847.

23. Franklin J, Rosenberg T, Paulos L, France E. (1991): Radiographic assessment of instability of the knee due to rupture of the anterior cruciate ligament. *J Bone Joint Surg [Am],* 73A:365–372.

24. Fukubayashi T, Torzilli P, Sherman M, Warren R. (1982): An *in vitro* biomechanical evaluation of anterior-posterior motion of the knee: tibial displacement, rotation and torque. *J Bone Joint Surg [Am],* 64A:258–264.

25. Galway R, Beaupre A, MacIntosh D. (1972): Pivot shift: a clinical sign of symptomatic anterior cruciate insufficiency. *J Bone Joint Surg [Br],* 54B:762–763.

26. Gurtler R, Stine R, Torg J. (1987): Lachman test evaluated: quantification of a clinical observation. *Clin Orthop,* 216:141–150.

27. Hanten W, Pace M. (1987): Reliability of measuring anterior laxity of the knee joint using a knee ligament arthrometer. *Phys Ther,* 67:357–359.

28. Highgenboten C, Jackson A, Meske N. (1989): Genucom, KT-1000, and Stryker knee laxity measuring device comparisons: device reproducibility and inter-device comparison in asymptomatic subjects. *Am J Sports Med,* 17:743–746.

29. Hooper G. (1986): Radiological assessment of anterior cruciate ligament deficiency: a new technique. *J Bone Joint Surg [Br],* 68B:292–296.

30. Howe J, Johnson R, Kaplan M, Fleming B, Jarvinen M. (1991): Anterior cruciate ligament reconstruction using quadriceps patellar tendon graft: Part 1. Long-term follow-up. *Am J Sports Med,* 19:447–457.

31. Hughston J, Andrews J, Cross M, Moshi A. (1976): Classification of knee ligament instabilities: Part 1. The medial compartment and cruciate ligaments. *J Bone Joint Surg [Am],* 58A:159–172.

32. Hughston J, Andrews J, Cross M, Moshi A. (1976): Classification of knee ligament instabilities: Part 2. The lateral compartment. *J Bone Joint Surg [Am],* 58A:173–179.

33. Jacob R. (1981): Observations on rotatory instability of the lateral compartment of the knee. *Acta Orthop Scand,* 52[Suppl 1]:1–31.

34. Jacobsen K. (1976): Stress radiological measurement of anteroposterior, medial and lateral stability of the knee. *Acta Orthop Scand,* 47:335–344.

35. Jacobsen K. (1981): Gonylaxometry: stress radiographic measurement of passive stability in the knee joints of normal subjects and patients with ligament injuries. *Acta Orthop Scand,* 52[Suppl 194]:13–255.

36. Johnson RJ, Eriksson E, Haggmark T, Pope M. (1984): Five to ten year follow-up evaluation after reconstruction of the anterior cruciate ligament. *Clin Orthop,* 183:122–140.

37. Jonsson T, Althoff B, Peterson L, Renstrom P. (1982): Clinical

38. Jonsson H, Elmqvist L-G, Karrholm J. (1990): Anterior-posterior laxity measurement of the knee joint: a comparison between KT-1000 and roentgen stereophotogrammetry. *Acta Orthop Scand,* 61[Suppl 237]:73.

39. Karrholm J, Selvik G, Elmqvist L-G, Hansson L, Johsson H. (1988): Three-dimensional instability of the anterior cruciate deficient knee. *J Bone Joint Surg [Br],* 70B:777–783.

40. Katz J, Fingeroth R. (1986): The diagnostic accuracy of ruptures of the anterior cruciate ligament comparing Lachman test, the anterior drawer sign, and the pivot shift tests in acute and chronic knee injuries. *Am J Sports Med,* 14:88–91.

41. Kennedy J, Fowler P. (1971): Medial and anterior instability of the knee: an anatomical and clinical study using stress machines. *J Bone Joint Surg [Am],* 53A:1257–1270.

42. King J, Kumar S. (1989): The Stryker knee arthrometer in clinical practice. *Am J Sports Med,* 17:649–650.

43. Leven H. (1977): Determination of sagittal instability of the knee joint. *Acta Radiol,* 18:689–697.

44. Losee R, Ennis T, Johnson R, Southwick W. (1978): Anterior subluxation of the lateral tibial plateau: a diagnostic test and operative review. *J Bone Joint Surg [Am],* 60A:1015–1030.

45. Malcom L, Daniel D, Stone M, Sachs R. (1985): The measurement of anterior knee laxity after ACL reconstructive surgery. *Clin Orthop,* 196:35–41.

46. Markolf K, Graff-Radford A, Amstutz H. (1978): *In vivo* knee stability: a quantitative assessment using an instrumented clinical testing. *J Bone Joint Surg [Am],* 60A:664–674.

47. Markolf K, Kochan A, Amstutz H. (1984): Measurement of knee stiffness and laxity in patients with documented absence of the anterior cruciate ligament. *J Bone Joint Surg [Am],* 66A:242–253.

48. Markolf K, Amstutz H. (1987): The clinical relevance of instrumented testing for ACL insufficiency: experience with the UCLA clinical testing apparatus. *Clin Orthop,* 233:198–207.

49. Marks J, Palmer M, Burke M, Smith P. (1978): Observer variation in the examination of knee joints. *Ann Rheum Dis,* 37:376–377.

50. McPhee I, Fraser J. (1981): Stress radiography in acute ligamentous injuries of the knee. *Injury,* 12:383–388.

51. McQuade K, Sidles J, Larson R. (1989): Reliability of the Genucom knee analysis system: a pilot study. *Clin Orthop,* 245:216–219.

52. Mononen T, Alaranta H, Harilainen A, Sandelin J, Vanhanen I, Osterman K. (1991): Instrumented measurements of anteroposterior knee translation in patients with old anterior cruciate ligament ruptures. Unpublished data.

53. Neuschwander D, Drez D, Paine R, Young J. (1990): Comparison of anterior laxity measurements in anterior cruciate deficient knees with two instrumented testing devices. *Orthopedics,* 13:299–302.

54. Noyes F, Grood E, Butler D, Malek M. (1980): Clinical laxity tests and functional stability of the knee: biomechanical concepts. *Clin Orthop,* 146:84–89.

55. Noyes R, Grood E, Torzilli P. (1989): Current concepts review: The definitions or terms and position of the knee and injuries of the ligaments. *J Bone Joint Surg [Am],* 71A:465–472.

56. Oliver J, Coughlin L. (1987): Objective knee evaluation using the Genucom knee analysis system: clinical implications. *Am J Sports Med,* 15:571–578.

57. Ouellet R, L'Evesque H, Laurin C. (1969): The ligamentous stability of the knee: an experimental investigation. *Can Med Assoc J,* 100:45–50.

58. Pope M, Johnson RJ, Lavalette R, Kristiansen T. (1987): Variations in the examination of the medial collateral ligament of the knee. *Clin Biomech,* 2:71–73.

59. Riederman R, Wroble R, Grood E, VanGinkel L, Shaffer B. (1991): Reproducibility of the knee signature system. *Am J Sports Med,* 19:660–664.

60. Sherman O, Markolf K, Ferkel R. (1987): Measurements of anterior laxity in normal and anterior cruciate absent knees with two instrumented test devices. *Clin Orthop,* 215:156–161.

61. Shino K, Inoue M, Horibe S, Nakamura H, Ono K. (1987): Mea-

surement of anterior instability of the knee: a new apparatus for clinical testing. *J Bone Joint Surg [Br]*, 69B:608–613.

62. Slocum D, James S, Larson R, Singer K. (1976): Clinical test for anterolateral rotatory instability of the knee. *Clin Orthop*, 118:63–69.

63. Staubli H-U, Jakob R. (1991): Anterior knee motion analysis: measurement and simultaneous radiography. *Am J Sports Med*, 19:172–177.

64. Steiner M, Brown C, Zarins B, Brownstein B, Koval P, Stone P. (1990): Measurement of anterior-posterior displacement of the knee: a comparison of the results with instrumented devices and with clinical examination. *J Bone Joint Surg [Am]*, 72A:1307–1315.

65. Sullivan D, Levy I, Sheskier S, Torzilli P, Warren R. (1984): Medial restrains to anterior-posterior motion of the knee. *J Bone Joint Surg [Am]*, 66A:930–936.

66. Torg J, Conrad W, Kalen V. (1976): Clinical diagnosis of anterior cruciate ligament instability in the athlete. *Am J Sports Med*, 4:84–93.

67. Torzilli P, Greenberg R, Insall J. (1981): An *in vivo* biomechanical evaluation of anterior-posterior motion of the knee. *J Bone Joint Surg [Am]*, 63A:960–968.

68. Torzilli P, Panariello R, Forbes A, Santner T, Warren R. (1991): Measurement reproducibility of two commercial knee test devices. *J Orthop Res*, 9:730–737.

69. White B, Brown D, Johnson R, Pope M. (1979): *In vivo* laxity testing of the knee: anterior displacement tests. *Trans Orthop Res Soc*, 4:255.

70. Wroble R, Grood E, Noyes F, Schmitt D. (1990): Reproducibility of Genucom knee analysis system testing. *Am J Sports Med*, 18:387–395.

71. Wroble R, VanGinkel L, Grood E, Noyes F, Shaffer B. (1990): Repeatability of the KT-1000 arthrometer in a normal population. *Am J Sports Med*, 18:396–399.

The Anterior Cruciate Ligament: Current and Future Concepts, edited by D.W. Jackson, et al. Raven Press, Ltd., New York © 1993.

CHAPTER 22

Selecting Patients for ACL Surgery

Dale M. Daniel

THE NATURAL HISTORY OF THE ACL-INJURED KNEE

To answer the question "Who needs ACL surgery?" we must first ask the question What is the fate of the ACL-injured knee treated without surgery? The ideal natural history study would identify all the patients who sustained the injury within the study group. It would document definitively the presence of the injury and exclude or subcategorize patients with additional injuries (including other ligament injuries, fractures, chondral injuries, and meniscal injuries). It would follow these patients over a long period without intervention and finally definitively assess the status of all these patients objectively, subjectively, and functionally. Of course, no such study has been done. Most of the literature on the unoperated ACL disruption is retrospective and has analyzed patients with chronic ACL disruptions presenting with knee symptoms (33,64), mixed patient populations presenting with acute or chronic injuries (30), patients with failed ACL repairs (28), and patient populations gleaned from surgical logs (9,58,69) or hospital records (50,61,73). Three prospective studies have been reported with a 4-year or more follow-up. Clancy (16) reported a 48-month follow-up of 22 patients, Hawkins (41) a 45-month follow-up of 40 patients, and Andersson (5,6) a 58-month follow-up of 59 patients. All of the patients in the Clancy and Andersson studies were surgically evaluated. Clancy treated 92 patients with an acute ACL disruption. He reconstructed 70 patients (those with a "moderate or severe" pivot shift), and treated nonoperatively 22 patients (those with an "absent, trace, or mild" pivot shift). Andersson randomized 156 patients into three treatment groups: ACL repair, ACL repair plus augmentation, and associated injury repair without ACL repair, which is the ACL not repaired population. Fifteen of the non-ACL surgery patients had medial collateral ligament repairs, 10 had posterior oblique ligament repairs, and 1 had an arcuate ligament complex repair. Hawkins did not report on what basis it was decided to treat the 40 ACL-injured patients in his study without ACL ligament surgery or what percentage of his ACL-injured patients the nonoperative group represented. Twenty-five of the Hawkins patients were evaluated surgically. The remainder of the patients were not examined surgically as "examination without anesthesia was sufficient for diagnosis in 15 of the patients, all of whom had a positive Lachman test, anterior drawer and pivot shift maneuver" (41).

At the Kaiser Hospital in San Diego we have recently completed a 5-year follow-up study on 236 patients presenting to us with an acute traumatic hemarthrosis who meet the study admission criteria presented in Table 1. Patients were entered into the study between 1981 and 1986. One hundred ninety of the patients had an arthroscopic examination within 90 days of injury, 90% of those within 21 days of injury (Table 2). One hundred eighty-eight of those patients had an ACL injury; thus, a KT unstable grade (injured − normal ≥3 mm) in this study was 99% diagnostic of an ACL disruption. The manual maximum test was the most sensitive test (Fig. 1). The sensitivity by test to diagnose a complete ACL disruption in the clinic on the first examination was 96% (89 Newton test = 68%, manual maximum = 96%). A histogram of the manual maximum measurements on the first clinical examination is presented in Fig. 2. Under anesthesia 95 patients with a complete ACL disruption were tested; 96% were KT unstable (89 Newton test = 76%, manual maximum test = 96%). Forty-five of the patients elected to have ACL surgery within 90 days of injury. One hundred ninety-one patients de-

D. M. Daniel: Kaiser Permanente and University of California at San Diego, San Diego, California 92020.

TABLE 1. *Study admission criteria*

Inclusion criteria
    Acute traumatic hemarthrosis
    Examination within 14 days of index injury
    Lower limb injuries limited to the index knee
    KT-1000 injured minus normal knee displacement difference of ≥3 mm on the 89
        Newton test, manual maximum test or quadriceps active test within 90 days of injury
Exclusion criteria
    History of injury or ailment in either knee before index injury
    Diagnosis of an acute patellar dislocation
    Soft "end point" to varus/valgus stress indicating a Grade III collateral ligament injury
    Positive quadriceps active test indicating a posterior cruciate ligament injury
    Standard knee radiographs reveal abnormal bone structures

cided to see if they could cope with their ACL-injured knee without ACL surgery (Fig. 3).

There are a number of differences between the Kaiser study population and the patient populations in the three previously published prospective studies (6,16,41). The Kaiser study included all patients that met the study admission criteria over a 5-year period. The Kaiser study includes patients who did not choose to have a surgical evaluation of the knee and patients with a wide range of joint instability. No collateral ligament surgery or extraarticular repairs were performed on the Kaiser patients. Though all four studies fall short of being an ideal natural history, there is much that we can learn from these prospective studies concerning the incidence of occupation and sports impairment, secondary surgery for meniscus tears and joint instability, and the incidence of postinjury arthritis.

Occupation and Sports

Only the Kaiser study reported on occupational history. No patient in the Kaiser study stated they changed work due to the knee injury. In the Hawkins study (41), 90% of the patients with a nonreconstructed knee were still playing sports, but 75% were playing at a decreased level. Andersson (5) reported that 23% of the nonreconstructed patients returned to their former level of sports activity. In the Kaiser study sports were documented as hours per year of participation in sports by sports level (Table 3). Prior to injury 92% of patients played a sport at least 50 hours a year, at follow-up the number was 50%. The average hours of sports participation had reduced from 322 hours a year to 223 hours a year. The patients had discontinued 33 Level I or II sports due to the knee injury.

Secondary Meniscus or Ligament Surgery

Surgery performed after the patient recovered from the index injury is termed late surgery. In the Kaiser study, all surgery greater than 90 days after the index injury is termed late surgery. The previously reported incidence of late meniscectomy in the ACL-injured knee/years of follow-up are as follows: 16%/12 years (79), 10%/4 years (41), 24%/5 years (6). The incidence in the Kaiser study was 20%/5 years. The reported incidence of late reconstruction in the ACL injured knee ranges from 25% to 38% (6,24,41). In the Kaiser study,

TABLE 2. *KT unstable knees arthroscopic findings (n = 190)*

Tissue	Condition	n	%
Anterior cruciate ligament	Normal	2	1
	Partial tear	27	14
	Complete tear	161	85
Medial meniscus	Normal	143	75
	Tear, no surgery	21	11
	Tear, repair	9	5
Lateral meniscus	Normal	124	65
	Tear, no surgery	32	17
	Tear, repaired	1	1
	Tear, excised	33	17
Meniscus surgery	Yes	54	28
Chondral pathology	Any chondral pathology	44	23
	Medial compartment	24	13
	Lateral compartment	16	8
	Patellofemoral	25	13

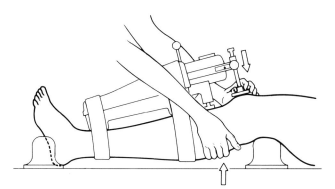

FIG. 1. KT-1000 manual maximum test. The relaxed limbs are supported in about 30° of flexion. The patellar sensor pad is stabilized, the testing reference position is established by pushing with an 89-N load posteriorly and then releasing the force. While the patellar sensor is stabilized with one hand, the other hand applies a strong anterior displacement force directly to the proximal calf to produce the maximum anterior displacement. Care is taken that the knee is not extended. The proximal load application allows forces of 30 to 50 lb while not extending the knee. Tibial displacement is read off the dial.

44 of the 191 KT unstable knees were reconstructed late (23%).

Most authors agree that there is a "high-risk" patient who should be treated with early surgery and a "low-risk" patient who should be treated nonsurgically

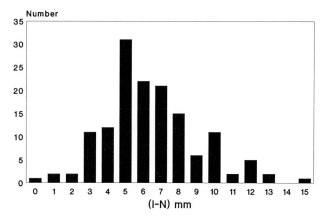

FIG. 2. Manual maximum displacement on the first clinical examination. Frequency distribution of the injured-minus-normal displacement difference in 144 patients with a complete ACL disruption examined in the clinic within 14 days of injury. The examination was performed before surgery.

(20,62,83,87). There is general agreement that the patient's risk is dependent on age, sports activity, and degree of joint instability (20,62,83,87). In the Kaiser study a number of factors correlated with patients who had late surgery for a meniscus tear or an ACL reconstruction ($p < 0.05$): patient age, preinjury hours of sports participation, arthrometer measurements at 0, 3, and 12 months after injury, and pivot shift test at 12 months.

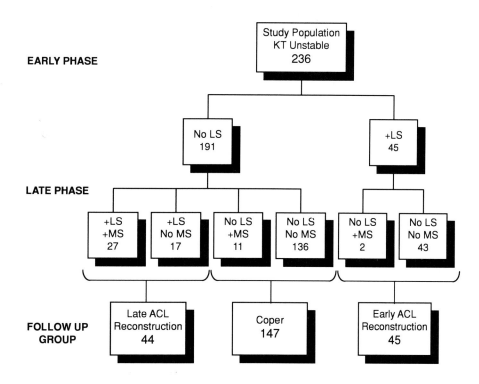

No LS= No ligament surgery, +LS= Ligament surgery, No MS= No meniscus surgery, +MS= Meniscus surgery

FIG. 3. Kaiser San Diego ACL Injury Study. *Early phase,* surgery within 90 days of injury; *late phase,* surgery >90 days after injury; *Coper,* ACL-injured patient who did not have ACL surgery; *early ACL reconstruction,* ACL surgery in the early phase; *late ACL reconstruction,* ACL surgery in the late phase.

TABLE 3. *Sports functional level*

Level	Activity
I	Jumping, pivoting, hard cutting (basketball, football, soccer)
II	Lateral motion; less jumping or hard cutting than Level I (baseball, racket sports, skiing)
III	Other sports (jogging, running, swimming)

Factors of interest which did not correlate with who had late surgery ($p > 0.1$): sex, mechanism of injury, hyperextension of the contralateral normal knee, A-P displacement of the contralateral normal knee, pivot shift tests under anesthesia during the early phase examination, and associated collateral ligament injuries. Stepwise discriminant analysis was performed to identify the factors in combination which were most predictive of which KT unstable patient not reconstructed during the early phase would require late meniscus surgery. The analysis was then performed to predict late ligament surgery. The most important single variable for predicting meniscus surgery or ligament surgery was total hours per year of sport Level I and II participation before injury. Because of the correlation between age and sports participation, once sports participation was placed into the formula, age added no additional predictive value. The second variable added to the equation was the manual maximum displacement difference. No additional variables improved the ability to predict which patient would have late meniscus or ligament surgery. The sensitivity and specificity of the formula to predict late surgery was tested in 158 patients who had a manual maximum displacement measurement in the clinic within 14 days of injury. Thirty-seven of the patients had late ligament surgery, and 30 had late meniscus surgery. A total of 45 patients had late ligament and/or meniscus surgery (28%). The percent sensitivity/specificity of the formula for meniscus surgery was 53/75, for ligament surgery 46/78, and for late meniscus or ligament surgery 47/76. Thus the equation is better at predicting who did not have late surgery than who did have late surgery. A guide to the patients surgical risk factor (SURF) is presented in Table 4.

Previous reports have documented that radiographic changes (15,35,41,57,64,73,79) and bone scan changes (23) occur in the chronic ACL-disrupted knee. The

Kaiser study is the first report that presents the results of imaging studies in a large ACL-injured population prospectively studied. Many patients had mild degenerative changes in the index knee. Some of the changes on x-ray and bone scan may be secondary to occult bone lesions sustained at the time of injury (70). In the Kaiser study meniscus surgery correlated with increased degenerative changes which supports the findings of previous authors (64,73,77,79). The relationship between osteoarthritis and meniscectomy has been previously documented (25,48,81). This is the first report to correlate degenerative changes with displacement measurements. The manual maximum and quadriceps active tests correlated with an increase in imaging scores ($p < 0.05$).

THE ACL-RECONSTRUCTED KNEE

The patient with the ACL-disrupted knee is at risk of functional impairment, secondary meniscus tear, and the development of joint arthrosis. What is the effect of ACL reconstructive surgery on this process? The only prospective studies that compare the outcome of a reconstructed group of patients with a nonoperative group of patients are those by Andersson (5), Clancy (16), and the Kaiser study. All three studies are flawed. The Andersson study is randomized, but includes patients with collateral ligament surgery. Clancy divided patients into surgical and nonsurgical patients based on the patients' instability examination. In the Kaiser study 45 patients elected to have early ACL surgery, 44 late ACL surgery, and 147 were treated without ACL surgery (Fig. 3).

What did the follow-up evaluation in the three studies show? In the Andersson study the level of activity was higher in the reconstructed patients, though the mean knee score was not significantly different. In the Clancy study 44% of the nonreconstructed patients had a good or excellent result versus 97% with an ACL reconstruction. In the Kaiser study 90% of the patients who had late ACL reconstructive surgery stated they were improved by the ligament surgery, and in most their hours of sports participation increased over their ACL-disrupted condition. The follow-up evaluation in the Kaiser study revealed the symptoms of giving way, swelling, and pain were not different between the nonreconstructed and reconstructed groups. The impairment inventory was not different between the two groups with the exception that the reconstructed patients had more trouble kneeling. The sports participation was similar for the two groups of patients.

The Kaiser study documented that ACL surgery decreased the measured joint instability. Both the Andersson and the Kaiser study showed a higher incidence of late meniscus tears in the ACL-disrupted knee versus the ACL-reconstructed knee. DeHaven has reported the incidence of meniscus tear after meniscus repair is higher

TABLE 4. *Surgical risk factor*

KT-1000 Man Max I-N	Sports hours per year (Level I or II)		
	<50	50–199	≥200
<5	Low	Low	Moderate
5–7	Low	Moderate	High
>7	Moderate	High	High

in the ACL-disrupted knee than the ACL-reconstructed knee (21). Hanks (38) and Sommerlath (78) have reported a high success rate with meniscus repair in patients with an ACL-deficient knee as well as patients with an ACL-competent knee.

The effect of ligament surgery on degenerative arthritis has not been reported. The Kaiser follow-up evaluation included radiographs (30° standing A-P, 30° lateral, and tunnel views) and bone scans of both knees. All imaging studies were evaluated by an examiner blinded as to the diagnosis and which knee was injured. A disturbing finding in the Kaiser study is an increased incidence of degenerative joint disease in the reconstructed patients, compared to the patient treated without ACL surgery, which could be explained only in part to a higher incidence of meniscus injury in the ACL-reconstructed patients prior to their reconstruction. The following are some possible explanations for this occurrence: (a) greater injury in the reconstructed knees prior to surgery than in the patients who did not choose reconstruction, (b) joint injury occurring at the time of surgery, (c) joint response to stress deprivation after surgery (2), (d) prolonged joint inflammation after surgery (4,71), and (e) abnormal joint mechanics after surgery (71). We hope that recent advances in ligament surgery technique (18) and earlier postoperative mobilization programs will decrease the incidence of degenerative changes after ligament surgery.

MANAGEMENT OF THE ACL-INJURED KNEE

The management goal of the ACL-injured patient is to prevent recurrent knee injury while allowing the patient to return to their desired work and level of sports participation. The cascade of events from ACL disruption to secondary injuries with meniscus tears to joint arthrosis is well documented (30,43,47,64,73,77). It is clear that some patients are able to cope with their ACL disrupted knee without sustaining secondary injuries (31,35,43,63, 73,82). Some cope without modifying their lifestyle, others modify their athletic participation, and others cope by discontinuing athletic participation. As demonstrated in the Kaiser study, the level of arthrosis is mild if the menisci are intact. The ACL cascade is presented in Fig. 4. At this time there is no evidence to support the thesis that ACL reconstructive surgery prevents arthritis in the ACL-injured knee status post meniscectomy. ACL surgery does protect the meniscus and thereby spares the knee from the arthritis that develops after meniscectomy. Management of the ACL-injured knee in a number of circumstances will be discussed.

ACL single ligament tear without a repairable meniscus tear evaluated within 90 days of injury. Until the patient has healed associated injuries, obtained a full range of motion, full limb strength, and learned how to adapt to the injured knee, neither the patient nor the

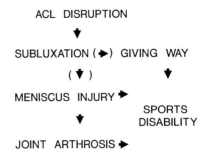

FIG. 4. The ACL injury cascade. The *arrows in parentheses* indicate that this will not always happen. This paradigm states that significant joint arthrosis will develop in an ACL-injured knee only after a meniscus injury. This does not include the possible role of ligament surgery as a cause of arthosis.

surgeon is sure of the level of disability the patient will experience. A decision to perform ACL surgery within the first three months is based on the patient's surgical risk factor (Table 4). I recommend high-risk patients have early ACL surgery and low-risk patients have a trial of activity after joint rehabilitation prior to deciding on surgery. More study is needed to determine the preferable early management of the moderate-risk patient. To minimize the incidence of postoperative joint stiffness, surgery is delayed 3 to 6 weeks until much of the acute injury inflammation is resolved (40,60,71,76).

ACL single ligament tear with a repairable meniscus tear. I recommend ACL surgery in combination with the meniscus repair if the patient is a moderate or high-risk patient (Table 4). If the patient is a low-risk patient, the meniscus is repaired, and the ACL is not reconstructed.

Patient with an acute partial ACL tear. The term "partial" ACL tear has not been clearly defined in the literature. The term implies that some of the ligament is torn and some is intact. The reported incidence of partial ACL tears is 10% to 42% of all ACL tears (13,14,20,34, 39,62). The reported clinical outcome of partial ACL tears diagnosed by direct inspection or arthroscopy is variable (13,26,32,52,56,65,67,72). Animal studies have demonstrated that partial ACL tears have little potential for healing (3,8,42). At the Kaiser Hospital in San Diego we have followed 34 patients with an arthroscopic diagnosis of a partial ACL tear. Arthrometer measurements within 90 days of injury revealed 7 patients were KT stable and 27 were KT unstable. The 5-year follow-up study revealed that none of the patients had early ACL surgery. Three of the 27 early KT-unstable patients had late ligament surgery. None of the early KT stable patients had late ligament surgery.

Acute ACL injury with associated Grade III MCL injury. The isolated medial collateral ligament heals satisfactorily without surgical repair (29,45,46,84,85). For many, disruption of the ACL and MCL in combination has been an indication for surgical repair. Some authors have repaired both structures (1,29,68), some only the MCL (44), some only the ACL (1,11,19,75). The combined injury has also been treated without surgical repair (49). There are no controlled studies or studies reported using a sufficiently standard protocol to document which of the treatment options is preferable. To minimize the risk of postoperative arthrofibrosis, I usually delay surgery. Patients are placed in a range of motion brace for 4 to 8 weeks to protect the MCL while regaining knee motion. I then reconstruct the ACL in the moderate and high-risk patients (Table 3). The low-risk patient is treated without ACL surgery. Depending on the patient's symptoms, an MRI may be performed to evaluate the menisci.

ACL disruption in a patient with open growth plates. Prior to age 12 the majority of the disruptions result from avulsion of the tibial insertion (12,22,53). Reattachment of the tibial tubercle avulsion results in good restoration of knee function (59,86), though normal joint laxity may not be obtained (17). It is likely in some cases there is a partial midsubstance ACL tear prior to the tibial tubercle avulsion. In the adolescent patient the injury is usually a midsubstance ACL tear. The results of suturing the midsubstance ACL tear have been disappointing in children (12,17,22,54,55), as they have been in adults (10,27,66). In the active patient with open growth plates, the natural history of the ACL deficient knee appears to be similar to the adult (7,51,55). However, tunnels placed through the knee with a standard intraarticular ACL reconstruction will cross both the distal femoral and proximal tibial growth plates with the risk of growth plate injury resulting in a limb length discrepancy or a limb alignment deformity. The assessment of the ACL-injured patient with open growth plates should include an estimation of remaining growth by determining bone age from a wrist film (37), a historic review of family growth characteristics, and evaluation of puberty signs (80). Some authors suggest that if "significant growth remains" an intraarticular reconstruction should not be performed (36,55,74). To date, what "significant growth" is has not been clearly defined.

I delay ACL reconstruction in the patient with an open growth plate until proximal tibial and distal femoral growth plates are closed or until little growth remains from these epiphysis (<1.5 cm). This usually corresponds to a bone age of 14 in females and 15 in males. Until the ACL is reconstructed the patient is advised not to participate in hard cutting or jumping sports activities. The risk of meniscus and joint surface injury secondary to repeated giving-way episodes in the ACL-disrupted knee must be balanced against the risk of limb length discrepancy or limb alignment deformity secondary to growth plate arrest, secondary to surgery. The patient and the patient's family must be clearly informed of the treatment options. If repeated knee injury requires surgery when significant growth remains, a surgical procedure is planned that will not cross growth plates.

Patient with chronic ACL disruption, no meniscus tear, and normal limb strength who is experiencing significant disability for work or sports activities and/or has recurrent giving-way episodes. If there is a reasonable chance that an ACL reconstruction will stabilize the patient's knee and the patient is willing to participate in the recommended postoperative rehabilitation program, ACL surgery is performed.

Patient with chronic ACL disruption who has been functioning satisfactorily, develops symptoms after sustaining a nonrepairable meniscus tear. Simple excision of the torn meniscus may return the patient to acceptable function (15). The decision to do ACL surgery should be delayed until the patient has a trial of activity after recovering from the meniscus surgery. A similar situation is that of the patient who has been having recurrent giving-way episodes and has both an ACL tear and an unstable nonrepairable meniscus tear. Which is causing the functional impairment: the unstable meniscus fragment or the ACL instability? The potential for function with the ACL disrupted knee cannot be known with certainty until the meniscus problem is resolved.

Symptomatic chronic ACL disruption with degenerative arthritis. The clinician must carefully define the symptoms, impairments, and knee pathology of the chronic ACL-injured knee. In addition to the ACL disruption the patient may have other ligament pathology, meniscus injury, patellofemoral or tibiofemoral arthrosis, and an alignment deformity. An attempt is made to relate specific symptoms or impairments to specific knee pathology. "Lack of confidence" in the knee may be due to any of the above items. "Giving-way" may be due to joint instability, meniscus pathology, or joint arthrosis. Giving-way episodes with postinjury swelling suggest a meniscus tear. Aching with activity may be due to meniscus disease or joint arthrosis. Anterior knee pain suggests patellofemoral disease. The patient's evaluation begins with a careful consideration of the history, a complete knee examination including strength testing, and radiologic evaluation. The degree of A-P instability is further documented with instrumented testing. Meniscus pathology may be delineated prior to surgery with an arthrogram or MRI, however if surgery is planned, the menisci may be evaluated more economically by arthroscopy at the time of surgery. There are many ACL-injured patients who present with symptoms of meniscus tears who can be managed adequately by caring for the meniscus pathology alone (57). There are other patients who present with symptoms of patellofemoral disease or tibiofemoral arthrosis who will need surgery of the patellofemoral joint or an alignment osteotomy. Not all patients with a chronic ACL disruption will benefit from ACL reconstruction surgery.

ACKNOWLEDGMENTS

San Diego Kaiser Hospital studies presented in this paper were funded by grants from the Southern California Kaiser Permanente Research Foundation and NIH grant AR 39359-03.

REFERENCES

1. Aglietti P, Buzzi R, Zaccherotti G, D'Andria S. (1991): Operative treatment of acute complete lesions of the anterior cruciate and medial collateral ligaments: a 4- to 7-year follow-up study. *Am J Knee Surg*, 4:186–194.
2. Akeson WH. (1991): The response of ligaments to stress modulation and overview of the ligament healing responses. In: Daniel DM, Akeson WH, O'Connor JJ, eds. *Knee ligaments: structure, function, injury, and repair.* New York: Raven Press, pp 315–327.
3. Amiel D, Kuiper S, Akeson WH. (1991): Cruciate ligaments: response to injury. In: Daniel DM, Akeson WH, O'Connor JJ, eds. *Knee ligaments: structure, function, injury, and repair.* New York: Raven Press, pp 365–377.
4. Amiel D, Kuiper S. (1991): Experimental studies on anterior cruciate ligament grafts: histology and biochemistry. In: Daniel DM, Akeson WH, O'Connor JJ, eds. *Knee ligaments: structure, function, injury, and repair.* New York: Raven Press, pp 379–388.
5. Andersson C, Odensten M, Gillquist J. (1991): Knee function after surgical or nonsurgical treatment of acute rupture of the anterior cruciate ligament: a randomized study with a long-term follow-up period. *Clin Orthop*, 264:255–263.
6. Andersson C, Odensten M, Good L, Gillquist J. (1989): Surgical or nonsurgical treatment of acute rupture of the anterior cruciate ligament: a randomized study with long term follow-up. *J Bone Joint Surg [Am]*, 71A:965–974.
7. Angel KR, Hall DJ. (1989): Anterior cruciate ligament injury in children and adolescents. *Arthroscopy*, 5:197–200.
8. Arnoczky SP, Rubin RM, Marshall JL. (1979): Microvasculature of the cruciate ligaments and its response to injury. *J Bone Joint Surg [Am]*, 61A:1221–1229.
9. Arnold JA, Coker TP, Heaton LM, Park JP, Harris WD. (1979): Natural history of anterior cruciate tears. *Am J Sports Med*, 6:305–313.
10. Balkfors B. (1982): The course of knee ligament injuries. *Acta Orthop Scand*, 198:1–99.
11. Ballmer PM, Ballmer FT, Jakob RP. (1991): Reconstruction of the anterior cruciate ligament alone in the treatment of a combined instability with complete rupture of the medial collateral ligament: a prospective study. *Acta Orthop Trauma Scand*, 110:139–141.
12. Bradley GW, Shives TC, Samuelson KM. (1979): Ligament injuries in the knees of children. *J Bone Joint Surg [Am]*, 61A:588–591.
13. Buckley SL, Barrack RL, Alexander AH. (1989): The natural history of conservatively treated partial anterior cruciate ligament tears. *Am J Sports Med*, 17:221–225.
14. Butler JC, Andrews JR. (1988): The role of arthroscopic surgery in the evaluation of acute traumatic hemarthrosis of the knee. *Clin Orthop*, 228:150–152.
15. Chick RR, Jackson DW. (1978): Tears of the anterior cruciate ligament in young athletes. *J Bone Joint Surg [Am]*, 60A:970–973.
16. Clancy WG, Ray JM, Zoltan DJ. (1988): Acute tears of the anterior cruciate ligament. *J Bone Joint Surg [Am]*, 70A:1483–1488.
17. Clanton TO, DeLee JC, Sanders B, Neidre A. (1979): Knee ligament injuries in children. *J Bone Joint Surg [Am]*, 61A:1195–1201.
18. Daniel DM. (1991): Principles of knee ligament surgery. In: Daniel DM, Akeson WH, O'Connor JJ, eds. *Knee ligaments: structure, function, injury, and repair.* New York: Raven Press, pp 11–29.
19. Daniel DM, Teitge RA, Grana WA, Brody DM. (1990): Knee and leg: soft tissue trauma. Presented at the OKU III Update, AAOS, Park Ridge, IL, pp 557–573.
20. DeHaven KE. (1980): Diagnosis of acute knee injuries with hemarthrosis. *Am J Sports Med*, 8:901–914.
21. DeHaven KE. (1985): Meniscus repair in the athlete. *Clin Orthop*, 198:31–35.
22. DeLee JC, Curtis R. (1983): Anterior cruciate ligament insufficiency in children. *Clin Orthop*, 172:112–118.
23. Dye SF, Andersen CT, Stowell MT. (1987): Unrecognized abnormal osseous metabolic activity about the knee of patients with symptomatic anterior cruciate ligament deficiencies. *Orthop Trans*, 11:492.
24. Engerbretsen L, Tegnander A. (1990): Short-term results of the nonoperated isolated anterior cruciate ligament tear. *J Orthop Trauma*, 4:406–410.
25. Fairbank TJ. (1948): Knee joint changes after meniscectomy. *J Bone Joint Surg [Br]*, 30B:664–670.
26. Farquharson-Roberts MA, Osborne AH. (1983): Partial rupture of the anterior cruciate ligament of the knee. *J Bone Joint Surg [Br]*, 65B:32–34.
27. Feagin JA, Curl WW. (1976): Isolated tear of the anterior cruciate ligament: 5-year follow-up study. *Am J Sports Med*, 4:95–100.
28. Feagin JA Jr, Lambert KL, Cunningham RR, Anderson LM, Riegel J, King PH, VanGenderen L. (1987): Consideration of the anterior cruciate ligament injury in skiing. *Clin Orthop*, 216:13–18.
29. Fetto JF, Marshall JL. (1978): Medial collateral ligament injuries of the knee: a rationale for treatment. *Clin Orthop*, 132:206–218.
30. Fetto JF, Marshall JL. (1980): The natural history and diagnosis of anterior cruciate ligament insufficiency. *Clin Orthop*, 147:29–38.
31. Fowler PJ, Regan WD. (1987): The patient with symptomatic chronic anterior cruciate ligament insufficiency: results of minimal arthroscopic surgery and rehabilitation. *Am J Sports Med*, 15:321–325.
32. Fruensgaard S, Johannsen HV. (1989): Incomplete ruptures of the anterior cruciate ligament. *J Bone Joint Surg [Br]*, 71B:526–530.
33. Funk FJ Jr. (1983): Osteoarthritis of the knee following ligamentous injury. *Clin Orthop*, 172:154–157.
34. Gillquist J, Hagberg G, Oretorp N. (1977): Arthroscopy in acute injuries of the knee Joint. *Acta Orthop Scand*, 48:190–196.
35. Giove TP, Miller SJ III, Kent BE, Sanford TL, Garrick JG. (1983): Nonoperative treatment of the torn anterior cruciate ligament. *J Bone Joint Surg [Am]*, 65A:184–192.
36. Graf BK, Lange RH, Fujisaki CK, Landry GL, Saluja RK: Anterior cruciate ligament tears in the skeletally immature patient. Personal communication.
37. Greulich WW, Pyle SL. (1959): *Radiographic atlas of skeletal development of the hand and wrist.* Stanford, CA: Stanford University Press.
38. Hanks GA, Gause TM, Sebastianelli WJ, O'Donnell CS, Kalenak A. (1991): Repair of peripheral meniscal tears: open versus arthroscopic technique. *Arthroscopy*, 7:72–77.
39. Hardacker WT, Garrett WE Jr, Bassett FH III. (1990): Evaluation of acute traumatic hemarthrosis of the knee joint. *South Med J*, 83:640–644.
40. Harner CD, Fu FH, Irrgang JJ, Silbey MB, DiGiacomo R. (1992): Recognition and management of the stiff knee following arthroscopic anterior cruciate ligament reconstruction: recent experience. Scientific exhibit presented at the meeting of the AAOS, Washington, DC, February 20–25.
41. Hawkins RJ, Misamore GW, Merritt TR. (1986): Follow up of acute nonoperated isolated anterior cruciate ligament tears. *Am J Sports Med*, 14:205–210.
42. Hefti FL, Kress A, Fasel J, Morscher EW. (1991): Healing of the transected anterior cruciate ligament in the rabbit. *J Bone Joint Surg [Am]*, 73A:373–383.
43. Hirshman HP, Daniel DM, Miyasaka K. (1991): The fate of unoperated knee ligament injuries. In: Daniel DM, Akeson WH, O'Connor JJ (eds). *Knee ligaments: structure, function, injury, and repair.* New York: Raven Press, pp 481–503.
44. Hughston JC, Barrett GR. (1983): Acute anteromedial rotatory instability. *J Bone Joint Surg [Am]*, 65A:145–153.
45. Indelicato PA. (1989): Nonoperative management of complete tears of the medial collateral ligament. *Orthop Rev*, 18:947–952.
46. Indelicato PA, Bittar ES. (1985): A perspective of lesions asso-

ciated with ACL insufficiency of the knee. *Clin Orthop,* 198:77–80.

47. Jacobsen K. (1977): Osteoarthrosis following insufficiency of the cruciate ligaments in man: a clinical study. *Acta Orthop Scand,* 48:520–526.

48. Johnson RJ, Kettelkamp DB, Clark W, Leaverton P. (1974): Factors affecting late results after meniscectomy. *J Bone Joint Surg [Am],* 56A:719.

49. Jokl P, Kaplan N, Stovell P, Keggi K. (1984): Nonoperative treatment of severe injuries to the medial and anterior cruciate ligaments of the knee. *J Bone Joint Surg [Am],* 66A:741–744.

50. Kannus P, Jarvinen M. (1987): Conservatively treated tears of the anterior cruciate ligament: long-term results. *J Bone Joint Surg [Am],* 69A:1007–1012.

51. Kannus P, Jarvinen M. (1988): Knee ligament injuries in adolescents. *J Bone Joint Surg [Br],* 70B:772–776.

52. Kannus P, Jarvinen M. (1990): Nonoperative treatment of acute knee ligament injuries: a review with special reference to indications and methods. *Sports Med,* 9:244–260.

53. Kellenberger R, VonLaer L. (1990): Nonosseous lesions of the anterior cruciate ligaments in childhood and adolescence. *Prog Pediatr Surg,* 25:123–131.

54. Lipscomb AB, Anderson AF. (1986): Tears of the anterior cruciate ligament in adolescents. *J Bone Joint Surg [Am],* 68A:19–28.

55. McCarroll JR, Rettig AC, Shelbourne KD. (1988): Anterior cruciate ligament injuries in the young athlete with open physes. *Am J Sports Med,* 16:44–47.

56. McDaniel WJ. (1976): Isolated partial tear of the anterior cruciate ligament. *Clin Orthop,* 115:209–212.

57. McDaniel WJ Jr, Dameron TB Jr. (1980): Untreated ruptures of the anterior cruciate ligament. *J Bone Joint Surg [Am],* 62A:696–705.

58. McDaniel WJ, Dameron TB Jr. (1983): The untreated anterior cruciate ligament rupture. *Clin Orthop,* 172:158–163.

59. Meyers MH, McKeever FM. (1970): Fracture of the intercondylar eminence of the tibia. *J Bone Joint Surg [Am],* 52A:1677–1684.

60. Mohtadi NG, Webster-Bogaert S, Fowler PJ. (1991): Limitation of motion following anterior cruciate ligament reconstruction: a case-control study. *Am J Sports Med,* 19:620–625.

61. Ngoi SS, Satku K, Kumar VP. (1987): The natural history of anterior cruciate ligament injuries. *Singapore Med J,* 28:311–313.

62. Noyes FR, Bassett RW, Grood ES, Butler DL. (1980): Arthroscopy in acute traumatic hemarthrosis of the knee: incidence of anterior cruciate tears and other injuries. *J Bone Joint Surg [Am],* 62A:687–695.

63. Noyes FR, Matthews DS, Mooar PA, Grood ES. (1983): The symptomatic anterior cruciate deficient knee: Part 2. The results of rehabilitation, activity modification, and counseling on functional disability. *J Bone Joint Surg [Am],* 65A:163–174.

64. Noyes FR, Mooar PA, Matthews DA, Butler DL. (1983): The symptomatic anterior cruciate deficient knee: Part 1. The long-term functional disability in athletically active individuals. *J Bone Joint Surg [Am],* 65A:154–162.

65. Noyes FR, Mooar LA, Moorman CT, McGinniss GH. (1989): Partial tears of the anterior cruciate ligament. *J Bone Joint Surg [Br],* 71B:825–833.

66. Odensten M, Lysholm J, Gillquist J. (1984): Suture of fresh ruptures of the ACL. *Acta Orthop Scand,* 55:270–272.

67. Odensten M, Lysholm J, Gillquist J. (1985): The course of partial anterior cruciate ligament ruptures. *Am J Sports Med,* 13:183–186.

68. O'Donoghue D. (1955): An analysis of end results of surgical treatment of major injuries to the ligaments of the knee. *J Bone Joint Surg [Am],* 37A:1.

69. Pattee GA, Fox JM, DelPizzo W, Friedman MJ. (1989): Four to ten-year follow up of unreconstructed anterior cruciate ligament tears. *Am J Sports Med,* 17:430–435.

70. Rosen MA, Jackson DW, Burger PE. (1991): Occult osseous lesions documented by magnetic resonance imaging associated with ACL ruptures. *Arthroscopy,* 7:45–51.

71. Sachs RA, Reznik A, Daniel D, Stone ML. (1991): Complications of knee ligament surgery. In: Daniel DM, Akeson WH, O'Connor JJ, eds. *Knee ligaments: structure, function, injury, and repair.* New York: Raven Press, pp 505–520.

72. Sandberg R, Balkfors B. (1987): Partial rupture of the anterior cruciate ligament: natural course. *Clin Orthop,* 220:176–178.

73. Satku K, Kumar VP, Ngoi SS. (1986): Anterior cruciate ligament injuries: to counsel or to operate? *J Bone Joint Surg [Br],* 68B:458–461.

74. Shelbourne KD, Nitz PA. (1990): Anterior cruciate ligament injuries in school-aged athletes. In: Reider B, ed. *Sports medicine: the school age athlete.* Philadelphia: Saunders.

75. Shelbourne KD, Porter DA. (1992): Anterior cruciate ligament–medial collateral ligament injury: nonoperative management of medial collateral ligament tears with anterior cruciate ligament reconstruction. A preliminary report. *Am J Sports Med,* 20:283–287.

76. Shelbourne KD, Wilckens JH, Mollabashy A, DeCarlo M. (1991): Arthrofibrosis in acute anterior cruciate ligament reconstruction: the effect of timing of reconstruction and rehabilitation. *Am J Sports Med,* 19:332–336.

77. Sherman MF, Warren RF, Marshall JL, Savatsky GJ: A clinical and radiographical analysis of 127 anterior cruciate insufficient knees. *Clin Orthop,* 227:229–237.

78. Sommerlath K, Hamberg P. (1989): Healed meniscal tears in unstable knees: a long term follow up of seven years. *Am J Sports Med,* 17:161–163.

79. Sommerlath K, Lysholm J, Gillquist J. (1991): The long-term course after treatment of acute anterior cruciate ligament ruptures: a 9 to 16-year follow up. *Am J Sports Med,* 19:156–162.

80. Tanner JM. (1956): *Growth at adolescence.* Springfield, IL, Charles C Thomas.

81. Tapper EM, Hoover NW. (1969): Late results after meniscectomy. *J Bone Joint Surg [Am],* 51A:517.

82. Walla DJ, Albright JP, McAuley E, Martin RD, Eldridge V, El-Khoury G. (1985): Hamstring control and the unstable anterior cruciate ligament deficient knee. *Am J Sports Med,* 13:34–39.

83. Warner JJP, Warren RF, Cooper DE. (1990): Management of acute anterior cruciate ligament injury. *Instr Course Lect,* 40:219–232.

84. Woo SL-Y, Horibe S, Ohland KJ, Amiel D. (1991): The response of ligaments to injury. In: Daniel DM, Akeson WH, O'Connor JJ, eds. *Knee ligaments: structure, function, injury, and repair.* New York: Raven Press, pp 351–364.

85. Woo SL-Y, Orlando CA, Frank CB, Gomez MA, Akeson WH. (1986): Tensile properties of the medial collateral ligament as a function of age. *J Orthop Res,* 4:133–141.

86. Zaricznyj B. (1977): Avulsion fracture of the tibial eminence: treatment by opening reduction and pinning. *J Bone Joint Surg [Am],* 59A:1111–1115.

87. Zarins B, Adams M. (1988): Medical progress: knee injuries in sports. *N Engl J Med,* 318:950–961.

The Anterior Cruciate Ligament: Current and Future Concepts, edited by D.W. Jackson, et al. Raven Press, Ltd., New York © 1993.

CHAPTER 23

The Mechanics of Anterior Cruciate Ligament Reconstruction

Bruce D. Beynnon, Robert J. Johnson, and Braden C. Fleming

The anterior cruciate ligament is the most frequently totally disrupted ligament within the knee (67). A surprising proportion of active young people sustain the injury, the consequences of which are potentially debilitating (77). Left untreated, a torn ACL can cause an increased incidence of meniscal tears, in addition to increased anterior and rotatory instabilities (101). McDaniel and Dameron have reported radiographic measurements of joint space narrowing, and demonstrated evidence of osteoarthrosis in one-third of the patients with disrupted ACLs (87,88). Many others report that disruption of the ACL results in severe functional problems for the subject (6,22,26,38,41,47,48,50,52,69,82,86,118). From these observations many orthopaedic surgeons have advocated repair or reconstruction of the ACL in patients who have a "high-risk lifestyle" or who have demonstrated functional disability after disruption of this structure. Operative procedures have been advocated including repair of the ACL, repair plus augmentation using various autogenous grafts (116), and reconstruction using autogenous materials, allografts, or prosthetic devices (67,69). Although allografts and prosthetic devices offer some theoretical advantages over autogenous grafts, these operations should probably be relegated to the category of investigational procedures. It has been reported that primary repair of a torn ACL (suturing the torn structure back in place) often results in an unsatisfactory outcome (39,49). Of the autogenous intraarticular reconstructions, it appears that the bone-patellar tendon-bone graft has become the ACL substitute to which all others are being compared (1,5,15,27–29,31,40,64,

67,71,73,81,84,97,106). Although several investigators report a high degree of success, it is clear that universally satisfactory results are not obtained using this graft (31,64,71). It has become apparent that many variables affect the final outcome of an ACL reconstruction procedure. Among the important variables are the structural and material properties of the graft, the intraarticular position of the graft (2,4,22,23,53,55,56,59,60,91,108, 120,121,130), initial tensioning of the graft during implantation (3,11,45,136), fixation of the graft (80,112), and the postoperative rehabilitation regimen (13,64,70, 100,101,105,107,109,111,120,122). This chapter will present a review of the latest investigations on these topics as they pertain to autogenous ACL reconstruction.

GRAFT BIOMECHANICS

Before reconstructing the ACL, an appropriate soft tissue replacement must be chosen (i.e., patellar tendon, semitendinosus, gracilis, iliotibial band, or a combination of these tissues). To fully describe the biomechanical behavior of the normal ACL or a soft tissue replacement, both structural and mechanical (sometimes referred to as material) properties must be appreciated and understood. Structural properties describe the behavior of an ACL bone-ligament-bone complex or a graft, such as the bone-patellar tendon-bone preparation, and are measured from the load-displacement response of a soft tissue tensile loading test. They include the linear stiffness, ultimate load, and energy absorbed at failure (132). Mechanical properties characterize the behavior of the ligament substance isolated from insertion site effects, and are measured from the stress-strain response of a soft tissue tensile load to failure test. They include the tangent modulus, ultimate stress, and ultimate strain at failure (131). Different soft tissue replacements have dif-

B. D. Beynnon, R. J. Johnson, and B. C. Fleming: McClure Musculoskeletal Research Center, Department of Orthopaedics, University of Vermont Medical School, Burlington, Vermont 05405.

ferent structural stiffness and ultimate failure load values (21). Consequently, once implanted, each soft tissue replacement will have a different effect on knee joint kinematics. For example, Butler (21) has reported that the peak failure strength of the semitendinosus is only 70% that of the ACL. In addition, this substitute has a longer length between attachment sites in comparison to the ACL. Many surgeons, because of these observations, either double this structure, or augment it with the gracilis tendon in an attempt to increase the graft strength and stiffness. There is controversy in the literature regarding the normal structural properties of the ACL to be used as a control for reconstructions. Noyes and Grood (99) originally set the standard for ACL linear stiffness as 182 N/mm; however, in a recent study Woo and associates have found this value to be 242 N/mm (132). Woo et al. (132) have demonstrated that the experimental technique used to evaluate the structural ultimate failure strength of the ACL is important, and have reported strength values as high as 2500 N, rather than the original 1725 N standard presented by Noyes et al. (98). This divergence in structural properties emphasizes the importance of reporting the methods used in the biomechanical evaluation of soft tissue structures. Tensile failure testing with the loading direction applied along a bony axis will produce different results in comparison to similar tests performed with load application directed along the length of the ligament fibers (132). This should be recognized in animal studies that use an inappropriate failure test technique, and report a low failure strength value for the normal control ACL. Low control ACL failure strength values will produce a graft to control ACL failure strength ratio, which is inappropriately high.

Butler and colleagues have performed failure tests of ACL subbundles dissected from human cadavers. They reported that spatial variations in strain biomechanics exist along the length of the ACL, with greater values of strain occurring near the insertion sites (24). In a later investigation Butler and associates used similar methodology to show that the anterior ACL subbundles have significantly larger strain energy density and maximum stress values at failure in comparison to the posterior ACL subbundles (20). All ACL subbundles had similar maximum strain values at failure, indicating that each bundle fails by a strain dependent mechanism (20).

Many different autogenous tissues have been used for reconstruction of the ACL. Some of the more popular tissues have included the iliotibial track (ITT) (62,104,123,128), the semitendinosus tendon (83,92), gracilis tendon (98), and the central or medial third of the patellar tendon (5,18,30,65,72,90,113,135). One of the primary biomechanical criteria used in the selection of an autogenous ACL replacement should be the reproduction of the structural and material properties of the normal ACL. This is not only a consideration at the time

of implantation but also during the process of inflammation, repair, and remodeling which results in significant changes in the structural properties of the graft with time after surgery. The temporal remodeling behavior of the different autografts and allografts used for ACL reconstruction has been investigated using the primate, canine, goat, and rabbit models. Newton, Horibe, and Woo have published a comprehensive literature review of the ACL reconstruction studies which have involved different animal models (93).

O'Donoghue et al. (104) reported that the free ITT graft used to replace the ACL in canines had a mean ultimate failure strength of 160 N, which was found to be 23% of the control ACL 4 years after implantation. Van Rens and colleagues (128) also used the canine model to study the biomechanical behavior of the ITT autograft. They reported that the ultimate failure load and graft stiffness were 40% and 45% of the normal control ACL 1 year after surgical reconstruction. Holden et al. (62) investigated the ITT autograft combined with the double belt buckle staple fixation technique using the goat model. They reported that the linear stiffness and ultimate failure load were 10% and 15% of the normal control ACL respectively 2 months postoperative reconstruction.

Of all the autogenous tissues available for ACL reconstruction, Noyes and coworkers (18,98) have reported that a 14 mm wide bone-patellar tendon-bone preparation has the highest ultimate failure strength, reported to range between 159% and 168% of the ultimate failure strength of the human ACL at the time of harvesting. In comparison, whole semitendinosus and gracilis tendons were reported to only have 70% and 49% of the normal ACL strength correspondingly (18,98). Although the studies performed by Noyes and associates have presented important data regarding the relative strengths of autogenous graft tissues, it should be mentioned that in clinical practice the usual width of a patellar tendon graft ranges between 9 mm and 11 mm, while only a portion of the semitendinosus and gracilis are usually harvested. Therefore, the ultimate failure strengths of these graft materials may be considerably less than the previously reported values. This observation has led some to use a combination of tendons (i.e., semitendinosus and gracilis tendons), or to double the semitendinosus. However, no one has shown that adding additional tendons or doubling a single tendon actually increases the ultimate failure strength and linear stiffness of the graft, or determined if they are proportionally additive. An additional advantage of the bone-patellar tendon-bone graft is the bone-to-bone opposition provided for fixation of the graft. This allows secure fixation initially and is thought by some to be an advantage in allowing early joint motion after surgery. As a result, the bone-patellar tendon-bone graft, as originally described by Jones (72), has become the most commonly used ACL graft material.

Even though at the time of implantation the bone-patellar tendon-bone graft may have a superior ultimate failure strength in comparison to the normal ACL, many studies have demonstrated that there is a considerable decrease in the structural properties of the graft (18,19) and changes in the diameter of the collagen fibrils through the time course of healing.

Clancy et al. (30) have shown that patellar tendon autografts used to replace the ACL of the rhesus monkey maintain 80% of their original tensile strength at 1 year following reconstruction. However, the tensile strength of one-third of the patellar tendon used in this procedure was approximately 50% of the strength of the normal ACL in these monkeys.

For a time it was hoped that the structural properties of the patellar tendon graft could be enhanced by maintaining the vascular supply. However, Butler and co-workers demonstrated in cynomolgus monkeys that the structural properties of free grafts were not inferior to similar vascularized patellar tendon grafts (19,23). Therefore, Butler and associates pooled the vascularized and nonvascularized graft data from their primate studies to describe the behavior of both graft types over time. At seven weeks postimplantation the graft stiffness and ultimate failure load was 24% and 16% of the ACL control respectively. At 1 year after surgery the graft stiffness had reached 57% of the normal ACL, while the ultimate failure strength reached 39% of the control ACL (18).

Yoshiya et al. (135,136) used the canine model to demonstrate that the bone-patellar tendon-bone graft had an ultimate failure load and stiffness value which were 20% and 22% of the normal control ACL respectively three months postimplantation. At 20 months the ultimate failure load was only 30% of the control value.

McFarland and associates reported that the patellar tendon autograft used to replace the canine ACL developed an increased vascular response, were more hydrated, while stiffness and ultimate failure strength decreased at a period one month postsurgical reconstruction in comparison to the contralateral control ACLs (89). By 4 months postreconstruction the graft regained only 40% of the normal control ACL failure strength (89). The decrease in strength was found to correlate with the increase in graft water content. This result led the authors to suggest that the change in the ACL graft strength through the healing process may be related to changes in the collagen fiber profile and rearrangement of the graft ultrastructural morphometry.

Shino and colleagues studied the free central patellar tendon autograft and allograft in the canine model (119). At 30 weeks postsurgical reconstruction they reported that the ultimate failure loads of both graft types were 30% of the control ACL. For the autograft the mean energy to failure was 36% of the control ACL, while this figure was 41% for the allografts. The authors reported no significant differences between the mechanical properties of the allografts and the autografts, however, the linear stiffness values for the two different graft types were not compared (119).

At periods up to 1 year the animal studies which have investigated the ITT autograft indicate the ultimate failure load values range between 23% and 40% of the control ACL, while the stiffness was 45% of the normal ACL a year or more postreconstruction. For the patellar tendon autograft the ultimate failure load values have been reported to range between 30% and 45% of the control ACL, while the stiffness has been reported to range between 35% and 57% of the normal ACL, a year or more postreconstruction.

From the biomechanics perspective it is not enough to just evaluate the structural or material properties of an ACL graft. In addition to having adequate strength and stiffness an ACL graft must also control anterior translation of the tibia relative to femur, and to a lesser degree internal-external and varus-valgus laxity of the knee joint. There are, however, very few ACL reconstruction investigations which have reported measurements of knee A-P load-displacement behavior. In one such study Butler has used the canine model to investigate the anterior-posterior displacement response of the knee joint with a combined fascia lata and lateral one-third of the patellar tendon graft at four time intervals (18). At implantation the A-P translation of the operated side was 154% of control, while 4 weeks after reconstruction this ratio increased to 306% (18). By 12 and 26 weeks the A-P translation had decreased to 209% and 153% of the control limb respectively (18). These results demonstrate that anterior translation of the tibia relative to the femur initially increases after surgery, reaching a maximum 1 month postreconstruction, and then decreases approaching the normal joint laxity at a time 6 months postsurgical reconstruction.

In an effort to describe the graft maturation process Yasuda and coworkers (134) made arthroscopic observations of autogenous quadriceps and patellar tendon grafts at various time intervals postsurgical reconstruction in human subjects. Oakes and associates (102) have performed quantitative ultrastructural morphometric analysis of collagen fibril populations in the ACL and patellar tendon grafts using the goat model. The graft remodeling process was found to change the ultrastructural profile of the original patellar tendon at the time of harvest to one containing a larger number of small diameter fibrils (<100 nm). A rapid decrease in the number of large diameter collagen fibers (>100 nm) was found at 12 weeks postsurgical reconstruction. Remodeling was found to begin from the outside of the graft and then move toward the graft center as the remodeling progressed over time. The authors found this remodeling behavior to be consistent with synovial revascularization, demonstrating the importance of not only investigating the surface and central portions of the graft, but also studying different regions along the graft length. Remodeling was found to continue for up to 52 weeks after surgical reconstruction (102). Arnockzy et al. (4) evaluated the temporal revascularization behavior of the patellar tendon graft using a canine model. The authors demonstrated that even when the tibial insertion of the graft was left intact, the patellar tendon graft behaved as an avascular free graft at transplantation. Revascularization of the graft progressed from the proximal and distal regions to the central portion of the graft and was reported to be complete 5 months postsurgical reconstruction.

Experimental studies cited in this review using animal knee joint models are limited with respect to the lack of similarity of the human knee joint. In addition, the animals have an uncontrolled postoperative rehabilitation regimen. Direct application of these results to current clinical practice must be done carefully, however these animal investigations have provided the clinical community with some insight into the graft remodeling process and biomechanical behavior.

POSITIONING OF THE ACL RECONSTRUCTION

Appropriate selection of the intraarticular insertion sites is undoubtedly very important for the successful outcome of ACL reconstruction surgery. However, a thorough review of the literature has revealed many different recommendations for the femoral insertion site of the graft. Some of these positions have included anatomical positioning (103), postero-superior placement (31), posterior placement (36,40), and anterior to the normal ACLs femoral insertion (72). Likewise, there are similar divergent reports in the literature which define appropriate attachment sites for the tibial insertion of the ACL replacement. However, one unique and optimal position exists for the ACL replacement in a given patient. Even though there are many studies which have investigated how knee movement affects the ACL elongation pattern (2,10,32,37,50,79,91,126,127,129), there have been no studies reported which directly describe the appropriate intraarticular position of an ACL replacement required to restore "normal" tibiofemoral kinematics. Previous experimental studies performed by Hefzy et al. (59,60) have used indirect approaches in their effort to describe the appropriate intraarticular position of a cruciate ligament replacement. The objective of their experimental study was to characterize the displacement patterns of various regions of the normal cruciate ligaments *in vitro*. They revealed that the displacement patterns of the ACLs bundle fibers are very sensitive to their precise intraarticular position during knee motion, and determined which regions of the cruciate ligaments underwent a minimum relative change in length throughout knee flexion. The femoral attachment that produced the smallest relative change in length, 2 mm or less, formed a region that was oriented in a proximal distal direction at the anatomical center of the ACL's femoral insertion (60). This region was described as an appropriate choice for cruciate replacement attachment. This work is founded on the premise that attachment of the ligament replacement to this region will allow the graft to undergo a minimal change in length and associated load (clinically termed "isometric" placement) during knee function. Even though this premise is founded on sound reasoning, it may only be true for reattachment of the normal anterior cruciate ligament, and not a replacement which has material and geometrical properties that are dissimilar to the normal cruciate ligament. Another limitation to this approach is that the actual insertion sites of the cruciate ligaments were not varied, but instead displacement patterns of the different pseudofibers of the normal cruciate ligaments were measured. Attachment of a cruciate ligament replacement at this potential site may not reproduce normal knee kinematics. Performing predictive measurements while actually moving potential ligament insertion sites should simulate the interaction between joint geometry and the cruciate ligaments which result once the ACL replacement is implanted *in vivo*.

The morphology of the normal ACL cannot be reproduced by any of the graft materials currently used (68). Consequently, the biomechanical behavior of the normal ACL cannot be completely reproduced. There are no fibers within the ACL that are isometric (60,69, 114,120). Therefore, it is impossible to identify positions of attachment that would allow no change in length of the graft during a range of knee motion. The anteromedial band has been characterized as the portion of the normal ACL which demonstrates the least amount of length change during knee flexion, and therefore is closest to demonstrating "isometric" or constant length behavior (114). Thus, autogenous grafting procedures should probably strive to reproduce the function of the anteromedial band of the ACL (69). Placement of the graft at the center of the tibial and femoral attachment of the anteromedial band results in the least amount of strain during knee flexion-extension motion (69).

Research at the University of Vermont has focused on the measurement of ACL biomechanics in subjects with normal knee joints (10), and ACL graft behavior at the time of surgical reconstruction in the *in vivo* environment (7,8,42). A comparison between the normal ACL and the bone-patellar tendon-bone graft behaviors have shown similarities in the magnitude and pattern of elongation (Fig. 1). This finding indicates restoration of normal ligament behavior, and indirectly suggests restoration of normal knee kinematics. This finding also demonstrates that reproducing the function of the anteromedial portion of the ACL is possible.

In an effort to aid in the identification of the centers of

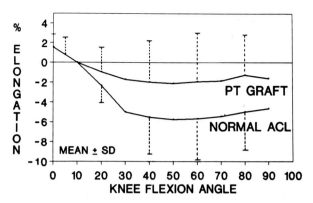

FIG. 1. The passive range of motion activity. Average strain data for patients with normal anterior cruciate ligaments (n = 10) and for patients immediately after ACL reconstruction with a bone-patellar tendon-bone graft (n = 10). (From ref. 8, with permission.)

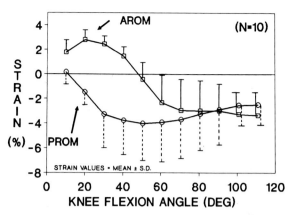

FIG. 2. Average data for 10 subjects for active and passive motion of the knee joint (AROM and PROM, correspondingly). Graph of anteromedial band strain (%) versus knee angle. (From ref. 10, with permission.)

graft attachment points, isometers (53) and tension/isometers (34) have been developed. Isometers have been designed to measure the displacement pattern between potential tibial and femoral graft attachment sites. Fixation of one end of the suture to the femoral attachment site and fixation of the compliant isometer spring-loaded scale to the suture extending from the trial tunnel in the tibia allows the operator to determine if the potential tunnel sites are in the optimal position. The clinician performs the isometer measurement by coursing the knee through a full range of motion while observing the maximum change in displacement magnitude and pattern of the isometer. Common clinical criteria indicates that if the change in displacement is less than 2 mm, then the proposed attachment sites are in the proper position (53,108). The Medmetric tension/isometer (Medmetric Corp, San Diego, California) is similar in design to compliant isometer spring-loaded scales, but is calibrated to measure both force and displacement. The tension/isometer is applied using a different protocol in comparison to the standard isometer systems. With the knee positioned at 90°, a suture which has been placed through the trial tunnels is tensioned (6 N is recommended) and the position on the displacement scale is recorded. The knee is then moved into extension where the tension magnitude developed along the suture line is readjusted to the initial tension (6 N). The change in displacement relative to 90° is then documented. As with the isometer measurement technique, if the change in displacement is less than 2 mm then the trial tunnels are considered to be in the proper position (34).

The decision to accept or reject the isometer or tension/isometer measurements should be based on whether the measured displacement pattern and maximum change in displacement are similar to that described for the normal anteromedial bundle of the ACL in vivo during passive knee flexion-extension (Fig. 2) (10). For passive flexion-extension motion of the knee

the difference in ACL strain between mean peak and mean minimum values was found to be 4.2% (range 3.0 to 7.2%). If this difference is assumed to occur uniformly over the anteromedial bundle length, (the mean length of the anteromedial band is 36 mm) (95), there would be an average change in anteromedial bundle length of 1.5 mm (range 1.1 – to – 2.6 mm). In addition, the clinician should strive to match the pattern of ACL strain versus knee flexion measured in vivo (Fig. 2) with that measured by the isometer. This would require the isometer to measure elongation ranging between 1.1 and 2.5 mm, indicating an increase in strain or developed tension, as the joint is brought from 50° (where it should be at a minimum), out to extension. Likewise, as the knee is flexed from 50° to near full flexion, the isometer should demonstrate some increase in elongation. If the isometer measurement does not duplicate the normal ACL displacement magnitude and pattern, new tunnel sites should be selected.

Caution must be used in the interpretation of isometer or tension/isometer measurements because they are made in a knee with a torn ACL. The kinematics in such a knee are abnormal, and therefore the isometer measurement may be misleading. Fleming and associates have studied the O.S.I. CA-5000 drill guide isometer in vivo in subjects with acute and chronic ACL disruptions, comparing the predictive isometer elongation measurement with the resulting graft elongation pattern (44,46). With passive knee extension from 30° to 10°, both the isometer measurement prediction and implanted graft exhibit elongation, suggesting that the replacement gets taut as the knee is extended from 30° of flexion (Fig. 3). However, with flexion of the knee from 40° the isometer demonstrates a greater elongation between the trial tunnel attachment sites relative to full extension, predicting the graft to get even more taut in flexion relative to 10°. This finding is contrary to the resulting graft behavior after fixation. A linear correlation between the predictive

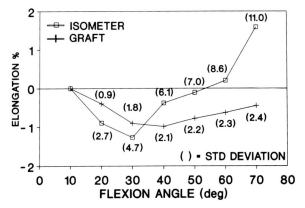

FIG. 3. Mean elongation data for the predictive OSI CA-5000 isometer measurement system and resulting bone-patellar tendon-bone graft elongation pattern (n = 10). The standard deviations are presented in parentheses. (From ref. 44, with permission.)

isometer elongation measure and the resulting patellar tendon graft elongation pattern has been shown (Fig. 4) (44). Even though there was a significant correlation between predictive isometer measurement and resulting graft behavior, the coefficient of determination (r^2) value was only .09. This coefficient indicates that only 9% of the total variability is explained by the linear relationship of the predictive isometer elongation measurement on resulting graft elongation. This low coefficient of determination indicates a variable regression. The standard error of the y-estimate, which indicates the error in the actual graft elongation prediction, was relatively high (1.8%) considering the average maximum graft elongation was 2%. A regression analysis was also performed on each individual patient (46). This analysis showed that the isometer prediction of graft elongation was not significant in 44% of the subjects (46). Considering this finding, the low coefficient of determination, and the high

standard error value, isometer measurement systems may not provide an accurate prediction of graft elongation behavior, and thus graft tunnel position.

There are several possible explanations for the discrepancies between isometer measurement systems and the graft biomechanics after implantation. One possible source for the unexplained variability may be attributed to an insufficient accuracy of the isometer systems. The resolution of the OSI CA-5000 device and the other commercially available isometer systems is no better than .5 mm. In clinical application of the isometer systems, trial tunnel positions are considered "near isometric" if the change in displacement with repeated flexion of the knee is less than or equal to 2 mm (53,108). Therefore, a resolution error of 25% must be associated with the application of current commercially available isometer measurement systems. A second possible source of the unexplained variability may result from performing the isometry measurement in an ACL deficient knee which may have abnormal kinematics in comparison to the normal or reconstructed knee. The isometer spring-scale stiffness is orders of magnitude less than that of the normal ACL or graft substitute. Therefore, near normal kinematics cannot be restored to the knee at the time the predictive measurement is made. A third source of variability may be attributed to the increased variability in tibiofemoral kinematics associated with an ACL deficient knee. To reduce this variability, application of a compressive joint force (114) or an anterior shear force (60) has been recommended while the knee is passively flexed during the isometry measurement. To date, this effect has not been confirmed through *in vivo* measurements.

The approach used at the University of Vermont in choosing ACL insertion sites is to restore knee kinematics with a trial ACL substitute, and then perform the predictive tunnel placement measurement (43). To accomplish this task we have developed a system where the ACL substitute is positioned at the potential femoral tunnel while the tibial end is fixed to a load cell positioned at the tunnel entrance (Fig. 5). With this technique, an initial ACL substitute tension which restores joint kinematics or, in this application, A-P plane load-displacement behavior, may be applied prior to making the predictive tunnel position measurement. This approach reduces the abnormal and variable kinematics associated with the ACL deficient knee, and the tunnel position measurement is then made under conditions similar to those which exist once the graft is positioned and fixed in place. The highly compliant isometer and tension/isometer displacement measurement systems are not designed to restore normal kinematics to the knee joint. Fleming and colleagues have demonstrated that the compliant spring isometer measurement correlates poorly with the tension measurement made along the ACL substitute after it was fixed in the tunnels (43).

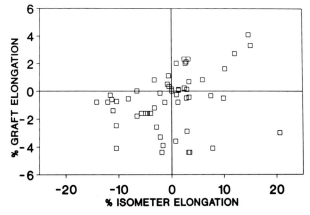

FIG. 4. The passive range of motion activity. Linear correlation between predictive isometer measurement and graft elongation (n = 10). A significant correlation was found (p ≤ .01); however, the coefficient of determination was only .09, indicating a variable correlation. (From ref. 44, with permission.)

extended position. Placement of the tibial tunnel is not considered as important as the femoral. However, the tibial tunnel should be positioned so that the graft does not impinge against the roof of the intercondylar notch when the knee is fully extended (17,59,60).

INITIAL TENSIONING OF THE GRAFT DURING FIXATION

After proper intraarticular positioning of the graft is achieved, an appropriate initial tension which restores joint kinematics to within normal limits must be developed. This concept not only involves developing a tension along the graft once positioned in the knee, but also includes the concept of preconditioning the graft prior to insertion and fixation. Graf et al. (54) have shown that preconditioning a previously frozen patellar tendon-tibia complex will significantly reduce acute load relaxation after implantation. Preconditioning by applying a fixed amount of deformation was more effective in reducing acute load relaxation in comparison to preconditioning with cyclic loading. Daniel and associates recommend preconditioning of the graft with the Medmetric Tension/isometer system (34).

The initial tension developed along an ACL graft at the time of fixation has a direct effect on restoration of normal knee kinematics. An initial tension which is too high may overconstrain the knee, compromise the ability of the graft to survive, permanently elongate the graft, or cause fixation failure (11). Insufficient initial tension may not provide enough joint stability and produce a lax knee (11). Consequently, there is a complex link between initial graft tension and tibiofemoral joint kinematics.

The initial load and strain on an ACL graft at the time of fixation has also been shown to affect the healing and remodeling process (3,136). Previous work performed at The University of Vermont has studied the effect of initial strain developed in the canine bone-patellar tendon-bone preparation in vivo (3). In this investigation, the strain biomechanics of the ACL graft were measured at the time of implantation and correlated against the ultimate failure strength of the graft 1 year postimplantation. The results suggest a trend in which grafts with high strain values at the time of implantation produce a substantially lower ultimate failure strength 1 year postimplantation (3). Yoshiya et al. (136) studied the effect of initial bone-patellar tendon-bone graft tension set at 1 N and 39 N using an in vivo canine model. They demonstrated that patellar tendon grafts tensioned to 39 N at the time of fixation had poor vascularity and focal myxoid degeneration in comparison to grafts with a 1 N initial tension. A comparison of A-P knee displacement at the load limits of 20 N, made between the two initial graft tension settings, did not demonstrate a significant

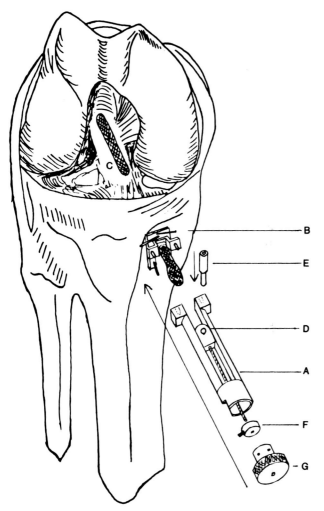

FIG. 5. Tension measurement system used to determine ACL graft tunnel positions. (From ref. 43, with permission.)

This evidence further questions the accuracy of current commercially available isometer measurement systems.

Because of the high degree of variability, identification of optimal ACL graft attachment sites should not be based only on isometer or tension/isometer measurements. Attention to proper three-dimensional anatomy of the tunnels is necessary. Accurate position of the femoral tunnel is critical (60,69). Anterior placement of the graft tunnel, relative to the normal anatomical insertion of the ACL, will result in high strain along the graft as the knee is flexed (25,63,108,115). Knee flexion may be restricted if the graft remains intact, or if normal range of motion is restored the graft may stretch out and permanently elongate (69). Graft placement posterior or distal to the normal attachment site of the ACL may result in excessive tightening of the graft as the knee is extended (14,25,59,120). The over-the-top position results in this anatomical variation. Therefore, some surgeons create a trough in the femur to bring the graft closer to the anatomical position, or they fix the graft with the knee in the difference three months postreconstruction. The ultimate failure load and stiffness values for the two initial graft tensions were also found to be similar (136). Burks and Leland (16) measured the graft tension required to restore normal tibiofemoral A-P load-displacement behavior in human cadaver specimens. To restore normal A-P load-displacement behavior they found that the following initial tensions were required at the time of soft tissue fixation: the patellar tendon 16 N, the semitendinosus 38 N, and the iliotibial band required 60 N of tension (16). This study demonstrated that the graft replacement pretension was specific to the graft material and the free length of the graft between fixation sites. Hefzy et al. (60) used a steel cable to replace the ACL in human cadavers and revealed that joint kinematics were restored when the cable was set at loads ranging between 4.5 and 9.0 N with the knee positioned at 90° of flexion. Noyes and colleagues have arbitrarily advocated adjusting ACL graft tension to allow 5 mm of "normal" anteroposterior translation with the knee flexed to 20° (97). The authors termed this clinical procedure as "building laxity into the knee joint."

It is currently unknown what initial graft tension will restore knee kinematics to within "normal" limits in sagittal, transverse, and coronal reference planes. It should be recognized that the loads on the ACL *in vivo* are currently unknown. Consequently, it is impossible to accurately recommend an appropriate graft tension at the time of fixation. In addition, it should be recognized that all grafts will exhibit a viscoelastic response. Therefore, after the graft is tensioned to the desired level and fixed to bone, the graft-fixation construct may undergo stress relaxation. Consequently, the effect of the initial graft tension on knee kinematics may decrease over time. Restoring the strain biomechanics of the normal ACL, or the normal contralateral knee A-P plane load-displacement behavior may be the best indirect measure currently available to assess proper initial tension of the graft, and restoration of normal knee kinematics at the time of reconstruction.

FIXATION OF THE GRAFT

The long-term success of any anterior cruciate ligament graft is also dependent on the type and integrity of graft fixation to the host bone. It has been shown by some investigators that the initial weak-link in the tibia-graft-femur construct is the fixation of the graft to bone, and not the isolated strength of the graft material (80,112). Robertson and associates (112), along with Kurosaka and coworkers (80), have demonstrated that placement of large major diameter interference-fit screws between the patellar tendon graft bone plugs and the tunnel wall, and fixation of soft tissue with a screw and spiked washer, produced higher initial fixation strength in comparison to fixation with staples and sutures. While the interference fit screw is the standard for bone-patellar tendon-bone fixation there is no consensus regarding optimal fixation for semitendinosus grafts. In a recent investigation we have compared the double staple belt-buckle with the double spiked washer in a figure-8 fixation technique using the bovine model (110). The double staple belt-buckle technique was found to be the stronger of the two methods in maximum load and yield point for single cycle failure testing. The mechanism of failure was different for each technique. For the figure 8 technique the tendons pulled through the spiked washers shredding the tendon, while for the belt buckle method a partial rupture occurred at the proximal staple where the tendons turned 180°.

Not all fixation techniques have been studied. Additional investigations are necessary before the ideal method of fixation can be identified. The relative ability of any fixation technique to resist repetitive physiological loads while maintaining strength and integrity over time needs to be evaluated before definitive recommendations can be made. Objective planning of postoperative rehabilitation programs should recognize that even though the ultimate failure strength of graft fixation is initially weaker than the graft material itself, this may be a relatively unimportant measure of the integrity of graft fixation over time. For example, the primary failure mechanism of a free tendon graft such as the semitendinosus may be a relative slip between the graft and fixation.

POSTOPERATIVE REHABILITATION REGIMEN

Innumerable investigations have documented the deleterious effects of knee immobilization on leg muscles, articular cartilage, periarticular bone, ligaments, and capsular structures (58,74–76,78,96). Yet it is possible that early unprotected motion may result in permanent elongation, if not destruction of reconstructed ligaments or capsular tissues. Thus, many clinicians advocate immobilization immediately following ACL reconstruction, while others believe that early mobilization may avoid many of the disadvantages while not significantly endangering the healing tissues (117). Since the loads developed along an ACL graft *in vivo* are currently unknown for all rehabilitation exercises, the relative risk of overloading and permanently elongating a reconstruction is unknown. Consequently, it is not surprising that a number of different rehabilitation protocols, ranging from low to high risk, have been advocated. This discussion demonstrates the controversy surrounding cruciate ligament rehabilitation.

Recent work performed at the University of Vermont

has established a scientific basis for the various means of protection and mobilization of the knee following ACL reconstruction by measuring the strain biomechanics of the normal ACL *in vivo* (7,9,10). This work involved arthroscopic implantation of the Hall Effect Strain Transducer (Microstrain Co., Burlington, Vermont) into the anteromedial band (AMB) of the normal ACL after partial meniscectomy or other minor procedure was performed under local anesthesia. This allowed the study patients full control of their lower limb musculature. The objective of these studies was to provide data for the clinical management of patients who have had ACL ruptures.

It was revealed that anterior shear loads of 150 N applied at 30° of flexion (the Lachman test) produced more strain within the normal AMB than did shear testing at 90° (the anterior drawer test) (10). Henning et al. (61) directly measured the displacement pattern of the anteromedial aspect of the ACL *in vivo* under anterior shear load conditions and demonstrated that the Lachman test produced greater elongation of the anteromedial band in comparison to the anterior drawer test. These *in vivo* results (10) are in agreement with previously published studies which either used instrumented knee laxity testing or clinical impressions to assess the behavior of the ACL under clinical examination conditions and confirm that the Lachman test is the clinical examination of choice to evaluate the integrity of the ACL (35,66, 67,85,124,125).

The *in vivo* study revealed that there was no significant change in AMB strain during isometric quadriceps contraction when the knee was maintained at either 60 or 90° of flexion (9,10). At these flexion angles, across all study patients, the AMB remained unstrained (or slack) as quadriceps activity increased. Isometric quadriceps strengthening should, therefore, be safe in the ACL injured or reconstructed knee if the flexion angle is maintained between 60° and 90°. At 30° of knee flexion, isometric quadriceps activity produced a large increase in AMB strain, and should be carefully controlled especially during the early stages of rehabilitation where soft tissue fixation may be tenuous (10), or the graft strength has diminished during remodeling (18). Nisell, Németh, and Ohlsén developed a two-dimensional analytic model of the knee (94). They predicted that isometric quadriceps extension against a fixed resistance produced an anterior directed shear force on the tibia with the knee positioned between 0° and 60°. An isometric quadriceps extension effort between 60° and full flexion produced posterior directed forces on the tibia which would strain the posterior cruciate ligament or its replacement, and not the ACL. Using a similar modeling approach, Yasuda and Sasaki (133) developed a two-dimensional sagittal plane equilibrium model of the knee with input parameters obtained from roentgenographic films and electromyographic measurements made on 20 healthy male subjects. Model predictions suggested that all subjects had a posterior directed shear force acting on the tibia between 70° and 90°. Between 70° and full extension the shear force was oriented in the anterior direction. This finding lead the authors to recommend that isometric quadriceps extension activities which are prescribed after an ACL reconstruction procedure should begin with the knee at or greater than 70° of flexion (133). For isometric hamstrings activity, the predicted shear force was posteriorly directed at all knee angles. As a result of these findings, the authors considered this a safe activity to be performed immediately following ACL surgery (133). The *in vivo* ACL strain study indicated that the knee flexion angle at which isometric quadriceps activity produced an increase in ACL strain, and may become unsafe for the injured or reconstructed ACL, is somewhere between 60° and 30° and remains to be determined (9,10). The model predictions presented by Yasuda and Sasaki (133) and Nisell et al. (94) suggest that isometric quadriceps extension efforts at knee angles between 60° and 0° may become unsafe for a newly reconstructed ACL, while with the knee positioned between 60° and full flexion this activity would produce minimal or no loading along the ACL reconstruction and would be safe.

In vivo strain measured within the AMB when a seated subject performed an isotonic quadriceps contraction (active range of motion) consistently produced a positive region of strain values between 10° and 48°, and an unstrained region between 48° and 110° of flexion (10) (Fig. 2). Active range of motion rehabilitation programs may now be prescribed with these two flexion angle regions adapted to the clinicians' requirements. In the unstrained region, quadriceps activity associated with active range of motion did not produce significantly different AMB strain values in comparison to the same knee motion without contraction of the leg musculature (flexion-extension motion of the subject's knee performed by an investigator and termed passive range of motion) (10). This suggests that active range of motion between the limits of 50° and 100° may be performed safely immediately following ACL reconstruction. The active range of motion activity may then move to the positive strain region when the reconstruction and fixation will tolerate this level of strain (*a time as yet not determined*). The maximum active range of motion strain values were greater (ranging between 4.1% and 1.5%) in comparison to the maximum passive range of motion strain values (10). Application of a 10 lb weight boot to the subject's foot during the active range of motion activity increased the AMB strain in comparison to the same activity without a weight boot (9). Grood et al. (57) have demonstrated in an *in vitro* model that leg extension exercises (in the range of 0°–30°) produce load-

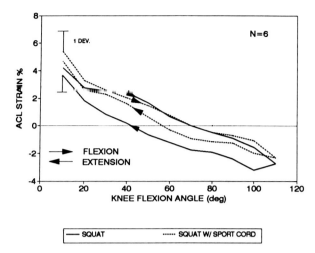

FIG. 6. The free squat and squat with Sport Cord (Sport Cord, Sandy, Utah) average strain data for patients with normal anterior cruciate ligaments (*n* = 6). A graph of ACL strain (%) plotted as a function of knee angle. (From ref. 9, with permission.)

ings which are potentially destructive to the repaired or reconstructed ACL. Further investigation is required to determine if the active range of motion strain values between 10° and 48° are large enough to produce permanent elongation of the reconstructed tissue or failure of the fixation construct. Our findings illustrate that both muscle activity and knee position determine AMB strain at rest and with joint motion (7,9,10). It appears that for active range of motion the AMB is strained between the limits of full extension and 48° (10). These findings are consistent with Henning's *in vivo* study of two patients with injured ligaments (61) and the findings of Markolf and associates (84).

Investigation of ACL strain *in vivo* during the squatting activity has revealed positive AMB strain values between 70° and full extension (9) (Fig. 6). The mean peak strain value for the free squat occurred at 10° of flexion and was a value of 4.2%. Elevated strain values were found during the squatting activities with application of the Sport Cord (Sport Cord Inc., Sandy, Utah), an elastic resistive device used in ACL rehabilitation programs (9). For this activity the peak strain value was also reached at 10° and was 5.4% (Fig. 6). A smaller hysteresis loop response was measured during the squat with the sport cord in comparison to that recorded during the free squat. This may be attributed to the increased tibiofemoral compressive force produced by the sport cord and leg musculature.

In vivo strain measured within the AMB for passive range of motion between 110° and full extension revealed that the ACL reaches positive strain values as the joint is brought into extension, and remains at or below the zero strain level between the limits of 11° and 110° of flexion using thigh and distal leg support during motion (10) (Fig. 2). Therefore, continuous passive motion of the knee within these limits should be safe for an ACL graft immediately following surgery when the leg is supported throughout flexion-extension motion without applied varus/valgus loading, internal/external torques, or anterior shear forces. The limits near extension (0° to 10°), however, can cause small magnitudes of strain (1% or less on average) (10). We feel this should be viewed as a relatively mild constraint to bracing a patient's knee in 0° of extension, or to the use of CPM during a rehabilitation program. A ranked comparison of the different activities evaluated in subjects with normal ACLs, ordered from high to low risk based on peak AMB strain values, is presented in Table 1. These *in vivo* data may be used in the development of objective ACL reconstruction rehabilitation programs.

TABLE 1. *Rank comparison of activities based on peak strain measurements during activity*

Activity	Peak *in vivo* ACL[a] strain	Test subjects (n)
Squat with sport cord	5.4 ± 1.6 @ 10° flexion	6
Squat without sport cord	4.2 ± 2.0 @ 10° flexion	6
AROM[b] with 10-lb weight boot	4.0% @ 10° flexion	8
Lachman test @ 150 (N) anterior shear	3.7%	10
AROM	3.1% @ 20° flexion	15
Isometric quadriceps contraction at 30° to 30 N-m exterior torque	3.0%	14
Anterior drawer @ 150 (N)	1.8%	10
PROM[c]	0.1% @ 0° flexion	10
Isometric quadriceps contraction at 90° and 60° to 30 N-m exterior torque	0.0%	14

[a] ACL, anterior cruciate ligament.
[b] AROM, active flexion-extension of the knee.
[c] PROM, passive flexion-extension of the knee.

FUTURE STUDIES

Future research endeavors in ACL biomechanics should recognize the complex behavior of the ACL and graft substitutes. The complex morphometry and different biomechanical properties of the ACL subbundles require that they be studied individually, and not grouped together as one structure. Therefore, it is probably not enough to just study the resultant ACL or graft substitute load. The ACL and graft substitute should be considered to have a stress and strain distribution across a transverse cross section. The strain distribution is probably dependent on joint position, joint loading, and will vary along the length of the ACL with higher strain values occurring near the insertions of the ligament to bone. The *in vivo* strain measurements as described in this chapter have attempted to accomplish this task through highly specific measurements (7–10). These studies, however, have only focused on the midsubstance and anteromedial portion of the ACL. The other ACL subbundles, and regions across the ligament insertions need to be investigated *in vivo* to describe this structure fully. ACL biomechanics research should continue to perform *in vivo* strain measurements of the soft tissues surrounding the knee, and establish new *in vivo* measurement techniques such as pressure or force sensors (12,33,51). In addition, the development of an analytic model that includes both patellofemoral and tibiofemoral articulations will permit the study of the complex ACL subbundle structure, investigation of injury mechanisms, allow the study of soft tissue reconstruction procedures, and permit the research of commonly prescribed rehabilitation activities. Application of the *in vivo* experimental techniques and analytical models to ACL reconstruction procedures should strive to reproduce normal ACL biomechanics, knee kinematics, and establish the relation between the biomechanical behavior of an ACL graft and the resulting biological properties. Methodology, such as an implantable, telemeterized load sensor, need to be designed to allow an optimal match between a rehabilitation regimen and the biological-mechanical behavior of the graft. Research efforts in biomechanics should strive to establish intraoperative techniques and measurements which can accurately provide the surgeon with the ability to reestablish normal joint kinematics during a soft tissue reconstruction procedure. Future clinical investigations of surgical procedures should include prospective, randomized, well-controlled, long-term studies which use standardized outcome evaluation techniques to assess the relative effectiveness of the many different soft tissue reconstruction techniques.

ACKNOWLEDGMENT

The authors acknowledge support from National Institute of Health Grants R01 AR39213 and R01 AR40174.

REFERENCES

1. AAOS Faculty Course. (1988): The knee: current concepts, New Orleans, November 3–5.
2. Arms SW, Pope MH, Johnson RJ, et al. (1984): The biomechanics of anterior cruciate ligament rehabilitation and reconstruction. *Am J Sports Med,* 12:8–18.
3. Arms SW, Pope MH, Johnson, RJ, Renström PA, Fischer RA, Jarvinen M, Beynnon BD. (1990): Analysis of ACL failure strength and initial strains in the canine model. In: *Proceedings of the 36th Annual Meeting of the Orthopaedics Research Society, New Orleans, LA, February.* Trans Orthop Res Soc: Park Ridge, Ill. 15:524.
4. Arnoczky SP, Tarvin GB, Marshall JL. (1982): Anterior cruciate ligament replacement using patellar tendon: an evaluation of graft revascularization in the dog. *J Bone Joint Surg [Am],* 64A:217–224.
5. Arnoczky SP, Warren RF, Ashlock MA. (1986): Replacement of the anterior cruciate ligament using a patellar tendon allograft. *J Bone Joint Surg [Am],* 68A:376–385.
6. Arnold JA, Coker TP, Heaton LM, Park JP, Harris WD. (1979): Natural history of anterior cruciate tears. *Am J Sports Med,* 7:305–313.
7. Beynnon BD. (1991): *The in-vivo biomechanics of the anterior cruciate ligament, reconstruction, and application of a mathematical model to the knee joint* [Dissertation]. Burlington, VT: University of Vermont.
8. Beynnon BD, Fleming BC, Johnson RJ, Renström PA, Nichols CE, Pope MH. (1992): The measurement of anterior cruciate ligament graft biomechanics in-vivo. Submitted for publication.
9. Beynnon BD, Fleming BC, Johnson RJ, Renström PA, Nichols CE, Pope MH. (1992): ACL strain behavior during rehabilitation activities. Submitted for publication.
10. Beynnon BD, Howe JG, Pope MH, Johnson RJ, Fleming BC. (1992): The measurement of anterior cruciate ligament strain *in vivo. Int Orthop,* 16:1–12.
11. Beynnon BD, Huston DR, Pope MH, Fleming BC, Johnson RJ, Nichols CE, Renström PA. (1992): The effect of ACL reconstruction tension on the knee and cruciate ligaments. *Trans Orthop Res,* 17:657.
12. Beynnon BD, Stankewich CJ, Fleming BC, Pope MH, Johnson RJ. (1991): The development and initial testing of a new sensor to simultaneously measure strain and pressure in tendons and ligaments. In: *Transactions of the Combined Orthopaedics Research Society of USA, Japan, and Canada, Banff, Alberta, Canada, October 21–23,* p 104.
13. Blackburn TA. (1985): Rehabilitation of ACL injuries. *Orthop Clin North Am,* 16:241–269.
14. Bradley J, Fitzpatrick D, Daniel D, et al. (1988): Orientation of the cruciate ligament in the sagittal plane. *J Bone Joint Surg [Br],* 70B:94–99.
15. Brostrom L, Gillquist J, Liljedahl SO, Lindvall N. (1968): Treatment of old ruptures of the anterior cruciate ligament. *Lakartidningen,* 65:4479–4486.
16. Burks RT, Leland R. (1988): Determination of graft tension before fixation in ACL reconstruction. *Arthroscopy,* 4:260–266.
17. Burns GS, Howell SM. (1992): The effect of tibial hole placement and roofplasty on impingement of anterior cruciate ligament reconstructions. *Trans Orthop Res,* 17:656.
18. Butler DL. (1989): The anterior cruciate ligament: its normal response and replacement. *J Orthop Res,* 7:910–921.
19. Butler DL, Grood ES, Noyes FR, Olmstead ML, Hohn RB, Arnoczky SP, Siegel MG. (1989): Mechanical properties of primate vascularized vs. nonvascularized patellar tendon grafts: changes over time. *J Orthop Res,* 7:68–79.
20. Butler DL, Guan Y, Kay MD, Feder SM, Cummings FJ. (1991): Location-dependent variations in the material properties of anterior cruciate ligament subunits. *Trans Orthop Res Soc,* 16:234.
21. Butler DL, Kay MD, Stouffer DC. (1986): Comparison of material properties in fascicle-bone units from human patellar tendon and knee ligaments. *J Biomech,* 19:425–432.
22. Butler DL, Noyes FR, Grood ES, Miller ES, Malek M. (1979): Mechanical properties of transplants for the anterior cruciate ligament. *Trans Orthop Res Soc,* 4:81.

23. Butler DL, Noyes FR, Grood ES, Olmstead ML, Hohn RB. (1983): The effects of vascularity on the mechanical properties of primate anterior cruciate ligament replacements. *Trans Orthop Res Soc*, 8:93.

24. Butler DL, Sheh MY, Stouffer DC, Samaranayake VA, Levy MS. (1990): Surface strain variation in human patellar tendon and knee cruciate ligaments. *J Biomech Eng*, 112:38–45.

25. Bylski-Austrow D, Grood E, Hefzy M, et al. (1990): Anterior cruciate ligament replacements: a mechanical study of femoral attachment location, flexion angle at tensioning, and initial tension. *J Orthop Res*, 8:522–531.

26. Cabaud HE, Feagin JA. (1979): Experimental studies of acute anterior cruciate ligament injury and repair. *Am J Sports Med*, 7:18–22.

27. Cabaud HE, Feagin JA, Rodkey WG. (1980): Acute anterior cruciate ligament injury and augmental repair. *Am J Sports Med*, 8:395–401.

28. Clancy WG. (1983): A static intra-articular and dynamic extra-articular procedure. *Clin Orthop*, 172:102–106.

29. Clancy WG. (1988): Arthroscopic anterior cruciate reconstruction with patellar tendon. *Techn Orthop*, 2:13–22.

30. Clancy WG, Narechania RG, Rosenberg TD, Gmeiner JG, Wisnefske D, Lange TA. (1981): Anterior and posterior cruciate ligament reconstruction in rhesus monkeys. *J Bone Joint Surg [Am]*, 63A:1270–1284.

31. Clancy WG, Nelson DA, Reider B, Narechania RG. (1982): Anterior cruciate ligament reconstruction using one-third of the patellar ligament augmented by extra-articular tendon transfers. *J Bone Joint Surg [Am]*, 64A:352–359.

32. Crowninshield R, Pope MH, Johnson RJ. (1976): An analytical model of the knee. *J Biomech*, 9:397–405.

33. Cummings JF, Holden JP, Grood ES, Wroble RR, Butler DL, Schafer JA. (1991): *In-vivo* measurement of patella tendon forces and joint position in the goat model. *Trans Orthop Res Soc*, 16:601.

34. Daniel D. (1990): Principles of knee ligament surgery. In: Daniel DM, Akeson WH, O'Connor JJ, eds. *Knee ligaments: structure, function, injury and repair*. New York: Raven Press, pp 11–29.

35. Daniel D, Malcolm L, Losse G, Stone M, Sachs R, Barks R. (1985): Instrumented measurement of anterior laxity of the knee. *J Bone Joint Surg [Am]*, 67A:720–725.

36. Drez DJ. (1978): Modified Eriksson procedure for chronic anterior cruciate instability. *Orthopedics*, 1:30–36.

37. Edwards RG, Lafferty JF, Lange KD. (1970): Ligament strain in the human knee. *J Basic Eng*, 92:131–136.

38. Ellison AE. (1979): Distal iliotibial band transfer for anterolateral rotatory instability of the knee. *J Bone Joint Surg [Am]*, 61A:320–337.

39. Engebretsen L, Renum P, Sundalsvoll S. (1989): Primary suture of the anterior cruciate ligament: a 6-year follow up of 74 cases. *Acta Orthop Scand*, 60:561–564.

40. Eriksson E. (1976): Reconstruction of the anterior cruciate ligament. *Orthop Clin North Am*, 7:167–169.

41. Fetto JW, Marshall JL. (1980): The natural history and diagnosis of the anterior cruciate ligament insufficiency. *Clin Orthop*, 147:29–38.

42. Fleming BC, Beynnon BD, Erickson AE, Pope MH, Johnson RJ, Nichols CE, Howe JG. (1990): An *in vivo* study of the reconstructed anterior cruciate ligament at the time of implantation. In: *Proceedings of the 36th Annual Meeting of the Orthopaedics Research Society, New Orleans, LA, February 15*, p 84.

43. Fleming BC, Beynnon BD, Johnson RJ, McLeod W, Pope MH. (1993): Isometers versus tensiometers: a comparison for the reconstruction of the anterior cruciate ligament. *Am J Sports Med*, 21:82–88.

44. Fleming BC, Beynnon BD, Nichols CE, Renström PA, Erickson AE, Johnson RJ, Pope MH. (1992): *In-vivo* comparison between predictive isometry measurement and elongation in the reconstructed ACL. *Trans Orthop Res Soc*, 17:222.

45. Fleming BC, Beynnon BD, Howe JG, McLeod W, Pope MH. (1992): Effect of tension and placement of a prosthetic anterior cruciate ligament on anteroposterior laxity of the knee. *J Orthop Res*, 10:177–186.

46. Fleming BC, Beynnon BD, Johnson RJ, Nichols CE, Renström PA, Pope MH. (1992): A comparison between isometry measurements and reconstructed ACL elongation *in-vivo*. Submitted for publication.

47. Furman W, Marshall JL, Girgis FC. (1976): The anterior cruciate ligament—a functional analysis based on post-mortem studies. *J Bone Joint Surg [Am]*, 58A:179–185.

48. Galway RD, Beaupre A, MacIntosh DL. (1972): The lateral pivot shift: a clinical sign of symptomatic anterior cruciate insufficiency. *J Bone Joint Surg [Br]*, 54B:762–763.

49. Gerber C, Matter P. (1983): Biomechanical analysis of the knee after rupture of the anterior cruciate ligament and its primary repair: an instant-centre analysis of function. *J Bone Joint Surg [Br]*, 65B:392–399.

50. Girgis FG, Marshall JL, Al Monajem RSH. (1975): The cruciate ligaments of the knee joint. *Clin Orthop*, 106:216–231.

51. Glos DL, Holden JP, Butler DL, Grood ES. (1990): Pressure versus deflected beam force measurement in the human patella tendon. *Trans Orthop Res Soc*, 15:490.

52. Gollehan DL, Warren RF, Wickiewicz TL. (1985): Acute repairs of the ACL past and present. *Orthop Clin North Am*, 16:111–125.

53. Graf BK. (1987): Isometric placement of substitutes for the anterior cruciate ligament. In: Jackson DW, Drez D Jr, eds. *The anterior cruciate deficient knee*. St. Louis: CV Mosby, pp 102–113.

54. Graf BK, Ulm MJ, Rogalski RP, Vanderby R. (1992): Effect of preconditioning on the viscoelastic response of the primate patella tendon. *Trans Orthop Res Soc*, 17:147.

55. Grood ES, Hefzy MS, Butler DL, et al. (1983): On the placement and initial tension of anterior cruciate ligament substitutes. *Trans Orthop Res Soc*, 8:92.

56. Grood ES, Hefzy MS, Butler DL, Noyes FR. (1986): Intra-articular vs. over the top placement of anterior cruciate ligament substitute. *Trans Orthop Res Soc*, 11:79.

57. Grood ES, Suntay WJ, Noyes FR, Butler DL. (1984): Biomechanics of the knee-extension exercise. *J Bone Joint Surg [Am]*, 66A:725–734.

58. Häggmark T, Eriksson E. (1979): Cylinder or mobile cast brace after knee ligament surgery: a clinical analysis and morphological and enzymatic study of changes in quadriceps muscle. *Am J Sports Med*, 7:48–56.

59. Hefzy MS, Grood ES. (1986): Sensitivity of insertion locations on length patterns of anterior cruciate ligament fibers. *J Biomech Eng*, 108:73–82.

60. Hefzy MS, Grood ES, Noyes FR. (1989): Factors affecting the region of most isometric femoral attachments: part 2. The anterior cruciate ligament. *Am J Sports Med*, 17:208–216.

61. Henning CE, Lynch MA, Glick KR. (1985): An *in-vivo* strain gauge study of elongation of the anterior cruciate ligament. *Am J Sports Med*, 13:22–26.

62. Holden JP, Grood ES, Butler DL, Noyes FR, Mendenhall HV, VanKampen CL, Neidich RL. (1988): Biomechanics of fascia lata ligament replacements—early postoperative changes in the goat. *J Orthop Res*, 6:639–647.

63. Hoogland T, Hillen B. (1984): Intra-articular reconstruction of the anterior cruciate ligament: an experimental study of length changes in different ligament reconstructions. *Clin Orthop*, 185:197–202.

64. Howe JG, Johnson RJ, Kaplan MK, Fleming BC, Jarvinen M. (1991): Anterior cruciate ligament reconstruction using quadricep patellar tendon graft: Part 1. Long-term follow-up. *Am J Sports Med*, 19:447–457.

65. Hurley PB, Andrish JT, Yoshiya S, Manley M, Kurosaka M. (1987): Tensile strength of the reconstructed canine anterior cruciate ligament—a long term evaluation of the modified Jones technique. *Am J Sports Med*, 14:393.

66. Jacob RP. (1981): Observations on rotary instability of the lateral compartment of the knee. *Acta Orthop Scand*, 52[Suppl 1]:1–31.

67. Johnson RJ. (1982): The anterior cruciate: a dilemma in sports medicine. *Int J Sports Med*, 3:71–79.

68. Johnson RJ. (1988): Anatomy and biomechanics of the knee. In: Chapman MW, ed. *Operative orthopaedics*. Philadelphia: Lippincott, pp 1617–1631.

69. Johnson RJ, Beynnon BD, Nichols CE, Renström PA. (1992): Current concepts review: the treatment of injuries to the anterior cruciate ligament. *J Bone Joint Surg [Am]*, 74A:140–151.

70. Johnson RJ, Eriksson E. (1982): Rehabilitation of the unstable knee. *Instr Course Lect*, 31:114–125.

71. Johnson RJ, Eriksson E, Haggmark T, Pope MH. (1984): A 5–10 year follow-up after reconstruction of the anterior cruciate ligament. *Clin Orthop*, 183:122–140.

72. Jones KG. (1963): Reconstruction of the anterior cruciate ligament: a technique using the central one-third of the patella ligament. *J Bone Joint Surg [Am]*, 45A:925–932.

73. Jones KG. (1970): Reconstruction of the anterior cruciate ligament using the central one-third of the patellar ligament. *J Bone Joint Surg [Am]*, 52A:1302–1308.

74. Jozsa L, Jarvinen M, Kannus P, Reffy A. (1987): Fine structural changes in the articular cartilage of the rat's knee following short-term immobilization in various positions: a scanning electron microscopical study. *Int Orthop*, 11:129–133.

75. Jozsa L, Reffy A, Jarvinen M, Kannus P, Lehto M, Kvist M. (1988): Cortical and trabecular osteopenia after immobilization —a quantitative histological study in rats. *Int Orthop*, 12:169–172.

76. Jozsa L, Thöring J, Jarvinen M, Kannus P, Lehto M, Kvist M. (1988): Quantitative alterations in intramuscular connective tissue following immobilization: an experimental study in rat calf muscle. *Exp Mol Pathol*, 49:267–278.

77. Kannus P. (1988): *Conservative treatment of acute knee distortions—long term results and their evaluation methods* [Dissertation]. Tampere, Finland: University of Tampere. *Acta Univ Tamperensis Ser A*, 250:1–110.

78. Kennedy JC. (1982): Symposium: current concepts in the management of knee instability. *Contemp Orthop*, 5:59–78.

79. Kennedy JC, Haskins RJ, Willis RB. (1977): Strain gauge analysis of knee ligaments. *Clin Orthop Rel Res*, 129:225–229.

80. Kurosaka M, Yoshia S, Andrish JT. (1987): A biomechanical comparison of different surgical techniques of graft fixation in anterior cruciate ligament reconstructions. *Am J Sports Med*, 15:225–229.

81. Lambert KL. (1983): Vascularized patellar tendon graft with rigid internal fixation for ACL insufficiency. *Clin Orthop*, 172:85–89.

82. Liljedahl SO, Nordstrand A. (1969): Injuries to the ligaments of the knee. *Injury*, 2:17–24.

83. Lipscomb AB, Johnston RK, Snyder RB, Brothers JC. (1979): Secondary reconstruction of anterior cruciate ligament in athletes by using the semitendinosus tendon. *Am J Sports Med*, 7:81–84.

84. Markolf KL, Gorek JF, Kabo M, Shapiro MS. (1990): Direct measurement of resultant forces in the anterior cruciate ligament: an *in-vitro* study performed with a new experimental technique. *J Bone Joint Surg [Am]*, 72A:557.

85. Markolf KL, Graff-Radford A, Amstutz HC. (1978): *In-vivo* stability—a quantitative assessment using an instrumented clinical testing apparatus. *J Bone Joint Surg [Am]*, 60A:664–674.

86. Marshall JL, Johnson RJ. (1977): Mechanism of the most common ski injuries. *Physician Sportsmed*, 5:49–54.

87. McDaniel WJ, Dameron TB. (1980): Untreated ruptures of the anterior cruciate ligament: a follow-up. *J Bone Joint Surg [Am]*, 62:696–705.

88. McDaniel WJ, Dameron TB. (1983): The untreated anterior cruciate ligament rupture. *Clin Orthop*, 172:158.

89. McFarland EG, Morrey BF, An KN, Wood MB. (1986): The relationship of vascularity and water content to tensile strength in a patellar tendon replacement of the anterior cruciate in dogs. *Am J Sports Med*, 14:436–448.

90. McPherson GK, Mendenhall HV, Gibbons DF, Plenk H, Rottmann W, Sanford JB, Kennedy JC, Roth JH. (1985): Experimental, mechanical and histologic evaluation of the Kennedy ligament augmentation device. *Clin Orthop*, 196:186–195.

91. Melhorn JM, Henning CE. (1987): The relationship of the femoral attachment site to the isometric tracking of the anterior cruciate ligament graft. *Am J Sports Med*, 15:539–542.

92. Mott HW. (1983): Semitendinosus anatomic reconstruction for cruciate ligament insufficiency. *Clin Orthop*, 172:90–92.

93. Newton PO, Horibe S, Woo SL-Y. (1990): Experimental studies on anterior cruciate ligament autografts and allografts. In: Daniel DM, Akeson WH, O'Connor JJ, eds. *Knee ligaments: structure, function, injury and repair.* New York: Raven Press, pp 389–399.

94. Nisell R, Nemeth G, Ohlsen H. (1986): Joint forces in extension of the knee. *Acta Orthop Scand*, 57:41–46.

95. Norwood LA, Cross MJ. (1979): Anterior cruciate ligament: functional anatomy and its bundles in rotatory instabilities. *Am J Sports Med*, 7:23–26.

96. Noyes FR. (1977): Functional properties of knee ligaments and alterations induced by immobilization. *Clin Orthop Rel Res*, 123:210–242.

97. Noyes FR, Butler DL, Paulos LE, Grood ES. (1983): Intra-articular cruciate reconstruction: 1. Perspectives on graft strength, vascularization and immediate motion after replacement. *Clin Orthop*, 172:71–77.

98. Noyes F, Butler D, Grood E, Zernicke R, Hefzy M. (1984): Biomechanical analysis of human ligament grafts used in knee ligament repairs and reconstruction. *J Bone Joint Surg [Am]*, 66A:344–352.

99. Noyes FR, Grood ES. (1976): The strength of the anterior cruciate ligament in humans and rhesus monkeys: age-related and species-related changes. *J Bone Joint Surg [Am]*, 58A:1074–1082.

100. Noyes FR, Mangine RE, Barber S. (1987): Early knee motion after open and arthroscopic ACL reconstruction. *Am J Sports Med*, 15:149–160.

101. Noyes FR, Matthews DS, Mooar PA, Grood ES. (1983): The symptomatic anterior cruciate-deficient knee: 2. The results of rehabilitation activity modification and counseling on functional disability. *J Bone Joint Surg [Am]*, 65A:163–174.

102. Oakes BW, Knight M, McLean ID, Deacon OW. (1991): Goat ACL autograft collagen remodelling—quantitative collagen fibril analysis over 1 year. In: *Proceedings of the Combined Meeting of the Orthopaedics Research Society of USA, Japan, and Canada, Oct 21–23*, p 60.

103. O'Donoghue DH. (1963): A method for replacement of the anterior cruciate ligament of the knee. *J Bone Joint Surg [Am]*, 45A:905–924.

104. O'Donoghue DH, Frank GR, Jeter GL, Johnson W, Zeiders JW, Kenyon R. (1971): Repair and reconstruction of the anterior cruciate ligament in dogs—factors influencing long term results. *J Bone Joint Surg [Am]*, 53A:710–718.

105. Ogata K, Whiteside LA, Andersen DA. (1980): The intra-articular effect of various postoperative managements following knee ligament repair: an experimental study in dogs. *Clin Orthop*, 150:271–276.

106. Paulos LE, Butler DL, Noyes FR. (1983): Intra-articular cruciate reconstruction: 2. Replacement with vascularized patellar tendon. *Clin Orthop*, 172:78–84.

107. Paulos LE, Noyes FR, Grood E, Butler DL. (1981): Knee rehabilitation after ACL reconstruction and repair. *Am J Sports Med*, 9:140–149.

108. Penner DA, Daniel DM, Wood P, Mishra D. (1988): An *in-vitro* study of anterior cruciate ligament graft orientation and isometry. *Am J Sports Med*, 16:238–243.

109. Piper TL, Whiteside LA. (1980): Early mobilization after knee ligament repair in dogs. *Clin Orthop*, 150:227–282.

110. Pyne J, Gottlieb D, Beynnon BD, Nichols CE, Johnson RJ, Renstrom PA. (1992): Semitendinous and gracilis, tendon graft fixation in ACL reconstruction. *Trans Orthop Res Soc*, 17:245.

111. Renström P, Arms SW, Stanwyck TS, Johnson RJ, Pope MH. (1986): Strain within the anterior cruciate ligament during hamstring and quadriceps activity. *Am J Sports Med*, 14:83–87.

112. Robertson DB, Daniel DM, Biden E. (1987): Soft tissue fixation to bone. *Am J Sports Med*, 15:225–229.

113. Ryan JR, Droupp BW. (1966): Evaluation of tensile strength of reconstructions of the anterior cruciate ligament using the patellar tendon in dogs. *South Med J*, 59:129–134.

114. Sapega AA, Moyer RJ, Schneck C, Komalahiranya N. (1990): Testing for isometry during reconstruction of the anterior cruciate ligament. *J Bone Joint Surg [Am]*, 72A:259–267.

115. Schutzer S, Christen S, Jakob R. (1989): Further observations on the isometricity of the anterior cruciate ligament: an anatomical study using a 6-mm diameter replacement. *Clin Orthop*, 242:245–255.

116. Sgaglione NA, Warren RF, Wickiewicz TL, Gold DA, Panariello

RA. (1990): Primary repair with semitendinosus tendon augmentation of acute anterior cruciate ligament injuries. *Am J Sports Med*, 18:64–73.

117. Shelbourne KD, Nitz P. (1990): Accelerated rehabilitation after ACL reconstruction. *Am J Sports Med*, 18:292–299.

118. Sherman MF, Warren RF, Marshall JL, Savatsky GJ. (1988): A clinical and radiographical analysis of 127 anterior cruciate insufficient knees. *Clin Orthop*, 227:229–237.

119. Shino K, Kawasaki T, Hirose H, Gotoh I, Inoue M, Ono R. (1984): Reconstruction of the anterior cruciate ligament by allogenic tendon graft: an experimental study in the dog. *J Bone Joint Surg [Br]*, 66B:672–681.

120. Sidles JA, Larson RV, Garbini JL, Downey DJ, Matsen FA. (1988): Ligament length relationships in the moving knee. *J Orthop Res*, 6:593–610.

121. Siegel MG, Grood ES, Hefzy MS. (1984): Analysis and placement of the ACL substitute. *Orthop Trans*, 8:69.

122. Skylar MJ, Danzig LA, Hargens AR, Akenson WH. (1985): Nutrition of the ACL, effects of continuous passive motion. *Am J Sports Med*, 13:415–418.

123. Thorsen EP, Rodrigo JJ, Vasseur PB, Sharkey NA, Heitter DO. (1987): Comparison of frozen allograft versus fresh autogenous anterior cruciate ligament replacement in the dog. *Trans Orthop Res Soc*, 12:65.

124. Torg J, Conrad W, Kalen V. (1976): Clinical diagnosis of ACL instability. *Am J Sports Med*, 4:84–92.

125. Torzilli P, Greenberg R, Hood R, Pavlov H, Insall J. (1984): Measurement of anterior-posterior motion of the knee in injured patients using a biomechanical stress technique. *J Bone Joint Surg [Am]*, 66A:1438–1442.

126. Trent PS, Walker PS, Wolf B. (1976): Ligament length patterns, strength, and rotational axis of the knee joint. *Clin Orthop*, 117:263–270.

127. Van Dijk R, Huiskes R, Selvik G. (1979): Roentgen stereophotogrammetric methods for the evaluation of the three dimensional kinematic behavior and cruciate ligament length patterns of the human knee joint. *J Biomech*, 12:727–731.

128. van Rens TJG, van den Berg AF, Huiskes R, Kuypers W. (1986): Substitution of the anterior cruciate ligament—a long term histologic and biomechanical study with autogenous pedicled grafts of iliotibial band in dogs. *Arthroscopy*, 2:139–154.

129. Wang CJ, Walker PS, Wolf B. (1973): The effects of flexion and rotation on the length patterns of the ligaments of the knee. *J Biomech*, 6:587–596.

130. Wilcox PG, Jackson DW. (1987): Arthroscopic anterior cruciate ligament reconstruction. In: Minkoff J, Sherman EH, eds. *Clinical and Sports Medical Arthroscopy*. Philadelphia: Saunders, pp 513–524.

131. Woo SL-Y, Gomez MA, Seguchi Y, Endo CM, Akeson WH. (1983): Measurement of mechanical properties of ligament substance from a bone-ligament-bone preparation. *J Orthop Res*, 1:22–29.

132. Woo SL-Y, Hollis MJ, Adams DJ, Lyon RM, Takai S. (1991): Tensile properties of the human femur-anterior cruciate ligament-tibia complex: the effects of specimen age and orientation. *Am J Sports Med*, 19:217–225.

133. Yasuda K, Sasaki T. (1987): Exercise after anterior cruciate ligament reconstruction—the force exerted on the tibia by separate isometric contractions of the quadriceps or the hamstrings. *Clin Orthop*, 220:275–283.

134. Yasuda K, Tomiyama Y, Ohkoshi Y, Kaneda K. (1989): Arthroscopic observations of autogenetic quadriceps and patellar tendon grafts after anterior cruciate ligament reconstruction of the knee. *Clin Orthop*, 246:217–224.

135. Yoshiya S, Andrish JT, Manley MT, Kurosaka M. (1986): Augmentation of anterior cruciate ligament reconstruction in dogs with prostheses of different studies. *J Orthop Res*, 4:475–485.

136. Yoshiya S, Andrish JT, Manley MT, et al. (1987): Graft tension in anterior cruciate ligament reconstruction. *Am J Sports Med*, 15:464–470.

The Anterior Cruciate Ligament: Current and Future Concepts, edited by D.W. Jackson, et al. Raven Press, Ltd., New York © 1993.

CHAPTER 24

The Acute Repair of Anterior Cruciate Ligament Tears

Lars Engebretsen

In his monograph, "On the Injuries to the Ligaments of the Knee Joint," Ivar Palmer (27) made an extensive description of the anatomy, the biomechanics including injury mechanisms, the pathology, and the treatment of knee ligament injuries. He emphasized the importance of early diagnosis and advocated primary repair, but he concluded that clinical observations were based on too few patients and the follow-up was too short to allow general recommendations concerning treatment. Later surgeons have followed his rationale and emphasized the need for early stabilization to avoid stretching out the secondary restraints. Additionally, the concept of acute repair today is based upon the hypotheses suggested by animal studies (3,33–36) that preserving the torn ligament would lead to better proprioception and thereby function. This chapter outlines the biomechanics, surgical techniques, and results of anterior cruciate ligament (ACL) repair and augmented repair.

ANIMAL STUDIES

The healing potential for the acutely torn ACL is still being debated. Although O'Donoghue et al. (25) found that the divided ACL in thirty dogs healed with surgical repair apposing the severed ends under proper tension, tensile strength remained substantially less than that of the normal ligament at ten weeks. A follow-up study (26) showed that ultimate resorption of the repaired ligament was not uncommon, occurring in 14 of 36 repairs. Cabaud et al. (7) found similar results in dogs and monkeys; none of the repaired cruciate ligaments were functionally competent to protect the knee joint from developing

rapid degenerative changes. In a later study (6) Cabaud obtained significantly better results when the repair was augmented with a vascularized patellar tendon graft in dogs and suggested that the results were encouraging enough for clinical trials to begin. Frank et al. (15) have also suggested some reasons for the observed poor healing potential of ACL repairs in their experimental studies.

BIOMECHANICAL CADAVERIC STUDIES

The subject of initial pretension in the repaired ACL has been cause for discussion. Jones (17) stated that the initial pretension in a repair should be sufficient to eliminate the anterior drawer sign, but still allow a full range of motion. Noyes et al. (22) proposed that the normal 5-mm anterior posterior translation should be preserved during pretensioning. In an experimental study using the Palmer repair technique and pretension according to Noyes, Engebretsen et al. (10) showed that the average of the forces seen by the repaired ACL exceeded those seen by a normal ACL when the tibia was subjected to a 20-lb anterior load in four of seven knees. The repair forces were always higher than normal at 60° and 90° of flexion. If these abnormally high forces occur *in vivo,* they could potentially lead to suture failure, loosening of the fixation and stretching of the repair. This situation could, in turn, produce increased loads in the secondary restraints, gradually stretching these tissues. Moreover, this study showed that although the A-P configuration of the tibia returned to within normal limits in the repaired state, the tibia was always externally rotated when compared to the normal knee in both an unloaded and an anterior loaded state. Thus, the normal kinematics were not restored by the repair.

L. Engebretsen: Department of Orthopaedic Surgery, Trondheim University Hospital, Trondheim, 7000 Norway.

PROTECTION OF THE REPAIR

The high loads seen by the repaired ligament could lead to early failure. This has been the rationale behind augmentation procedures. The augmentation is supposed to protect the repair while remodeling and growth takes place. It has been shown (10) that the use of a synthetic augmentation device placed in the over-the-top position could protect the repair tissue at extension. Although the total forces in a composite repair were considerably higher than in the intact ligament at extension, the forces in the repair tissue segment itself approached normal when the augmentation device was positioned anatomically through the condyle, and were lower than normal when it was positioned over-the-top. Thus it has been shown experimentally that synthetic intraarticular augmentation may protect the repair at least in extension when the augmentation is placed in the over-the-top position. There are so far no identical studies on the protective effect of the numerous biologic augmentation—procedures described in recent years.

In addition to an intraarticular "splint" the repair may be protected with an extraarticular tenodesis. These extraarticular "backups" serve to reinforce the secondary restraints and protect the intraarticular repair. In a study describing the effect of an iliotibial tenodesis fixed with a pretension of 27 Newton at Krackow's F-9 position with the tibia manually externally rotated on an intraarticular graft and knee joint kinematics, it was shown that the tenodesis will reduce the forces in the repair by 43% when the tibia is subjected to 90 Newton anteriorly directed load (11).

SURGICAL TECHNIQUE

Below are descriptions of the most common repair and augmented repair techniques. To obtain good ACL remnants, the surgery should probably be carried out within two weeks of injury. These techniques may be indicated when a proximal or distal tear in the ACL occurs.

Repair According to Palmer/Marshall (20)

Multiple loop sutures (Ethibond 2-0) are placed in the ACL remnants anteromedial to posterolateral in the distal stump (i.e. proximal stump when a distal rupture is detected) A 7/64-inch Steinmann pin is used to drill two holes in the anatomic insertion sites through the lateral femoral condyle. The sutures are passed with a suture passer and tied over the bone bridge with the knee in 30 degrees of flexion and a pretension sufficient to prevent >5 mm anterior drawer when the Lachman test is performed (Fig. 1).

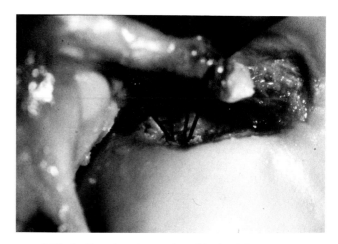

FIG. 1. Repair sutures placed in the ACL stump.

Repair with Synthetic Ligament Augmentation Devices

Two different techniques have been used—both will be described (12,32).

A 7/64-inch Steinmann Pin Placed in the Anteromedial Part of the Tibial ACL Insertion Site and Overdrilled with a Reamer (4.5 to 6 mm)

The posterior part of the tibial tunnel is chamfered in order to prevent the protrusion. A small notchplasty is carried out. The over-the-top position is identified and prepared with a curved rasp to obtain a small groove. The ligament augmentation device (LAD) is then passed through the tibial tunnel and sutured to the tibial periosteum with 6 to 8 interrupted nonresorbable sutures. The ACL remnants are sutured to the LAD with 2-0 Vicryl. The LAD with the ACL remnants is then routed through the over-the-top position and tensioned at 30° of flexion with pretension as for the repair. The LAD is secured to the lateral femoral condyle with the belt buckle technique (Figs. 2 and 3).

The Present LAD Technique Used by the Author When the ACL Is Torn in the Proximal Part

Through a central incision, 4 nonabsorbable sutures are placed in the ACL in the anteromedial to posterolateral direction. A 7/64 Steinmann pin is placed through the lateral femoral condyle, emerging in the anterior part of the ACL insertion site. The posterolateral suture bundle is passed through this tunnel. A LAD is passed through a 4.5-mm-wide tibial tunnel, entering the joint on the anteromedial part of the tibial insertion site. A small notchplasty is performed, and the over-the-top position is prepared with a curved rasp to obtain a small groove. The LAD is then routed with the anteromedial suture bundle from the ACL remnants through the over-the-top position. The LAD is fixed with the belt buckle

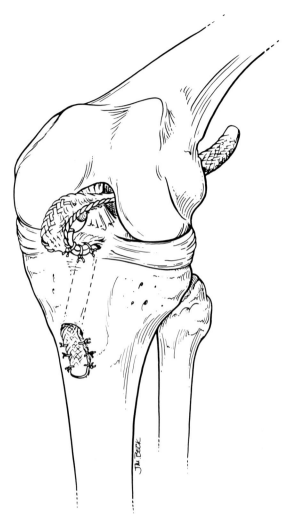

FIG. 2. LAD suture technique. The ACL remnants are sutured to the LAD with 2-0 Vicryl.

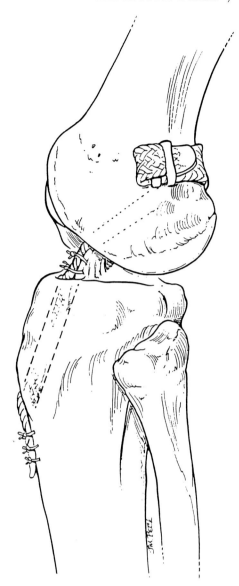

FIG. 3. The LAD with the ACL remnants is routed through the over-the-top position and secured with the belt-buckle technique.

staple technique on the tibial side. The ACL sutures are tied over the bone bridge with the knee in approximately 30° of flexion. The knee is then extended and the LAD fixed on the lateral femoral condyle with the belt buckle technique. The composite graft is pretensioned to prevent a Lachman >5 mm (Fig. 4).

Repair with Patellar Tendon Augmentation

A variant of the procedure proposed by Clancy (8) is currently used by the author. A free graft is harvested from the central one-third of the patellar tendon with the bone blocks measuring 25 × 10 × 5 mm. The procedure is carried out through the central patellar tendon incision. The drill holes are made in the usual fashion with a Steinmann pin on a drill guide entering the joint on the anteromedial part of the ACL insertion on the tibia and in the posterior part of the insertion site on the lateral femoral condyle. Four nonabsorbable sutures are placed in the ACL remnants anteromedially to posterolaterally.

The graft is passed with the posterolateral suture bundle through the femoral tunnel, while the anteromedial bundle is passed through the over the top position. The ACL sutures are tied over the bone bridge at 30° of flexion, while the graft is fixed with an interference screw at full extension.

In an alternative technique, the ACL remnants are sutured to the patellar tendon graft, being pulled toward the femoral insertion site when the graft is pretensioned.

Repair with Semitendinosus Augmentation (31)

The semitendinosus graft is passed proximally through tibial drill holes entering the joint anteromedial

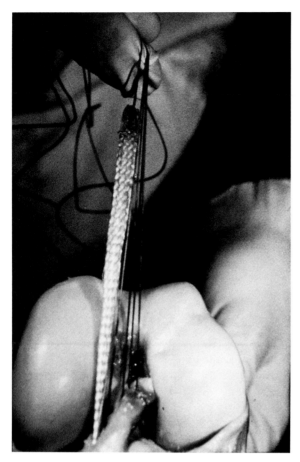

FIG. 4. Four nonabsorbable sutures are placed in the ACL in the anteromedial to posterolateral position. The LAD is passed through a 4.5-mm-wide tibial tunnel, entering the joint on the anteromedial part of the tibial insertion site of the ACL.

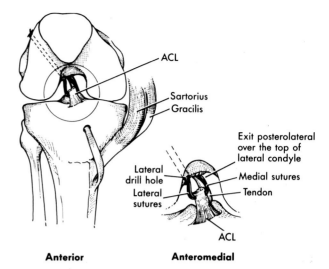

FIG. 5. Semitendinosus augmentation technique. The distally placed anteromedial suture bundle in the ACL remnants, along with the semitendinousus graft, is passed proximally and laterally using the over-the-top position. The posterolateral group of sutures are passed through a femoral drill hole.

to the tibial insertion of the ACL. After subperiosteal midlateral femoral condyle dissection is completed, the distally placed anteromedial suture bundle in the ACL remnants along with the semitendinosus graft is passed proximally and laterally using the over-the-top position. The second posterior grouping of distal stump sutures are passed through a femoral drill-hole placed 5 to 6 mm anterior to the over-the-top position. The sutures are tied over bone and a barbed staple fixation of the semitendinosus graft is achieved (Fig. 5).

Repair with Patellar Retinaculum Augmentation (18)

The medial or lateral retinaculum is used as the augmentation strip, at least 10 mm wide, starting at the superior margin of the patella and moving to its attachment at the tibia. A channel from the medial aspect of the tibia, just proximal to the tibial attachment of the strip, is drilled slightly anterior and medial to the tibia attachment of the ACL. The opening of the joint is achieved with a semilunar osteotome. Another channel is drilled through the lateral femoral condyle just posterior to the

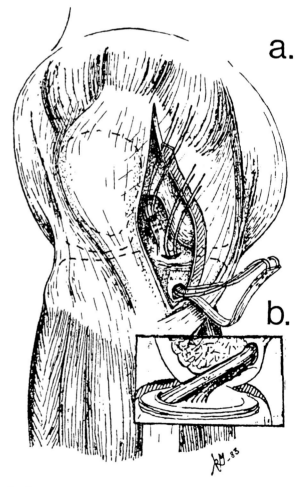

FIG. 6. Patellar retinaculum augmentation technique. The medial longitudinal retinaculum is prepared for augmentation of the sutured ACL (**A**), covering its anteromedial part (**B**).

femoral attachment. The strip is pulled through the channel in the tibia, through the joint covering the repaired ligament, and then through the channel in the femur. The sutures from the strip and the repaired ligament are tightened separately over a button after conditioning, i.e., prestretching the sutures by repeated flexion-extension movements (Fig. 6).

Repair with Iliotibial Band Augmentation (1)

Of the two limbs of the sutures in the distal portion of the ruptured ACL, one is passed posteriorly over the top of the lateral femoral condyle, while the other is passed through a hole drilled through the lateral condyle at the site of attachment of the ACL. The two limbs are tied together on the posterosuperior aspect of the condyle. A 1.5-cm distally based strip of the iliotibial band is passed through the hole in the lateral femoral condyle and then through a hole in the tibia, and is secured to the tibia with a staple.

Comments on These Surgical Techniques

ACL repair is presently used primarily for proximal ruptures of the ACL. The augmentation procedures are all described for use in the same patient population; midsubstance ruptures are specifically not suited for these techniques.

RESULTS AFTER ACUTE REPAIR AND REPAIR WITH AUGMENTATION

The literature contains many conflicting reports concerning the various modes of treatment of an acute ACL injury. Most studies are retrospective, nonrandomized, using different techniques, immobilization, rehabilita-

tion and follow-up protocols. In general, North American studies characteristically include young men highly active in sports, whereas Scandinavian studies cover relatively more women and a generally older patient population participating in recreational sports (Table 1).

The first reports on ACL repair in the English literature were by Battle in 1900 (5) and Mayo Robson in 1903 (29) who in a single patient with a 6-year follow-up found good function and no abnormal motility. In 1919 Hey Groves (16) discouraged further attempts at repair, stating that direct suture of the ligament was "utterly impossible." When Ivar Palmer in 1937 reported on ten cases of repair of the ACL and subsequently published his thesis in 1938, interest in repair was renewed, and in short term follow-up O'Donoghue (24) and Liljedahl et al. (19) both had good results. Liljedahl, reporting on 33 knees 6 to 18 months following surgery, showed all knees to be stable and all patients had resumed their sports activities. In 1977 Marshall (20) reported on a modification of the Palmer suture technique, using varying depth multiple loop sutures to reapproximate both cruciate stumps. He found that 48 of 61 patients returned fully to preinjury sports level participation. However, 25% displayed a positive pivot shift after 29 months. Subsequently, another 15% of these patients were reported to display "giving way." At a mean 6.5-year follow-up of 50 of these patients, 30% had a positive pivot shift and KT-1000 laxity data revealed that 40% had >3 mm side-to-side difference. The recent experimental data suggesting poor results after ACL repair in general have found support in newer clinical studies. Feagin and Curl (13), after reporting promising results 2 years after surgery, found 30 of 32 patients to have symptoms of instability after 5 years. Arnold et al. (2) reported on 75 patients treated with direct repair. At an average of 5-year follow-up, 84% had a positive pivot shift and overall results were no better than in knees with no surgical treatment. Balkfors (4) in a 10-year retrospective study found 50% of re-

TABLE 1. *Studies on knee injury*

Study	Follow-up (yr)	Design	No.	Age	Sex or F/M ratio	Sport injury	Coll. ligament injury	Meniscus injury
Feagin	5	Retro[a]	32	20	Male	<100%	None	
Strand	5–10	Retro	68	36	47/53%	2/3	94%	48%
Balkfors	>5	Retro	86	28		64%		
Arnold	5	Retro	75	22		100%	25%	
Odensten	5	Prosp[b]	41	28	21/79%	83%	78%	59%
Marshall	3	Retro	70	26	20/80%	100%	66%	37%
Sandberg	3	Retro	100	28	50/50%	90%	19%	
Straub	2	Retro	42	22	30/70%	95%	None	35%
Shields	6	Retro	21	28		100%		
Andersson	4	Prosp	23	25		83%		
Engebretsen	5	Retro	74	34	41/59%	70%	73%	53%
Engebretsen	2	Prosp	50	29	42/58%	83%	52%	38%
Raunest	3.5	Retro	51	33		51%	49%	15%

[a] Retro, retrospective.
[b] Prosp, prospective.

paired knees to have a positive pivot shift. He concluded that early repair "cannot be demonstrated to alter significantly the course of the ACL injured knee." Marshall et al. (20,21) found a positive pivot shift in only 25%, and 89% were participating fully at their preinjury sports level. He could show little deterioration with time. This is contradicted by Feagin (13), Odensten (23), and Strand (34), who all found a decrease in function and stability with time. Engebretsen (9) found good functional and objective results in 3/4 of 84 patients, but the good results are explained by low activity level and in particular less contact sport participation than similar studies. Raunest (28) followed 51 selected patients with proximal lesions of the ACL for 1 to 7 years. Thirty-eight patients had a very good or good result. His results suggest that primary repair of proximal tears without accompanying collateral ligament injuries may give reasonable results.

Three recent prospective, randomized studies have addressed this issue. Sandberg (30) followed 157 patients for 2 years randomized to nonsurgical treatment or repair. He found no difference between the groups and concluded that primary suturing of ACL tears is an insufficient procedure.

Engebretsen (12) randomized 150 patients to treatment with repair, patellar tendon augmentation or LAD augmentation. There were no differences between the 50 patients in each group concerning additional ligament or meniscal injuries. The repair group had a decreased activity level at 1 year and stayed at this level. Every third patient had a Lachman 2+ at 1 year increasing to 53% at 2 years. Thirty-eight percent had a 2+ pivot shift at 2 years. This trend has continued at the 5-year follow-up. In general the results both in function and in objective stability is inferior to both types of augmentation.

Andersson (1) followed 111 patients for 47 months and concluded that simple repair of the ACL gave inferior results compared to augmented repairs and resulted in lower level of activity.

Currently, there are no long-term reports on arthroscopically sutured ACL tears, although Fox et al. (14) reported a pilot study on 5 arthroscopically repaired ACLs. The authors question the feasibility of arthroscopic repair with the current technical resources.

THE RESULTS OF AUGMENTATION

Synthetic (LAD) Augmentation

Schabus (32) has published a 3-year follow-up of 50 patients using the LAD technique previously described in addition to loop sutures in the ACL remnants. After 3 years, 46 of the patients had a KT-1000 difference of <3

mm and a negative pivot shift. The average Lysholm score was 94. Engebretsen et al. (12) followed 50 patients for 2 years using the technique where the ACL remnants were sutured to the LAD. The average Lysholm score was 90 after 1 year, and this did not deteriorate at 2 years as opposed to the nonaugmented 50 patients. Nineteen percent had a 2+ Lachman and 13% a positive pivot shift at 1 year with no deterioration at 2 years. Thirteen of 43 LAD patients had a side difference of >3 mm after 2 years. During the follow-up, three LAD patients underwent reoperations due to LAD breakage. This group of patients is currently undergoing a 5-year follow-up.

Biological Augmentation with Bone Patellar Tendon Bone

Clancy (8) reported 90% good/excellent results in his patellar tendon augmented group in a prospective study which included 70 patients followed at an average of 48 months. There were no failures and only two patients with a fair result. Clancy suggests that the method might improve further when the arthroscopic technique is used. Engebretsen (12) found four patients with a 2+ Lachman and none with a positive pivot shift after 2 years in a prospective, randomized study. The Lysholm functional score increased from 91 to 94 even though the activity level was increased in this group. However, four patients were reoperated on due to flexion contractures. These studies, both being prospective and one randomized suggest that the good results on function and stability reported in similar retrospective studies are valid.

Biological Augmentation with the Patellar Retinaculum

Jonsson et al. (18) has reported a 7-year follow-up of acutely torn ACLs randomized between repair alone or retinaculum augmented repairs. In the repair group, 6/22 had unchanged activity and intensity levels compared with 24/29 in the augmentation group. Lysholm's functional score was higher in the augmentation group. All the clinical tests and all the objective measurements except Lachman's test showed better stability in the augmented group.

Biological Augmentation with the Semitendinosus

Scaglione et al. (31) reported good to excellent results in 82%, and 77% returned to preinjury sports participation without limitation in a follow-up of 38 months. Objective examination revealed 93% to have a 1+ or less Lachman test and 86% to have a negative pivot shift. Of 60 knees tested, 93% had KT-1000 side-to-side difference of <3 mm.

Biological Augmentation with the Iliotibial Band

Andersson (1) reported a 48-month follow-up of 29 patients. The mean Lysholm score was 92 and 20 of the patients had a high activity level. However, 16 of the knees did not have a normal Lachman test when compared to the noninjured knee. The augmented knees had fewer subsequent meniscal tears than the nonoperated knees. Instability which was felt to necessitate late reconstruction was also less frequent in the patients who had an augmented repair.

CONCLUSION

The hypothesis of regaining normal proprioception when the ACL is repaired has not been proven clinically. In addition, there is so far no evidence of the repair rendering a more kinematically normal knee. Based on experimental and clinical research, there is currently no place for ACL repair alone. If one believes in the proprioception hypothesis, an augmentation of the repair should be carried out. The technique is feasible through a small central incision if a patellar tendon or a LAD is used and allows for early rehabilitation. However, the technique will undoubtedly be improved when better arthroscopic equipment is available.

REFERENCES

1. Andersson C, Odensten M, Good L, Gillquist J. (1989): Surgical or nonsurgical treatment of acute rupture of the anterior cruciate ligament. *J Bone Joint Surg [Am]*, 71A:965–974.
2. Arnold JA, Coher TP, Heaton LM, et al. (1979): Natural history of anterior cruciate tears. *Am J Sports Med*, 7:305–313.
3. Arnoczky SP. (1983): Anatomy of the anterior cruciate ligament. *Clin Orthop*, 172:19–25.
4. Balkfors B. (1982): The course of knee ligament injuries. *Acta Orthop Scand Suppl*, 198.
5. Battle WH. (1900): A case after open section of the knee joint for irreducible traumatic dislocation. *Trans Clin Soc Lond*, 33:232–238.
6. Cabaud HE, Feagin JA, Roley WG. (1980): Acute anterior cruciate ligament injury and augmented repair: experimental studies. *Am J Sports Med*, 8:395–401.
7. Cabaud HE, Roley WG, Feagin JA. (1979): Experimental studies of acute anterior cruciate ligament injuries and repair. *Am J Sports Med*, 7:18–22.
8. Clancy WG, Ray M, Zoltan J. (1988): Nonoperative or operative treatment of acute anterior cruciate ligament tears. *J Bone Joint Surg [Am]*, 70A:1483–1486.
9. Engebretsen L, Benum P, Sundalsfold S. (1989): Primary suture of the anterior cruciate ligament: a 6-year follow-up of 74 cases. *Acta Orthop Scand*, 60:561–564.
10. Engebretsen L, Lew WD, Lewis JL, Hunter RE. (1989): Knee mechanics after repair of the anterior cruciate ligament: a cadaver study of ligament augmentation. *Acta Orthop Scand*, 60:703–709.
11. Engebretsen L, Lew WD, Lewis JL, Hunter RE. (1990): The effect of an iliotibial tenodesis on intra-articular graft forces and knee joint motion. *Am J Sports Med*, 18:169–176.
12. Engebretsen L, Benum P, Fasting O, Moelster A, Strand T. (1990): A prospective randomized study on three surgical techniques for treatment of acute rupture of the anterior cruciate ligament. *Am J Sports Med*, 18:585–590.
13. Feagin JA, Curl WW. (1976): Isolated tear of the anterior cruciate ligament: 5 year follow-up study. *Am J Sports Med*, 4(3):95–100.
14. Fox JM, Sherman OH, Markolf K. (1985): Arthroscopic ACL repair: preliminary results. *Arthroscopy*, 1(3):175–181.
15. Frank C, Amiel D, Woo SL-Y, Akeson W. (1985): Normal ligament properties and ligament healing. *Clin Orthop*, 196:15–25.
16. Hey Groves EW. (1917): Operation for the repair of the cruciate ligaments. *Lancet*, 3:674–675.
17. Jones KG. (1963): Reconstruction of the anterior cruciate ligament: a technique using the central one-third of the patellar ligament. *J Bone Joint Surg [Am]*, 45A:925–932.
18. Jonsson T, Peterson C, Renström P. (1990): Anterior cruciate ligament repair with and without augmentation. *Acta Orthop Scand*, 61:562–566.
19. Liljedahl SO, Lindvall N, Wetterfors J. (1965): Early diagnosis and treatment of acute rupture of the anterior cruciate ligament: a clinical and arthrographic study of forty eight cases. *J Bone Joint Surg [Am]*, 47A:1503–1513.
20. Marshall JL, Warren RF, Wickiewicz TL. (1979): The anterior cruciate ligament: a technique of repair and reconstruction. *Clin Orthop*, 143:97–106.
21. Marshall JL, Warren RF, Wickiewicz TL. (1982): Primary surgical treatment of anterior cruciate ligament lesion. *Am J Sports Med*, 10:103–107.
22. Noyes FR, Butler DL, Paulos LE, Grood ES. (1983): Intra-articular cruciate reconstruction: perspectives on graft strength, vascularization and immediate motion after replacement. *Clin Orthop*, 172:71–77.
23. Odensten M, Lysholm J, Gillquist J. (1984): Suture of fresh ruptures of the anterior cruciate ligament: a 5-year follow-up. *Acta Orthop Scand*, 55:270–272.
24. O'Donoghue DH. (1980): Surgical treatment of injuries to the knee. *Clin Orthop*, 18:11.
25. O'Donoghue DH, Rockwood CA, Frank GR, Jack S, Kenyon R. (1966): Repair of the anterior cruciate ligament in dogs. *J Bone Joint Surg [Am]*, 48A:503–519.
26. O'Donoghue DH, Frank GR, Grady LJ, Johnson W, Zeiders JW, Kenyon R. (1971): Repair and reconstruction of the anterior cruciate ligament in dogs. *J Bone Joint Surg [Am]*, 53A:710–718.
27. Palmer I. (1938): On the injuries to the ligament of the knee joint: a clinical study. *Acta Chir Scand Suppl*, 53.
28. Raunest J, Derra E, Oliman C. (1991): Klinische Ergebnisse der primären Kreuzbanderinsertion nach Palmer ohne Augmentation. *Unfallchirurgie*, 17:166–174.
29. Robson AWM. (1903): Ruptured cruciate ligaments and their repair by operation. *Ann Surg*, 37:716–718.
30. Sandberg R. (1987): *Knee ligament injuries: a plan of action* [Dissertation]. Sweden: Lund University.
31. Scaglione AA, Warren RF, Wickiewicz TH, Gold DA, Panoriello RA. (1990): Primary repair with semitendinosus tendon augmentation of acute anterior cruciate ligament injuries. *Am J Sports Med*, 18:64–73.
32. Schabus R. (1985): Die Bedeutung der Augmentation fur die Rekonstruktion des vorderes Kreuzbandes. *Acta Chir Aust Suppl*, 77.
33. Schultz RA, Miller DC, Kerr CS, Mickeli L. (1984): Mechanoreceptors in human cruciate ligaments. *J Bone Joint Surg [Am]*, 66A:1072–1076.
34. Sjölander P. (1990): A sensory role for the cruciate ligaments: regulation of joint stability via reflexes into the muscle spindle system. *Acta Orthop Scand*, 61[Suppl 235].
35. Strand T, Engesaeter LB, Moelster AO, et al. (1984): Knee function following suture of fresh tear of the anterior cruciate ligament. *Acta Orthop Scand*, 55:181–184.
36. Zimmy ML, Schuttle M, Dabezies E. (1986): Mechanoreceptors in the human anterior cruciate ligament. *Anat Rec*, 214:204–209.

The Anterior Cruciate Ligament: Current and Future Concepts, edited by D.W. Jackson, et al. Raven Press, Ltd., New York © 1993.

CHAPTER 25

Autograft Reconstruction of the Anterior Cruciate Ligament

Placement, Tensioning, and Preconditioning

Ben K. Graf and Ray Vanderby, Jr.

Despite a decade of clinical and basic research on graft placement and tensioning, definitive guidelines for ideal attachment sites and optimal graft tension remain elusive. Recommended femoral attachment sites range from over-the-top to positions in the center of the anterior cruciate ligament's (ACL) femoral origin, locations that are nearly 1 cm apart (8,33). Similarly, placement of the tibial tunnel has been recommended for both the anteromedial (eccentric) and posterior regions of the normal ACL's tibial insertion (6,19). The recognition of notch impingement as a factor in postoperative knee motion, and perhaps in graft maturation, has further complicated the placement issue (18,19). Finally, new techniques such as endoscopic ACL reconstruction have placed new constraints on the selection and creation of attachment sites.

Recommendations for ideal graft tension have also been less than consistent. Cadaveric and clinical research has demonstrated a complex interrelationship between graft tension, graft placement, weight bearing and muscular forces across the knee, and knee stability and kinematics (1,4,5,15,20–22,27–29,32,38,43). To further complicate this issue, the viscoelastic nature of tendons and ligaments implies that graft tension will change over time even when all the factors listed above are controlled (14,26,31). This chapter will cite previous work relating to graft placement and tensioning, present relevant data from our laboratory, and make some suggestions for future areas of research.

B. K. Graf and R. Vanderby, Jr.: Division of Orthopedic Surgery, University of Wisconsin, Madison, Wisconsin 53792.

GRAFT PLACEMENT

Selection of femoral and tibial attachment sites during ACL reconstruction is generally based on a visual, radiographic, or drill guide–assisted assessment of local anatomy. In addition, a functional assessment of proposed femoral and tibial sites may be obtained with various devices to estimate graft stresses or strains (7,11). These devices commonly use a suture to measure changes in attachment site separation distance or suture tension as the knee is put through a range of motion. The pattern of these length or tension changes with respect to knee flexion angle can identify an attachment site as functionally posterior, anterior, or near isometric. The accuracy of these devices in predicting actual graft stresses and strains in the ACL graft remains open to question. Nonetheless, current surgical techniques depend on anatomic clues and/or intraoperative functional assessment to define the attachment sites for an ACL replacement.

Anatomic Guides to Graft Placement

The anatomic landmarks for placement of the femoral attachment site are the lateral wall and roof of the intercondylar notch, the posterior cruciate ligament, and the over-the-top position. The latter is often difficult to visualize but can be palpated with a probe through the intercondylar notch. With these landmarks in mind, the surgeon can choose an attachment site that is over-the-top (i.e., no femoral tunnel), central (i.e., in the presumed center of the femoral ACL origin), or eccentric (i.e., a tunnel posterior and superior to the center of the ACL origin in the region where the anteromedial bundle of the ACL originates). Of these commonly recommended sites, only the over-the-top position is well defined on an anatomic basis. This fact is reflected in the smaller variability in length or tension changes with this location compared with osseous tunnels (5,8).

Identification of central or posterosuperior attachment sites can be difficult. At the time of ACL reconstruction there is generally little remaining of the femoral ACL stump, and the size and shape of the intercondylar notch are variable. The limited visual clues make definition of the normal ACL origin difficult. In recognition of this problem, several drill guides have been designed that use the over-the-top position as a reference point (Fig. 1). These guides have a foot that slips over the top of the lateral femoral condyle and are cannulated to place a small pilot hole at a desired distance from the posterior cortex. Use of these guides does not completely define the femoral tunnel location because rotation of the guide will alternately place the tunnel on the roof of the intercondylar notch or low on the lateral

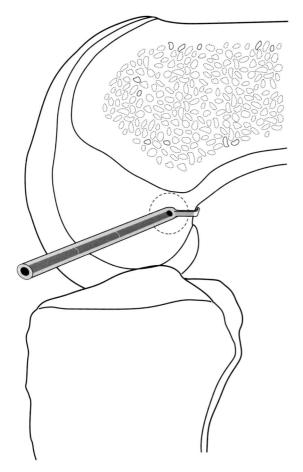

FIG. 1. Schematic showing a prototype guide (courtesy of D.W. Jackson, M.D.) that facilitates placement of a pilot hole 7 mm anterior to the over-the-top position so that the resulting 10-mm femoral tunnel will have a 2-mm thick posterior wall.

wall. Furthermore, the knee flexion angle at the time the guide is used has a significant effect on placement. Nonetheless, these guides are an aid in defining femoral tunnel placement, being most effective in preventing the creation of tunnels that break through the posterior cortex of the femur. This is important, because a loss of posterior wall integrity makes endoscopic techniques with interference screws impossible.

Tibial tunnel placement also has been traditionally defined by local anatomy. The two available reference points are the anterior slope of the anterior tibial spine, which represents the posterior extent of the ACL's tibial insertion, and the roof of the intercondylar notch with the knee in full extension. With a probe or drill guide the spine can be palpated and used as a landmark for placement, and once a Kirshner wire (K-wire) is inserted, the knee can be brought into full extension to examine the relationship between this K-wire and the roof of the intercondylar notch. Considering the radius of the tibial tunnel to be 5 to 6 mm, 5 to 6 mm of clearance must exist between the K-wire and the roof at full extension if the entire tunnel is to lie within the confines of the roof. Here again, new devices are becoming available to strengthen the relationship between local anatomy and placement. One such guide designed by Howell uses the roof of the intercondylar notch to define both the angle of the tibial tunnel and its anterior-to-posterior position (Fig. 2). With this technique a transverse pin is placed just below the roof and 10 mm from the articular margin. When the tibial guide is hooked over this pin and the knee brought into full extension, a K-wire can be inserted parallel and approximately 5 mm posterior to the roof. In spite of this guides-fixed relationship between the roof and the tibial tunnel, placement in the medial-to-lateral direction is less well defined. Furthermore, orientation of the tunnel parallel to the roof of the intercondylar notch may not always be desired. For example, when a patellar tendon graft is placed endoscopically, it is often longer than the tibial tunnel can accommodate. In such circumstances, by increasing the angle of inclination of the tibial tunnel, its length can be increased, allowing the distal bone block to be fixed within an osseous tunnel. Guides with fixed angles do not accommodate this.

Anatomic factors come into play in more ways than just to provide landmarks for tunnel placement. Howell et al. has shown (Fig. 3A and B) that placement of grafts in excessively anterior tibial tunnels causes graft impingement, which can be documented on magnetic resonance imaging (MRI) (18,19). Such impinged grafts demonstrate increased signal intensity on MRI, suggesting increased water content, whereas unimpinged grafts retain the low signal intensity associated with dense connective tissues. In addition to MRI abnormalities, impinged grafts were reported to be associated with restricted motion or increased knee laxity. In another

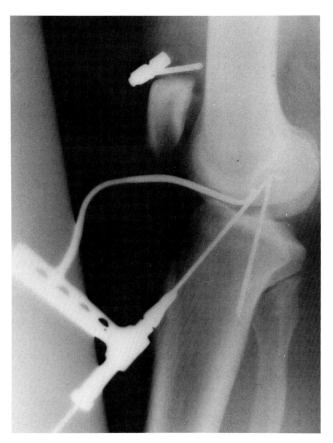

FIG. 2. Radiograph demonstrating the use of a prototype guide (courtesy of S. Howell, M.D.) to direct placement of a tibial K-wire approximately 5 mm posterior and parallel to the intercondylar roof with the knee in full extension.

study, Romano et al. (37) reviewed the postoperative x-rays on 111 patients after ACL reconstruction. Excessive anterior tibial tunnel placement was correlated with a loss of both flexion and extension postoperatively, and excessive medial tunnel placement was associated with restricted knee flexion.

The current recommendation of Howell et al. (19) for tibial tunnel placement is that when a lateral x-ray is taken of the knee in full extension, the anterior edge of the tibial tunnel should be posterior to a line drawn along the roof of the intercondylar notch and extended to the tibia. Such a tunnel lies posterior to the insertion of the anteromedial bundle (a part of the ACL position that many surgeons have recommended be recreated with ACL reconstruction). Further studies will be necessary to identify all the consequences of this proposed posterior shift in the placement of the tibial tunnel.

Functional Assessment as a Guide to Tunnel Placement

The concept of ACL isometry arose out of the work of Mueller (30), who showed that the complex kinematics

of the knee could be modeled in two dimensions with a four-bar linkage. Such a model suggested that attachment sites should exist that do not cause the fibers of the ACL to change in length as the knee moves through a full range of motion. In an attempt to help the surgeon identify such points, a number of different devices have been constructed to allow testing of a suture placed through small pilot holes or attached to a threaded tack at the identified sites for tibial and femoral attachment (7,11). As the knee is placed through a range of motion, changes in separation distance between these sites can be measured. Some devices also allow the length of the suture to be fixed and the tension to be measured through a range of motion. Whereas Odensten and Gillquist (33) found that the distance between central points in the ACL's femoral origin and tibial insertion resulted in a separation distance that did not change with motion, other investigators have been unsuccessful in finding truly isometric attachment sites (11,15,28,38,40). Sapega et al. (38), for example, found that even for the attachments of the most isometric ACL fibers (the anteromedial bundle), separation distances may change by as much as 3 mm with knee motion. Thus, the concept of isometry has evolved from one of identifying isometric attachment sites to a technique where an isometer or tensiometer is used to map out the functional anatomy of the presumed ACL insertions. The goal is not to identify a pair of sites with less than a predetermined amount (e.g., 2 mm) of change in separation distance or change in tension, but to use the pattern of these changes to identify potential attachment sites as anteriorly, posteriorly, or centrally located.

How are anatomic sites differentiated by functional assessment? Data from the Noyes Giannestras Biomechanics Laboratories (5) showed that placement is the major determinant of the pattern of length or tension changes with knee motion. Therefore, either tension or length (separation distance) measurements help distinguish functionally between different attachment sites.

The patterns of changes in separation distance with knee motion have been widely reported (5,8,11,31,35). In a study of 10 cadaveric knees (13), changes in attachment site separation distance for 12 different femoral sites spaced 5 mm apart were measured with a commercially available isometer. The pooled data from these knees are shown in Fig. 4. As noted by others, anterior sites can be identified by their characteristic increase in separation distance with flexion, whereas posterior sites produce a characteristic increase in separation distance with extension. The effect of three different tibial locations is shown in Fig. 4C. These data suggest that although the location of the femoral attachment has the greatest effect on separation distance, the location of the tibial site is also important. For example, an anterior femoral point (F3) produces a greater increase in separation distance with flexion when combined with an ante-

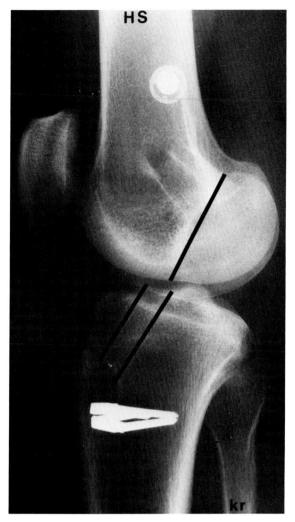

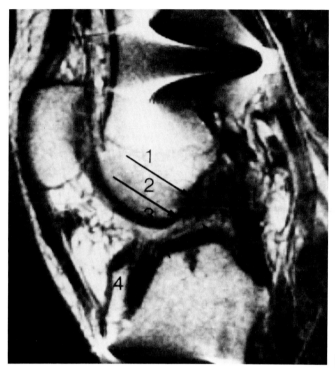

FIG. 3. A: Radiograph showing an impinged graft with the tibial tunnel anterior to the roof of the intercondylar notch. **B:** MRI of the same patient, with increased signal intensity in the middle and distal thirds of the graft (courtesy of S. Howell, M.D.).

rior tibial point (T3) than when paired with a posterior tibial point (T1).

The changes in tension with knee flexion are similar to the separation distance changes. As shown by Penner et al. (35), a posterior femoral point such as OT produces the largest increases in tension with knee extension, whereas an anterior femoral point produces the largest tension increases in flexion (Fig. 5). Similar results have been found by Fleming et al. (9) and Bylski-Austrow (5). Therefore, it is the authors' opinion that either separation distance or tension measurements at various knee flexion angles can provide a functional assessment of attachment sites. Such information can supplement the surgeon's visual or tactile evaluation of the local anatomy, especially when that anatomy is atypical or has been distorted by arthritis or prior surgery.

Although attachment sites can be analyzed and carefully selected, the location of ideal sites has not been

determined. Recommendations that the anteromedial bundle be recreated are based on the small length and tension changes associated with these attachments, and on the similarity of the patterns with that of the ACL (25) (Fig. 6). However, no long-term, adequately controlled clinical study has shown one placement to be superior to all the others.

Femoral Tunnel Orientation

Although a great deal of attention has been directed toward the placement of the femoral tunnel, there has been less study of the importance of the tunnel orientation. As the knee is flexed from 0 to 140 degrees the ACL rotates approximately 100 degrees about its femoral attachment. Before achieving biologic fixation at the tunnel orifice, an ACL graft is free to move within its femo-

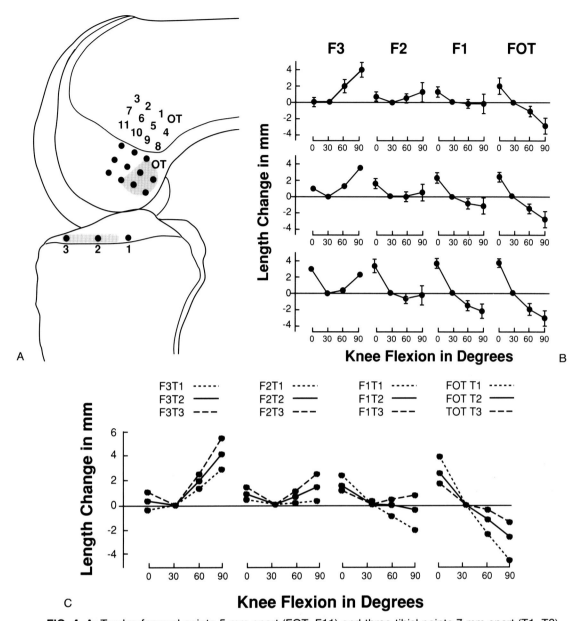

FIG. 4. A: Twelve femoral points 5 mm apart (FOT–F11) and three tibial points 7 mm apart (T1–T3) were evaluated. For reference, the origin and insertion of the ACL are shaded. **B:** The effects of femoral placement: changes in length (attachment site separation distance) in mm as determined with a spring-loaded isometer for the 12 femoral points paired with tibial point T2. **C:** The effects of tibial placement: length changes for femoral points FOT, F1, F2, and F3 when paired with the three tibial points T1, T2, and T3.

ral tunnel. The edges of the tunnel may subject the graft to contact forces and abrasion as the knee flexes and extends. Studies of synthetic grafts have shown them to be sensitive to such abrasion with failure commonly occurring at the femoral notch or femoral tunnel (2,23,24,36,42). Biologic materials may also be subject to contact forces and abrasion. Burkes et al. (3) investigated the effects of continuous passive motion (CPM) on ACL reconstructions in cadaveric knees. After 43,200 cycles of knee flexion from 20 to 70 degrees, loss of knee stability was common for grafts inserted in a femoral

tunnel. In three of the four cases where graft rupture occurred, the site of failure was at the edge of the femoral tunnel. Failure was much less common with placement over the top, where no tunnel was created. O'Meara et al. (34) also noted failure of grafts in femoral tunnels after CPM. Whereas in the past CPM has been clinically demonstrated to be safe after ACL reconstruction, current aggressive rehabilitation may subject the graft to thousands of knee flexion extension cycles in the immediate postoperative period. The potential for damage to the graft with this rehabilitation protocol remains unknown.

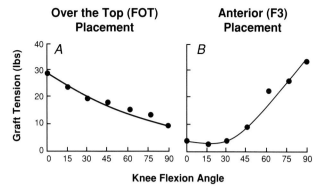

FIG. 5. The over-the-top femoral position produces maximal graft tension in extension (pattern similar to FOT in Fig. 4B), whereas an anterior femoral position produces maximal graft tension in flexion (pattern similar to F3 in Fig. 4B). (From ref. 35, with permission.)

To study the effects of tunnel orientation, chamfering the edge of the femoral tunnel, and graft loading on abrasion and failure, we studied 25 calf knees in our laboratory (12). Instrumentation was developed to allow reproducible placement of femoral tunnels 1 cm in diameter within the normal origin of the ACL. These tunnels were either oriented parallel to the long axis of the ACL (simulating the straight-line tunnels common with endoscopic techniques) or 45 degrees off axis (simulating the more transverse tunnels possible with external drill guides). The intraarticular edges of tunnels were either left unchanged after reaming or chamfered with a commercially available hand rasp. Patellar tendon grafts 1 cm in diameter were inserted in these tunnels and loaded to 2, 5, or 10 pounds as a mechanical device rotated the femur through an arc of 80 degrees in a saline bath.

Results of this experiment are as follows. All five specimens with straight-line femoral tunnels and an applied load of 5 pounds survived greater than 125,000 cycles. All five 5-pound unchamfered transverse tunnels failed at an average of 19,869 cycles. Chamfering transverse tunnels resulted in survival of four of five specimens loaded to 5 pounds. Decreasing the load for transverse

unchamfered tunnels to 2 pounds increased survival to one of five specimens and cycles to failure to 75,132.

From these data we concluded that if patellar tendon grafts used to reconstruct the ACL are subjected to large numbers of flexion-extension cycles, the risk of wear-related damage and early failure may be decreased with straight-line femoral tunnel orientation, by chamfering of more transverse tunnels, or by avoiding large graft preloads. These results are consistent with the three-dimensional kinematic modeling of knee motion used by Gely et al. (10) to investigate the torsion and bending imposed on an ACL prosthesis during knee flexion. In that study the magnitude of both torsion and bending was most affected by the orientation of the femoral tunnel. Similarly, Sidles et al. (39) used pressure-sensitive film to measure pressures applied to a human Achilles tendon graft as it exited a tunnel drilled in a block of lucite. They found that forces increased as the angle between the tunnel and ligament increased.

Is the wear-related damage caused by femoral tunnels in the laboratory clinically relevant? Although graft fail-

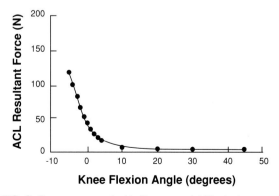

FIG. 6. Forces generated in the normal ACL during passive extension. (From ref. 25, with permission.)

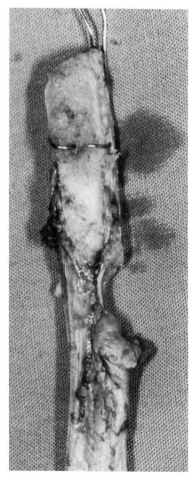

FIG. 7. Patellar tendon graft after 125,000 cycles of simulated knee motion. This specimen did not fail, yet demonstrates significant wear-related damage.

ure after ACL reconstruction is an uncommon event, graft damage may occur. In our experiments we noted that many of the grafts still in continuity at the completion of the experiment nonetheless showed signs of wear and abrasion (Fig. 7). Furthermore, our preliminary data raised concerns that graft elongation may accompany the wear-related damage that occurs before failure. It is clear that further work will be necessary to determine the importance of tunnel orientation in ACL surgery. However, these data suggest that there may be some advantage to either creating straight-line tunnels or carefully chamfering the edges of more transverse tunnels.

GRAFT TENSIONING

It is now apparent that graft tension is among the many factors in surgical technique and postoperative management that affect the ultimate result of ACL reconstruction. Graft tension plays an important role in knee kinematics and perhaps in ligament remodeling (44). Beginning with Grood et al. in 1983 (7), many investigators have shown that joint laxity is related to graft tension (1,4,5,8,20–22,27,29). In cadaveric knees, Burks and Leland (4) investigated ACL reconstruction with bony tunnels at "isometric" points on the femur and tibia. Using a KT-1000 to measure anteroposterior translation at 25 degrees of knee flexion, Burks and Leland found that the amount of graft tension needed to restore normal anteroposterior laxity to the knee appeared to be tissue specific. That is, the required tensions for patellar tendon, semitendinosus, and iliotibial bands were significantly different. Studies from the University of Minnesota (20–22) found that graft force or graft tension was highly sensitive to the length of the graft at the time of fixation. Furthermore, it was noted that even small changes in position of the femoral tunnel resulted in changes in graft tension. Bylski-Austrow et al. (5) further defined the complex interrelationship between placement and graft tension. Using a cable to represent the reconstructed ACL, Bylski-Wustrow et al. investigated over-the-top femoral placement and three potential femoral tunnel locations. They also evaluated initial graft tensions of 22 and 44 N with knees at either 0 or 30 degrees at the time of fixation. Under these conditions, graft (cable) tension was measured at various flexion angles under a 100-N anterior load applied to the tibia. Both the initial tension applied to the graft and the flexion angle at tensioning affected the magnitude of graft tension but did not affect the pattern of tension changes throughout the range of knee motion (Fig. 8). Bylski-Wustrow et al. also noted that the anteroposterior position of the tibia was related to graft tension. They concluded that although over-the-top placement provided the most reproducible results, placement of the graft in the isometric region with 44 N of tension applied to the

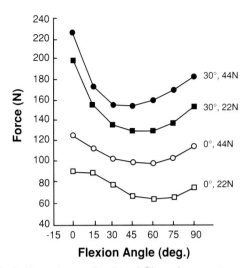

FIG. 8. Force transmitted by ACL replacement as a function of flexion: effect of flexion angle at tensioning and initial tension. Anterior load 100 N; distal placement for the four combinations of flexion angle at tensioning (0 degrees, 30 degrees) and initial applied tension (22 N, 44 N). (From ref. 5, with permission.)

graft with the knee at full extension best reproduced the normal restraints to anteroposterior translation of the knee.

Graft tension may also have an effect on the remodeling that occurs when autologous tissue is used to reconstruct the ACL. In a study of dogs reconstructed with patellar tendon grafts subjected to 1 or 39 N of pretensioning, Yoshiya et al. (44) suggested that revascularization of autogenous grafts may be adversely affected by excessive pretensioning. However, statistically significant differences in graft strength were not noted.

If graft tension is important, then the time-dependent mechanical behavior of ligaments and tendons must be considered. Patellar tendon, like other tendons and ligaments, is a viscoelastic material (14,16,17,41), meaning that the relationship between graft stress and strain is time dependent. This time dependency can manifest itself in several ways. If a fixed load in the physiologic range is applied to patellar tendon, its length will increase over time (creep). On the other hand, if a fixed deformation is applied, the load will decrease over time (relaxation). Therefore, if a patellar tendon is used to reconstruct the ACL, the desired initial tension applied, and the graft fixed, graft tension can be expected to decrease over time. Furthermore, the amount of tension that is lost will depend on the load history of the graft, because it is well known that preconditioning of viscoelastic materials affects their mechanical properties. Fredrich et al. (31) investigated this phenomenon by reconstructing the ACL in cadaveric knees with patellar tendon grafts. They noted a 42% drop in a 22-N preload over 15 minutes and a 35% drop in a 66-N preload over 15 minutes. They also reported that preconditioning the graft before fixation could decrease the amount of stress

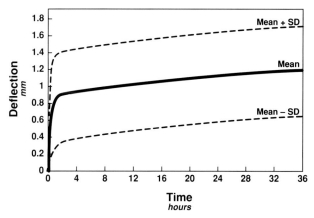

FIG. 9. Changes in length for a patellar tendon graft maintained in a saline bath under a constant 5-pound load.

relaxation, but that the effect was short-lived. McPherson et al. (26), on the other hand, found a significant preconditioning effect even after 60 minutes of recovery time in rabbit medial collateral ligaments.

To investigate the effect of preconditioning on a viscoelastic response of patellar tendon, our laboratory conducted a study of 35 primate patella/patellar tendon/tibia complexes (14). Specimens were divided into five groups of seven and subjected to 10-minute relaxation tests at 2.5% strain with and without preconditioning.

The results of these tests showed that significant relaxation occurs in unpreconditioned specimens. Ten minutes after application of a 2.5% strain, the patellar tendon tension had decreased to an average of only 30% of the peak tension. After preconditioning, significantly more of the peak tension was maintained over time. When the interval between preconditioning and the relaxation test was only 1 minute, 68.8% of peak tension was maintained through 10 minutes, compared with 49% with a 10-minute unloaded interval and 49% with a 30-minute unloaded interval. In addition, cyclic preconditioning was found to be no more or less effective than static preconditioning.

In another experiment we subjected five (frozen, then thawed), nonpreconditioned human patellar tendon grafts, 10 mm in width, to a 5-pound load in a saline bath. After 36 hours, mean length changes of 1 mm were observed, with the greatest changes occurring in the first 4 hours (Fig. 9). If a length change of this magnitude were to occur in the clinical situation, significant changes in knee laxity or graft tension could result. However, the *in vivo* situation differs in that neither length nor tension is held constant. Furthermore, with knee motion, periods of both high and low graft tension will occur. The intervals of low tension will allow recovery from the viscous effects. Therefore, despite the viscoelastic nature of the ACL grafts, overconstraint of the joint caused by excessive graft loading remains a concern.

SUMMARY

The knee is a complex mechanical system with an interdependency of its constituents. In reconstructing the ACL, any change in structural properties (stiffness, strength, viscosity, length, cross-section, fiber direction, points of attachment, etc.) will inevitably alter knee mechanics. Optimal points of attachment can be identified in a knee with normal kinematics, but the abnormal kinematics of the ACL-deficient knee make attachment site selection difficult. The surgeon can rely entirely on anatomic clues, or can perform a functional assessment before selecting points of attachment.

Although the pattern of the changes in tension with knee motion is determined by the placement of the graft, the magnitude of the tension is very much affected by the pretension applied to the graft, the flexion angle at tensioning, the load history of the graft, and time. In addition, preliminary data suggest that postoperative impingement and abrasion at the tunnel margin can damage the graft. Reproducible techniques must be developed to control all of these variables. Only then can we evaluate the relative sensitivity of the surgical outcome to these parameters and determine their optimal values.

The complex interrelationships between structure, kinematics, and joint loads suggest that *in vitro* experiments that single out one or two variables at a time for study may be necessary to gain a more complete understanding of the problem. Cell and organ culture techniques allow good control of the mechanical and biochemical environment of connective tissues, but the artificial nature of the environment may alter the cellular response to mechanical challenges. *In vivo* monitoring of tendon stresses and strains offers another avenue to investigate the relationship between the mechanical environment and cellular activity in both normal and remodeling tissues. The greatest advances will probably be made by conducting experiments of both types.

REFERENCES

1. Amis AA. (1989): Anterior cruciate ligament replacement. Knee stability and the effects of implants. *J Bone Joint Surg* 71B:819–824.
2. Andersen HN, Bruun C, Sondergard-Peterson PE (1992): Reconstruction of chronic insufficient anterior cruciate ligament in the knee using a synthetic Dacron prosthesis. A prospective study of 57 cases. *Am J Sports Med* 20:20–23.
3. Burks R, Daniel D, Losse G. (1984): The effect of continuous passive motion on anterior cruciate ligament reconstruction stability. *Am J Sports Med* 12:323–327.
4. Burks RT, Leland R. (1988): Determination of graft tension before fixation in anterior cruciate ligament reconstruction. *Arthroscopy* 4:260–266.
5. Bylski-Austrow DI, Grood ES, Hefzy MS, Holden JP, Butler DL. (1990): Anterior cruciate ligament replacements: a mechanical study of femoral attachment location, flexion angle at tensioning, and initial tension. *J Orthop Res* 8:522–531.
6. Clancy WG Jr, Nelson DA, Reider B, Narechania RG. (1982):

Anterior cruciate ligament reconstruction using one-third of the patellar ligament, augmented by extra-articular tendon transfers. *J Bone Joint Surg* 64A:352–359.

7. Daniel DM. (1990): Principles of knee ligament surgery. In: Daniel DM, Akeson WH, O'Connor JJ, eds. *Knee ligaments: structure, function, injury, and repair.* New York: Raven, pp. 11–29.

8. Fleming B, Beynnon B, Howe J, McLeod W, Pope M. (1992): Effect of tension and placement of a prosthetic anterior cruciate ligament on the anteroposterior laxity of the knee. *J Orthop Res* 10:177–186.

9. Fleming B, Beynnon B, Johnson R, McLeod W, Pope M. (1992): Isometric versus tension measurements: a comparison for the reconstruction of the anterior cruciate ligament. *Am J Sports Med* [*in press*].

10. Gely P, Drouin G, Thiry PS, Tremblay GR. (1984): Torsion and bending imposed on a new anterior cruciate ligament prosthesis during knee flexion: an evaluation method. *J Biomech Eng* 106:285–294.

11. Graf BK. (1987): Isometric placement of substitutes for the anterior cruciate ligament. In: Jackson DW, ed. *The anterior cruciate deficient knee.* St. Louis: Mosby, pp. 102–113.

12. Graf BK, Henry J, Rothenberg M, Vanderby R Jr. (1992): Anterior cruciate ligament reconstruction with patellar tendon: an *ex vivo* study of wear-related damage and failure at the femoral tunnel. Presented at the American Orthopaedic Society of Sports Medicine meeting, July.

13. Graf BK, Simon T, Jackson D. (1985): Isometric placement of cruciate ligament substitutes: a new technique. Presented in part at the Annual Meeting of the International Society of the Knee, Salzburg, Austria, May.

14. Graf BK, Vanderby R Jr, Ulm MJ, Rogalski RP, Thielke RJ. (1992): The effect of preconditioning on the viscoelastic response of primate patellar tendon. *Transactions of the 38th Annual ORS,* Washington DC, February 17–20, 38:147.

15. Grood ES, Hefzy MS, Butler DL, Suntay WJ, Siegel MG, Noyes FR. (1983): On the placement and the initial tension of anterior cruciate ligament substitutes. *Transactions of the 29th annual ORS,* Anaheim, CA, March 8–10, 29:92.

16. Haut RC, Powlison AC. (1990): The effects of test environment and cyclic stretching on the failure properties of human patellar tendons. *J Orthop Res* 8:532–540.

17. Hooley CJ, McCrum NG, Cohen RE. (1980): The viscoelastic deformation of tendon. *J Biomech* 13:521–528.

18. Howell SM, Clark JA, Blasier RD. (1991): Serial magnetic resonance imaging of hamstring anterior cruciate ligament autografts during the first year of implantation. A preliminary study. *Am J Sports Med* 19:42–47.

19. Howell SM, Clark JA, Farley TE. (1991): A rationale for predicting anterior cruciate graft impingement by the intercondylar roof. A magnetic resonance imaging study. *Am J Sports Med* 19:276–282.

20. Hunter RE, Lew WD, Lewis JL, Kowalczyk C, Settle W. (1990): Graft force-setting technique in reconstruction of the anterior cruciate ligament. *Am J Sports Med* 18:12–19.

21. Lew WD, Engebretsen L, Lewis JL, Hunter RE, Kowalczyk C. (1990): Method for setting total graft force and load sharing in augmented ACL grafts. *J Orthop Res* 8:702–711.

22. Lewis JL, Lew WD, Engebretsen L, Hunter RE, Kowalczyk C. (1990): Factors affecting graft force in surgical reconstruction of the anterior cruciate ligament. *J Orthop Res* 8:514–521.

23. Lopez-Vazquez E, Juan JA, Vila E, Debon J. (1991): Reconstruction of the anterior cruciate ligament with a Dacron prosthesis. *J Bone Joint Surg* 73A:1294–1300.

24. Lukianov AV, Richmond JC, Barrett GR, Gillquist J. (1989): A multicenter study on the results of anterior cruciate ligament re-

construction using a Dacron ligament prosthesis in "salvage" cases. *Am J Sports Med* 17:380–386.

25. Markolf KL, Gorek JF, Kabo JM, Shapiro MS. (1990): Direct measurement of resultant forces in the anterior cruciate ligament. *J Bone Joint Surg* 72A:557–567.

26. McPherson R, King G, Shrive N, Frank C (1992): Extension rate alters load relaxation in the rabbit MCL. *Transactions of the 38th Annual ORS,* Washington, DC, February 17–20, 38:126.

27. Melby A III, Noble JS, Askew MJ, Boom AA, Hurst FW. (1991): The effects of graft tensioning on the laxity and kinematics of the anterior cruciate ligament reconstructed knee. *Arthroscopy* 7:257–266.

28. Melhorn JM, Henning CE. (1987): The relationship of the femoral attachment site to the isometric tracking of the anterior cruciate ligament graft. *Am J Sports Med* 15:539–542.

29. More RC, Markolf KL. (1988): Measurement of stability of the knee and ligament force after implantation of a synthetic anterior cruciate ligament. *J Bone Joint Surg* 70A:1020–1031.

30. Muller W. (1988): *The knee: form, function and ligament reconstruction.* New York: Springer Verlag.

31. O'Brien WR, Friederich NF, Muller W, Henning CE. (1992): The effects of stress relaxation on initial graft loads during anterior cruciate ligament reconstruction. *Trans Orthop* 13:316–317.

32. O'Brien WR, Henning CE. (1987): Anterior cruciate ligament substitute load versus tibial positioning: an *in vitro* study. *Am J Sports Med* 15:398.

33. Odensten M, Gillquist J. (1985): Functional anatomy of the anterior cruciate ligament and a rationale for reconstruction. *J Bone Joint Surg* 67A:257–262.

34. O'Meara PM, O'Brien WR, Henning CE. (1992): Anterior cruciate ligament reconstruction stability with continuous passive motion. The role of isometric graft placement. *Clin Orthop* 277:201–209.

35. Penner DA, Daniel DM, Wood P, Mishra D. (1988): An *in vitro* study of anterior cruciate ligament graft placement and isometry. *Am J Sports Med* 16:238–243.

36. Richmond JC, Manseau CJ, Patz R, McConville O. (1992): Anterior cruciate reconstruction using a Dacron ligament prosthesis. A long-term study. *Am J Sports Med* 20:24–28.

37. Romano VM, Graf BK, Keene JS, Lange RH. (1992): Anterior cruciate ligament reconstruction: the effect of tibial tunnel placement on range of motion. *Am J Sports Med* [*in press*].

38. Sapega AA, Moyer RA, Schneck C, Komalahiranya N. (1990): Testing for isometry during reconstruction of the anterior cruciate ligament. *J Bone Joint Surg* 72A:259–267.

39. Sidles JA, Clark JM, Huber JD. (1990): Large internal pressures occur in ligament grafts at bone tunnels. *Transactions of the 36th Annual ORS Meeting,* New Orleans, Louisiana, February 5–8, 36:81.

40. Sidles JA, Larson RV, Garbini JL, Downey DJ, Matsen FA (1988): Ligament length relationships in the moving knee. *J Orthop Res* 6:593–610.

41. Woo SL-Y. (1982): Mechanical properties of tendons and ligaments. I. Quasi-static and nonlinear viscoelasticproperties. *Biorheology* 19:385–396.

42. Woods GA, Indelicato PA, Prevot TJ. (1991): The Gore-Tex anterior cruciate ligament prosthesis. Two versus three-year results. *Am J Sports Med* 19:48–55.

43. Yaru NC, Daniel DM, Penner D. (1992): The effect of tibial attachment site on graft impingement in an anterior cruciate ligament reconstruction. *Am J Sports Med* 20:217–220.

44. Yoshiya S, Andrish JT, Manley MT, Bauer TW. (1987): Graft tension in anterior cruciate ligament reconstruction. An *in vivo* study in dogs. *Am J Sports Med* 15:464–470.

The Anterior Cruciate Ligament: Current and Future Concepts, edited by D.W. Jackson, et al. Raven Press, Ltd., New York © 1993.

CHAPTER 26

Autograft Reconstruction of the Anterior Cruciate Ligament

Bone–Patellar Tendon– Bone

Douglas W. Jackson and Mark J. Lemos

A patella tendon autograft with bone plugs at each end is presently the most commonly used graft to reconstruct the anterior cruciate ligament (ACL). Its popularity among surgeons is related to its time zero maximum load to failure strength (15) and its bone-to-bone fixation capabilities. Although the initial fixation of the bone plugs with interference screws gives the highest pull-out values, other methods of fixation include sutures tied over screw posts, buttons, or staples (11). Other sections of this text (Section II) have discussed in detail the mechanical and structural properties of patella tendon autografts. In addition, our current understandings of the biological incorporation (Chapter 14) and eventual mechanical and structural properties of the autograft have been presented (Chapter 20).

Whether using an autograft, allograft, or prosthetic substitute, reconstructions of the ACL have many common steps. The evaluation and documentation of the ACL-deficient knee under anesthesia and the treatment of other associated intraarticular pathology is common to all reconstructions. This chapter will concentrate on those principles and techniques unique to using the patella tendon autograft to reconstruct an ACL. Special considerations will be given to harvesting and preparation of the bone–patella tendon–bone autograft, position and length of the tunnels, graft placement in the osseous tunnels, tensioning and fixation of the autograft, and bone grafting of the residual patellar defect.

D. W. Jackson and M. J. Lemos: Southern California Center for Sports Medicine, Long Beach, California 90806.

HARVEST AND PREPARATION OF PATELLAR TENDON AUTOGRAFT WITH BONE PLUGS

Timing for harvesting the autograft during the surgical reconstruction is the surgeon's preference. If there is a question of whether the ACL is incompetent after the examination under anesthesia, an arthroscopic evaluation of the ACL should be performed before harvesting the graft. If the preoperative examination of the knee documents a deficient ACL, then harvesting the graft before arthroscopy offers several advantages. Harvested initially, there is no soft tissue swelling associated with the arthroscopy portals, and the dissection of the soft tissue planes is easier. It also allows the final trimming and placement of sutures in the graft to be accomplished simultaneously by an assistant while the surgeon is doing the arthroscopic intraarticular surgery and tunnel preparation. The graft is then ready for passage when the surgeon has prepared the tibial and femoral tunnels, reducing the overall surgical time.

The skin exposure for harvesting the graft may be through two small transverse incisions overlying the bony insertions of the patella tendon or through one vertical incision exposing the entire length of the tendon. The vertical incision allows for direct visualization of the patellar tendon during graft harvesting. The vertical approach is a more utilitarian exposure that can be extended for possible subsequent surgical procedures. It extends along the medial border of the patellar tendon, from the inferior pole of the patella to a point just medial to the tibial tubercle. The overlying soft tissue should be meticulously dissected and mobilized in a layer fashion from the tendon. This will facilitate soft tissue closure over the remaining patella tendon defect. Similar attention to the soft tissue elevation over the distal patella allows for a closure that uses soft tissue to assist in holding the bone graft in place in the patellar defect. Many surgeons elect not to bone graft the defect. If the donor site from the patella is not grafted, the osseous defect usually does not fill in, but this does not appear to have significant additional morbidity.

Tendon Harvesting

Harvesting of the middle third of the patella tendon is the current choice of most surgeons. The most commonly used width is a 9-, 10-, or 11-mm graft (Fig. 1). This varies according to the surgeon's preference (15). The upper limits in the width of the graft are also determined in consideration of the strength of the remaining tendon. A consensus rule of thumb is that the graft probably should not exceed 40% of the overall patella tendon width. This has been a clinical observation and is not based on human studies. No correlation has been reported between graft size and a propensity for rupture of the remaining patellar tendon after graft removal. We have recently shown in the goat model that the remaining tendon is weakened by 50% when a central third graft of 40% the width of the patellar tendon is harvested. There is evidence that the tendon regains strength with

time, and tendon rupture has been a rare complication after graft harvesting (9,14).

The tendon is incised between the bone–tendon junctions by pushing the scalpel blade or a specialized knife in line with the collagen fibers. The incisions in the patella tendon are facilitated by keeping the tendon fibers under tension with retraction of the patella proximally and some degree of knee flexion. Care should be taken not to damage the fiber insertion at the bone junctions.

Bone Plug Harvesting

The object in harvesting the bone plugs is to reproducibly obtain a plug that fills the osseous tunnel, requires minimal additional time to trim, allows secure fixation, and does not predispose the remaining patella to subsequent fractures. The most commonly used bone plug widths are 9, 10, or 11 mm. The dimensions of the bone plugs are determined by the diameter of the femoral and tibial tunnels. We use harvesting plug cutters (Fig. 2) powered by an oscillating saw to uniformly obtain cylindrical bone plugs. The potential advantages of cylindrical bone plugs are: (a) decreased patella stress riser at the graft harvest site; (b) ease of graft insertion due to uniform sizing; and (c) a reproducible cylindrical bone plug 1 mm in diameter smaller than the corresponding circular osseous tunnel (8). The bone plug filling the osseous tunnel optimizes the interference screw fixation and

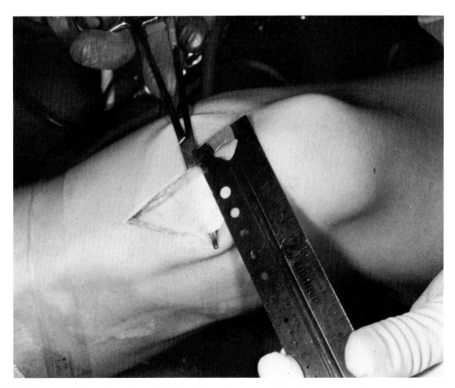

FIG. 1. A clamp is placed underneath the dissected middle third of the patella tendon and its width measured with a ruler. The central 11 mm is marked with the bovie.

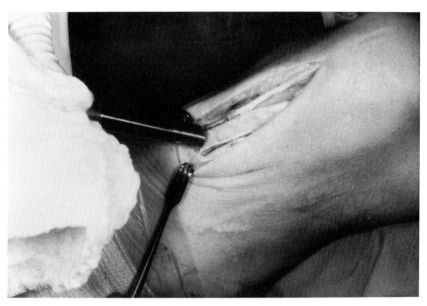

FIG. 2. Harvesting plug cutters are available in diameters of 9, 10, and 11 mm. They provide semicylindrical bone plugs. This tibial bone plug was harvested with an 11-mm plug cutter.

bone incorporation. The advantages of a uniformly shaped plug can be obtained by strict adherence to several techniques while harvesting the graft, whether using a saw, gouge, or osteotome.

If the tibial bone plug is harvested first and mobilized, it then may be grasped and pulled distally with a towel clip, drawing the patella distally into the wound. This allows a smaller skin incision to be used (Fig. 3).

Bone–Patellar Tendon–Bone Graft Preparation

The autograft may be trimmed to the surgeon's specification on a side table by an assistant. Our preference for instruments on this side table work station include (a) four bone plug sizers in diameters of 9, 10, 11, and 12 mm; (b) a bone rongeur; (c) Mayo scissors, (d) a bone plug holder; (e) a drill guide for drilling holes to accept

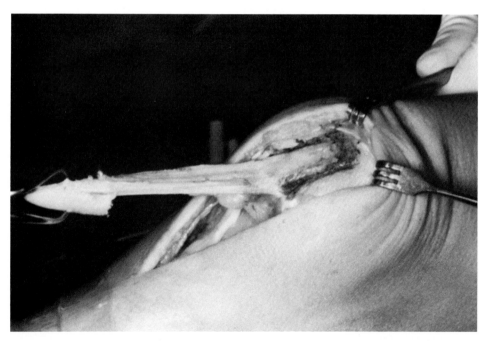

FIG. 3. A shorter skin incision can be made by harvesting the tibial bone plug first, then placing a towel clamp on it to pull the patella into the wound. The dimensions of the patella bone plug have been outlined with electrocautery.

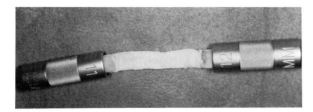

FIG. 4. The patella/lesser diameter bone plug, obtained with the 10-mm harvesting plug cutter, easily slides through the 11-mm sizer with minimal trimming. The tibial/larger diameter end was harvested with the 11-mm plug cutter and slides through the 12-mm sizer.

sutures; (f) a spring-loaded device to hold the ligament under tension, facilitating final trimming of the graft; and (g) a measuring device to determine the length of the overall graft and bone plugs.

The assistant simulates the size and the ease of passing the graft through the desired tibial and femoral osseous tunnels (Fig. 4). The eventual tunnel and sizer should be 1 mm larger in diameter than the bone plug. The bone plug is trimmed as necessary until it easily passes through the appropriate sizer. The width and length of the bone plugs are the surgeon's preference and relate to selection of a fixation technique; if necessary, the length and shape of the bone plugs can be altered using a rongeur. We prefer the bone plug harvested from the tibia to measure 25 mm and the bone plug harvested from the patella to measure 20 to 22 mm in length.

If the endoscopic technique of ACL reconstruction is used, a single drill hole is made through the cortical sur-face of one bone plug fairly close to its end. We prefer to use the patella bone plug for this. This placement provides better directional control of the plug when pulling it into the osseous tunnels. Three evenly spaced drill holes are made in the tibial bone plug. These sutures will be used for tensioning of the graft after the endoscopic fixation of the femoral bone plug. For the three tensioning sutures, one drill hole is made from the cortical bone surface, and then the plug is rotated 90 degrees and two holes are drilled perpendicular to the first. This will minimize the possibility of an interference screw cutting all three sutures at the time of insertion. If a two-incision technique (distal lateral femoral incision) is used instead of the endoscopic technique, three #5 Tevdek sutures are placed in each bone plug, as described for the tibia.

With the graft under tension it is rotated, and a curved Mayo scissor is used to remove excess tissue. The patella bone–tendon junction is marked with a marking pen (Fig. 5). This marking assists in determining the desired positioning and rotational alignment of the bone plug in the femoral osseous tunnel. Once the graft is prepared, it can be wrapped with an antibiotic-soaked sponge until the surgeon is ready to place it into the joint.

TIBIAL OSSEOUS TUNNEL PREPARATION

Calculating Tibial Osseous Tunnel Length

When using a bone–patellar tendon–bone autograft, if it is the desire of the surgeon to have both of the bone

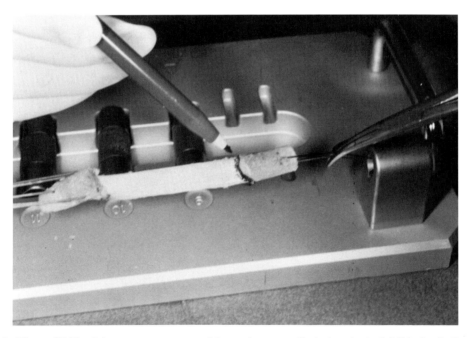

FIG. 5. Three #5 Tevdek sutures are passed through perpendicularly oriented drill holes in the tibial/larger diameter bone plug. A 30-inch long #2 Dermalon suture is passed through a single drill hole in the patella/lesser diameter plug. The graft is placed under 8 to 10 pounds of tension, and final trimming of the fat and extraneous tissue is performed. The patella bone–tendon junction is marked with a marking pen.

plugs contained in the osseous tunnels, special consideration must be given to the length of the tibial osseous tunnel.

The total length of the typical bone–patella tendon-bone autograft after harvesting usually measures 90 to 105 mm. The length of the tibial tunnel is determined from the overall length of the graft minus the length of the femoral tunnel and 30 mm for the intraarticular portion of the graft (Fig. 6). This usually leaves a desired tibial tunnel length of 35 to 50 mm to accommodate most grafts. Most tibial guides have measurements that allow the length of the tibial tunnel to be determined. We

prefer making the tibial tunnel 5 mm longer than projected to accommodate the resultant oblique opening of the tunnel at the tibial cortical surface.

For example, a graft with an overall length of 100 mm might consist of a 20 mm long patella bone plug, a 55 mm long patella tendon, and a 25 mm long tibial bone plug. If the endoscopic technique is being used, we would use the 20 mm long patella bone plug placed within a 25 mm deep femoral osseous tunnel. The remaining graft length must fit into the combined length of the intraarticular distance (30 mm) and the tibial osseous tunnel length. Preparing the appropriate length

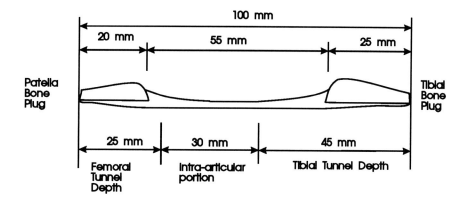

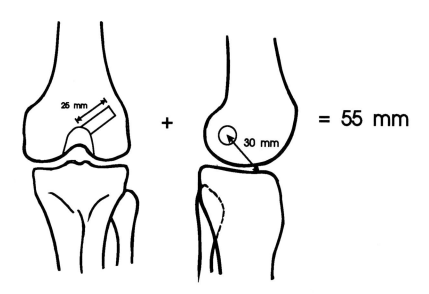

100 mm (Total Grft Length) - 55 mm = 45 mm (Tibial Tunnel Length)

FIG. 6. The length of the tibial tunnel is calculated by subtracting total graft length from the sum of the length of the femoral tunnel (25 mm) and the intraarticular distance between the tunnel openings (30 mm). Another 5 mm should be added to the difference to accommodate for the obliquity of the tibial tunnel.

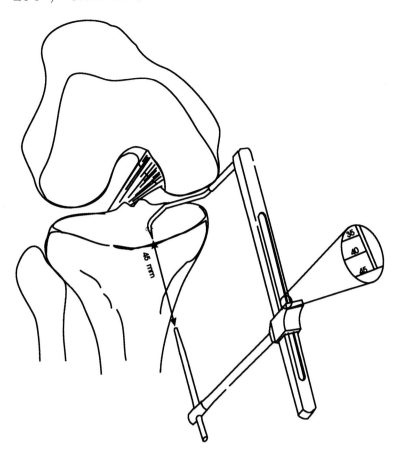

FIG. 7. Calculation of the tibial tunnel length for a 100-mm graft with bone plugs of 20 and 25 mm. Assuming a femoral tunnel length of 25 mm (not yet drilled) and an intraarticular distance of 30 mm (the average length of an ACL), the tibial tunnel would have to be at least 45 mm in length to accommodate the graft. In this case a tunnel of 50 mm would be preferable.

for the tibial tunnel to use interference fixation results in the tip of the tibial bone plug being flush with the tibial cortex when it is tensioned (Fig. 7).

Drilling the Tibial Osseous Tunnel

With the knee at 90 degrees of flexion, the tip of the tibial drill guide is passed through the anteromedial portal and seated in the center of the tibial insertion of the ACL. For the selection of the tibial insertion site, identification of the center of the ACL tibial insertion footprint uses several landmarks. These include continuation of a line from the inner rim of the anterior horn of the lateral meniscus, the midpoint of the medial intercondylar eminence, and a distance of 1 to 2 mm plus the radius of the desired tibial osseous tunnel anterior to the fibers of the posterior cruciate ligament (Fig. 8). In addition, this point selected for the placement of the tibial osseous tunnel should allow clearance of the graft under the roof of the intercondylar notch on full knee extension. Care must be taken to avoid placing the tibial tunnel too anteriorly. Roof impingement of the graft will contribute to difficulty obtaining extension and is a risk to graft survival (7,18). Using a posterior wall within 1 to 2 mm of the posterior cruciate ligament assures not being too anterior. The other consideration is the angle the tibial tunnel will enter the joint. The tibial tunnel length

should not exceed 50 mm or the angle becomes too vertical.

The skin incision is retracted medially and distally to allow placement of the drill sleeve medial to the tibial tubercle. The length of the drill guide is adjusted to give the predetermined desired tibial osseous tunnel length (Fig. 9). The length of the tibial osseous tunnel is verified and a guide pin is passed through the drill guide. As the drill is started, attention should be given to prevent it from walking along the tibial surface. This can be facili-

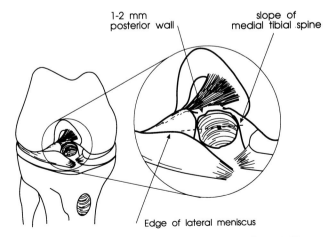

FIG. 8. The tibial footprint, selection of the graft's tibial insertion site using the anatomic landmarks described in the text.

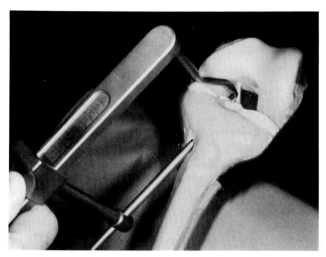

FIG. 9. A calibrated drill guide is used to make the tibial tunnel the desired predetermined length. The point of entry should not interfere with the insertion of the patella tendon.

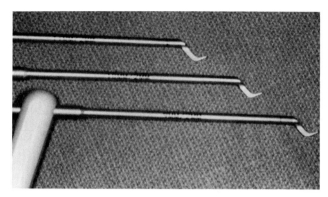

FIG. 10. The femoral tunnel placement guide. The end slips over the top, and a drill, passed through the drill sleeve, marks the center of the femoral tunnel. Guides have been made for 9-, 10-, and 11-mm tunnels, each leaving a 2-mm posterior cortical rim.

tated by using a tapping action as the drill bit starts to cut into the cortex.

We prefer to use a cannulated core drill that cuts a dowel plug of bone from the tibia, which we use for bone grafting the patella. As it enters the joint, it produces a well-marginated tunnel. If a drill is used, a curette is placed over the tip of the guide pin. This helps to prevent the drill and guide pin from plunging into the joint at the completion of drilling the tibial osseous tunnel. The tibial osseous tunnel entrance into the joint is debrided of excess soft tissue and bony debris. Meticulous care is taken to prevent any debris from being left anterior to the graft exit site on the tibia. This bone, cartilage, and soft tissue debris may result in impingement and is thought to contribute to the development of a postoperative "cyclops" lesion (10). Plugging the outflow of fluid through the tibial tunnel maintains joint distention while this work is being done.

LOCATION OF THE FEMORAL TUNNEL SITE

Identification of the superolateral aspect of the intercondylar notch and the over-the-top position are integral to selecting the location of the center of the femoral osseous tunnel. These landmarks are best visualized and prepared with the knee flexed at 70 degrees or more. There are three commonly used methods to locate the desired center of the femoral osseous tunnel. It may be selected by direct visualization, by using an "isometric" device, or by using a guide that keys off anatomic landmarks. We have developed an endoscopic femoral osseous tunnel placement guide that consists of a handle, a drill sleeve, and a locator (Fig. 10). The selection of the center of the osseous tunnel is separate from determining the trajectory of the femoral osseous tunnel. The trajectory is determined by which portal is used to drill the

femoral tunnel. Our preference is to drill the femoral tunnel through the tibial osseous tunnel.

Selection of the femoral tunnel should reproducibly result in a femoral osseous tunnel with 1 to 2 mm thick posterior cortical wall if interference fixation is to be used on the femoral side. This provides a margin of safety for fixation, as well as protection of posterior vessels and nerves. The use of the placement guide, which measures from the posterior cortex, prevents putting the femoral osseous tunnel too far anterior. Similarly, it ensures the most posterior position of the osseous tunnel without destroying the posterior wall of the tunnel. Isometry of the center of the osseous tunnel remains a method used by many surgeons. It is our impression that the most valued contribution of these devices is to prevent excessive anterior placement of the femoral osseous tunnel. Some surgeons feel they can consistently choose this site visually. The desired diameter of the femoral tunnel is generally 1 mm greater in diameter than the corresponding bone plug. This facilitates the passage and placement of the graft. The size of the femoral tunnel should be determined after the final trimming and sizing of the corresponding bone plug.

If an 11-mm femoral osseous tunnel is desired, the center of the osseous tunnel should be approximately 7.5 mm anterior to the over-the-top position. This results in a tunnel with a 5.5-mm radius and a thickness of 2 mm of bone at the posterior wall of the osseous tunnel.

FEMORAL OSSEOUS TUNNEL PREPARATION

Determining Femoral Osseous Tunnel Trajectory

A small drill or guide pin may be used as a guide for the cannulated reamer that creates the femoral osseous tunnel. To achieve the desired trajectory for placement of the femoral tunnel, we prefer to have the knee flexed 60 to 80 degrees. With the knee flexed at approximately 70 degrees, the femoral drill guide can be passed through the tibial osseous tunnel. It is then drilled to a prechosen depth of approximately 25 to 30 mm. The trajectory is changed if the femoral tunnel is drilled through the anteromedial arthroscopic portal or an accessory portal. The femoral tunnel can be drilled as a straight line or less dependent of the tibial osseous tunnel trajectory. This variation in the trajectory can be achieved by using a larger diameter tibial osseous tunnel, by varying the desired knee flexion angle, or by using a specialized drill that allows a smaller shaft than tip, which allows the shaft to rest against the posterior lateral aspect of the tibial osseous tunnel.

Drilling the Femoral Osseous Tunnel

The cannulated drill is passed over the guide pin. Care must be taken in passing the femoral reamer's cutting blades through the tibial osseous tunnel and joint to avoid damage to the posterior cruciate ligament. The reamer is advanced under arthroscopic visualization without power until it is flush with the bone in the notch. Power is then applied to the reamer, and it is advanced slowly to the desired depth. The exact depth depends on the length of the patella bone plug and is generally at least 5 mm deeper than the length of the bone plug. The depth is arthroscopically read from the markings on the cannulated reamer at the opening of the femoral osseous tunnel. The reamer is backed out carefully after drilling the osseous tunnel. The tunnel and joint are debrided of residual bone fragments and inspected to ensure that they are clear of any bone or soft tissue debris.

The surgeon may desire to initially make a smaller femoral osseous tunnel and progressively enlarge it. Starting with a small size allows some manipulation in position if necessary. The other option is to drill the desired tunnel diameter in one step.

The overall end-to-end length between the two osseous tunnels is measured by reading the distance off the calibrated shaft of the reamer as it exits the tibial osseous tunnel (Fig. 9). The total length we desire is 5 mm longer than the overall graft length. If the graft length is too long, the length of the bone plugs may be shortened. Another option is to deepen the femoral osseous tunnel, which increases the end-to-end tunnel distance to accommodate the length of the graft.

An eyeloop drill is advanced through the tibial and femoral tunnels with the knee flexed 90 to 110 degrees. It is drilled out the anterolateral aspect of the thigh. To assist the drill exiting through the skin, an instrument is placed proximal to the exit point of the pin on the skin and pressure is applied. Once the drill is through the skin, a drill puller may be placed over the tip of the exposed drill. This is used to stabilize the drill, cover its sharp tip, and assist in passing the sutures attached to the graft.

GRAFT PLACEMENT AND FIXATION

Graft Placement

The graft is passed to the surgeon, and if an endoscopic technique is to be used, the single suture through the patella bone plug is passed through the eyelet of the previously placed femoral drill. Using a drill puller, the eyeloop drill is pulled cranially until the suture exits through the skin. A hemostat is attached to both ends of the exposed suture and used to draw the graft through the tibial osseous tunnel into the joint. Under arthroscopic visualization, the graft is then rotated to orient the cancellous surface of the patella bone superolaterally (Fig. 11). The tibial bone plug is rotated to orient the cancellous bone surface posteriorly. With the graft bone plug surfaces oriented to the surgeon's preference, the graft is pulled into place. The marking at the bone tendon junction should assist in determining its depth in the femoral osseous tunnel. Positioning the bone plug with the cancellous surface facing anteriorly holds the collagen posteriorly in the femoral tunnel. Similarly, rotation of the tibial plug in the tibial tunnel determines the collagen placement. The graft position is important to minimize impingement of the roof of the femoral notch with knee extension. If it does impinge, the tibial bone plug

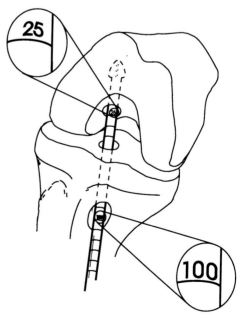

FIG. 11. The calibrated reamer demonstrates that the femoral tunnel has been drilled to a depth of 25 mm, while the end-to-end length between the tunnels is 100 mm. The prepared graft should not be longer than this length.

may be rotated, a larger notchplasty performed, or the tibial tunnel moved more posteriorly.

Graft Fixation

Our preference at the present time is to use a guide wire passed through the accessory inferomedial portal and slid between the superolateral cancellous surfaces of the bone plug into the femoral osseous tunnel (Fig. 12). The guide wire is inserted no more than 10 mm. This allows for easier removal once the interference screw is in place. A 7 mm diameter by 20 mm length cannulated interference screw is our preference and is placed on the cannulated screwdriver. With the knee flexed up to 110 degrees, the interference screw is advanced through the portal until it is visualized at the entrance of the femoral tunnel. The screw is advanced until the proximal end is just beyond the marking of the bone tendon junction. The screwdriver and guide wire are removed. The strength of the femoral fixation is tested by pulling the three sutures in the tibial plug manually with a force of approximately 40 pounds.

The knee is cycled through a full range of motion several times while maintaining tension on the three sutures to see that femoral fixation is adequate. The tibial bone plug is visualized during the range of motion to see if there is excursion of the bone plug in the tibial osseous tunnel. The excursion should ideally be less than 3 mm. Tibial fixation should take into consideration the point during range of motion that requires the greatest excursion of the graft. Ideally, the greatest length of the graft is as the knee approaches extension. The interference screw is placed fixing the tibial bone plug in the tibial osseous tunnel at this position. The preferable pull on the sutures at the time of graft fixation is approximately 5 to 10 pounds. One concern is overtensioning the graft and capturing the joint (2,19). Aspects of tensioning are

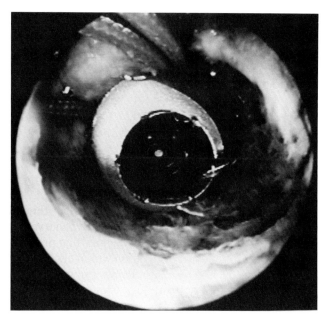

FIG. 13. The tip of the arthroscope can be inserted into the opening of the tibial tunnel, demonstrating that the end of the screw is flush with the tibial bone plug. The #5 Tevdek sutures are also seen.

discussed in Chapter 22. We prefer a 9 mm diameter by 25 mm long noncannulated interference screw introduced on the posterior aspect of the tibial plug between the cancellous surfaces of the tibial osseous tunnel and tibial bone plug. The screw is advanced until its end is just below the tibial cortex or flush with the tip of the plug (Fig. 13). If a tourniquet is used, we prefer to deflate it at this point. With an experienced operative team, harvesting of the graft, tunnel preparation, and fixation of the graft usually takes under 1 hour. The knee is moved through a full range of motion, and the graft is once again observed arthroscopically for position in the intercondylar notch. The knee is manually evaluated for anterior laxity and instrumented for stability before the patient leaves the operating room.

INTERFERENCE SCREW FIXATION

Kurosaka et al. compared different methods of fixation of various autogenous tissues used in anterior cruciate ligament reconstruction (11). Patellar bone–patellar tendon–tibial specimens fixed with either a 6.5-mm A-O cancellous screw or a custom 9.0-mm screw had greater strengths with greater linear load to failure compared with staples or sutures over buttons for fixation. This method of fixation as described by Lambert involve interference fit of a bone plug with a 30-mm length, 6.5-mm A-O cancellous screw inserted extraarticularly through the exit of the 10-mm femoral tunnel (12).

Interference fit is dependent on the geometry of the

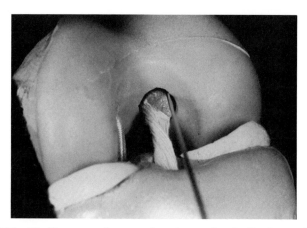

FIG. 12. The cancellous surface bone plug in the femoral osseous tunnel is positioned superolaterally, holding the collagen posteriorly. The guide wire is placed superolaterally, which will keep the screw away from collagen.

bone plug in addition to methods of fixation (17). Traditionally, bone plugs have been obtained with an oscillating saw using straight fine blades yielding triangular bone plugs. Clancy has described a technique that produces a thin rectangular bone plug measuring 10 mm wide and 4 mm deep (3). Recently, templates have been developed to produce trapezoidal grafts to enhance interference fit and decrease the stress concentration in the remaining patella (Concept, Inc., Largo, FL). These grafts often require manipulation of the bone plugs to allow passage through circular tunnels in the femur and tibia. Excess reshaping has the potential to alter the biomechanical strength and produces stress risers within the bone plugs. We have described a technique of harvesting bone plugs using a circular oscillating saw that produces cylindrical bone anchors for fixation within circular tunnels (8). The technique reproducibly provides consistently shaped and sized bone plugs. Compared with trapezoidal bone plugs, circular bone plugs secured with interference fit fixation showed higher maximum tensile strength to failure (17). The interference fit obtained with circular grafts and 9-mm screws is significantly stronger than the values reported by Kurosaka et al. using an identical strain rate (11).

Although interference screw fixation gives significantly stronger initial fixation, it has not been shown to give superior clinical results, even with aggressive early rehabilitation. Clancy has reported excellent results with bone–patella tendon–bone autografts using sutures tied over a button for fixation (4).

BONE GRAFTING AND CLOSURE

Bone–patella tendon–bone autografts raise concern for alterations in patellofemoral tracking, rupture of the patellar tendon, patellofemoral pain, patellar tendinitis, and patellar fracture as potential problems (1,5,14,16). Intraoperative and postoperative patella fracture associated with or following the harvesting of the patella bone plug has been rarely reported in literature (5,14). In an artificial bone composite, circular defects are found to require greater forces to fracture in four-point bending compared with triangular and trapezoidal configurations (17). These findings were reproduced in fresh frozen patella comparing circular and trapezoidal defects in three-point bending. In obtaining triangular or trapezoidal bone plugs, saw penetration to variable depths beyond the desired geometry should be avoided to minimize potential stress risers. Clinical results have not indicated that any one shape of the defect in the patella has been correlated with complications. The fractures of the patella that have occurred in the postoperative phase have been transverse in nature (14).

Filling of Graft Harvest Defect Sites

A core of bone or bone meal may be placed into the patella bone plug graft defect site (Fig. 14). The overlying tissue is closed over the graft. If desired, the remaining bone can be used to graft the tibial bone plug harvest site.

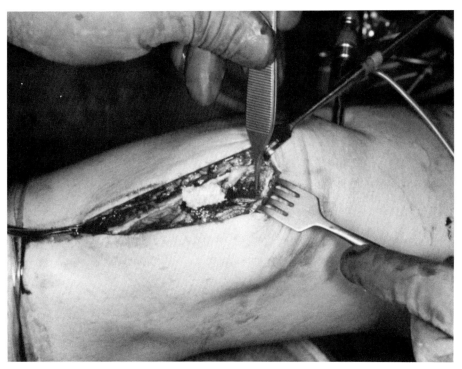

FIG. 14. The dowel plug obtained from the tibial core drill is split in half. This bone graft is about to be placed in the defect (shown with forceps) created from harvesting the patella bone plug.

If a reamer or drill is used, the bone meal from the tibial tunnel or local bone may be a source to graft the defect.

Closure of Patella Tendon

We prefer that the patellar tendon be loosely reapproximated with several sutures. This closure should not shorten the remaining patella tendon. The peritendinous tissue is closed as a layer over the underlying tendon.

ENDOSCOPIC ACL RECONSTRUCTION VERSUS THE TWO-INCISION TECHNIQUE

The learning curve for a surgeon to reproducibly perform the endoscopic technique is longer than the two-incision technique. We have found at the time of surgery that it is still necessary to convert, intraoperatively, from the endoscopic interference technique to the open technique in fewer than 5% of our anterior cruciate ligament reconstructive procedures. This is because we are unable to obtain femoral fixation that will resist 40 pounds of pull after cyclic loading. Because of the inability to uniformly (less than 5% failure at these values) achieve the high pull-out femoral interference fixation values by endoscopic fixation, we compared this method of interference screw placement to our previous open lateral femoral approach.

DIVERGENCE OF INTERFERENCE SCREW FIXATION

The anterior-posterior and lateral screw angles are different when comparing the open technique with the endoscopic technique. The screws diverge greater than 5 degrees on roentgenograms in the endoscopic group in one third of our cases, as seen in Figs. 15 and 16.

That differences exist in the radiographic appearance of these two techniques is not surprising, but that there is actual screw divergence in greater than a third of those placed endoscopically is of concern. Unlike the open technique, where direct visualization and control are easily maintained, the endoscopic technique makes it more difficult to consistently place the femoral screws parallel

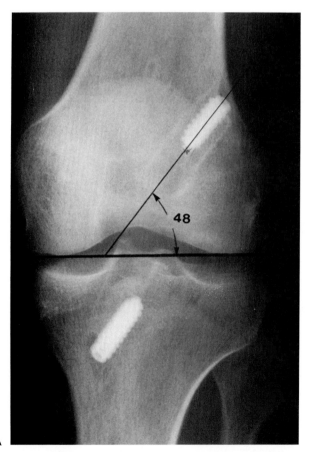
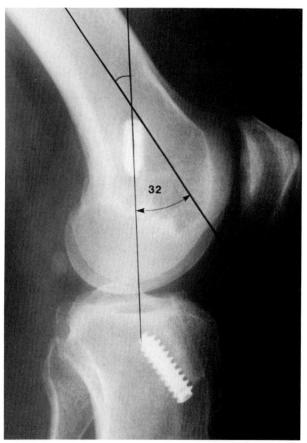

FIG. 15. Interference screw measurements were made directly from the roentgenograms. Representative roentgenograms after femoral interference screw placement using the distal femoral incision (open technique): anteroposterior (**A**) and lateral views (**B**).

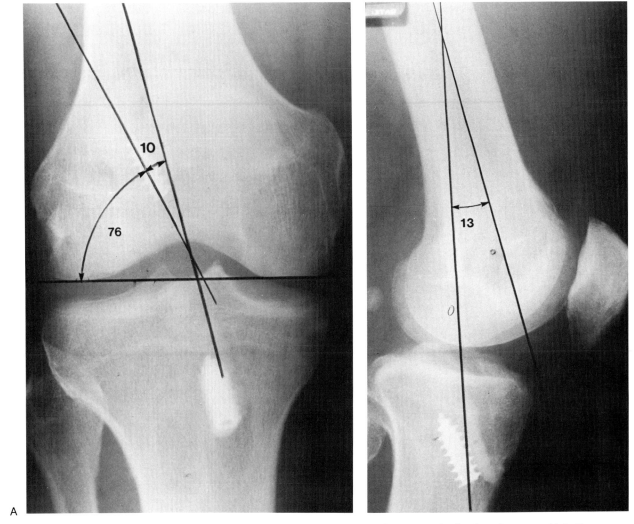

FIG. 16. Anteroposterior (**A**) and lateral (**B**) roentgenograms of endoscopically placed screws. Note the 10 degrees of divergence of the screw from the bone plug in **A**.

to the bone plug. It was our concern that this radiographic finding may result in weaker initial fixation.

Three current endoscopic portals are clinically used for placement of the interference screw with arthroscopic assistance. The screw fixation may be passed through the anteromedial portal via an accessory anteromedial portal just over the upper tibial plateau or through the tibial tunnel. The placement of the interference screw through the anteromedial portal theoretically would give the most divergence and the tibial tunnel the least divergence. The disadvantage of passing the interference screw through the tibial tunnel is the need for additional space in the osseous tunnel for instrumentation and the graft. We have used the accessory medial portal, which allows a more parallel placement of the screw relative to the graft and femoral tunnel when the knee is flexed over 110 degrees. Even with this portal we have a significant incidence of divergence, because true parallelism is not achieved even with the knee maximally flexed.

Previously reported endoscopically placed interfer-ence screws in cadavers without divergence showed high pull-out values. These values approached those of the ultimate load to failure strength of the tendon. Fulkerson and Cautilli (6) presented data on pull-out of divergent screws with ultimate strength of failure increasing significantly when screw divergence increased from 15 to 30 degrees. Their study used adult bovine knees (fresh). They had three groups: group I with no divergence, group II with 15 degrees of divergence, and group III with 30 degrees of divergence. In groups I and II, failure occurred at approximately 20 N/mm^2 when compared with 4.88 N/mm^2 for group III. Mode of failure for groups I and II was bone fracture and midsubstance when compared with group III, which all failed with graft pull-out.

Only one of 25 consecutive patients' radiographs we evaluated had divergence greater than 15 degrees (13). This degree of divergence occurred in fewer than 5% (1 of 25). This correlates with our own experience, in which radiographic differences exist between femoral interference screws placed for fixation of an ACL graft using the open approach and those placed endoscopically. Although the clinical significance of these differences have not been reported as contributing to surgical failures, the propensity for greater divergence in femoral interference screw placement using the newer endoscopic interference techniques does exist. The level for pull-out values for fixation of the bone–patella tendon–bone by various techniques has ranged from 50 to 1,000 N. Authors are reporting excellent long-term clinical results, with a wide variation of initial fixation values. The initial fixation values become less of a factor with bone-to-bone healing after 6 weeks. There are many factors important in the ultimate clinical result, and as yet the strength required for the initial fixation remains controversial.

SUMMARY

We have presented and discussed our preferred techniques of ACL reconstruction when using a bone–patella tendon–bone autograft. Similar clinical results are being obtained by clinicians using a small arthrotomy or two-incision techniques. Surgeons must integrate the knowledge gained from the basic science laboratories and from clinical studies and apply it to their preference for ACL reconstruction. These applications will continue to evolve. The present use of bone–patella–bone autografts will represent a historic milestone when advances in anterior cruciate surgery are described in the future.

REFERENCES

1. Bonamo J, Krinick R, Spain A. (1984): Rupture of the patellar ligament after use of its central third for ACL reconstruction. A report of two cases. *J Bone Joint Surg* 66A:1294–1297.
2. Bylski-Austrow DI, Grood ES, Hefzy MS, Holden JP, Butler DL. (1990): Anterior cruciate ligament replacements: a mechanical study of femoral attachment location, flexion angle at tensioning, and initial tension. *J Orthop Res* 8:522–531.
3. Clancy WG. (1988): Arthroscopic anterior cruciate ligament reconstruction with patellar tendon. *Technique Orthop* 2:13–22.
4. Clancy WG, Narchania RG, Rosenberg TD, et al. (1981): Anterior and posterior cruciate ligament reconstruction in rhesus monkeys. *J Bone Joint Surg* 63A:1270–1284.
5. DeLee J, Craviotta D. (1991): Rupture of the quadriceps tendon after a central third patellar tendon anterior cruciate ligament reconstruction. *Am J Sports Med* 19:415–416.
6. Fulkerson JP, Cautilli R, Hosick WB, Wright J. (1992): Divergence angles and their effect on the fixation strength of the Kurosaka screw. Presented at the AOSSM Annual Meeting, July 1992.
7. Howell SM, Clark JA, Farley TE. (1991): A rationale for predicting anterior cruciate graft impingement by the intercondylar roof. A magnetic resonance imaging study. *Am J Sports Med* 19:276–282.
8. Jackson DW, Cohn BT, Morrison DS. (1990): A new technique for harvesting the patella tendon in patients undergoing anterior cruciate ligament reconstruction. *Orthopaedics* 13:165–167.
9. Jackson DW, Grood ES, Goldstein J, et al. (1992): A comparison of patellar tendon autograft and allograft used for anterior cruciate ligament reconstruction in the goat model. Read at the AOSSM Annual Meeting, July 1992.
10. Jackson DW, Schaefer RK. (1990): Cyclops syndrome: loss of extension following intra-articular ACL reconstruction. *Arthroscopy* 6:171–178.
11. Kurosaka M, Yoshiya S, Andrish JT. (1987): A biomechanical comparison of different surgical techniques of graft fixation in anterior cruciate ligament reconstruction. *Am J Sport Med* 15:225–229.
12. Lambert KL. (1983): Vascularized patellar tendon graft with rigid internal fixation for anterior cruciate ligament insufficiency. *Clin Orthop* 172:85–89.
13. Lemos MJ, Jeffrey A, Simon TM, Jackson DW. (1992): Radiographic analysis of femoral interference screw placement during anterior cruciate ligament reconstruction: endoscopic versus open technique. *Arthroscopy* 9:2.
14. McCarroll JR. (1983): Fracture of the patella during a golfswing following reconstruction of the anterior cruciate ligament: a case report. *Am J Sports Med* 11:26–27.
15. Noyes FR, Butler DL, Grood ES, et al. (1984): Biomechanical analysis of human ligament grafts used in knee ligament repairs and reconstructions. *J Bone Joint Surg* 61A:344–352.
16. Roberts T, Drez D Jr, Banta MC. (1989): Complications of ACL ligament reconstruction. In: Sprague N III, ed. *Complications of ACL reconstruction.* New York: Raven Press, pp. 169–177.
17. Shapiro JD, Cohn BT, Jackson DW, Greenwald AS, Parker R, Postak P. (1992): The biomechanical effects of geometric configuration of bone–tendon–bone autografts in anterior cruciate ligament reconstruction. *J Arthroscopy Rel Surg* 8:453–458.
18. Yaru NC, Daniel DM, Penner D. (1992): The effect of tibial attachment site on graft impingement in an anterior cruciate ligament reconstruction. *Am J Sports Med* 20:217–220.
19. Yoshiya S, Andrish JT, Manley MT, Banes TW. (1987): Graft tension in anterior cruciate ligament reconstruction. An in vivo study in dogs. *Am J Sports Med* 15:464–470.

The Anterior Cruciate Ligament: Current and Future Concepts, edited by D.W. Jackson, et al.
Raven Press, Ltd., New York © 1993.

CHAPTER 27

Autograft Reconstruction of the Anterior Cruciate Ligament

Semitendinosus Reconstruction

Brad S. Tolin and Marc J. Friedman

The treatment of the anterior cruciate ligament (ACL) remains controversial (63). Recent studies have demonstrated that the ACL-deficient knee is at risk for meniscal injury and the development of degenerative changes as a result of abnormal kinematics (21,22,28,42,55,59). The complexity of surgically reproducing the natural biomechanical and anatomical function of the ACL has led to a diversity of reconstructive procedures.

Controversy continues to exist regarding the best graft substitute for the ACL-deficient knee. The ideal graft for the anterior cruciate ligament reconstruction should have (a) sufficient tensile strength to withstand the forces during knee function, (b) minimal morbidity with no significant functional loss associated with harvesting the graft, and (c) no source of disease transmission, and should be nonimmunogenic and nonmutagenic (77). No single graft material currently available meets all these criteria. Each graft type has its own inherent advantages and disadvantages. Graft substitutes used have been either autogenous tissue, synthetic ACL prosthesis, or allografts. Autografts such as the patellar tendon (1,11,12,16,17,39,40,41,66,72), semitendinosus tendon (3,4,10,19,22–24,29,30,46–52,62,66–68,74–76,80,86–88), gracilis tendons (15,54,78), quadriceps tendon (57), iliotibial band (31,34,58,60,73), or meniscus (18,79,80,82,83) have been previously used in ACL reconstruction surgery with varying success. For an overview of autogenous ACL reconstruction, several summary articles have recently appeared in the literature (7,24,64). The central

third of the patellar tendon used as a graft has been advocated by many investigators, although its use may contribute to dysfunction in certain patients. The primary advantage of the use of the bone–patellar ligament–bone graft is its biomechanical strength and the ability to obtain rigid fixation of the bone plugs on each end of the graft within the tibial and femoral tunnels. Complications, including patellofemoral pain, patellar fracture, ligament rupture, infrapatellar contracture syndrome, arthrofibrosis, osteoarthrosis, and biomechanical alterations of the extensor mechanism have all been reported after ACL reconstruction using the patellar tendon (5,6,36,43,53,65,69,70). Avoiding patellofemoral complications with the extensor mechanism has caused surgeons to consider alternative graft choices. The semitendinosus tendon with or without the gracilis tendon provides an accessible autograft that is technically simple to harvest and is associated with less dissection and subsequent morbidity (22,74,84). Another advantage is that the same incision for obtaining the graft is used for placement of the proximal tibial tunnel when performing an intraarticular reconstruction.

Biomechanical analysis of human graft substitutes has demonstrated that a single strand of the semitendinosus tendon is approximately 70% as strong as the normal ACL (59). Doubling the semitendinosus tendon and/or adding the gracilis tendon, which can withstand approximately 50% of the normal ACL load, has been proposed to increase the cross-sectional area of the graft, as well as the graft's tensile strength. The tensile strength of the semitendinosus and gracilis tendons in terms of load capacity per unit cross-sectional area is almost twice that of

B. S. Tolin and M. J. Friedman: Southern California Orthopedic Institute, Van Nuys, California 91405.

patellar tendon tissue (59), thus a considerable overall tensile strength can be placed into an osseous tunnel of limited diameter. This allows precise selective ACL reconstruction and theoretically minimizes inhomogeneous loading within the graft caused by differential fiber length behavior within the graft as the knee moves through a range of motion (71). The maximum strength of the graft is an important factor in graft selection, because it must be able to withstand the force of normal and athletic activities, but many other factors (e.g., isometric positioning of the graft, graft tensioning and fixation, and postoperative rehabilitation) also determine the ultimate success or failure of the reconstruction.

All autogenous substitutes for the ACL have been shown to undergo the process of necrosis, revascularization, and maturation. Kennedy et al. (42) demonstrated that the normal semitendinosus tendon in a rabbit model failed at 10 kg, but after intraarticular transplantation it failed at 4 to 5 kg. Similarly, Clancy et al. (11) showed that a patellar tendon graft at 1 year after ACL reconstruction performed in rhesus monkeys had 81% of its original tensile strength and only 52% of the strength of the normal ACL. The functional integrity and fate of the grafts used in the reconstructions can be further investigated with second-look surgeries. Puddu and Ippolito (68) examined a ruptured intraarticular semitendinosus tendon ACL reconstruction 16 months after the initial reconstruction. Structural changes occurred in the transferred tendon, which appeared grossly viable, and was contained circumferentially within a synovial lining. Collagen fiber bundles were oriented similar to a normal ACL. The transferred tendon was thought to be undergoing structural transformation into a ligament. Zaricznyj (86) performed a biopsy of an intraarticular semitendinosus tendon ACL reconstruction $7\frac{1}{2}$ years postoperatively and noted well-organized fibrous bundles and cells histologically. Lipscomb et al. (48) examined seven reconstructed patients 11 to 42 months postoperatively. In five cases, the intraarticular semitendinosus tendon reconstructions were viable and functional without evidence of attenuation. The other two cases had intrasubstance tears during the first postoperative year. Tendon healing in all cases at the tibial and femoral bony tunnels was complete. The ruptured tendons grossly appeared similar to an acute intrasubstance tear of the ACL. Microscopic examination of the ruptured intraarticular semitendinosus tendon showed viable tissue with normal appearing collagen and nuclei and few chronic inflammatory cells present. Cho (9) reoperated on a patient's knee 8 months after semitendinosus tendon ACL reconstruction and noted a hypertrophic tendon covered with synovium without gross evidence of necrosis or attenuation. Likewise, Johnson (38) performed second-look arthroscopies in 20 patients 3.5 weeks to 42 months after ACL reconstruction with the semitendinosus tendon. Initially, he found tendon in-

jury from the surgical transplantation, but by 3 months the tendon had normal gross and histological appearances. From these studies, the intraarticular transferred tendon graft appears to undergo a process of "ligamentatization" in an attempt to grossly and histologically resemble the normal ACL.

Using the semitendinosus and/or gracilis tendons for ACL reconstruction generally has not led to clinically perceptible weakness of the hamstrings (9,25). Lipscomb et al. (49) studied 51 patients who had undergone semitendinosus tendon or semitendinosus and gracilis tendon intraarticular ACL reconstruction. They averaged 22.6 months follow-up before testing. Cybex testing at slow and fast speeds found no significant loss of hamstring strength when these tendons were used to reconstruct the ACL. However, Marder et al. (51) noted significant weakness in peak hamstring torque at 60 degrees per second when the reconstruction was performed using doubled semitendinosus and gracilis tendons. Potential factors contributing to the hamstring weakness observed in their study included failure to repair the sartorial fascia incision, lack of slow speed of isokinetic training in their postoperative rehabilitation program, and a less motivated patient population. Cross et al. (14) have actually demonstrated anatomic and functional regeneration of the semitendinosus and gracilis tendons after their use for grafting.

HISTORY AND LITERATURE REVIEW OF SEMITENDINOSUS/GRACILIS TENDON ACL RECONSTRUCTIONS

The semitendinosus tendon has been used extensively to reconstruct the ACL-deficient knee, either alone or with the gracilis tendon. Various procedures have been described using the semitendinosus tendon as a single strand or a double loop, as an intraarticular reconstruction alone or with an extraarticular reinforcement, or as an augmentation of a primary repair of the ACL. The semitendinosus tendon also has been used as a free graft or left at its anatomic attachment, either proximally or distally. Current techniques of ACL reconstruction have focused on arthroscopically-assisted methods. No consensus of opinion exists as to the best technique of ACL reconstruction using the semitendinosus (and/or gracilis) tendon as evidenced by the multitude of existing procedures.

Macey (50) in 1939 first described a new procedure for intraarticular ACL reconstruction using the semitendinosus tendon. He left the semitendinosus tendon attached distally at its anatomic insertion, then routed the tendon intraarticularly through tibial and femoral bone tunnels, creating a "normal anatomical reconstruction." Most current semitendinosus tendon ACL reconstructions are modifications of this original description. Cho (9), used a similar technique of semitendinosus tendon ACL reconstruction with the free end of the graft fixed on the femoral side, with sutures placed over the iliotibial band (Fig. 1). He reported on five patients, with a follow-up of 21.4 months. Objectively, two of the five patients had a residual anterior drawer and associated recurvatum. All patients had functional improvement without subjective instability, although no pivot shift test was performed. Vandendriessche et al. (81) combined this procedure with reefing of the posterior medial capsule and a modified Mueller procedure. Lipscomb et al. (48), reported on 78 cases with an 11-month follow-up using Cho's technique of semitendinosus tendon tenodesis combined with posterior medial capsular reefing (in 35 knees). Subjectively, 90% of the patients were satisfied with the procedure. Objectively, 86% demonstrated a 0 to 1+ anterior drawer and 14%

had a residual 2 to 3+ anterior drawer. In a subsequent study, Lipscomb et al. (47) modified this technique to use both the semitendinosus and gracilis tendons through bony tunnels in the proximal tibial and lateral femoral condyle. Both tendons were left attached distally at their anatomic insertion and fixed to the femur with sutures tied subperiosteally on the lateral femoral condyle (Fig. 2). They reported reconstruction of the chronically torn ACL in 284 patients. Initially, a single semitendinosus tendon with reefing of the posterior medial capsule was performed in 88 cases. The next 97 cases were performed using both semitendinosus and gracilis tendons in addition to reefing of the posterior medial capsule. In the last 99 cases, both the semitendinosus and gracilis tendons were used, with reefing of the posterior medial capsule in combination with either an Ellison or Losee extra-articular reconstruction added to

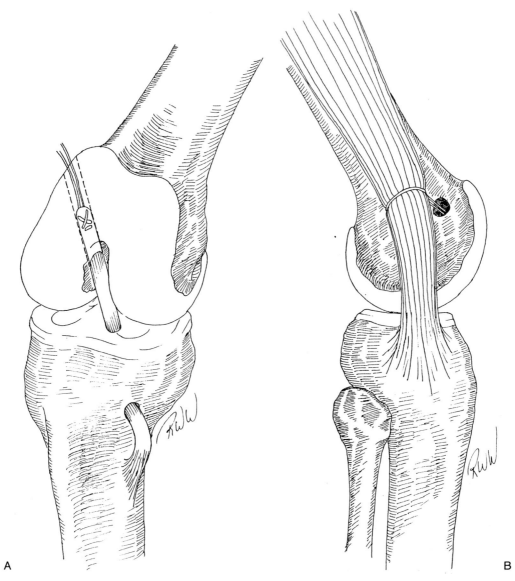

FIG. 1. Cho's technique of semitendinosus tendon tenodesis ACL reconstruction.

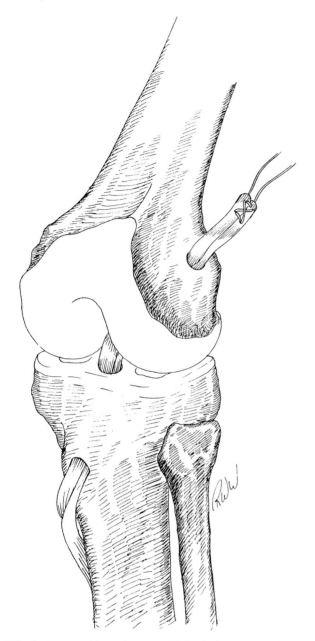

FIG. 2. Lipscomb's technique with both the semitendinosus and gracilis tendons placed through tibial and femoral tunnels.

acute reconstruction group was found to generally result in a more stable knee joint than was the chronic reconstruction group, but again, no objective data are presented to compare these two groups of patients.

Puddu (66) in 1980 described a procedure in which the semitendinosus tendon is detached at its tibial insertion, passed through drill holes of the tibia and femur, and secured to the iliotibial band. The musculotendinous unit proximally is left intact. The tibial drill hole is placed through the anterior portion of the medial collateral ligament 2 to 3 cm below the joint line in an attempt to preserve the flexion and internal rotation function of the semitendinosus tendon (Fig. 3). Twelve cases of chronic combined anteromedial and anterolateral rotatory instability were reviewed with a follow-up of 8

correct rotatory instability. Overall, 84% of the reconstructions had good results (0 to 1+ anterior drawer) and had an average follow-up of 22 months (range 1 to 5 years). No subjective evaluation was included. Most of the poor results occurred in the initial two groups, where an extraarticular procedure was not performed, although no data are presented to support this contention. A second reason the investigators found a poor outcome was error in intraarticular placement of the graft of the lateral femoral condyle. Evaluation of reconstruction of acute ACL tears with both the semitendinosus and gracilis tendons demonstrated 85% good results in 58 patients. The

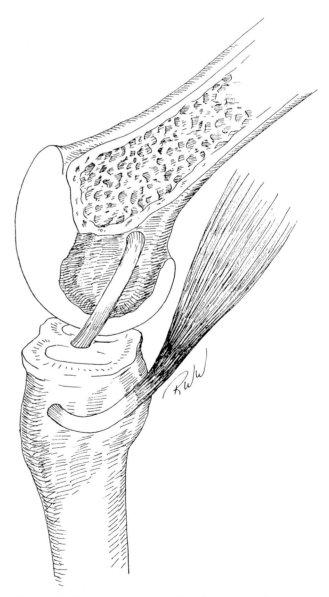

FIG. 3. Puddu's procedure routing the semitendinosus tendon from a medial tibial drill hole to preserve function of the muscle.

months. All reconstructions were combined with an extraarticular procedure. All patients had less than a 1+ anterior drawer at follow-up. Ferretti et al. (19) modified Puddu's technique to include the use of the gracilis tendon with the semitendinosus tendon in acute ACL ruptures. Some knees were also augmented with an extraarticular reconstruction. Fifty-five cases were reported, of which 35 had semitendinosus tendon reconstruction only and 20 had both semitendinosus and gracilis tendon reconstructions. The results of each group were not evaluated independently. Subjectively, only 5% were not satisfied with the procedure. Seventy-eight percent of the patients had a negative Lachman test and the jerk test was <1+ in 96% of the cases. Ferretti et al. (20) also reported on results of reconstructions using the semitendinosus and gracilis tendons in the chronic ACL-deficient knee. Eight-eight patients were followed an average of 41 months, and 64% had a negative Lachman <1+ and 98% had a <1+ jerk test. Ninety-six percent of the patients who were satisfied with the procedures subjectively and overall 82% of the patients were classified as excellent or good, and 18% fair or poor. Likewise, Puddu et al. (67) clinically evaluated 88 patients with chronic ACL deficiency reconstructed with the semitendinosus tendon in combination with an extraarticular procedure. The Lachman was negative in 67% of the cases with a jerk test <1+ in 92%. Seventy-five percent of full-time professional athletes have returned to sports. There was marked discrepancy in the results of objective testing and patient satisfaction based on resumption of full athletic activity. Those patients who were unable to resume their prior level of sports activity had poor overall results. Barber et al. (3), also using Puddu's technique, compared reconstructions with the semitendinosus and gracilis tendons in acute and chronically deficient ACL knees with a mean follow-up of 52 months. The Lachman test was improved in 87% of the acute reconstructions and in 62% of the chronic reconstructions. The pivot shift was eliminated in all patients in the acutely reconstructed group compared with only 71% in the chronic group. Overall, 87% of the acute reconstructions and only 76% of the chronic group had excellent/good results.

Zaricznyj (86) reported on using a free semitendinosus tendon graft stapled to both the distal femur and proximal tibia in 15 of 22 patients undergoing ACL reconstruction while the other 7 patients had a semitendinosus tendon graft left attached to its anatomic insertion distally. He found no difference in the clinical results in these two groups with an average follow-up of 5.4 years. He later modified this technique, reporting on 14 patients using a double semitendinosus tendon graft placed through a single hole in the femur and two separate tibial holes in an attempt to increase the strength of the tendon graft and duplicate the anatomic insertion of the ACL (87). The graft was secured proximally by tying sutures over the drill hole in the lateral femoral condyle and distally at the tibia by suturing the graft to itself and the adjacent soft tissue (Fig. 4). The Lachman test was 0 to 1+ and the pivot shift test absent in all patients. Subjectively, 12 patients were rated excellent/good and 2 fair. Gomes and Marczyk (24) also used a free graft of a loop of double thickness semitendinosus tendon in combination with an extraarticular procedure to reconstruct the ACL in 26 patients. A trephine was used to create the tibial and lateral femoral condylar tunnels for graft placement. The bone plugs obtained from the trephine were then used to fix the graft in position after passage through the tunnels (Fig. 5). The patients were then immobilized for 7 weeks. Twenty-four patients were satisfied with the procedure and asymptomatic, the Lach-

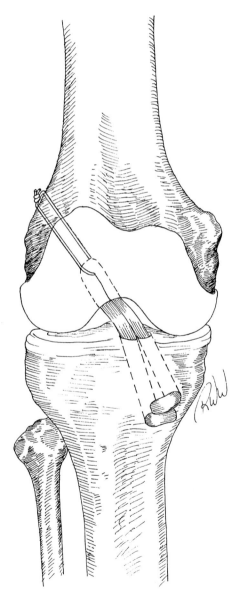

FIG. 4. Zaricznyj's reconstruction whereby the double-looped semitendinosus tendon is passed through two different tibial holes.

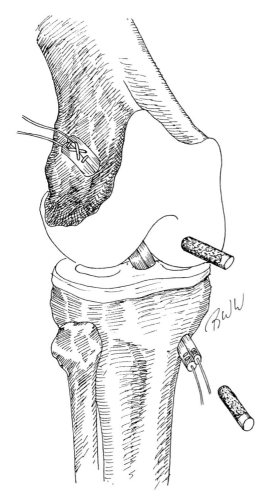

FIG. 5. A double-looped semitendinosus tendon graft is fixed with bone plugs.

man test was 0 to 1+ and the pivot shift negative in all patients. Twenty-three patients were classified as good and three as fair.

Mott (56) has devised a technique of ACL reconstruction called the semitendinosus anatomic reconstruction (STAR) in an attempt to rebuild the major anatomic bands of the ACL and restore isometric ligamentous relationships. In this technique, two tibial and two femoral tunnels are made, each at the anatomic origin and insertion of the anterior medial posterior lateral bands of the ACL. According to Mott, this technique has been a reliable method for reconstruction in augmentation of repairs of the ACL and the chronically ACL-deficient knee, although no results are given. Horne and Parsons (33) developed a technique in which the semitendinosus tendon was passed through a tibial drill hole and placed in the over-the-top position of the lateral femoral condyle through the posterior capsule. They reasoned that a graft passed through the lateral femoral condyle tunnel would fail secondary to abrasion at the tendon/bone interface. Modifications of this technique have been used in other series. Zarins and Rowe (88) used the semitendinosus tendon and iliotibial band in a combined intra-

articular and extraarticular ACL reconstruction. The combined method passes both grafts in opposite directions through the same proximal tibial tunnel and over the top of the lateral femoral condyle. Both grafts are tensioned, then sutured to one another proximally at the lateral femoral condyle and distally at the proximal tibia. The posterior medial and lateral capsule were advanced, and the semitendinosus tendon was left attached to its distal insertion. The initial 106 consecutive patients with chronic instability were evaluated with a minimum 3-year follow-up, during which 6 patients were excluded due to incomplete follow-up. The Lachman and pivot shift tests were reduced to <1+ in 80% and 91% of the knees, respectively. Thirty-five patients were able to return to their preinjury athletic activity without limitations, and 55% of patients were able to return to moderate athletic activity. Overall, there was an excellent/good result in 88 patients, fair in 8, and poor in 3, with 1 failure. Follow-up arthroscopy in 16 knees performed 1 to 7½ years postreconstruction demonstrated 6 of the 16 ligament reconstructions to be either significantly lax or disrupted. There was noted to be more tension in the reconstructed graft when the knee was in full extension rather than at 90 degrees of flexion, which was the result of nonisometric placement of the graft in the over-the-top position. Wilson and Scranton (85) similarly used a combined reconstruction of the ACL using the semitendinosus tendon for the intraarticular portion of the reconstruction and an extraarticular modified MacIntosh technique in 58 professional and competitive athletes. The semitendinosus tendon graft was also placed in an over-the-top position, and in the last 25 patients the graft was doubled and fixed at both the lateral femoral condyle and proximal tibia with a 6.5 AO screw (Fig. 6). Only 30 patients (32 knees) could be evaluated an average of 4 years postoperatively. Twenty-eight of these 30 patients were able to return to their full athletic activity. All patients had a Lachman test of <1+, and of the 27 knees tested by arthrometry, 18 demonstrated anterior tibial translation of <2 mm and 9 had 2 to 5 mm of excursion compared with the normal contralateral knee. The overall results were graded 20% excellent, 73% good, and 7% fair.

The hamstring tendons also have been used in surgical procedures, creating a dynamic intraarticular ACL reconstruction. Augustine (2) in 1956 described such a procedure whereby the semitendinosus tendon was detached distally and routed through the intercondylar notch and tibial tunnel, then fixed distally with a boat nail. Later, DuToit (15) reported on the Lindmann procedure, which was initially described in the German literature in 1950. With this technique, the ACL is substituted by a proximally based, free-sliding gracilis tendon passed through the posterior lateral capsule and intercondylar notch, then through a proximal tibial bony tunnel (Fig. 7). DuToit reasoned that the success of the procedure would be a result of maintaining the

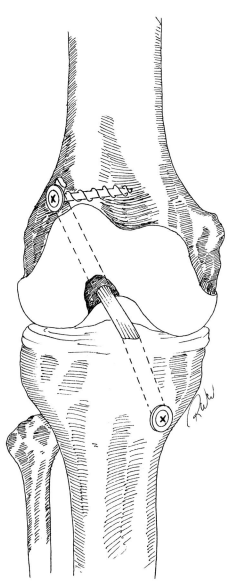

FIG. 6. The double-looped semitendinosus tendon graft is fixed with a screw and washer technique at both the tibial and femoral ends.

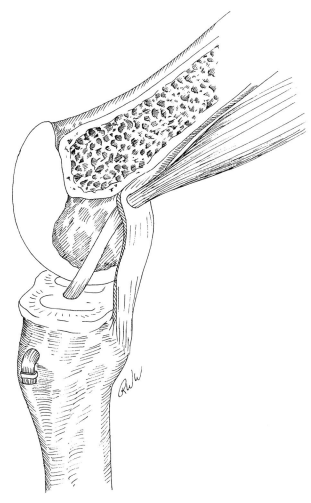

FIG. 7. The Lindmann procedure. The semitendinosus or gracilis tendon, detached distally, is routed through the posterior capsule in an over-the-top position, then through a tibial bone tunnel.

proprioceptors of the viable tendon and keeping its attachment to active muscle, which would act to preserve the tension in the transfer. No objective data were presented, but improved subjective stability was noted in all 12 patients. Lange (44) preferred to use the semitendinosus tendon in a procedure similar to Lindmann's. In 1978, Thompson et al. (79) presented the results of eight patients who had undergone the Lindmann operation. Seven of the eight patients were subjectively improved and returned to sports activities, although evidence of a clinical instability persisted.

Augmentation of acute ACL ruptures has been another circumstance where the semitendinosus tendon commonly has been used. Studies have demonstrated by histological and mechanical testing that augmentation was superior to repair of the ruptured ACL alone (8).

Augmentation theoretically allows for protection of the repair, while the graft provides stability and acts as a stent for the repaired ligament. The repaired ACL stump is thought to enhance revascularization of the graft and preserve some proprioceptive function of the ligament. The surgical procedures used for augmentation of the ACL repairs are based on these concepts. Larson (45) has attempted to repair the torn ACL, if possible, by passing the semitendinosus tendon through a proximal tibial hole just posterior to the ACL stump, then placing the graft in the over-the-top position of the lateral femoral condyle. A preliminary report showed an 87% successful result, but no objective data or follow-up were given. Gomez et al. (25) used a similar technique with over-the-top placement of the graft. Thirty-seven patients with an acute ACL rupture were retrospectively reviewed with an average follow-up time of 37.9 months. No subjective evaluation was presented. The operated knee demonstrated some residual laxity on KT-1000 arthrometer testing, although all had <3 mm side-to-side difference.

The calculated compliance index was not significantly different than the normal knee, suggesting that the mechanical properties of the reconstructive ligament approximated that of the normal ligament. In another series, Sgaglione et al. (76), evaluated 72 acute ACL injuries that had been treated with primary semitendinosus tendon augmentation. Seventy-one percent of the patients had undergone an extraarticular procedure consisting of an iliotibial band lateral sling reinforcement. Objective examination showed 86% to have a negative pivot shift and 93% to have a ≤1+ Lachman test. E17E-1000 arthrometer testing showed a side-to-side difference of <3 mm of anterior displacement. Excellent/good results were reported in 82% of the patients, and 77% returned to their preinjury athletic level. Analysis of the results of patients with or without an additional extraarticular procedure showed no difference in objective outcome.

Attempts to improve the strength and reinforce the intraarticular semitendinosus tendon graft used in ACL reconstruction, especially during its susceptible revascularization process, has led to the development of a synthetic augmentation device. Kennedy developed the Ligament Augmentation Device (LAD; 3M, Minneapolis, Minnesota) for this purpose after he noted that the intraarticular transfer of the semitendinosus tendon in rabbits was associated with a marked decrease in graft tensile strength at 6 months (42). The LAD is used to construct a composite graft by suturing the autogenous graft to the polypropylene braid. The composite graft theoretically promotes optimal load and stress sharing, which protects the autogenous graft in the early postoperative period (26).

Sgaglione et al. (75) retrospectively reviewed and compared two groups of patients with chronic ACL deficiency that underwent arthroscopically-assisted reconstruction with a semitendinosus tendon/polypropylene augmented composite graft (STP) and a semitendinosus tendon without augmentation (ST). In all cases, the diameter of the biological graft was approximately 7 mm. No standard method of graft fixation was used. Excellent/good subjective results were reported in 86% of the STP patients, and 78% of the ST patients had a mean follow-up of 31 and 34 months, respectively. In both groups, >85% were able to return to sports activities. Objectively, 73% of the STP group and 82% of the ST group had a 0 to 1+ Lachman test. The pivot shift was negative in 80% of the STP group and in 82% of the ST group. KT-1000 arthrometer testing showed <3 mm side-to-side differences in 60% of the STP patients and in 61% of the ST patients. Subjective and functional results tended to be uniformly better than objective results in both groups, with an overall difference between the augmented and nonaugmented groups. Others have noted accelerated rehabilitation and slightly improved functional results at 18 months' follow-up (13). The semiten-

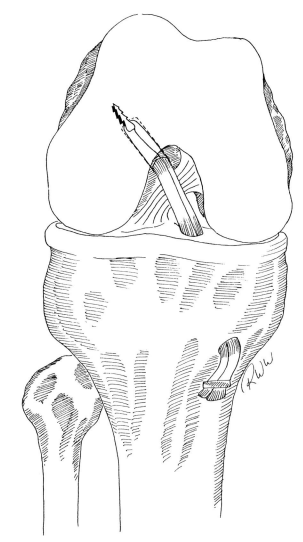

FIG. 8. Endoscopic fixation of the intraarticular graft with an arthroscopic staple.

Quadruple Semitendinosus

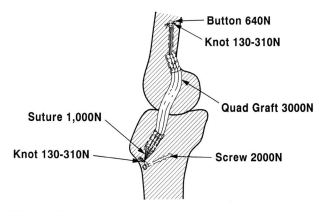

FIG. 9. Rosenberg's technique of semitendinosus/gracilis tendon ACL reconstruction with approximate biomechanical strength of each component of the reconstruction. (Courtesy of Tom Rosenberg, M.D.)

dinosus tendon has also been used for ACL reconstruction in combination with the Gore-Tex ligament with encouraging preliminary results (12).

ARTHROSCOPICALLY ASSISTED RECONSTRUCTION

Recently, arthroscopically assisted techniques of semitendinosus tendon ACL reconstruction have been developed with the advantage of avoiding the morbidity associated with an open procedure. Moyer et al. (57) reported on 31 patients who had undergone combined semitendinosus and gracilis tendon ACL reconstruction, 50% having had an arthroscopically-assisted reconstruction. Overall, the arthroscopically-assisted group had less pain, a shorter hospitalization, and fewer complaints of patellofemoral pain compared with those patients who had undergone the traditional open method of ACL reconstruction.

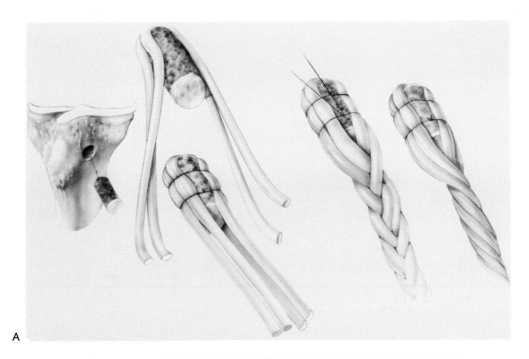

A

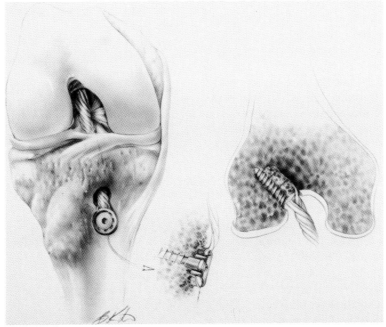

B

FIG. 10. Endoscopic fixation of the semitendinosus/gracilis tendons and bone plug composite with an interference screw. (Courtesy of John C. Garrett, M.D.)

With the advent of arthroscopically assisted reconstructions, endoscopic methods of graft fixation have subsequently been devised. Johnson (37) has used a loop of semitendinosus tendon placed through two tibial bony tunnels and fixed the graft endoscopically to the lateral femoral condyle with an arthroscopic staple. Hendler (29) described a unitunnel technique to create a single tibiofemoral tunnel for graft placement in which the central axis of the graft coincides with the anatomic center of the normal ACL. With this technique, the lateral femoral condyle tunnel is drilled to a depth of only 1 cm so that fixation of the graft with an intraarticular staple can be used (Fig. 8). Hendler has performed the procedure in 40 cases with an average follow-up of 20 months without evidence of subjective instability symptoms. No patient has demonstrated a pivot shift postoperatively, although most have had some residual laxity present. Wainer et al. (82) also have used an endoscopic staple to fix allograft tendons in the lateral femoral condyle tunnel in 65 patients. Only 1 patient had failure of the staple, which was revised 2 weeks postoperatively. The pull-out strength of the endoscopic staple was found to be only 100 N (Harry Alexander, PhD, personal communication), so the postoperative rehabilitation program in these patients must be adjusted accordingly to avoid excessive forces on the graft and pull-out of the staple fixation.

Friedman (22) reported using a double loop of free semitendinosus and gracilis tendons placed through separate tibial and femoral drill holes. The loop of the graft was fixed distally around a screw and washer, with the thinner portion of the graft fixed at the lateral femoral condyle with a double-staple technique. Rosenberg used four separate strands of semitendinosus and gracilis tendons reinforced with sutures at the ends of the grafts (Rosenberg T: personal communication, 1992). He fixed the graft at the distal femur by tying the sutures over a button, and at the tibial side with the sutures tied around a screw and washer (Fig. 9). Garrett used an innovative technique to perform an endoscopic semitendinosus/gracilis tendon ACL reconstruction (Garrett W: personal communication, 1992) (Fig. 10A,B). He wove the tendon grafts around a bone plug, and placed the composite in the lateral femoral condylar tunnel, fixing the graft and bone plug with an interference screw. On the tibial side, the graft was secured with a screw and spiked washer. Marder et al. (51) tied sutures placed on both ends of the graft around a cancellous screw and smooth washer, adjacent to both the tibial and femoral tunnels. Sisk (78) left the insertion of the semitendinosus and gracilis tendons attached distally, then routed the tendon(s) through the tibial and femoral tunnels. The proximal graft was secured to the lateral femoral condyle with a screw and washer (Fig. 11). Boden et al. (4) used a comparable technique in combination with an extra-articular iliotibial band tenodesis. In their study, 80% of the 20 athletes studied had returned to their preinjury

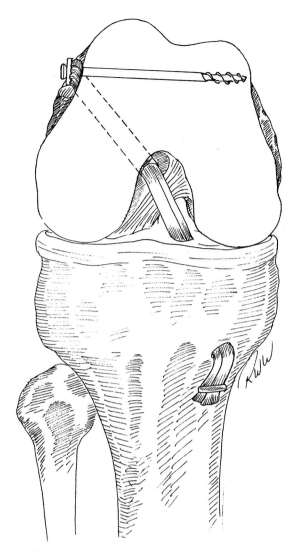

FIG. 11. Arthroscopic technique used by Sisk.

activity level. No pivot shift was present on clinical examination, and 65% had a 0 to 1+ Lachman test at 26 months' follow-up. Likewise, Larsen (46) used an arthroscopically-assisted procedure, but placed the semitendinosus tendon in the over-the-top position instead of through a lateral femoral condyle tunnel.

PATELLAR TENDON VERSUS SEMITENDINOSUS/GRACILIS TENDON ACL RECONSTRUCTIONS

Only recently have studies appeared in the literature directly comparing patellar tendon with semitendinosus and gracilis tendon ACL reconstructions. Prospective studies are necessary because interstudy comparisons are difficult due to differences in patient selection, study design, surgical technique, postoperative rehabilitation, subjective rating systems, and objective criteria used for evaluation. One recent study by Marder et al. (51) prospectively evaluated 80 consecutive patients with chronic ACL deficiency who had undergone either arthroscopically-assisted autologous patellar tendon or doubled semitendinosus and gracilis tendon reconstructions. Follow-up ranged from 24 to 40 months. The choice of the procedure performed was based on a strict alternating sequence. Both types of grafts were secured to the femoral and proximal tibia using a post and washer fixation, and both groups underwent the same postoperative rehabilitation regimen. Six patients in the patellar tendon showed a >5 degree loss of flexion or extension compared with only two in the semitendinosus/gracilis tendon reconstruction group. No significant differences were found between the groups in terms of functional level, subjective complaints, or objective laxity testing, although the mean KT-1000 measurements were 1.6 mm for the patellar tendon group and 1.9 mm for the semitendinosus and gracilis tendon groups. Eight-six percent of cases in the patellar tendon group and 74% in the semitendinosus and gracilis tendon group demonstrated <2 mm side-to-side differences. Harter et al. (27) also showed no significant differences in the results of instrumented Lachman tests in knees reconstructed with either the semitendinosus tendon or the central third of the patellar tendon.

Holmes et al. (32) retrospectively reviewed 75 of 90 consecutive patients with ACL-deficient knees who had undergone open reconstruction with either the central third of the patellar tendon or with the semitendinosus tendon. All patients had a minimum follow-up of 5 years. Three groups were evaluated: the chronic ACL-deficient knee reconstructed with either the central third of the patellar tendon or semitendinosus tendon, or an acute ACL-deficient group reconstructed with the semi-tendinosus tendon. All reconstructions were accompanied by a secondary extraarticular procedure, and all grafts were placed in the over-the-top position. Subjectively, only 50% of the chronic ACL-deficient group reconstructed with the semitendinosus tendon (double stranded) had excellent/good results compared with 85% of the chronic reconstructed patellar tendon group and the acutely reconstructed group with a single-stranded semitendinosus tendon. KT-1000 arthrometer testing demonstrated a mean 1.4-mm difference between the reconstructed and normal knee in the patellar tendon group, 2.0 mm in the chronic/semitendinosus tendon group, and 1.2 mm in the acute/semitendinosus tendon group. Based on their results, the investigators did not recommend the use of an intraarticular semitendinosus tendon reconstruction in the chronically ACL-deficient knee. It is interesting to note in this study that even a double-looped semitendinosus tendon graft did not provide adequate stabilization in the chronically deficient ACL knee. Various factors other than the retrospective study design may account for the findings reported, such as the methods of graft fixation used, the placement of the graft in the over-the-top position, and differences in postoperative rehabilitation between the groups that were not addressed in the study. It is clear that these factors can ultimately influence the success of ACL reconstruction, but the conclusions of this study cannot be ignored and should serve to stimulate further comparative prospective investigations.

Recently, Feagin et al. (17) reported no statistically significant differences in reconstruction either with the semitendinosus or patellar tendon, although the results with the patellar tendon graft reconstruction were per-

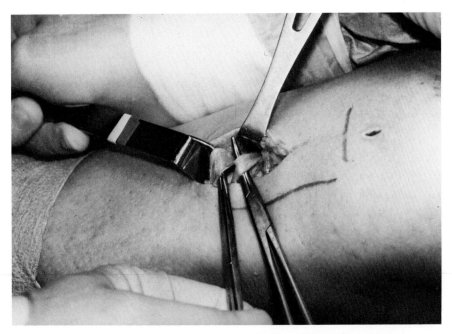

FIG. 12. Tibial insertion of the semitendinosus and gracilis tendons.

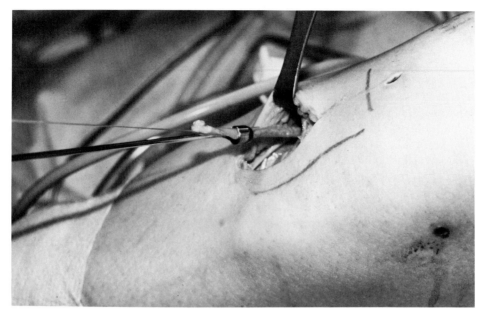

FIG. 13. A tendon stripper is applied over the semitendinosus tendon.

ceived both subjectively and objectively as slightly better than the semitendinosus tendon reconstructions. Oter et al. (61) directly compared doubled semitendinosus/gracilis tendon autograft reconstructions to the central third of the patellar tendon reconstructions. The hamstring grafts were secured both proximally and distally by tying sutures around a screw and washer. The patellar tendon grafts were fixed with interference screws at both ends. The postoperative rehabilitation regimen differed in terms of the time of immobilization between the groups. In both graft techniques, subjective and objective scores at 1 year were better in the acutely reconstructed group when compared with the chronic group using either the semitendinosus or patellar tendon. The investigators suggested that the double-stranded semitendinosus/gracilis tendon technique was slightly less successful than the patellar tendon graft technique,

although overall success appeared to be affected by other factors, such as chondromalacia and meniscal tissue loss, rather than by any specific graft type.

OUR TECHNIQUE OF SEMITENDINOSUS/ GRACILIS TENDON ACL RECONSTRUCTION

Under epidural or general anesthesia, a complete standard diagnostic arthroscopic evaluation is performed with specific attention to articular chondral defects and the presence of meniscal lesions. In the ACL-deficient knee, tears of the posterior horn of the lateral meniscus or periphery of the medial meniscus are not uncommon. If the meniscus is repairable, the repair is performed before the ligament reconstruction, but the sutures are not tied until the completion of the reconstruction. A notchplasty is performed to avoid impingement on the new

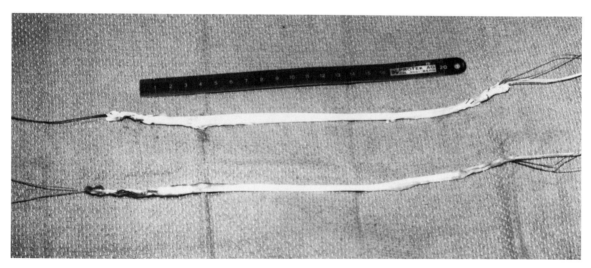

FIG. 14. The harvested tendon grafts.

graft if the intercondylar notch is significantly narrowed. We use a mechanical full radius resector to debride the soft tissue in the notch, then an arthroscopic burr for the notchplasty. Special attention is given to the apex of the notch and the lateral femoral condyle to assure that no impingement of the new graft will occur when the knee is extended. When the notchplasty is completed, the posterolateral capsule should be readily visualized so that a nerve hook can easily pass over the posterior edge of the lateral femoral condyle in the over-the-top position. If this area is not adequately seen, further resection of the soft tissue along the posterior notch is necessary.

Next, the semitendinosus and/or gracilis tendon is harvested. A 5-cm incision is made medial to the tibial tubercle vertically over the pes anserinus tendons, which can be palpated. The deep fascia overlying the tendons is incised longitudinally. The individual semitendinosus and gracilis tendons are then localized with a right-angle clamp (Fig. 12). Metzenbaum scissors are used to dissect each tendon free from its deep fascial attachments. Commonly, the inferior fibers of the semitendinosus tendon form an accessory insertion, which also needs to be transected (61). It is extremely important to excise all fascial attachments to the tendon(s), because the tendon stripper can follow an aberrant course along the tendon, causing amputation of the tendon graft short of its muscle body. Digital palpation can be used to assure that there are no residual fascial bands attached to the tendon being harvested. The tendons are then transected at their tibial insertion. If there is difficulty identifying or separating the semitendinosus and gracilis tendons, first the lower border of the pes anserinus must be identified, then the pes tendon group must be reflected proximally. By turning the pes over, the semitendinosus and gracilis tendons can be easily identified, because the individual tendons are more distinct on the undersurface. A #2 Tevdek suture is then applied in a whip stitch fashion at

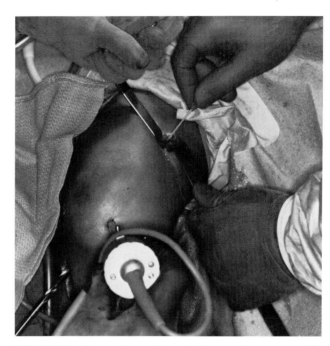

FIG. 16. The femoral tunnel is made by reaming over a guide wire retrograde.

the distal end of the semitendinosus and gracilis tendons and used to maintain tension on the graft(s) during harvesting. A tendon stripper is applied sequentially over each graft and advanced proximally to the distal thigh (Fig. 13). Semitendinosus and gracilis tendon grafts of 25 to 30 cm in length are usually obtained (Fig. 14). A #2 Tevdek suture is also placed in the proximal end of each tendon, and any extraneous muscular tissue is debrided from the grafts. The semitendinosus and gracilis tendons

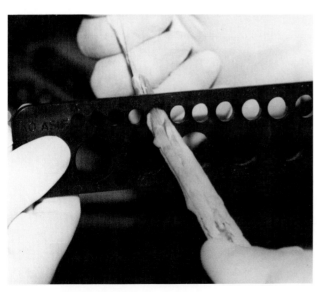

FIG. 15. Sizing the looped tendon grafts.

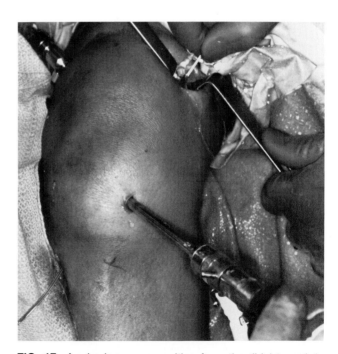

FIG. 17. A wire loop, seen exiting from the tibial tunnel, is used as a tendon passer.

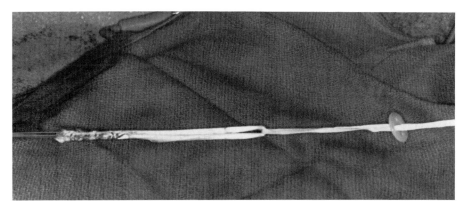

FIG. 18. The button, Dacron tape, and semitendinosus tendon graft composite.

can be double-looped, singly or in combination, creating two to four strands of tendon graft to be used in the intraarticular reconstruction. The graft is then sized to determine the corresponding reamer diameter for the tibial and femoral tunnels (Fig. 15).

The arthroscope is reinserted through the anterolateral portal. A tibial drill guide is used to drill a guide wire into the anatomic tibial insertion of the ACL. If necessary, small adjustments in position can be made using parallel drill guides. The prior tibial incision for harvesting the hamstring grafts is used as the starting site of the tibial tunnel. The guide pin is protected intraarticularly with a curette to prevent the pin from inadvertently being driven across the joint while reaming. The appropriate sized cannulated reamer is then drilled over the guide wire, creating the tibial bony tunnel. The internal edges of the tibial tunnel are chamfered, and any residual

soft tissue at the intraarticular margin of the tibial tunnel is removed. Next, the guide wire is reinserted through the tibial tunnel into the notch. The isometric point of graft placement on the lateral femoral condyle is identified. Various guide systems are available to aid the surgeon in defining the isometric point. Once this area is identified, the knee is flexed at least 90 degrees and the guide wire drilled from inside and then out the lateral femoral condyle. The pin should be palpable subcutaneously at the lateral femoral condyle. A 5-cm incision is then made over the guide wire at the lateral femoral condyle. The fascia lata is split longitudinally and the vastus lateralis musculature is elevated from the intermuscular septum. The guide pin exiting the lateral femoral condyle should be clearly identified. Next, the cannulated reamer is placed over the guide wire and through the tibial tunnel. The femoral tunnel is made by reaming over the guide wire inside-out (Fig. 16). The tunnel is

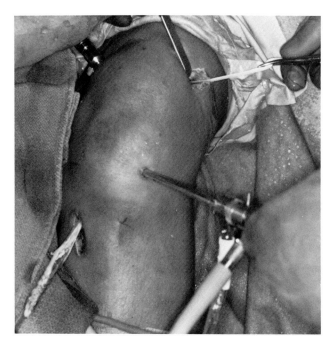

FIG. 19. Passing the graft with arthroscopic visualization.

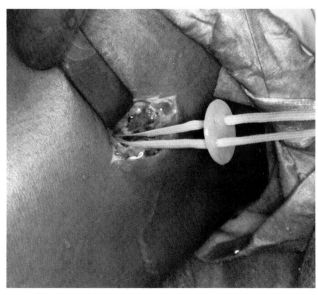

FIG. 20. The graft is fixed at the distal lateral femur by tying the Dacron tape over a button.

chamfered to remove any bony debris. A tendon passer is placed antegrade from the femoral tunnel and out the tibial tunnel (Fig. 17). A Dacron tape is looped around the doubled semitendinosus (and gracilis) tendon graft (Fig. 18) and the graft is then pulled intraarticularly through the tibial tunnel and out the femoral tunnel under arthroscopic visualization (Fig. 19). While maintaining tension on the graft distally, the Dacron tape is tied over a polyethylene button at the lateral femoral condyle (Fig. 20). The graft is pretensioned while repetitively moving the knee through a range of motion. The knee is placed at approximately 20 degrees of flexion and a posteriorly directed Lachman is then applied while the graft is securely fixed to the proximal tibia. Recently, we have been using a soft tissue plate and screw developed by Goble for fixation of the tendon graft(s) at the tibia (Figs. 21 and 22A–C). Biomechanical testing has

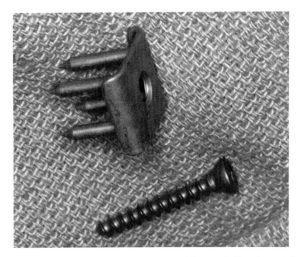

FIG. 21. Goble plate and screw used for graft fixation at the proximal tibia.

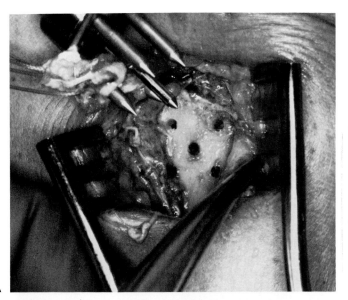

A

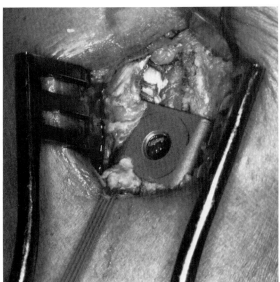

B

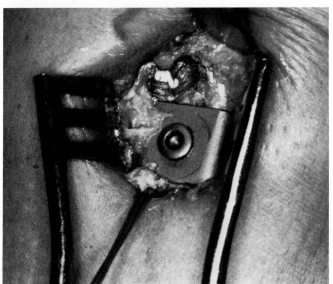

C

FIG. 22. A: A template for the plate is used to drill holes at the tibial fixation site. The holes correspond to the prongs of the plate. **B** and **C:** The plate fixes the graft to the proximal tibia. The central screw is inserted through the plate and graft for additional fixation.

demonstrated that this fixation method is approximately 400 N strong (Goble M: personal communication).

After final fixation of the graft, the knee again is taken through a range of motion while viewing arthroscopically to assure that there is no evidence of graft impingement on the intercondylar notch. The wounds are then copiously irrigated and closed in layers.

POSTOPERATIVE REGIMEN

The knee is placed in a TED compression dressing and ice packs are continually applied for 48 hours. These patients are generally discharged to home the same day of surgery or after 1 day of hospitalization. A physical therapist evaluates the patient before surgery and postoperatively, emphasizing maintenance of range of motion of the knee, specifically complete extension. Our goal is to restore a symmetrical range of motion of the knees, and if recurvatum is present in the nonoperated knee, we would like to regain the same hyperextension on the reconstructed knee. Weight-bearing as tolerated is begun immediately, with the use of crutches for support. Crutches are usually not necessary after 2 to 3 weeks. At this point, light bicycling is started followed by the Stairmaster at 3 to 4 weeks postoperatively. A hinged patellar brace is used only for prolonged ambulation or when additional support is needed. In addition, pool therapy, when available, can be initiated at 3 weeks. Light jogging on a treadmill is allowed at approximately 3 months postoperatively, and return to sports is at a minimum of 6 months after surgery. Our postoperative regimen does not differ in the event a meniscal repair was performed at the time of reconstruction.

A postoperative rehabilitation program must be carefully developed, with the mechanical strength of the graft and fixation methods used in the reconstruction taken into account. For instance, in Rosenberg's reconstruction (Fig. 9), the weak link in the reconstruction is the suture knot, which can be only 130 N strong, whereas full weight-bearing produces a force of approximately 160 N (Rosenberg T: personal communication). Also, leaving the semitendinosus tendon attached at its distal insertion, as many of the reconstructions previously described in this chapter have done, is one of the weaker techniques of graft fixation and is estimated to be only 80 N strong (35). In these cases, full weight-bearing may have to be delayed for 4 to 6 weeks until some additional graft fixation in the bony tunnels has occurred. On the other hand, if the tendon can be fixed with a screw and washer, which is on the order of 250 N, weight-bearing and rehabilitation can be more aggressive. Currently, newer techniques of graft fixation have been developed that supply significantly stronger fixation of the graft, but a detailed description is beyond the scope of this chapter. One technique, The Fastlok device (Neoliga-

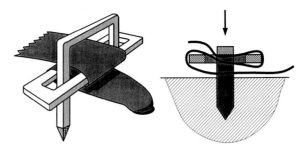

FIG. 23. The Fastlok Fixation System.

ments, Leeds, UK) is estimated to be 600 N strong using a double strand of semitendinosus tendon, and theoretically may allow an accelerated rehabilitation program (35) (Fig. 23).

OUR RESULTS (74)

We have reviewed our experience using the semitendinosus/ gracilis tendons in acute and chronic ACL reconstructions. Fifty ACL-deficient knees were consecutively reviewed with arthroscopically-assisted reconstruction using a pes anserine autograft. Twenty-eight patients underwent delayed reconstruction for chronic ACL deficiency, and 22 had reconstruction performed acutely (within 3 weeks of injury). A mean follow-up for the acutely reconstructed group was 39 months, whereas follow-up for the chronic reconstructed group was 34.1 months. The average age of the acute group was 23.4 years compared with 24.8 years in the chronic group. No attempts at primary repair of the torn ACL was performed in any case. Time from injury to surgery was 22.5 months in the group of patients with chronic ACL deficiency. In the chronic group, reconstruction was performed with the semitendinosus tendon doubled in 75% of the cases and as a single tendon strand combined with the gracilis tendon in 25% of the cases. The semitendinosus tendon was used in combination with the gracilis tendon when the semitendinosus tendon alone was of inadequate length to be doubled. The semitendinosus tendon was doubled in 86% of the reconstructions in the acute group; the tendon was used as a single strand in combination with the gracilis tendon in the remaining cases. In all cases, the diameter of the biologic graft approximated 7 mm and was composed of a double-stranded tendon graft. A similar postoperative regimen was used for both groups. The knee was placed into a postoperative hinge brace, allowing motion from −10 degrees of extension to 60 degrees of flexion with an early range of motion. Partial weight-bearing was allowed immediately and progressed to full weight-bearing by 4 to 6 weeks, at which time postoperative bracing was discontinued.

In the acutely reconstructed group, 77% reported excellent to good subjective results compared with 75% in the chronic reconstructed group. Ninety-five percent of the acutely reconstructed patients returned to sports participation, compared with 88% of the chronic group. Objective outcome was found to be more optimal in the acute group and was better than subjective outcome in either group. Seventy-one percent of the acute group patients were able to return to a preinjury sports level and participation without limitation, compared with only 63% of the chronic group. Clinical examination showed 95% of the acute group patients and 82% of the chronic group patients to have a ≤1+ Lachman test, and 96% of the acute group patients and 82% of the chronic group patients to have an absent pivot shift. Eighty-eight percent of the acute group patients had a KT-1000 result of <3 mm as compared with 61% of the chronic group patients. Range-of-motion impairment was significantly greater in the acutely reconstructed group. A strict rating system was used to obtain an overall grade, combining subjective, objective, and functional criteria. Eight variable criteria were used to access the overall grade. The lowest individual rating in any of the eight categories determined the highest overall grade the patient could be assigned. Using this rating system, patients reconstructed acutely had a better outcome, compared with the group that underwent delayed reconstruction. Meniscal injury and accumulative postmeniscectomy tissue loss appeared to be significant contributing factors in the overall success of the procedure.

Our results are similar to others that have demonstrated less optimal objective results using the semitendinosus/gracilis tendon grafts in chronic ACL reconstruction. Despite the conclusions of the studies, we do not entirely avoid use of the hamstring tendons to reconstruct the chronic ACL-deficient knee; the decision to use the semitendinosus and/or gracilis tendons is made on an individual basis. The surgical technique and graft choices for ACL reconstruction should be selected after careful consideration of several factors, which include the patient's age, size, level of activity, acuteness of injury, and other concomitant knee injuries, as well as the patient's level of expectation, degree of functional instability, and motivation and willingness to participate in a postoperative rehabilitation program. Over a 2-year period from 1988 to 1990 at the Southern California Orthopedic Institute, we have performed 532 ACL reconstructions. Approximately half of the reconstructions have been performed using the semitendinosus and/or gracilis tendons, whereas 27% have used the bone–patellar tendon–bone autograft and the additional 23% either Achilles tendon or patellar tendon allografts.

When choosing the type of graft to be used in ACL reconstruction, we consider a semitendinosus/gracilis tendon reconstruction in those patients who have an acute injury, mild to moderate laxity, and/or a significant history of patellofemoral symptoms. In the chronic ACL-deficient knee, or in an acute patient with moderate to severe laxity who is a high-level athlete, we would prefer reconstruction with the bone–patellar tendon-bone autogenous graft.

REFERENCES

1. Alm A, Gillquist J. (1974): Reconstruction of the anterior cruciate ligament by using the medial third of the patellar ligament. *Acta Chir Scand* 140:289–296.
2. Augustine RW. (1956): The unstable knee. *Am J Surg* 92:350–388.
3. Barber AF, Small NC, Click J. (1991): Anterior cruciate ligament reconstruction by semitendinosus and gracilis tendon autograft. *Am J Knee Surg* 4:84–93.
4. Boden BP, Moyer RA, Betz RR, Sapega AA. (1990): Arthroscopically-assisted anterior cruciate ligament reconstruction: a followup study. *Contemp Orthop* 20:187–194.
5. Bonamo JL, Krinick RM, Sporn AA. (1984): Rupture of the patellar ligament after use of its central third for anterior cruciate reconstruction. A report of 2 cases. *J Bone Joint Surg* 66A:1294–1297.
6. Burks RT, Haut RC, Lancaster RL. (1990): Biomechanical and histological observations on the dog patellar tendon after removal of its central one-third. *Am J Sports Med* 18:146–153.
7. Burnett QM, Fowler PJ. (1985): Reconstruction of the anterior cruciate ligament: historical overview. *Orthop Clin North Am* 16:143–157.
8. Cabaud HE, Feagin JA, Rodkey WG. (1980): Acute anterior cruciate ligament injury and augmented repair: experimental studies. *Am J Sports Med* 8:395–401.
9. Cho KO. (1975): Reconstruction of the anterior cruciate ligament by semitendinosus tenodesis. *J Bone Joint Surg* 57A:608–612.
10. Clancy WG. (1983): Anterior cruciate ligament functional instability. A static intra-articular and dynamic extra-articular procedure. *Clin Orthop* 172:102–106.
11. Clancy WG, Narechania RG, Rosenberg TD, et al. (1981): Anterior and posterior cruciate ligament reconstruction in rhesus monkeys. *J Bone Joint Surg* 64A:1270–1284.
12. Collins HR. (1990): Anterior cruciate ligament reconstruction using Gore-Tex. Presented at the 7th International Symposium: Advances in Anterior Cruciate Ligament Reconstruction of the Knee: Autogenous vs. Prosthetic. Palm Desert, California, March 1990.
13. Conteduca F, Ferretti A, Mariani PP. (1989): LAD augmentation of semitendinosus and gracilis in anterior cruciate reconstruction. Technique and preliminary results. *Am J Sports Med* 17:709–710.
14. Cross MJ, Anderson I, Roger G. (1989): Regeneration of the semitendinosus and gracilis following their transection for repair of the anterior cruciate ligament. *Am J Sports Med* 17:709.
15. DuToit GT. (1967): Knee joint cruciate ligament substitution. The Lindmann (Heidelberg) operation. *S Afr J Surg* 5:25–30.
16. Eriksson E. (1976): Reconstruction of the anterior cruciate ligament. *Orthop Clin North Am* 7:167.
17. Feagin JA, Wills RP, Van Meter CD, Lambert KL, Cunningham RR, Ruttle PE. (1990): Intraarticular anterior cruciate ligament reconstruction without extra-articular augmentation: 2-10 year followup. *Orthop Trans* 14:561–562.
18. Ferkel RD, Goodfellow D, Markolf K, et al. (1984): The ACL deficient knee: substitute or follow along? *Orthop Trans* 8:257.
19. Ferreti A, Conteduca F, DeCarly A, Fontana M, Mariani PP. (1990): Results of reconstructions of the anterior cruciate ligament with the tendons of semitendinosus and gracilis in acute capsuloligamentous lesions of the knee. *Ital J Orthop Traumatol* 16:451–458.
20. Ferreti A, DeCarly A, Conteduca F, Mariani PP, Fontana M. (1989): The results of reconstruction of the anterior cruciate ligament with semitendinosus and gracilis tendons in chronic laxity of the knee. *Ital J Orthop Traumatol* 15:415–424.
21. Fetto JF, Marshall JL. (1980): The natural history and diagnosis of anterior cruciate ligament insufficiency. *Clin Orthop* 147:29–38.
22. Friedman MJ. (1988): Arthroscopic semitendinosus (gracilis) reconstruction for anterior cruciate ligament deficiency. *Techniques Orthop* 2:74–80.
23. Friedman MJ, Sherman OH, Fox JM, Del Pizzo W, Snyder SJ,

Ferkel RD. (1985): Autogenic anterior cruciate ligament reconstruction of the knee: a review. *Clin Orthop* 96:914.

24. Gomes JL, Marczyk LR. (1984): Anterior cruciate ligament reconstruction with a loop or double thickness of semitendinosus tendon. *Am J Sports Med* 12:199–203.

25. Gomez T, Ratzlaff C, McConkey JP, Thompson JP. (1990): Semitendinosus repair augmentation of acute anterior cruciate ligament rupture. *Can J Sports Sci* 15:136–142.

26. Hanley P, Lew WD, Lewis JL, et al. (1989): Load sharing and graft fixation in the ACL reconstruction with the ligament augmentation device. *Am J Sports Med* 17:414–422.

27. Harter RA, Osternig LR, Singer KM. (1989): Instrumented Lachman tests for the evaluation of anterior laxity after reconstruction of the anterior cruciate ligament. *J Bone Joint Surg* 21A:975–983.

28. Hawkins RJ, Misamore GW, Merritt TR. (1986): Follow up of the acute nonoperated isolated ACL tear. *Am J Sports Med* 14:205–210.

29. Hendler RC. (1988): Unitunnel technique for arthroscopic anterior cruciate ligament reconstruction. *Techniques Orthop* 2:52–59.

30. Hendler RC. (1991): Total intra-articular semitendinosus anterior cruciate ligament reconstruction. In: Scott WN, ed. *Ligament and extensor mechanism injuries of the knee: diagnosis and treatment.* St. Louis, MO: Mosby Yearbook, pp. 285–300.

31. Hey Groves EW. (1920): The cruciate ligament of the knee joint: their function, rupture, and the operative treatment of the same. *Br J Surg* 7:505.

32. Holmes PF, James SL, Larson RL, Singer KM, Jones DC. (1991): Retrospective direct comparison of 3 intra-articular anterior cruciate ligament reconstructions. *Am J Sports Med* 19:596–600.

33. Horne JG, Parsons CJ. (1977): The anterior cruciate ligament: its anatomy and a new method of reconstruction. *Can J Surg* 20:214–220.

34. Insall JN, Joseph DM, Anglietti P, Campbell R. (1981): Bone block iliotibial band transfer for anterior cruciate insufficiency. *J Bone Joint Surg* 63A:560.

35. Ivey M, Li F. (1991): Tensile strength of soft tissue fixations about the knee. *Am J Knee Surg* 4:18–23.

36. Jackson DW, Schaefer RK. (1990): Cyclops syndrome: loss of extension following intraarticular anterior cruciate ligament reconstruction. *Arthroscopy* 6:171.

37. Johnson LL. (1986): Extra synovial knee conditions. In: *Arthroscopic surgery: principles and practice.* 3rd ed. St. Louis, MO: CV Mosby.

38. Johnson LL. (1992): Fate of semitendinosus autogenous grafts. Presented at Update 1992: New Perspectives in Arthroscopy and Sports Medicine, March 18–22, 1992, Palm Springs, California.

39. Johnson RJ, Eriksson E, Haggmark T, Pope MH. (1984): Five- to ten-year follow-up evaluation after reconstruction of the anterior cruciate ligament. *Clin Orthop* 183:122–140.

40. Jones KG. (1963): Reconstruction of the anterior cruciate ligament. A technique using the central one-third of the patellar ligaments. *J Bone Joint Surg* 45A:925–932.

41. Kannus P, Jarvinen M. (1987): Conservatively treated tears of the ACL. Long-term results. *J Bone Joint Surg* 69A:1007–1012.

42. Kennedy JC, Roth JH, Mendenhall I IV, Sanford JB. (1980): Intra-articular replacement of the anterior cruciate ligament deficient knee. *Am J Sports Med* 8:1–8.

43. Langan P, Fontanetta AP. (1987): Rupture of the patellar tendon after use of its central third. *Orthop Rev* 15:61.

44. Lange M. (1962): *Orthopadiche-Chirurgische Operationslehre.* 2nd ed. JF Bergmann, pp. 692–700.

45. Larsen RL. (1985): Augmentation of acute rupture of the anterior cruciate ligament. *Orthop Clin North Am* 16:135–142.

46. Larsen RL. (1987): Technique of arthroscopically aided anterior cruciate ligament reconstruction. In: Crenshaw AH, ed. *Campbells's operative orthopaedics.* 7th ed., Vol. 3. St. Louis, MO: CV Mosby, p. 2455.

47. Lipscomb AB, Johnston RK, Snider RB. (1981): Technique of cruciate ligament reconstruction. *Am J Sports Med* 9:77–81.

48. Lipscomb AB, Johnston RK, Snider RB, Brothers JC. (1979): Full and secondary reconstruction of the anterior cruciate ligament in athletes by using the semitendinosus tendon: preliminary report of 78 cases. *Am J Sports Med* 7:8184.

49. Lipscomb AB, Johnston K, Snider RB, Warburton MJ, Gilbert PP. (1982): Evaluation of hamstring strength following use of semitendinosus and gracilis tendons to reconstruct the anterior cruciate ligament. *Am J Sports Med* 10:340–342.

50. Macey HB. (1939): New operative procedures for the repair of ruptured cruciate ligaments of the knee joint. *Surg Gynecol Obstet* 69:108–109.

51. Marder RA, Raskind JR, Carroll M. (1991): Prospective evaluation of arthroscopically assisted anterior cruciate ligament reconstruction: patellar tendon vs. semitendinosus and gracilis tendons. *Am J Sports Med* 19:478–484.

52. Marshall JL, Warren RF. (1979): Reconstruction of functioning anterior cruciate ligament. Preliminary report using quadriceps tendon. *Orthop Rev* 6:49.

53. McCarroll JR. (1983): Fracture of the patellar during a golf swing following reconstruction of the anterior cruciate ligament. *Am J Sports Med* 11:26–27.

54. McDaniel WJ, Dameran TB. (1983): The untreated anterior cruciate ligament rupture. *Clin Orthop* 172:158–163.

55. McMaster JH, Weinert CR, Scranton P. (1974): Diagnosis and management of isolated anterior cruciate ligament tears: preliminary report of reconstruction with a gracilis tendon. *J Trauma* 14:230–235.

56. Mott HW. (1983): Semitendinosus anatomic reconstruction for cruciate ligament insufficiency. *Clin Orthop* 172:90–92.

57. Moyer RA, Betz RR, Iaquinto J, et al. (1986): Arthroscopic anterior cruciate reconstruction using the semitendinosus and gracilis tendons: a preliminary report. *Contemp Orthop* 12:17–23.

58. Nicholas JA, Minkoff J. (1978): Iliotibial band transfer through the intercondylar notch for combined anterior instability (ITBT Procedure). *Am J Sports Med* 6:341.

59. Noyes FR, Butler DL, Grood ES, Zernike RF, Hefzy MS. (1984): Biomechanical analysis of human ligament grafts used in the knee—ligament repairs and reconstructions. *J Bone Joint Surg* 66A:344–352.

60. O'Donoghue DH. (1963): A method for replacement of the anterior cruciate ligament of the knee. *J Bone Joint Surg* 45A:905.

61. Oter AL, McDermott KL, Hutcheson L. (1991): Arthroscopic anterior cruciate ligament reconstruction: a comparison of semitendinosus and gracilis vs. patellar tendon autografts. *Arthroscopy* 7:319.

62. Pagnami MJ, Warner JJP, O'Brien SJ, Warren RF. (1991): Anatomical considerations in harvesting the semitendinosus and gracilis tendons. Presented at the American Academy of Orthopaedic Surgeons Annual Meeting, Anaheim, California, March 1991.

63. Pattee GA, Friedman MJ. (1988): A review of autogenous intra-articular reconstruction of the anterior cruciate ligament. In: Friedman MJ, Ferkel RD, eds. *Prosthetic ligament reconstruction of the knee.* Philadelphia: WB Saunders, pp. 22–28.

64. Paulos LE, Butler DL, Noyes FR, Grood ES. (1983): Intra-articular cruciate reconstruction II: replacement with vascularized patellar tendon. *Clin Orthop* 172:78.

65. Paulos LE, Rosenberg TD, Drawbert J, et al. (1987): Intrapatellar contracture syndrome. *Am J Sports Med* 15:331–341.

66. Puddu G. (1980): Method for reconstruction of the anterior cruciate ligament using the semitendinosus tendon. *Am J Sports Med* 8:402–404.

67. Puddu G, Ferreti A, Conteduca F, Mariani PP. (1988): Reconstruction of the anterior cruciate ligament by semitendinosus transfer and chronic anterior instability of the knee. *Ital J Orthop Traumatol* 14:187–193.

68. Puddu J, Ippolioto E. (1983): Reconstruction of the anterior cruciate ligament using the semitendinosus tendon: histological study of a case. *Am J Sports Med* 11:1416.

69. Roberts TS, Drez D, Banta CJ. (1989): Complications of anterior cruciate ligament reconstruction. In: Brigg NF, ed. *Complications in arthroscopy.* New York: Raven Press, pp. 169–177.

70. Sachs RA, Daniel DM, Stone ML, Garfen RF. (1989): Patellofemoral problems after anterior cruciate ligament reconstruction. *Am J Sports Med* 17:760–765.

71. Sapega M. (1990): Arthroscopically assisted reconstruction of the anterior cruciate ligament. In: Torg JS, ed. *Current therapy in sports medicine—2.* Toronto: BC Decker, pp. 292–297.

72. Schaefer RK, Jackson DW. (1991): Arthroscopic management of the cruciate ligaments. In: McGinty JB, et al. eds. *Operative arthroscopy.* New York: Raven Press, pp. 389–416.

73. Scott WN, Schosheim PM. (1983): Intra-articular transfer of the iliotibial muscle-tendon unit. *Clin Orthop* 172:97–101.

74. Sgaglione NA, Del Pizzo W, Fox JM, Friedman MJ. (1991): Arthroscopic-assisted anterior cruciate ligament reconstruction with the pes anserine tendons: comparison of results in acute and chronic ligament deficiency. Presented at the American Academy of Orthopaedic Surgeons 58th Annual Meeting, Anaheim, California, March 1991.

75. Sgaglione NA, Del Pizzo W, Fox JM, Friedman MJ, Snyder SJ, Ferkel RD (1992): Arthroscopic assisted anterior cruciate ligament reconstruction with the semitendinosus tendon: comparison of results with and without braided propylene augmentation. *Arthroscopy.* 8:65–77.

76. Sgaglione NA, Warren RF, Wickiewicz TO, Gold DA, Panariello RA. (1990): Primary repair of semitendinosus tendon augmentation of acute anterior cruciate ligament injuries. *Am J Sports Med* 18:64–73.

77. Simon TM, Jackson DW. (1987): Anterior cruciate ligament allografts. In: Jackson DW, Drez D, eds. *The anterior cruciate deficient knee.* St. Louis, MO: CV Mosby.

78. Sisk TD. (1987): Knee injuries. In: Crenshaw AB, ed. *Campbell's operative orthopaedics.* 7th ed., Vol. 3. St. Louis, MO: CV Mosby, p. 2283.

79. Thompson SK, Calver R, Monk CJ. (1978): Anterior cruciate ligament repair for rotatory instability: the Lindmann dynamic muscle transfer procedure. *J Bone Joint Surg* 60A:917–920.

80. Tillberg B. (1977): The late repair of torn cruciate ligaments using the menisci. *J Bone Joint Surg* 59B:15–19.

81. Vandendriessche G, Gunst P, Rombouts J, et al. (1986): Reconstruction of the anterior cruciate ligament using the tendon of the semitendinosus muscle. *Acta Orthop Belg* 52:528–540.

82. Wainer RA, Clarke TJ, Poehling GG. (1988): Arthroscopic reconstruction on the anterior cruciate ligament using allograft tendon. *Arthroscopy* 4:199–205.

83. Walsh JJ. (1972): Meniscal reconstruction of the anterior cruciate ligament. *Clin Orthop* 89:171–177.

84. Warner JP, Warren RF, Cooper D. (1991): Management of acute anterior cruciate ligament injury. In: *Instructional course lectures, American Academy of Orthopaedic Surgeons.* Vol. 50. Park Ridge, IL: American Academy of Orthopaedic Surgeons, pp. 219–222.

85. Wilson WJ, Scranton PE. (1990): Combined reconstruction of the anterior cruciate ligament in competitive athletes. *J Bone Joint Surg* 72A:742–748.

86. Zaricznyj B. (1983): Reconstruction of the anterior cruciate ligament using free tendon graft. *Am J Sports Med* 11:164–176.

87. Zaricznyj B. (1987): Reconstruction of the anterior cruciate ligament of the knee using a double tendon graft. *Clin Orthop* 220:167–175.

88. Zarins B, Rowe CR. (1986): Combined anterior cruciate ligament reconstruction using semitendinosus tendon and iliotibial tract. *J Bone Joint Surg* 68A:160–177.

The Anterior Cruciate Ligament: Current and Future Concepts, edited by D.W. Jackson, et al. Raven Press, Ltd., New York © 1993.

CHAPTER 28

Allograft Reconstruction of the Anterior Cruciate Ligament

Freddie H. Fu, Douglas W. Jackson, James Jamison, Mark J. Lemos, and Timothy M. Simon

The use of musculoskeletal allografts in orthopedic surgery have included bone, articular cartilage, tendon, and ligaments. During the past decade, the specific use of allograft tissue for the reconstruction of the anterior cruciate ligament (ACL)-deficient knee has increased significantly. The most common sources of allograft tissue used for ACL reconstruction have included (a) bone–patellar tendon–bone, (b) iliotibial band, (c) Achilles tendon, (d) semitendinosus and gracilis tendons, and (e) ACL. Shino et al. have reported that 22 different grafts may be harvested from one human donor that are appropriate for ACL reconstruction (104).

The use of an allograft to reconstruct the ACL is appealing because there is no donor site morbidity for the recipient and it allows the harvesting of larger and more varied graft material. The disadvantage of an allograft includes limited availability, sterility considerations, and potential variations in the biologic response of the recipient in comparison with an autograft. Although the risk is extremely low, the greatest current concern among informed recipients is the potential for disease transmission (7,12,34,37,43,103,111).

Most of the allografts used to date for ACL reconstructions have been harvested and stored in either the fresh-frozen or freeze-dried state. Fresh-frozen ligament and tendon allografts can be stored for up to 5 years at −70°C (6 months at −20°C), and freeze-dried grafts are usable for at least 5 years. Fresh-frozen and freeze-dried allografts do not preserve living ligament or tendon cells. This differs from fresh tissue allografts such as organ transplants that contain living cells that are felt to be vital to their function. The desire to transplant living mature ACL fibroblasts, in addition to the collagen in an allograft, has caused some interest in fresh and cryopreserved allografts for ACL reconstruction. The use of grafts with living cells poses additional logistic considerations because they must be procured and transplanted into the recipient within hours of the harvest. Fresh grafts require the recipient, the tissue harvesting, and the surgical implantation all to be coordinated. In an attempt to achieve more time between harvesting and transplantation, cryopreservation (slow rate freezing) techniques have been proposed as a method of transplanting living cells with some longer term storage.

PROCUREMENT TECHNIQUES

The American Association of Tissue Banks (AATB) has been instrumental in standardizing approaches for safe and efficacious tissue procurement and banking (2–4). The AATB provides training and examinations for tissue bank technicians and coordinators, inspects tissue banks for accreditation, and has published a manual on tissue banking. The manual establishes guidelines that reduce the risk of disease transmission and neoplastic disorders from allografts. It provides appropriate methods for donor selection, tissue retrieval, processing, preservation, storage, labeling, and distribution (3). The nonurgent nature of musculoskeletal transplants for ACL reconstructions enables the tissue banks ample time to perform donor screening. This includes an extensive review of the donor's medical and social history,

F. H. Fu and J. Jamison: Department of Orthopaedics, University of Pittsburgh School of Medicine, Pittsburgh, Pennsylvania 15261.

D. W. Jackson, M. J. Lemos, and T. M. Simon: Southern California Center for Sports Medicine, Long Beach, California 90806.

laboratory testing of blood, and review of autopsy results with special attention to lymph node examination.

When a potential donor has been identified, and appropriate consent or approval has been obtained, the tissue bank coordinator or transplant donor coordinator verifies suitability of the donor using stringent screening criteria. It is the primary responsibility of the coordinator to select donors with the lowest risk of transmitting disease to the graft recipient.

The donated tissues should be surgically removed using aseptic techniques in an operating room environment. The tissues are cultured extensively during procurement to document any bacterial and fungal contamination. The use of disposable supplies also assists in reducing the risk of tissue contamination. The tissues are triple wrapped, with the innermost wrap placed in a sterile plastic bag to prevent seepage-borne contamination. The wrapped tissues are then labeled and transported on ice to the tissue bank for further processing.

At the tissue bank the tissue may be deep frozen at $-70°C$ or below until all laboratory testing, screening, and autopsy results are completed and reviewed. Any tissues that fail screening tests are discarded appropriately. All subsequent tissue processing is performed under aseptic conditions. The tissues are unwrapped and trimmed of extraneous tissue, then washed to remove blood and marrow elements. Tissues to be used for ACL reconstruction, such as patellar tendon, Achilles tendon, and fascia lata, are amenable to longer term processing steps, such as ethanol soaks, antibiotic soaks, or other disinfection or sterilization procedures (10,67,72,95).

If the grafts are going to be freeze dried for storage, the allografts are transferred to sterile bottles, partially capped, and placed in a sterile freeze-dry (lyophilizer) instrument and frozen under vacuum. The tissue is freeze dried over a span of days with gradual increases in temperature to ambient conditions. The bottle is then capped under vacuum, removed from the lyophilizer, checked for vacuum, and labeled. A representative number of coprocessed tissues are usually cultured after the freeze-drying cycle to verify sterility as part of the tissue bank's quality control protocol. The finished product, after passing all quality control testing, is inventoried, and all records relevant to the tissue are maintained by the tissue bank. Currently, donor blood samples are maintained for future laboratory testing. It has been recommended that the tissue banks maintain a record of where allografts have been shipped and, through a cooperative effort by the surgeon and hospital, the name of the allograft recipient maintained for "look back" purposes.

Since 1985, donors of organs or tissue transplantation in the United States have been screened for human immunodeficiency virus type I (HIV-I), and more than 60,000 organs and one million tissues have been trans-

planted. To date, one patient has developed an HIV infection following an ACL reconstruction (11,105). This graft was obtained from a donor in 1985, a 22-year-old man who died 32 hours after a gunshot wound. The donor had no known risk factors for HIV infection and was seronegative. In retrospective testing of the donor's stored lymphocytes for HIV by viral cultures and the polymerase chain reaction (PCR), HIV-I was detected. This particular case and the overall experience to date using allografts to reconstruct the ACL illustrates the following:

1. To date, one HIV-infected donor of tissue for ACL reconstruction has been missed using the 1985 screening techniques. These screening techniques have been significantly improved since that time.

2. Transmission of HIV through musculoskeletal allografts has occurred from this one donor. Three recipients of fresh-frozen bone from the same donor have acquired HIV from these grafts. During the time period since 1985, more than one million tissues have been distributed.

3. No HIV transmission to date has been documented from musculoskeletal tissues treated by lyophilization or from frozen bone with the marrow washed thoroughly during processing before transplantation.

4. The most effective control of the risk of HIV transmission remains associated with the donor screening process. The manner in which the tissue has been stored or processed may also reduce the risk.

5. Risk of HIV transmission with musculoskeletal allografts from seronegative donors is extremely small (14,15,22,105). The exact risk remains unknown.

These observations reinforce the need to acquire musculoskeletal allografts from sources that follow appropriate guidelines for donor selection and tissue processing. The use of musculoskeletal allografts are, as are most therapeutic approaches, associated with risks that must be weighed against their benefits.

ALLOGRAFT STERILITY

Tissue for use as fresh, cryopreserved, fresh-frozen, or freeze-dried allografts is usually harvested in an operating room under standard sterile surgical conditions (12,94). However, these procedures incur considerable time and financial expense.

The development of ethylene oxide sterilization seemed to provide a suitable alternative, enabling allograft tissue be harvested under clean, but not sterile, conditions and secondarily sterilized (94). When this technique is combined with freeze drying, the tissue can be stored at room temperature (115). However, France stressed the importance of adequate aeration to remove remaining ethylene oxide from the tissue so as to prevent possible toxic effects that could thwart the long-term success and incorporation of the tissue *in vivo* (37). Jackson reported intraarticular reactions after ethylene oxide sterilized allografts for ACL reconstruction and documented by-products of ethylene oxide in the grafts several months after transplantation (60). Some of the by-products of ethylene oxide appear to be removed by solvents and not entirely by aeration.

Gamma irradiation also has received considerable attention in efforts toward allograft sterilization (23,27, 106,107,109,116,125). A 2.5-Mrad dose of ^{60}Co irradiation has been considered to provide adequate sterilization with a good safety margin for medical products(116). However, many bacteria and viruses are radiation resistant and require higher doses. Viruses are recognized as being more resistant than fungi, bacterial spores, or bacteria, although the contamination load is important (23).

A 7.5×10^5 rad dose of gamma irradiation proved ineffective in deactivating the viral enzyme of lymphadenopathy-associated virus, a pathogen linked to HIV. However, 2.5×10^5 rad rendered viral samples noninfectious when administered before lymphocyte exposure (107). Wright and Trump (125) reviewed literature citing a minimum dose of 2.4 Mrad as adequate for the inactivation of almost all viruses, although their 1969 article was too early to include HIV. In their experience, doses greater than 3 Mrad resulted in vessel-wall destruction of aortic transplant grafts. This finding has implications for tendon and ligament allografts because, like aortic grafts, collagen is the primary structural component. Hiemstra et al. (49) investigated the inactivation of HIV in plasma by gamma irradiation. A dose of 5 to 10 Mrad was required to reduce the viral titer significantly in samples frozen to $-80°C$, whereas samples at $15°C$ required 2.5 Mrad for the same effect. Because it destroyed the biologic activity of the plasma components, irradiation was considered an unacceptable form of plasma sterilization.

Fideler et al. (35) recently assessed the ability of gamma irradiation to inactivate HIV in fresh-frozen bone–patellar tendon–bone allografts. Specimens were harvested from six cadavers in which death resulted from complications of acquired immunodeficiency syndrome. HIV positivity was confirmed in serum and tissue from each cadaver by PCR. The tissue was fresh frozen to $-70°C$ and exposed to 2.0, 2.5, 3.0, or 4.0 Mrad of irradiation. After irradiation, the tissue specimens were tested again by PCR. A dose of 3.0 Mrad was necessary to render the tissue HIV negative. The authors acknowledged the small sample size studied, and currently are conducting a larger study to provide more definitive information in this area.

Several authors have examined how the different methods of allograft sterilization affect the biomechanical properties of the specimen. In fresh-frozen patellar tendon–bone specimens, Butler et al. (17) found no significant difference in modulus and maximum stress between a group that was irradiated with 1.95 Mrad and a nonirradiated control group. In contrast, they found large differences after irradiation in freeze-dried specimens. It must be noted that 2.5 Mrad, the usual dose for sterilization, was not evaluated in this study. Nevertheless, several other investigators have found that irradiation significantly altered the biomechanical properties of freeze-dried allografts (37,58,89).

In response to the findings of Butler et al. (17) and Paulos et al. (89), Gibbons et al. (41) studied dose-dependent effects of gamma irradiation on the material properties of the goat patellar tendon, fresh frozen to $-30°C$. Significant differences were noted only in the maximum stress and strain energy density measurements of specimens irradiated with 3 Mrad as compared with nonirradiated fresh-frozen control tendons. The modulus and maximum strain values displayed a trend toward decreasing in these irradiated specimens, but the decrease was not statistically significant. No significant change in any of the four properties was associated with 2-Mrad doses of irradiation. They concluded that moderate irradiation doses could be used without deleterious effects.

The investigation of irradiation by Fideler et al. (35) also examined its effect on the material and mechanical properties of the bone–patellar tendon–bone allograft. They observed an obvious dose-dependent effect of irradiation on the graft's properties, finding a statistically significant loss of initial strength between doses of 2.0 and 3.0 Mrad. However, the clinical significance of this compromise could not be determined.

Haut and Powlison (47) examined the effects of the sequence of freezing and irradiation at 2 Mrad. A significant decrease in ultimate stress was noted after irradiation of fresh-frozen specimens. Freeze drying after irradiation did not affect the ultimate stress significantly, but freeze drying first caused a significant decrease in ultimate stress as compared with fresh-frozen specimens. In addition, inspection of the gross specimens showed separation of collagen fascicles. Haut and Powlison concluded that irradiation is most deleterious to dry tissue, and that collagen denaturation depends on radiation dose and the state of tissue hydration.

Gibbons et al. (40) reported that irradiation produced a trend toward compromise of fresh-frozen bone–patellar tendon–bone allograft biomechanical properties. These changes were of statistical significance only at 3 Mrad. Overall, the effect of gamma irradiation was determined to be dose dependent, but in a nonlinear fashion, indicating that more significant changes would occur at doses higher than those studied. Ruptures that were observed were mostly in the tendon midsubstance. The long-term significance of these time zero changes in allografts is yet to be defined. Butler et al. (18) found no significant difference in biomechanical properties between nonirradiated and 2 Mrad–irradiated fresh-frozen goat patellar tendon allografts that had been implanted for 6 months. Both sets of grafts provided substantial anterior stiffness, and Butler et al. concluded that irradiation at this dose produces no deleterious effects on the grafts after incorporation.

The information available on allograft sterility with secondary methods remains less well defined than state-of-the-science screening of donors. Screening remains the main prevention of transplanting potentially diseased allografts. Fresh freezing alone offers little additional protection in eliminating the potential for HIV transmission. The addition of irradiation may be helpful, but a dose low enough to prevent collagen degradation may not ensure viral inactivation.

IMMUNOGENICITY

The implantation of any foreign tissue causes concern regarding its potential immunogenicity. Solid organ transplantation with the recipient's immunologic response often presents a major hurdle to success. In osteochondral allografts, the recipient's response is thought to promote the rapid stimulation of osteoclasts and osteoblasts, resulting in allograft resorption and remodeling into viable bone (50). Collagen, which makes up 90% of the organic matrix of bone (50), provides the main structural component of the ACL allograft. Controversy surrounds the existence, stimulation, and significance of an immunologic response to collagen. The different types of collagen have been implicated as autoantigens in the arthritides (50,112–114), which suggests the possibility of a similar response to the collagen in allografts. Minami et al. (74) found that the Achilles tendon expresses major histocompatibility antigenicity in its cellular components, not in collagen, and that freezing reduces this antigenicity, whereas irradiation has little effect on the immune response. Other studies support the idea that the immune response is directed mainly toward the cellular components of transplanted tendon or bone (20,39,43,77,91,103).

Although fresh freezing and freeze drying apparently decreases the antigenicity of collagenous grafts, the exact mechanism of this action is unknown. It is speculated that the processing kills cells and damages or denatures the antigens on their surface, resulting in a vast reduction of the immunologic response (20,39,44,74). This theory was supported by the histological finding of maintenance of the normal collagen bundle framework in the graft (103). However, another theory is that thawing causes cell lysis, leading to the release of cell membranes, which then become available for phagocytosis by host macrophages. These membranes are believed to be processed by macrophages and expressed on their surface as foreign class I or class II antigens (50). Friedlaender et al. (39) suggested this same idea, finding freeze drying to be

somewhat more effective than fresh freezing in eliminating the immunologic response to cortical and corticocancellous bone allografts. Cryopreservation that preserves cellular viability does not decrease the immunologic response (64).

Debate surrounds not only the origin of the stimulus for a response, but the mode of its suppression. The components of the immune system that may participate in the response to transplanted collagenous tissue must be further delineated. *In vitro* assays have demonstrated collagen to be responsible for both humoral and cell-mediated responses (50,114). Lanzer et al. (69) reported that an immunologic host response to freeze-dried allograft tissue does occur in humans and that this response is humoral, involving the formation of immune complexes. In the canine model, several investigators have observed both humoral and cell-mediated responses to fresh-frozen patellar tendon (7), fresh-frozen bone (108), and snap-frozen (5-minute immersion in liquid nitrogen) bone–ACL–bone allografts (117). In addition, the detection of higher antibody titers in synovial fluid than in serum indicates that the response may be much more intense locally than systemically (108,117).

Despite these findings, numerous studies have observed no demonstrable immunologic response to allografts used for reconstruction of the ACL. Shino et al. (100,101,103,104) have conducted investigations of allograft ACL reconstruction in dogs and in humans. In dogs, fresh-frozen patellar tendon allografts resembled the normal ACL both microangiographically and histologically by 52 weeks, with no sign of rejection (103). Fresh-frozen tendon allografts used for ACL reconstruction in humans also yielded good results, with no evidence of effusion, synovial thickening, or skin necrosis that would suggest rejection by 24 to 40 months postoperatively (104). In an arthroscopic study of patients 6 weeks to 55 months after reconstruction with fresh-frozen allograft tissue, the grafts showed no gross or histologic evidence of an immune response (101). Long-term follow-up of these same patients (36 to 90 months postoperatively) showed similarly good gross and histologic results, 94% having good or excellent subjective and functional outcomes (100). Arnoczky et al. (7) compared fresh and fresh-frozen patellar tendon allografts for ACL replacement in the dog. They documented a marked rejection response in the fresh grafts, noting perivascular cuffing and lymphocytic invasion. In contrast, the fresh-frozen allografts appeared to undergo remodeling and revascularization in a manner similar to autografts, with no sign of rejection. In a study conducted by Indelicato et al. (51) of patients who received either freeze-dried or fresh-frozen patellar tendon allografts as ACL substitutes, none demonstrated clinical signs or histologic evidence of an immune reaction. Nonetheless, none of these studies evaluated serum or synovial fluid for the presence of immunologic factors.

In contrast, Vasseur et al. (117) performed immunologic analyses of serum and synovial fluid from dogs receiving snap-frozen bone–ACL–bone allografts. Systemic antibodies to donor lymphocyte antigens were present in two of six dogs at 6 weeks after surgery, but these persisted throughout the 9-month course of the study in only one dog. By comparison, antidonor antibody was found in the synovial fluid of four of the six dogs 4 months postoperatively and in all six by 9 months. However, the method of rapid freezing in this study was not the same as that used clinically, and probably did not decrease or eliminate allograft antigenicity to the extent that fresh freezing does. In addition, the significance of this antibody response to the success of the grafts could not be determined. Similarly, in another study, dogs that received frozen bone–ACL–bone allografts had a higher mean synovial leukocyte count than did autografted dogs at 16 weeks. In addition, four of eight dogs in the allograft group demonstrated donor-specific antibodies in the synovial fluid by 8 weeks, and three of these dogs displayed serum antibodies (110). Additionally, two reports suggest that the human immune response to freeze-dried bone–patellar tendon–bone allografts may be detrimental to the graft (93,97). Future studies of the human immune response to allografts used to reconstruct the ACL will need to assess preoperative and postoperative blood samples that can be compared for components of both the humoral and cellular immune responses. In addition, for patients requiring follow-up arthroscopy, synovial fluid and graft biopsies should be collected and tested for immune components to further clarify these issues.

ALLOGRAFTS TO RECONSTRUCT THE ACL

The first biologic ACL reconstruction was described in 1917 by Hey Groves (48), who used an iliotibial band autograft. Several subsequent autograft procedures were introduced with either a proximally or distally based graft that was used for replacement of the ACL (21,33,61,70,71,85). In 1976, Franke (38) reported the first use of a free patellar tendon autograft with patellar and tibial bone blocks. The concept of a biologic graft free of vascularity and potentially without living cells stimulated interest in using an allograft as an alternative.

The challenge in using either autograft or allograft collagen is to reconstruct a functional ACL. The ACL consists of fibers of different lengths and orientations. The fibers respond to the complex geometry of the knee joint, which changes with flexion and extension the orientation of the ACL, transferring load between different fiber groups during motion (42,63). The tissue selected to substitute for ACL must possess sufficient biomechanical properties to withstand the demands of the knee joint, both initially (24,25,45) and after remodeling (121). The

selected graft should be readily available, should be of sufficient size and length, and should have minimal morbidity associated with its harvesting (82).

Although several different grafts have been proposed to reconstruct the ACL, the autograft patellar tendon with proximal and distal bone blocks has been labeled the standard for ACL reconstructions (32). The initial biomechanical properties of the patellar tendon graft are felt to be superior to other potential grafts (81). Other desirable aspects of this particular graft include the integrity of the tendon–bone interface, the potential for bone-to-bone healing, and the initial rigid fixation at the time of implantation (88). The time zero mechanical and structural properties of bone–patella tendon–bone allografts and autografts are similar. The bone–patella tendon–bone autograft has been reported to give encouraging clinical results (26,62,87). The long-term clinical results of comparable allografts and autografts are what is not available at this time.

The interest in allograft tissue was stimulated also by the potential associated benefits of a shortened surgical time, smaller incisions (52,88), and less dissection, because there is no need to harvest the graft and sacrifice normal host tissue. The optimal size and shape of the graft for the procedure can be determined preoperatively and is not limited by tissue availability at the patient's donor site (40,119). With patellar tendon allografts, patellofemoral tracking is unaltered (40). Allografts provide an alternative when previous autograft reconstructions have failed and no autologous tissue is available (51,52). Other infrequent problems associated with using autografts to reconstruct the ACL have been reported (9,29–31,51,73,90,96,99,100,118,119). Allografts for ACL reconstruction continued to receive more attention as an alternative, particularly after their reported success as substitutes for other musculoskeletal tissues (5,12,13,20,78,92) and for ACL reconstruction in the dog (28,103,118).

REPLACING AN ACL WITH AN ACL ALLOGRAFT

In contrast to solid organ transplantation, in which the maintenance of cellular viability is critical to organ function, allografts and autografts are presently used as collagen struts that function as a check reign to anterior tibial translation. Cellular viability at the time of transplantation has not been felt to be required, and the allografts used in the past decade have been primarily fresh frozen or freeze dried (37,52,115). These techniques have allowed longer term preservation of the allografts before transplantation (52,54,79,103,118).

Replacement cells from the host that repopulate the transplanted allografts have not maintained their time zero structural and mechanical properties (55,57). An attempt to retain the preimplantation properties of the allograft stimulated interest in transplanting differentiated specialized ACL cells with the collagen in the graft. If these cells continue to populate the graft and function, they might retain the inherent properties of the normal ACL.

Transplanting the ACLs with living cells can be performed using fresh grafts (within 6 hours of death of the donor) or using cryopreserved ACL allografts. Cryopreservation is the process where the allograft is subjected to a very slow rate of freezing along with the use of a cryoprotectant (usually 7.5% to 15% glycerol or dimethyl sulfoxide). Cell survival rates with soft tissue allografts that have been cryopreserved vary (21). Transplantation of a differentiated cell line with the donor tissue has been suggested to be beneficial and is part of the justification

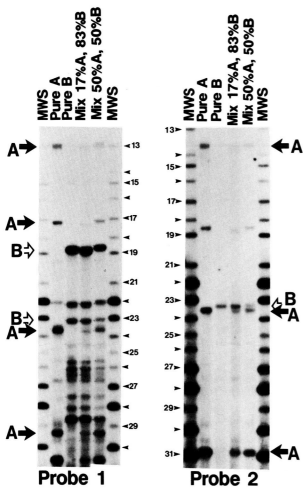

Probe 1   **Probe 2**

FIG. 1. DNA band patterns obtained from mixtures of tissue from the ACL from two different goats with use of DNA probes 1 and 2. Unique DNA bands form goat A (pure A), marked with closed arrows and an A, are shown with probe 1 at or between band numbers 13, 17, and 18; 23 and 24; and 29 and 30, and with probe 2 at band numbers 13 and 14; 23 and 24; and 31. Similarly, unique DNA bands from goat B (pure B), marked with open arrows and a B, are shown with probe 1 between band numbers 118 and 119, and 23 and 24, and with probe 2 between band numbers 23 and 24. The density of the unique DNA bands in the lanes marked Mix, compared with that in the corresponding bands in the pure A and pure B lanes, reflects the relative concentrations of A and B tissue that are present. The MWS lane contains the molecular weight sizing standard. The small arrowheads and numbers indicate the relative band positions and band numbers of the molecular weight sizing standard. (From ref. 59, with permission.)

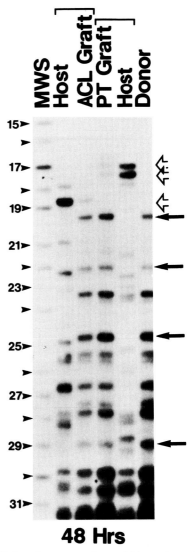

48 Hrs

FIG. 2. DNA band patterns from ACL and patellar tendon allografts, host goats (recipients of allografts), and donor goats 48 hours after transplantation, identified with the use of probe 1. Brackets indicate the same animal. The host tissue is from the contralateral ACL. The closed arrows indicate the positions of the unique donor bands (also present in the patellar and ACL allografts) between band numbers 19 and 21, 21 and 22, 24 and 25, and 28 and 29. Characteristic bands from the hosts are beginning to appear faintly in the patellar ligament allografts (open arrows) between band numbers 17 and 18, and in the ACL allografts between band numbers 18 and 19. The MWS lane contains the molecular weight sizing standard. (From ref. 59, with permission.)

for the use of cryopreserved heart valves (68,75,76,84). The transplantation of living fibroblasts (fresh or cryopreserved) from ACLs, which may synthesize and maintain collagen fibrils of the appropriate diameter and other extracellular components, is based on an assumption that the donor cells survive and maintain their phenotypic expression after transplantation. At the current time, cryopreservation to maintain living fibroblasts that replicate and contribute to maintaining the mechanical and structural properties of the ligament after transplantation has not been demonstrated.

CELL SURVIVAL WITH ACL ALLOGRAFTS

Survival of transplanted living donor fibroblasts in allografts had not been documented. The recent development of DNA probes has provided a method for identification of DNA from cells of different individuals. Jackson et al. used DNA probes to identify and demonstrate the presence and relative amounts of cellular DNA in fresh ACL and patellar tendon allografts that were used for reconstruction of the ACL in a goat model (Fig. 1)(59). The fate of the donor and recipient DNA in the

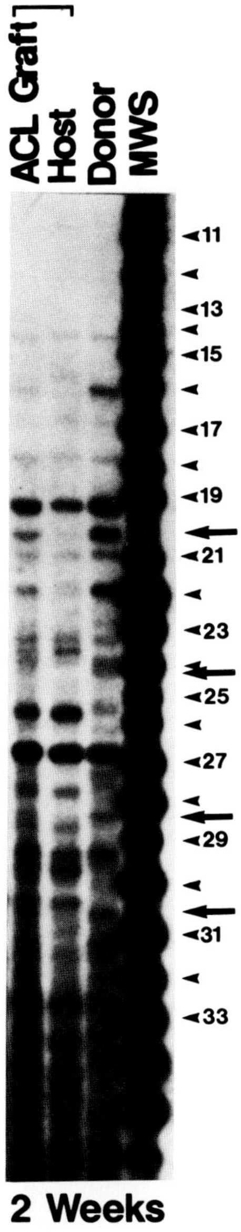

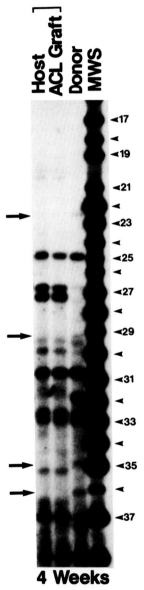

FIG. 3. DNA band patterns from ACL allografts, host goats (recipients of allografts), and donor goats 2 weeks after transplantation. Brackets indicate same animal. Long arrows indicate the position of donor bands that are also identified in the allograft, but at reduced levels; these appear between band numbers 19 and 21, 24 and 25, 28 and 29, and 30 and 31. Characteristic DNA bands seen in the host lane also are present in the allograft lane. (From ref. 59, with permission.)

FIG. 4. DNA band patterns from ACL allografts, hosts goats (recipients of allografts), and donor goats 4 weeks after transplantation. Brackets indicate same animal. Long arrows indicate the position of unique donor bands that are no longer present in the allograft lane. These DNA bands appear between band numbers 22 and 23, 29 and 30, 34 and 35, and 36 and 37. The band pattern of the allograft is identical to that of the host. (From ref. 59, with permission.)

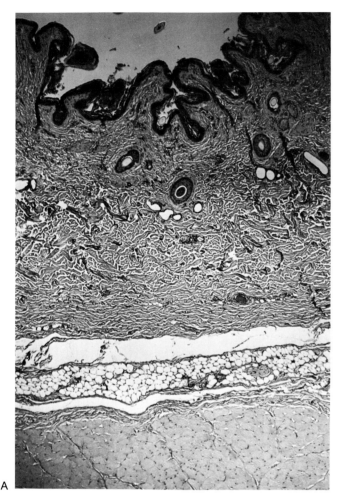
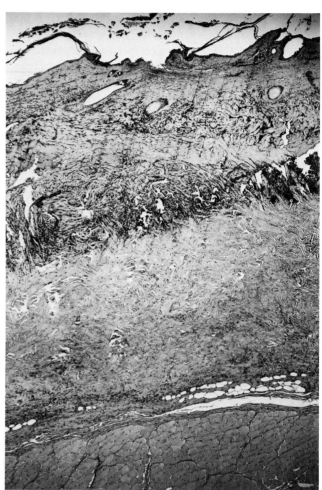

A

B

FIG 5. A: Photomicrograph showing the histological appearance of normal, healthy skin in the goat. The epidermal layer is seen at the top of the image. The dermal layers contain vessels and hair shafts. Hematoxylin and eosin; original magnification ×10. (From ref. 59, with permission.) **B:** Photomicrograph showing the histological appearance of the skin allograft 2 weeks after transplantation. A band of dark staining inflammatory cells (arrows) demarcates the edge of the graft. At 4 weeks, the skin graft is typically rejected due to the ensuing traditional immune response. The epidermal layer is seen toward the top of the image. Hematoxylin and eosin; original magnification ×10. (From ref. 59, with permission.)

transplanted allografts was then followed over time (Figs. 2–4).

In the 4-week interval after transplantation, the donor DNA dropped to 0% in fresh patellar tendon and fresh ACL allografts. At 2 weeks, donor DNA was still present in both types of allograft but was markedly reduced, whereas host DNA became apparent (Fig. 3). At 4 weeks, no donor DNA was demonstrated in the transplanted ligament allografts; however, host DNA in the graft was readily identified (Fig. 4), and the content of host DNA in the transplanted allografts approached that in the contralateral host ACL.

The histological appearance of the skin grafts 4 weeks after transplantation was that of normal rejection (Figs. 5A,B). There was no indication of a rapid rejection reaction that would suggest the presence of a preformed antibody to the donor tissue.

REMODELING IN ACL ALLOGRAFTS

Transmission electron microscopy has shown that the collagen present in tendons and ligaments has a tissue-specific ratio of small- and large-diameter fibrils. After transplantation and during incorporation of the allografts used to reconstruct the ACL, the collagen fibril profile is altered to primarily small-diameter (500-angstrom) collagen fibrils. Allografts, both patellar tendon and ACL, used to reconstruct the ACL have shown replacement with small-diameter collagen fibrils. The grafts demonstrate less tensile strength than their time zero values at transplantation. To evaluate some of the variables that might contribute to these changes in an allograft, Jackson et al. studied the ACL in the goat after devascularization and killing of the fibroblasts by an *in situ* freeze-thaw technique (55). It was the authors' premise that this model represented the ideal ACL replacement using a collagen graft. They reported a dramatic increase in small-diameter collagen fibrils within 6 months in the native ACL. Changes were similar to the autogenous grafts and allografts of the ACL and patellar tendons that demonstrated this alteration in the collagen-fibril pattern in the goat model at 6 months. The replacement cells in the devitalized and devascularized ACLs, as well as the allografts of the ACL and the patellar ligaments, were presumed to be responsible for the increase in small-diameter collagen fibrils. There is no evidence that the collagen fibril pattern of the ACL is ever reestablished over time using any allograft or autograft.

Replacing an ACL with living fibroblasts that would continue the production and maintenance of the larger sized collagen fibrils remains a challenge. It is not clear what accounts for the death of the transplanted fibroblasts in these allografts. This occurs after the graft is placed in an intraarticular environment. In addition to the question of cell survival, Jackson et al. have discussed other concerns to consider if one uses fresh or cryopreserved ACL allografts to replace an ACL in a human knee:

1. Sizing problems between the recipient and donor of the ACL allograft.

2. A decrease in the strength of allografts after implantation (23). Previously published ACL allograft results in the goat model after incorporation demonstrated a much weaker graft (25% to 50% of original maximum load to failure) (52,53). A tendon that starts inherently stronger than the ACL is presently preferred.

3. Present techniques do not allow for the precise positioning and tensioning of individual fibers of the ACL allograft. This fails to take advantage of the potential benefits of the complex orientation of the ACL collagen fibers.

BIOMECHANICAL CONSIDERATIONS IN ALLOGRAFTS USED FOR ACL RECONSTRUCTIONS

Evaluation of the normal properties of the ACL of humans has been limited by the scarcity of young cadaveric specimens for testing, as well as by the complexity of the ligament's anatomy and geometric alignment (121). Noyes and Grood (83) determined the linear stiffness and ultimate load of the femur–ACL–tibia complex (FATC) in young donors to be 182 N/mm and 1,730 N, respectively. These data for young specimens has served as a benchmark for the tensile properties of autografts and allografts (16,81,89). More recently, Woo et al. (121) measured higher strength and stiffness values for the FATC of young donors. The importance of studying the biomechanical properties of the human ACL in its normal anatomic orientation also was demonstrated by

Woo et al. (122). Other investigations have illustrated the effects of knee flexion angle, axial rotation, and the direction of tensile load application (1,36,46,124). Anatomic orientation resulted in higher values of linear stiffness, ultimate load, and energy absorbed at failure. In addition, younger specimens had the highest stiffness (242 N/mm), ultimate load (2,160 N), and energy absorbed at failure (11.6 N-m), as compared with those properties of the middle-aged and older specimens (122). These values for stiffness and ultimate load of the FATC were more than 30% higher than those reported by Noyes and Grood (83,122).

Noyes et al. (81) examined the various graft tissues used in knee ligament reconstruction. The central one third (14 mm) of the bone–patellar tendon–bone complex had an ultimate load at 2,900 N. This value was 168% of the value they obtained for the normal ACL (1,730 N). However, based on the finding by Woo et al. (122) that the ultimate load of the anatomically tested ACL was approximately 2,200 N, the ultimate load of the average patellar tendon autograft and allograft is closer to the normal ACL ultimate load. These findings must be considered in light of the inevitable decline in strength of graft materials after implantation. Ideally, the structural properties of the incorporated graft should equal, if not exceed, those of the normal ligament (19,81,119). In their review of ACL allograft biomechanics, France et al. (37) proposed that these tissues should provide stability at about two times the total strength at time zero of the normal ACL, because 50% of their initial strength is lost during healing.

Several investigators have compared the biomechanical properties of allografts and autografts. In dogs, Shino et al. (103) compared patellar tendon ACL autografts with fresh-frozen allografts, and also compared allografts of two different widths. For autografts 4 to 4.5 mm wide, the ultimate load was 150 N at 30 weeks, 30% of the opposite leg normal ACL control value of 505 N. Allografts 4 to 4.5 mm wide had an ultimate load of 127 N, 28% of control values, at the same time interval. In addition, patellar tendon allografts 8 to 9 mm wide had ultimate loads of 245 N (35% of controls) at 30 weeks and 227 N (36% of controls) at 52 weeks. In one study the ultimate load of the implanted canine patellar tendon graft was less than 15% of the normal femur–ACL–tibia complex 2 to 22 weeks after surgery (98). Nikolaou et al. (79) made comparisons using fresh-frozen bone–ACL–bone allografts in dogs. Their results are the most favorable comparisons reported in the literature, but their control values are much lower than that of other investigators.

Jackson et al. compared similar sized and shaped patellar tendon autografts and fresh-frozen allografts used for ACL reconstruction in the goat. At 6 months the strength of the autografts was 62% of normal control ACL strength and that of the allografts was 27% of the control measurement. The maximal load to failure at 6 months was significantly greater for autografts. The comparative weakness demonstrated in the allografts had no apparent effect on the animals' level of functioning. Their data suggested a slower period of maturation for the allograft tissue as compared with autografts (56,57). Long-term follow-up comparison studies are necessary to demonstrate if similar allografts ever approach autograft properties.

EFFECTS OF FREEZING ON ALLOGRAFTS USED FOR ACL RECONSTRUCTION

Many investigators have addressed concerns that freezing may compromise the structural properties of allografts. The ACLs of rhesus monkeys were fresh frozen to −80°C for 3 to 5 weeks, thawed, and compared with fresh ACLs stored at 4°C overnight in a study by Barad et al. (8). No differences of statistical significance were noted for any parameter tested, although ultimate load differences approached significance. Overall, the fresh tissue exhibited a slight trend toward being stronger and stiffer. Woo et al. (120) found little effect on the structural properties of the medial collateral ligament–bone complex or the mechanical properties of the ligament substance after specimens were fresh frozen at −20°C for 3 months. In a canine study, Nikolaou et al. (79) found that fresh freezing to −80°C for 2 to 12 weeks had no significant effect on allograft ACL tissue biomechanics as compared with autografts, both reaching 90% of control ultimate loads at 36 weeks.

Paulos et al. (89) examined the effects of preservation methods on material properties of the human patellar tendon, Achilles tendon, and fascia lata. They noted no significant difference between fresh-frozen and freeze-dried specimens in terms of ultimate stress, ultimate strain, or modulus, although a trend toward a slight decrease in ultimate stress was associated with freeze drying. Turner et al. (115) used the canine model to compare the structural properties of fresh-frozen bone–ACL–bone specimens stored at −70°C for 12 weeks with those freeze dried and sterilized with ethylene oxide. The opposite knee served as the control in each animal, and was tested fresh. The ultimate loads of the fresh-frozen and freeze-dried specimens were not significantly different from those of their fresh controls.

ALLOGRAFT REMODELING, REVASCULARIZATION, AND JOINT PATHOLOGY

Kleiner et al. (65,66) referred to the histological changes observed in rabbit patellar tendon autografts as "ligamentization." By this process, the grafts underwent apparent necrosis with central acellularity at 2 weeks and progressed to homogenous cellularity at 1 month. They suggested a rapid repopulation of the autograft with cells. Shino et al. demonstrated in fresh-frozen canine patellar tendon allografts a decreased cellularity after implantation (103). By 3 weeks, a vascular synovial membrane enveloped the graft, and spindle-shaped mesenchymal cells had reached the grafts' centers. Six-week specimens exhibited central acellularity with collagen bundle fragmentation and necrosis. At 15 weeks, acellularity persisted, although some invasion by viable cells was observed. The central area was normal in appearance by 30 weeks, having normal spindle-shaped nuclei and collagen orientation, but peripheral hypercellularity and disorganization. By 1 year, the allografts histologically resembled the normal ACL. Similar findings were noted by other investigators (7,28).

In comparing autograft and allograft bone–ACL–bone ACL reconstructions in dogs, Nikolaou et al. (79) described an initial massive and disorganized vascular and cellular proliferation, with subsequent alignment to the direction of force transmission and tissue deformation. Cellularity decreased with maturity, and a normal appearance was evident by 16 weeks in autografts and by 24 weeks in allografts.

Jackson et al. (56,57) examined the differences between bone–patellar tendon–bone autografts and fresh-frozen allografts after both 6 weeks and 6 months in the goat. Histologically, allografts showed a greater vascular and inflammatory response at 6 weeks, with a cellular sheath covering the graft. At 6 months, these grafts had a similar appearance, with good cellular alignment at the ligament–bone interface, bone plug incorporation, and collagen crimp orientation in both graft types. Allograft specimens in comparison with a similar autograft had a smaller cross-sectional area, more of the original large-diameter collagen fibrils, fewer small-diameter collagen fibrils, and a persistent inflammatory response at 6 months. In addition, the maximal load to failure at 6 months was significantly greater for autografts. Both graft types had greater anterior-posterior excursion than did controls, but the measurements for allografts were significantly greater than those for autografts at 6 months. Overall, the allografts appeared to be incorporated more slowly than the autografts.

Shino et al. (101,102) found a thick synovial sheath and spindle-shaped nuclei in the midsubstance at 3 months in fresh-frozen allografts implanted in humans. A regular collagen bundle alignment was seen at 6 months, although hypercellularity persisted. At 1 year, the synovial thickness had decreased to a one-cell layer, as in the normal ACL, but midsubstance hypercellularity was unchanged. A total of 18 to 55 months was required for the development of a normal-appearing graft with well-arranged collagen bundles, spindle-shaped nuclei, and normal cellularity.

In an investigation of graft revascularization, Shino et

al. (102) evaluated the surface blood flow of human fresh-frozen ACL allografts, observing a normal level of flow in grafts tested 12 to 89 months postoperatively. However, flow was significantly higher at 6 months. This result was thought to be consistent with the early hypercellularity of the grafts. Human graft revascularization was considered complete by 6 months, whereas this process required 6 weeks in their dog study (103). The blood flow results were consistent with the investigators' earlier observation of allograft morphologic and histologic stability at 18 months (101). Gross inspection via second-look arthroscopy at 12 to 30 months showed a normal synovial membrane and normal vascularity (104).

Arnoczky et al. (6) observed vascular buds within the allograft substance by 3 months in dogs. These arose from the infrapatellar fat pad and posterior synovial tissue and seemed to accompany cellular repopulation. Both responses were increased at 4 months and began to decrease at 5 months. The allografts resembled normal tissue at 1 year and closely approximated autograft results. The investigators suggested that the lag between transplantation and revascularization with cellular repopulation may contribute to the alteration of material properties of the graft (7). Nikolaou et al. (79) found nearly normal autograft revascularization in dogs from 16 weeks onward, whereas allografts required 24 weeks to reach normal vascularity. Likewise, autografts appeared normal histologically at 16 weeks, and allografts again required 24 weeks to normalize.

OUTCOME

The most important assessment of the success or failure of an allograft ACL reconstruction for both the physician and the patient is the postoperative clinical evaluation. Noyes and Barber (80) used both subjective and objective methods to evaluate the results of ACL allografts alone and combined with extraarticular augmentation. Both procedures succeeded in decreasing functional limitations and symptoms and in improving the patient's overall activity level. No significant difference was noted in the amount of anterior-posterior displacement, in symptoms of pain, swelling, and partial or full giving way, or in functional limitations. The ability to regain full knee extension was hindered by augmentation, although not significantly. Both groups had insignificant increases in patellofemoral crepitus. Noyes and Barber felt that the additional surgery of augmentation posed a risk for increased morbidity without certain benefit.

Shino et al. (100) reported good to excellent results in 94% of his patients at an average of 57 months after they received fresh-frozen allografts to reconstruct their ACLs. Results were evaluated by questionnaire, physical examination, and radiographs. Sixty-five percent of these patients could function normally without a brace, and 41% returned to competitive sports. Minimal joint effusions and quadriceps atrophy were noted, and only 2 of 81 patients failed to regain full knee extension. Lachman and pivot shift test findings were negative in 73 and 74 of 81 patients, respectively. No unsatisfactory measurements of joint laxity were obtained, and no statistically significant loss in muscle strength was noted by Cybex isokinetic analysis.

In their clinical comparison of fresh-frozen and freeze-dried patellar tendon allografts, Indelicato et al. (51) examined patients 2 to 3 years after surgery. Overall, subjective and objective results had improved markedly over their preoperative status in both groups, with fresh-frozen graft recipients doing slightly better. Of the 21 variables tested, only 3 showed statistically significant differences between groups. Freeze-dried graft recipients had less satisfactory results in terms of positive pivot shift tests, lower Lysholm knee instability scores, and more reports of giving way. Combined scores showed good to excellent results in 81% of patients with fresh-frozen allografts and in 64% of those with freeze-dried transplants.

Olson et al. (86) conducted a 4-year follow-up study of athletes who had undergone fresh-frozen allograft ACL reconstruction. They found results to be favorable with no problems such as significant effusions, intraarticular reactions, graft failures, or tunnel resorption seen previously with secondarily sterilized and freeze-dried allografts. Preoperatively, 86% of patients had reported a drop in their activity level after ACL disruption. Postoperatively, 73% returned to their former activity level. Of 33 patients evaluated, 73% could run competitively, but limitations during running were described by 54% and during jumping by 41%. Fifty-nine percent of the patients had pain and 32% had swelling after rigorous activity. In addition, 26% reported partial giving way postoperatively, whereas 9% noted full giving way. Patients averaged 87.3 on a 100-point knee rating scale emphasizing ACL function. Other findings included trace effusions in 18%, moderate effusions in 9%, and significantly decreased vertical and horizontal leaps in 32% and 27% of patients, respectively. KT-1000 testing showed a side-to-side difference in laxity of at least 3 mm in 32% of knees. Olsen et al. felt that although the laxity was somewhat greater than in normal knees, fresh-frozen allograft ACL reconstruction provided an acceptable level of function.

SUMMARY

Experience thus far suggests that allografts are an alternative graft choice for ACL reconstructive surgery. Although the time zero mechanical and structural properties of allografts used to reconstruct the ACL are similar to autografts in animal studies, they do not equal those of comparable autografts or the normal ACL after incorporation. The long-term result of ACL allografts in remodeling, revascularization, and incorporation remains to be clarified in the human. The early clinical results have been encouraging. In light of these findings, allograft ACL reconstruction should continue to be an area of great interest and concentration in orthopedic research. Careful screening of donors, as well as continued investigation into methods of tissue sterilization that prevent the possibility of disease transmission and have minimal impact on the graft itself, is needed. Allograft tissue can be used safely and effectively to reconstruct the ACL in carefully selected patients.

REFERENCES

1. Alm A, Ekstrom H, Stromberg B. (1974): Tensile strength of the anterior cruciate ligament in the dog. *Acta Chir Scand* 445:15–23.
2. American Association of Tissue Banks. (1987): *Standards for surgical bone banking.* Arlington, VA: American Association of Tissue Banks.
3. American Association of Tissue Banks. (1989): In: Mowe J, ed. *Standards for tissue banking.* McLean, VA: American Association of Tissue Banks.
4. American Association of Tissue Banks. (1991): *Technical manual musculoskeletal tissues.* Appendix 3. McLean, VA: American Association of Tissue Banks, p. M-40.
5. Andreeff L, Denioff G, Metscharski S. (1967): A comparative experimental study on transplantation of autogenous and homogenous tendon tissue. *Acta Orthop Scand* 38:35.
6. Arnoczky S, Tarvin G, Marshall J. (1982): Anterior cruciate ligament replacement using patellar tendon. An evaluation of graft revascularization in the dog. *J Bone Joint Surg* 64A:217–224.
7. Arnoczky S, Warren R, Ashlock M. (1986): Replacement of the anterior cruciate ligament using a patellar tendon allograft. An experimental study. *J Bone Joint Surg* 68A:376–385.
8. Barad S, Cabaud H, Rodrigo J. (1982): Effects of storage at −80°C as compared to 4°C on the strength of rhesus monkey anterior cruciate ligaments. *Trans Orthop Res Soc* 7:378.
9. Bonamo J, Krinick R, Sporn A. (1984): Rupture of the patellar ligament after use of its central third for anterior cruciate reconstruction. A report of two cases. *J Bone Joint Surg* 66A:1294–1297.
10. Bond WW, Favero MS, Peterson NJ, Ebert JW. (1983): Inactivation of hepatitis B virus by intermediate to high level disinfectant chemical. *J Clin Microbiol* 18:535–538.
11. Bottenfield S. (1991): HIV transmission incident. *Am Assoc Tissue Banks Newsletter* 14:1–2.
12. Bright R, Friedlaender G, Snell K. (1977): Tissue banking: the United States Navy Tissue Bank. *Milit Med* 142:503.
13. Bright R, Green W. (1981): Freeze-dried fascia lata allografts: a review of 47 cases. *J Pediatr Orthop* 1:13.
14. Buck B, Malinin T, Brown M. (1989): Bone transplantation and human immunodeficiency virus. An estimate of risk of acquired immunodeficiency syndrome (AIDS). *Clin Orthop* 240:129–136.
15. Buck B, Resnick L, Shah S, Malinin T. (1990): Human immunodeficiency virus cultured from bone. Implications for transplantation. *Clin Orthop* 251:249–253.
16. Butler D, Hulse D, Kay M, et al. (1983): Biomechanics of cranial cruciate ligament reconstruction in the dog. II. Mechanical properties. *Vet Surg* 12:113–118.
17. Butler D, Noyes F, Walz K, Gibbons M. (1987): Biomechanics of human knee ligament allograft treatment. *Trans Orthop Res Soc* 12:128.
18. Butler D, Oster D, Feder S, Grood E, Noyes F. (1991): Effects of gamma irradiation on the biomechanics of patellar tendon allografts of the ACL in the goat. *Trans Orthop Res Soc* 16:205.
19. Cabaud H, Feagin J, Rodkey W. (1980): Acute anterior cruciate ligament injury and augmented repair. Experimental studies. *Am J Sports Med* 8:395–401.
20. Cameron R, Conrad R, Sell K, Latham W. (1971): Freeze-dried composite tendon allografts: an experimental study. *Plast Reconstr Surg* 47:39–46.
21. Campbell W. (1939): Reconstruction of the knee ligaments. *Am J Surg* 43:473–480.
22. Centers for Disease Control. (1988): Transmission of HIV through bone transplantation: case report and public health recommendations. *Morbid Mortal Weekly Report* 37:597–599.
23. Christensen E, Kristensen H, Sehestad K. (1982): Radiation sterilization. In: Russel A, Huge W, Aycliffe G, eds. *Principles and practices of disinfection. Preservation and sterilization.* Oxford, England: Blackwell Scientific, pp. 513–533.
24. Clancy W. (1985): Advances in biologic substitution for cruciate deficiency. In: Finerman G, ed. *AAOS symposium on sports medicine: the knee.* St. Louis, MO: CV Mosby, pp. 222–229.
25. Clancy W, Narechania R, Rosenberg T, Gmeiner J, Wisnefske D, Lange T. (1981): Anterior and posterior cruciate ligament reconstruction in rhesus monkeys. A histological, microangiographic, and biomechanical analysis. *J Bone Joint Surg* 63A:1270–1284.
26. Clancy W, Nelson D, Reider B, Narechania R. (1982): Anterior cruciate ligament reconstruction using one-third of the patellar ligament, augmented by extra-articular tendon transfers. *J Bone Joint Surg* 64A:352–359.
27. Conway B, Tomford WW, Hirsch MS, Schooley RT, Mankin HJ. (1990): Effects of gamma irradiation on HIV-1 in a bone allograft model. *Trans Orthop Res Soc* 15:225.
28. Curtis R, DeLee J, Drez D. (1985): Reconstruction of the anterior cruciate ligament with freeze dried fascia lata allografts in dogs. A preliminary report. *Am J Sports Med* 13:408–414.
29. Daluga D, Johnson C, Bach B. (1990): Primary bone grafting following graft procurement for anterior cruciate ligament insufficiency. *Arthroscopy* 6:205–208.
30. Daniel D, Woodward E, Losse G, Stone M. (1988): The Marshal/MacIntosh anterior cruciate ligament reconstruction with the Kennedy ligament augmentation device: report of the United States clinical trials. In: Friedman M, Ferkel R, eds. *Prosthetic ligament reconstruction of the knee.* Philadelphia: WB Saunders, pp. 71–78.
31. DeLee J, Craviotto D. (1991): Rupture of the quadriceps tendon after a central third patellar tendon anterior cruciate ligament reconstruction. *Am J Sports Med* 19:415–416.
32. Drez D. (1987): Allograft reconstruction of the anterior cruciate ligament. *Orthop Today* 7:1–7.
33. DuToit G. (1967): Knee joint cruciate ligament substitution, the Lindemann (Heidelbert) operation. *S Afr J Surg* 5:25–30.
34. Eastland T. (1991): Infectious disease transmission through tissue transplantation: reducing the risk through donor selection. *J Transplant Coordination* 1:23–30.
35. Fideler B, Vangsness T, Moore T, Mekellop H, Rasheed S. The human bone–patellar tendon–bone allograft for anterior cruciate ligament reconstruction (submitted for publication).
36. Figgie H, Bahniuk E, Heiple K, Davy D. (1986): The effects of tibial femoral angle on the failure mechanics of the canine anterior cruciate ligament. *J Biomech* 19:89–91.
37. France E, Paulos L, Rosenberg T, Harner C. (1988): The biomechanics of anterior cruciate allografts. In: Friedman M, Ferkel R, eds. *Prosthetic ligament reconstruction of the knee.* Philadelphia: WB Saunders, pp. 180–185.
38. Franke K. (1976): Clinical experience in 130 cruciate ligament reconstructions. *Orthop Clin North Am* 7:191–193.
39. Friedlaender G, Strong D, Sells K. (1976): Studies on the antigenicity of bone. I. Freeze-dried and deep-frozen bone allografts in rabbits. *J Bone Joint Surg* 58A:854–858.
40. Gibbons M, Butler D, Grood E, Bylski-Austrow D, Levy M, Noyes F. (1991): Effects of gamma irradiation on the initial mechanical and material properties of goat bone-patellar tendon-bone allografts. *J Orthop Res* 9:209–218.
41. Gibbons M, Butler D, Grood E, Chun K, Noyes F, Bukovec D. (1989): Dose-dependent effects of gamma irradiation on the material properties of frozen bone-patellar tendon-bone allografts. *Trans Orthop Res Soc* 14:513.

42. Girgis F, Marshall J, Al-Monajem A. (1975): The cruciate ligaments of the knee joint. Anatomical, functional, and experimental analysis. *Clin Orthop* 106:216–231.

43. Gresham R. (1964): Freeze-drying of human tissue for clinical use. *Cryobiology* 1:150.

44. Gresham W, Smith D, McGuire M. (1955): The use of frozen stored tendons for grafting: an experimental study. *J Bone Joint Surg* 37A:624.

45. Grood E, Butler D, Noyes F. (1985): Models of ligament repairs and grafts. In: Finerman G, ed. *AAOS symposium on sports medicine: the knee.* St. Louis, MO: CV Mosby, pp. 169–181.

46. Gupta B, Subramanian K, Brinker W, Gupta A. (1971): Tensile strength of canine cranial cruciate ligaments. *Am J Vet Res* 32:183–190.

47. Haut R, Powlison A. (1989): Order of irradiation and lyophilization on the strength of patellar tendon allografts. *Trans Orthop Res Soc* 14:514.

48. Hey Groves E. (1917): Operation for the repair of the crucial ligaments. *Lancet* 2:674–675.

49. Hiemstra H, Tersmette M, Vos A, Over J, van Berkel M, de Bree H. (1991): Inactivation of human immunodeficiency virus by gamma radiation and its effect on plasma and coagulation factors. *Transfusion* 31:32–39.

50. Horowitz M, Friedlaender G. (1991): The immune response to bone grafts. In: Friedlaender G, Goldberg V, eds. *Bone and cartilage allografts: biology and clinical applications.* Park Ridge, IL: American Academy of Orthopaedic Surgery, pp. 85–101.

51. Indelicato P, Bittar E, Prevot T, Woods G, Branch T, Huegel M. (1990): Clinical comparison of freeze-dried and fresh frozen patellar tendon allografts for anterior cruciate ligament reconstruction of the knee. *Am J Sports Med* 18:335–342.

52. Jackson DW. (1992): Use of allografts for anterior cruciate ligament reconstruction. *Am Acad Orthop Surgeons Bull* 40:10–11.

53. Jackson DW, Grood ES, Arnoczky SP, Butler D, Simon TM. (1987): Cruciate reconstruction using freeze dried anterior cruciate ligament allograft and a ligament augmentation device (LAD). *Am J Sports Med* 15:528–538.

54. Jackson DW, Grood ES, Arnoczky SP, Butler D, Simon TM. (1987): Freeze dried anterior cruciate ligament allografts. Preliminary studies in a goat model. *Am J Sports Med* 15:295–313.

55. Jackson DW, Grood ES, Cohn BT, Arnoczky SP, Simon TM, Cummings JF. (1991): The effects of in situ freezing on the anterior cruciate ligament: an experimental study in goats. *J Bone Joint Surg* 73A:201–213.

56. Jackson DW, Grood EW, Goldstein J, et al. (1993): A comparison of patellar tendon autograft and allograft used for anterior cruciate ligament reconstruction in the goat model *Am J Sports Med* 21:176–185.

57. Jackson DW, Grood ES, Goldstein J, Rosen MA, Kurzweil PR, Simon TM. (1991): Anterior cruciate ligament reconstruction using patella tendon autograft and allograft—an experimental study in goats. *Trans Orthop Res Soc* 16:208.

58. Jackson DW, Grood ES, Wilcox P, Butler D, Simon TM, Holden J. (1988): The effects of processing techniques on the mechanical properties of bone–anterior cruciate ligament–bone allografts. *Am J Sports Med* 16:101–105.

59. Jackson DW, Simon TM, Kurzweil PR, Rosen MA. (1992): Survival of cells after intraarticular transplantation of fresh allografts of the patellar and anterior cruciate ligaments. DNA probe analysis in a goat model. *J Bone Joint Surgery* 74A:112–118.

60. Jackson DW, Windler GE, Simon TM. (1990): Intraarticular reactions associated with the use of freeze-dried, ethylene oxide sterilized bone–patellar tendon–bone allografts in the reconstruction of the anterior cruciate ligament. *Am J Sports Med* 18:1–11.

61. Jones K. (1963): Reconstruction of the anterior cruciate ligament. A technique using the central one-third of the patellar ligament. *J Bone Joint Surg* 45A:925–932.

62. Jones K. (1970): Reconstruction of the anterior cruciate ligament using the central one-third of the patellar ligament. A follow-up report. *J Bone Joint Surg* 52A:1302–1308.

63. Kennedy J, Weinberg H, Wilson A. (1974): The anatomy and function of the anterior cruciate ligament as described by clinical and morphologic studies. *J Bone Joint Surg* 56A:223–235.

64. Kirkpatrick J, Glisson R, Seaber A, Bassett MF. (1991): Biomechanical, histological, and microvascular properties of cryopreserved ACL allografts 9 months post-transplantation. *Trans Orthop Res Soc* 16:183.

65. Kleiner J, Amiel D, Harwood F, Akeson W. (1989): Early histologic, metabolic, and vascular assessment of anterior cruciate ligament autografts. *J Orthop Res* 7:235–242.

66. Kleiner J, Amiel D, Roux R, Akeson W. (1986): Origin of replacement cells for the anterior cruciate ligament autograft. *J Orthop Res* 4:466–474.

67. Kobayashi H, Tsuzuki M, Koshimizu K, et al. (1984): Susceptibility of hepatitis B to disinfectants and heat. *J Clin Microbiol* 20:214–216.

68. Kosek JC, Iben AB, Shumway ME, Angell WE. (1969): Morphology of fresh heart valve homografts. *Surgery* 66:269–274.

69. Lanzer W, Jackson D, Simon T, Ferguson M. (1988): Immune response in allograft reconstruction of the anterior cruciate ligament. *Trans Orthop Res Soc* 13:209.

70. Lindstrom N. (1959): Cruciate ligament plastics with meniscus. *Acta Orthop Scand* 29:150–151.

71. Macey H. (1939): A new operative procedure for repair of ruptured cruciate ligaments of the knee joint. *J Surg Gynecol Obstet* 69:108–109.

72. Martin L. (1985): Disinfection and inactivation of the human T lymphadenopathy associated virus. *J Infect Dis* 152:400.

73. McCarroll J. (1983): Fracture of the patella during a golfswing following reconstruction of the anterior cruciate ligament. A case report. *Am J Sports Med* 11:26–27.

74. Minami A, Ishii S, Ogino T, Oikawa T, Kobayashi H. (1982): Effect of the immunological antigenicity of the allogeneic tendons on tendon grafting. *Hand* 14:111–119.

75. Mohri H, Reichenbach DD, Barnes RW, Merendino KA. (1967): A biologic study of the homologous aortic valve in dogs. *J Thoracic Cardiovasc Surg* 54:622–629.

76. Mohri H, Reichenbach DD, Barnes RW, Merendino KA. (1968): Homologous aortic valve transplantation. Alterations in viable and nonviable valves. *J Thoracic Cardiovasc Surg* 56:767–774.

77. Muscolo D, Kawai S, Ray R. (1976): Cellular and humoral immune response analysis of bone-allografted rats. *J Bone Joint Surg* 58A:826–832.

78. Neviaser S, Neviaser R, Neviaser T. (1978): The repair of chronic massive ruptures of the rotator cuff of the shoulder by use of a freeze-dried rotator cuff. *J Bone Joint Surg* 60A:681–684.

79. Nikolaou P, Seaber A, Glisson R, Ribbeck B, Bassett F. (1986): Anterior cruciate ligament allograft transplantation. Long-term function, histology, revascularization, and operative technique. *Am J Sports Med* 14:348–360.

80. Noyes F, Barber S. (1991): The effect of an extra-articular procedure on allograft reconstructions for chronic ruptures of the anterior cruciate ligament. *J Bone Joint Surg* 73A:882–892.

81. Noyes F, Butler D, Grood E, Zemicke R, Hefzy M. (1984): Biomechanical analysis of human ligament grafts used in knee-ligament repairs and reconstructions. *J Bone Joint Surg* 66A:344–352.

82. Noyes F, Butler D, Paulos L, Grood E. (1983): Intra-articular cruciate reconstruction. I: Perspectives on graft strength, vascularization, and immediate motion after replacement. *Clin Orthop* 172:71–77.

83. Noyes F, Grood E. (1976): The strength of the anterior cruciate ligament in humans and rhesus monkeys. *J Bone Joint Surg* 58A:1074–1082.

84. O'Brien MF, Staffor G, Gardner M, Pohlner P, et al. (1987): The viable cryopreserved allograft aortic valve. *J Cardiac Surg* 2(Suppl):153–167.

85. O'Donoghue D. (1950): Surgical treatment of fresh injuries to the major ligaments of the knee. *J Bone Joint Surg* 32A:721–738.

86. Olson E, Harner C, Fu F, Irrgang J, Maday M. (1992): The use of fresh frozen allograft tissue in knee ligament reconstruction: indications, results, techniques and controversies (scientific exhibit). In: *American Academy of Orthopaedic Surgeons 59th Annual Meeting.* Washington, DC: American Academy of Orthopaedic Surgeons, p. 315.

87. Patterson F, Trickey E. (1986): Anterior cruciate ligament reconstruction using part of the patellar tendon as a free graft. *J Bone Joint Surg* 68B:453–457.

88. Paulos L, Cherf J, Rosenberg T, Beck C. (1991): Anterior cruciate ligament reconstruction with autografts. *Clin Sports Med* 10:469–485.

89. Paulos L, France E, Rosenberg T, et al. (1987): Comparative material properties of allograft tissues for ligament replacement: effects of type, age, sterilization and preservation. *Trans Orthop Res Soc* 12:129.

90. Paulos L, Rosenberg T, Drawbert J, Manning J, Abbott P. (1987): Infrapatellar contraction syndrome. An unrecognized cause of knee stiffness with patella entrapment and patella infera. *Am J Sports Med* 15:331–341.

91. Peacock E, Petty J. (1960): Antigenicity of tendon. *J Surg Gynecol Obstet* 110:187–192.

92. Peacock EJ, Madden J. (1967): Human composite flexor tendon allografts. *Ann. Surg* 166:624–629.

93. Pinkowski J, Reiman P, Chen S. (1989): Human lymphocyte reaction to freeze-dried allograft and xenograft ligamentous tissue. *Am J Sports Med* 17:595–600.

94. Prolo D, Pedrotti M, White D. (1980): Ethylene oxide sterilization of bone, dura mater, and fascia lata for human transplantation. *Neurosurgery* 6:529.

95. Resnik L, Veren K, Salahuddin SZ, Tondreau S, Markham PD. (1986): Stability and inactivation of HTLV-III/LAV under clinical and laboratory environments. *JAMA* 255:1887–1891.

96. Roberts T, Drez D Jr., Banta MC. (1989): Complications of anterior cruciate ligament reconstruction. In: Sprague N, ed. *Complications in arthroscopy.* New York: Raven Press, pp. 169–177.

97. Rodrigo J, Jackson D, Simon T, Muto K. (1988): The immune response to freeze dried bone–tendon–bone ACL allografts in humans. *Trans Orthop Res Soc* 13:105.

98. Ryan J, Drompp B. (1966): Evaluation of tensile strength of reconstruction of the anterior cruciate ligament using patellar tendon in dogs: a preliminary report. *South Med J* 59:129–134.

99. Shelbourne K, Wilckens J, Mollabashy A, DeCarlo M. (1991): Arthrofibrosis in acute anterior cruciate ligament reconstruction. The effect of timing of reconstruction and rehabilitation. *Am J Sports Med* 19:332–336.

100. Shino K, Inoue M, Horibe S, Harnada M, Ono K. (1990): Reconstruction of the anterior cruciate ligament using allogenic tendon. Long-term followup. *J Sports Med* 18:457–465.

101. Shino K, Inoue M, Horibe S, Nagano J, Ono K. (1988): Maturation of allograft tendons transplanted into the knee. An arthroscopic and histologic study. *J Bone Joint Surg* 70B:556–560.

102. Shino K, Inoue M, Horibe S, Nakata K, Maeda A, Ono K. (1991): Surface blood flow and histology of human anterior cruciate ligament allografts. *Arthroscopy* 7:171–176.

103. Shino K, Kawasaki T, Hirose H, Gotoh I, Inoue M, Ono K. (1984): Replacement of the anterior cruciate ligament by an allogenic tendon graft. An experimental study in the dog. *J Bone Joint Surg* 66B:672–681.

104. Shino K, Kimura T, Hirose H, Inoue M, Ono K. (1986): Reconstruction of the anterior cruciate ligament by allogenic tendon graft. An operation for chronic ligamentous insufficiency. *J Bone Joint Surg* 68B:739–746.

105. Simonds RJ, Holmberg SD, Hurwitz R, et al. (1992): Transmission of human immunodeficiency virus type 1 from a seronegative organ and tissue donor. *N Engl J Med* 326:726–732.

106. Sommer N. (1973): *The effects of ionizing radiation on fungi.* Vienna: International Atomic Energy Agency, Technical Report Series, No. 149.

107. Spire B, Barre-Sinoussi F, Dormont D, Montagnier L, Chermann J. (1985): Inactivation of lymphadenopathy-associated virus by heat, gamma rays, and ultraviolet light. *Lancet* 1:(8422) January 26:188–189.

108. Stevenson S. (1987): The immune response to osteochondral allografts in dogs. *J Bone Joint Surg* 69A:573.

109. Sullivan R, Fassolitis A, Larkin E, Read R Jr., Peeler J. (1971): Inactivation of thirty viruses by gamma radiation. *Appl Microbiol* 22:61–65.

110. Thorson E, Rodrigo J, Vasseur P, Sharkey N, Heitter D. (1987): Comparison of frozen allograft versus fresh autogenous anterior cruciate ligament replacement in the dog. *Trans Orthop Res Soc* 12:65.

111. Tomford W, (1991): Prepared statement to FDA. Human organ and tissue transplantation. Public Hearing Docket No. 91N-0318.

112. Trentham D, Dynesius R, Rocklin R, David J. (1978): Cellular sensitivity to collagen in rheumatoid arthritis. *N Engl J Med* 299:327–332.

113. Trentham D, Townes A, Kang A. (1977): Autoimmunity to type II collagen: an experimental model of arthritis. *J Exp Med* 146:857–868.

114. Trentham D, Townes A, Kang A, David J. (1978): Humoral and cellular sensitivity to collagen in type II collagen-induced arthritis in rats. *J Clin Invest* 61:89–96.

115. Turner W, Vasseur P, Gorek J, Rodrigo J, Wedell J. (1988): An *in vitro* study of the structural properties of deep-frozen versus freeze-dried, ethylene oxide sterilized canine anterior cruciate ligament bone–ligament–bone preparations. *Clin Orthop* 230: 251–256.

116. Van Winkle W Jr., Borick P, Fogarty M. (1967): Destruction of radiation resistant microorganisms on surgical sutures by 60Co irradiation under manufacturing conditions. In: *Symposium on radiosterilization of medical products.* Budapest: International Atomic Energy Agency, pp. 169–180.

117. Vasseur P, Rodrigo J, Stevenson S, Clark G, Sharkey N. (1987): Replacement of the anterior cruciate ligament with a bone–ligament–bone anterior cruciate ligament allograft in dogs. *Clin Orthop* 219:268–277.

118. Webster D, Werner F. (1983): Freeze-dried flexor tendons in anterior cruciate ligament reconstruction. *Clin Orthop* 181:238–243.

119. Webster D, Werner F. (1983): Mechanical and functional properties of implanted freeze-dried flexor tendons. *Clin Orthop* 180:301–309.

120. Woo S, Orlando C, Camp J, Akeson W. (1986): Effects of postmortem storage by freezing on ligament tensile behavior. *J Biomech* 19:399–404.

121. Woo SL-Y, Buckwalter J. (1991): Ligament and tendon autografts and allografts. In: Friedlaender G, Goldberg V, eds. *Bone and cartilage allografts: biology and clinical applications.* Park Ridge, IL: American Academy of Orthopaedic Surgeons, pp. 103–121.

122. Woo SL-Y, Hollis J, Adams D, Lyon R, Takai S. (1991): Tensile properties of the human femur–anterior cruciate ligament–tibia complex. The effects of specimen age and orientation. *Am J Sports Med* 19:217–225.

123. Woo S-Y, Hollis J, Lyon R, Lin H, Marcin J, Horibe S. (1987): On the structural properties of the human anterior cruciate ligament–bone complex from young donors. In: *Proceedings on the biomechanics of human knee ligaments.* Ulm, Germany: University of Ulm, p. 23.

124. Woo S-Y, Hollis J, Roux R, Gomez M, Inoue M, Kleiner J, Akeson W. (1987): Effects of knee flexion on the structural properties of the rabbit femur anterior cruciate ligament–tibia complex (FATC). *J Biomech* 20:557–563.

125. Wright K, Trump J. (1969): Co-operative studies in the use of ionizing radiation for sterilization and preservation of biologic tissues. Twenty years' experience. In: *Panel on radiation sterilization of biologic tissues for transplantation.* Budapest: International Atomic Energy Agency, pp. 107–118.

*The Anterior Cruciate Ligament: Current and
Future Concepts,* edited by D.W. Jackson, et al.
Raven Press, Ltd., New York © 1993.

CHAPTER 29

Synthetic Augmentation

Peter J. Fowler

Synthetic augmentation of the biological tissue used in an anterior cruciate ligament (ACL) reconstruction was proposed to address the posttransplantation decrease in strength of the biological graft. This dramatic weakness occurs 2 weeks to 4 months after transplantation, when the biological tissue is most vulnerable to stretching and rupturing. The augmentation device used in an ACL reconstruction should have distinctive characteristics. These may be grouped into three specific areas: (a) load sharing with the biologic graft, (b) structural and material characteristics that contribute to the composite ACL graft, and (c) biocompatibility and facilitation of the initial fixation of the composite graft. Clinical experience to date with synthetic augmentation has not involved as many devices as with prosthetic ligaments. The prosthetic ligament experience to date in comparison with augmentation devices has included increased numbers of materials and centers contributing to the data available.

Much of the experimental work related to synthetic augmentation has been based on the use of the Kennedy ligament augmentation device (LAD). This chapter will be confined primarily to this experience with synthetic augmentation.

Some of initial work with synthetic augmentation includes the experimental work performed in animals by Cabaud et al. using a Dexon graft, a braid of polyglycolic acid (2). In theory, the Dexon would degrade after providing immediate protection and allow a gradual transfer of stress to the autogenous tissue. However, full resorption of the material occurred at 5 weeks. This was too short a period for the stent to be of value in the human knee. Strum and Larson have reported on the use of a polylactic acid (PLA)-coated carbon fiber as augmentation of both the central third of the patellar tendon

and a double-loop semitendinosus tendon (7). A short-term review of this group of 10 patients offered no demonstrable benefits.

As mentioned, the most extensive experience to date with synthetic augmentation, both clinical and in the laboratory, has been with the Kennedy LAD, a flat braid of polypropylene yarn. Roth et al. reviewed the initial 43 patients of 143 LAD-augmented reconstructions performed by Kennedy using the Marshall-MacIntosh technique at a mean follow-up of 4 years (5). These were compared with 45 patients at the same follow-up period who had undergone the same procedure with no augmentation. Included in the evaluation were subjective assessment, clinical examination, anterior laxity measurement with the KT-1000 arthrometer, Cybex strength testing, and functional analysis by a one-legged hop test. On subjective evaluation, clinical examination and radiographic analysis patients in the augmented group had significantly better results. In addition, these patients demonstrated a trend toward better results in objective laxity and functional testing. A later subjective follow-up at 7.5 years showed no fall-off in results (3).

AUGMENTATION CONCEPT AND LOAD SHARING

The principle of load sharing is fundamental to the concept of synthetic augmentation, and load distribution between the device and the biological tissue is dependent on the relative stiffness of each. Van Kampen et al. (8) hypothesized a mathematical model demonstrating that as graft stiffness decreases, the load in the graft decreases and the load in the augmentation device increases; as graft stiffness increases, the load in the graft increases and the load in the device decreases. The model is summarized as follows:

1. During the immediate postoperative healing phase, the synthetic augmentation device carries the majority

P. J. Fowler: Department of Orthopaedic Surgery, University of Western Ontario, London, Ontario N6A 5A5, Canada.

of the load. The biological tissue is maximally protected during this initial period, but at the same time it carries a small portion of the load.

2. The ability to load share may be achieved by suturing together the augmentation material and the graft tissue.

3. Reorganization and remodeling of the biological tissue is stimulated by the load it carries.

4. Gradual transfer of the load from the augmentation device to the biological graft results in the development of a more functional structure.

BIOMECHANICAL PROPERTIES

The role of synthetic augmentation is temporary. At time zero, the augmentation device should carry the greatest portion of the load in the composite graft. In this setting, the biomechanical qualities should ideally approach those of a normally functioning ACL. Once regeneration of the biological graft occurs, the role of the device becomes passive.

Biocompatibility of the synthetic material is another important feature. The absence of particulate debris and resistance to abrasion in the augmentation device is essential. This is particularly true for any intraarticular material. In addition, bioabsorbability might be an additional desirable property if the other parameters needed for augmentation are met.

Strength and Fatigue Resistance

As the patient resumes activities of daily living, the augmentation device needs sufficient strength, as well as resistance to fatigue, to support normal stresses. Van Kampen et al. have estimated that a synthetic augmentation device will withstand loads of less than 500 N for a period of 12 to 18 months (8). This may be equal to approximately 5 million cycles, in contrast to the 250 million cycles at a full 500-N load that a prosthesis would be required to carry. Prosthetics of adequate strength exist; however, there are problems with meeting long-term fatigue requirements. In regard to the strength and fatigue demands of synthetic materials, those placed on an augmentation device appear to be more achievable.

With synthetic augmentation, it is important to consider the strength of the composite as a whole. This includes its initial fixation to bone and the suture connection between the synthetic and the graft. The augmentation device should have increased strength over that of the graft alone.

Stiffness and Load Sharing

In synthetic augmentation, stiffness (the amount of force required to elongate a structure to a certain length)

of both the device and the biological tissue are important. Hanley et al. measured load sharing in LAD-augmented semitendinosus and gracilis tendon grafts, as well as in bone–patellar tendon–bone composite grafts (4). The results of this work demonstrated that load sharing occurred and that the load shared between the biological tissue and the LAD is dependent on the relative stiffness of both substances. In the semitendinosus and gracilis tendon grafts, the LAD carried an average of 45% of the load; in the bone–patellar tendon–bone grafts, it carried 28% of the load. The more stiff the tissue, the less load was carried by the synthetic; the less stiff the tissue, the more load was carried by the synthetic. An augmentation device of excessive stiffness could prevent the biological tissue from carrying sufficient load. As with strength and fatigue resistance, the stiffness of a synthetic augmentation device should approximate that of the normal ACL. For further description of the measurement of ACL and segment composite graft forces see Chapters 7, 8, and 9.

Creep

Creep is unrecoverable elongation of a material over time after multiple cyclic loads. It is present in all synthetics to various extents, and because these materials cannot undergo repair, creep eventually will result in laxity of a device. Theoretically, the critical function of an augmentation device is during the first year; resistance to creep is not crucial over the long term, but remains important in the early healing phase, when the device is performing its protective role. The augmentation device should offer sufficient resistance to creep to prevent stretching out the device before the graft is adequately healed.

It is important that a synthetic augmentation device allow and facilitate remodeling of biological tissue. This was examined in an animal study by Amendola and Fowler (1). Using composite grafts of LAD-augmented bone–patellar tendon–bone allografts, biomechanical, histologic, and morphologic changes in the tissue were assessed at 0, 4, 16, and 52 weeks postimplantation. The results of this study showed that synthetic augmentation appears to improve initial strength in the composite graft and allows normal remodeling to occur.

SURGICAL TECHNIQUE

The experience from LAD synthetic augmentation has demonstrated some specific surgical considerations:

1. A composite graft of a synthetic and a biological tissue that are sutured together enhances the load sharing between these two components. Load transference occurs through these suture connections.

2. As the composite graft is prepared, the synthetic

material should be completely surrounded with biological tissue to diminish the risk of abrasion.

3. Absorbable sutures are desirable in the intraarticular segment of the composite because once they have absorbed, the joint is free of exposed nonbiological material.

4. It appears from analysis of load sharing and stress distribution that sutures near the bony attachment of soft tissue carry the highest loads (8). This emphasizes the suitability of a permanent suture connection in this extraarticular area.

5. Initial fixation of the composite graft involves fastening the synthetic to the bone at one end only. Rigid fixation of the augmentation device at both ends may result in increased stress shielding. With rigid fixation, the augmentation device becomes a prosthesis and could impair remodeling of the biological graft. It has been calculated that in the presence of fixation at both ends, the synthetic device would carry 10 times the load of the biological tissue (8). In addition to stress shielding the graft, the synthetic material may not tolerate the higher load.

The strength of the initial fixation of the graft is a consideration in early loading that occurs as part of the rehabilitation. Different means of fixation and their strength were studied by Shabus et al. (6). They attached the LAD to bone using spiked plates, screws, spiked washers, and various types of staples, used singly, two in parallel, and two in a belt buckle fashion. Screw and washer fixation demonstrated the highest mean fixation strength of 1,270 N. Belt buckle staple fixation was next, with a mean fixation strength of 843 N.

SUMMARY

Synthetic augmentation offers the potential advantages of a biological tissue ACL reconstruction and a temporary prosthetic replacement. The augmentation device offers potential protection to the transplanted bio-

logical tissue during its loss of strength while incorporation occurs. The long-term limitations of synthetic materials in prosthetics, particularly in the area of cyclic loading, are not the same in synthetic augmentation. Once the load transferral is made to the mature biological graft, the nonabsorbable augmentation device remains permanently, but should assume a passive and inert role. Many feel that once an implant has served its purpose, its presence is undesirable, regardless of biocompatibility. Bioabsorbabilty, added to the other required properties of an augmentation device, is a reasonable concept that merits further attention in the future. As with any synthetic device, implantation of an augmentation device requires meticulous attention to detail and an understanding of the principles of its function.

REFERENCES

1. Amendola A, Fowler PJ. (1992): Allograft anterior cruciate ligament reconstruction in a sheep model: the effect of synthetic augmentation. *Am J Sports Med* 20:336–346.
2. Cabaud EH, Feagin JA, Rodney WG. (1982): Acute anterior cruciate ligament injury and repair reinforced with a biodegradable intra-articular ligament. *Am J Sports Med* 10:259.
3. Fowler PJ, Mackinlay D, Roth JH. (1989): Long term review of intra-articular ACL reconstructions with braided polypropylene. Proceedings of the International Society of the Knee, Rome. Clinical Residents Day, University of Western Ontario, 1989.
4. Hanley P, Lew WD, Lewis JL, Hunter RE, Kirstkas S, Kowalczyk C. (1988): Load sharing and graft forces in anterior cruciate ligament reconstructions with the ligament augmentation device. *Am J Sports Med* 17:414.
5. Roth JH, Kennedy JC, Lockstadt H, McCallum CL, Cunning LA. (1985): Polypropylene braid augmented and nonaugmented intra-articular anterior cruciate ligament reconstruction. *Am J Sports Med* 13:321–336.
6. Schabus R, Fuchs M, Grundl S. (1988): *Experimental mechanical stability investigations of the LAD fixations.* Vienna: Technical Test and Research Institute of the Technical University.
7. Strum GM, Larson RL. (1985): Clinical experience and early results of carbon fibre augmentation of anterior cruciate reconstruction of the knee. *Clin Orthop Rel Res* 196:124–138.
8. Van Kampen CL, Mendenhall HV, McPherson GK. (1987): Synthetic Augmentation of biological anterior cruciate ligament substitutions. In: Jackson DW, Drez D, eds. *New concepts in ligament repair.* St. Louis, MO: CV Mosby.

*The Anterior Cruciate Ligament: Current and
Future Concepts,* edited by D.W. Jackson, et al.
Raven Press, Ltd., New York © 1993.

CHAPTER 30

Prosthetic Replacement for the Anterior Cruciate Ligament

Donal M. McCarthy, Brad S. Tolin, Les Schwendeman,
Marc J. Friedman, and Savio L-Y. Woo

In the past decade, clinical and biomechanical investigations of prosthetic anterior cruciate ligaments (ACLs) have dramatically increased. There are disadvantages with the use of autogenous tissue in ACL reconstructions, and this has stimulated the search for alternatives such as artificial ligaments. These disadvantages include complications related to harvesting the autogenous tissue, as well as the relative lack of strength of the autogenous ACL grafts compared with prosthetic implants. The average strength of the ACL taken from young cadavers was found to be 1,730 N (71). Of the autogenous grafts mechanically tested, only the bone–patellar tendon–bone specimens at time zero had a strength greater than the *in vivo* ACL. However, the bone–patellar tendon–bone specimen tested was a 14-mm graft, which is significantly larger than the 10-mm graft usually used in clinical practice. Other studies have suggested that the central third of the patellar tendon is stronger than previously reported, with the average strength of a 10-mm graft found to be 2,977 N (20). Also, rotating the graft 90 degrees was found to significantly increase its strength. When interpreting the biomechanical data, it is important to note that these results reflect strength in a static mode and immediately after harvesting. After the graft is implanted, the autogenous tissue, being a free graft, undergoes a process of revascularization and remodeling (72). The graft undergoes progressive weakening after implantation and continues to remain significantly weaker than the normal ACL.

The use of allograft and prosthetic implants have been stimulated in part to avoid sacrificing the patient's own tissues and to avoid the associated morbidity (16). Problems associated with allografts include the potential for disease transmission, the possibility of subclinical rejection, and that they require a longer revascularization period than autogenous substitutes (3,45,63). A prosthetic ligament has the advantages of a biomechanically stronger graft material, which allows for earlier range of motion of the knee, weight-bearing, and return to full activities. Despite these theoretical advantages, the prosthetic ligaments continue to have inherent problems.

HISTORICAL PERSPECTIVE

One of the earliest descriptions of prosthetic reconstruction of the ACL was by Corner (21) in 1914. He used a loop of silver wire to replace the torn ACL in a football player, with no long-term follow-up reported. In 1918, Smith (88) used multiple sutures through channels in the tibia and femur to reconstruct the torn ACL. The sutures were removed at 11 weeks postreconstruction due to a severe inflammatory reaction. Von Mironova (98) used a ligament composed of Lavsan, a type of polyester, to reconstruct the ACL. He claimed 91% satisfactory results in 262 patients in over 15 years of study.

The Proplast ligament substitute (Vitek Inc.) was originally intended to be used as a stent, or temporary internal splint, to provide stability while an associated extra-articular reconstruction was healing. This prosthesis was approved by the U.S. Food and Drug Administration (FDA) for implantation in 1973. James et al. (46) reported results of 15 patients in which the ligament was implanted as a salvage procedure for chronic anterior

D. M. McCarthy, L. Schwendeman, and S. L-Y. Woo: Musculoskeletal Research Laboratories, Department of Orthopaedic Surgery, University of Pittsburgh, Pittsburgh, Pennsylvania 15261.

B. S. Tolin and M. J. Friedman: Southern California Orthopaedic Institute, Van Nuys, California 91405.

laxity. Only 50% of the patients had satisfactory results, and ligament breakage occurred in 8 of the 15 patients. Most of the failures occurred during the first postoperative year.

In 1976, the Richards Polyflex System (Richards Manufacturing Co.) was the only prosthetic ligament marketed in the United States. The prosthesis was constructed of an ultra high molecular weight polyethylene and stainless steel tubes that were fixed with a threaded nut augmented with polymethylmethacrylate cement. Biomechanical and clinical studies using the Polyflex ligament raised concern over the ability of the implant to resist *in vivo* forces in the young active patient without sustaining any permanent deformation (17,30,40). The failure rate was over 50% within the first year of implantation. In November 1977, Richards ceased commercial production and distribution of the device. The experience with this ligament stimulated the FDA to form an advisory panel to develop guidelines to be used in the approval process for prosthetic ligaments (27).

Jenkins (47) in 1978, began to use flexible carbon fibers to reconstruct the ACL. The carbon was thought to act as a temporary scaffold that encouraged the ingrowth of fibroblastic tissue and subsequently produced new collagen. The clinical results reported by Rushton et al. (81) demonstrated that a high percentage of patients had persistent pain and effusions that necessitated removal of the carbon fiber implant. There was no ingrowth of organized fibroblastic tissue observed, and free carbon fibers were found within the joint. Denti et al. (24) also highlighted the problems with these uncoated carbon ligaments. Of further concern was the migration of the carbon fibers from the ligament to regional lymph nodes. In an attempt to reduce the shedding of the carbon particles and improve its handling characteristics, the carbon fiber implants were coated with a polylactate acid polymer. This ligament was known as the Integraft Stent (Osteonics Biomaterials, Livermore, CA). The composite allows for reabsorption of the copolymer shortly after implantation. The carbon fibers then underwent a more prolonged mechanical degradation while simultaneously gradually transferring the forces to the newly formed collagen tissue. This graft was used to augment standard autogenous ACL reconstruction and was designed to be completely covered by the autogenous grafted tissue when implanted. Initially, the Integraft ligament (Fig. 1) was woven through a strip of iliotibial band that had been detached distally, passed through the posterior capsule of the knee, and then through a tibial tunnel. The graft was fixed to the tibia with a carbon-polylactate acid fastener. Subsequent studies demonstrated that the carbon fiber was found in the lymph nodes after implantation of the uncoated carbon material, but coating the carbon decreased the fragmentation and particle migration (6). Preliminary clinical studies demonstrated satisfactory results in patients who

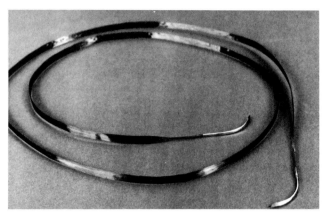

FIG. 1. The Integraft stent. (From ref. 80a, with permission.)

underwent reconstruction with this ligament as a salvage procedure (99). Another study showed no apparent difference at one year postsurgery between patients who had had ACL reconstruction with the central one third patellar tendon or semitendinosus tendon augmented with the Integraft prosthesis and those patients who had had a nonaugmented autogenous reconstruction. The ligament was never given market approval by the FDA.

In July 1981, clinical trials began using the ProCol Xenograft Bioprosthesis (Xenotech Laboratories, Irvine, CA), which was composed of bovine extensor tendons treated with glutaraldehyde (Fig. 2). The glutaraldehyde treatment protects the collagen bundles from proteolytic enzyme degradation by cross-linking adjacent molecules. This process produces an implant that has a greater modulus of elasticity and does not undergo remodeling; thus, the ligament is considered to be a permanent prosthesis. Results of implantation with the Xenograft have generally been disappointing. In patients in whom the ligament was implanted arthroscopically, the reconstruction failed in 31%, and 29% developed a sterile synovitis (100). Failure of the graft usually occurred in the first postoperative year. Tietge and Rojas (92) examined 18 patients after implantation over an 18-month period. Ten of the patients had recurrent effusions and only one patient was stable by KT-1000 testing. Nine grafts had been removed at the time of the report, and the majority had demonstrated a chronic inflammatory response with foreign body giant cell granulomatous reactions. The FDA in May 1987 reported that the ProCol

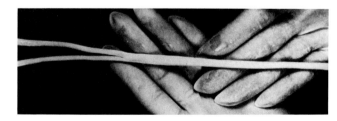

FIG. 2. Xenotech ACL prosthesis.

bioprosthesis was not approved for release, specifically citing concern over the high incidence of effusions.

CLASSIFICATION OF PROSTHETIC LIGAMENTS

Prosthetic ligaments are generally classified into three types: permanent ligaments, stents, or scaffolds. Permanent ligaments include the Gore-Tex and Stryker-Dacron ligaments and are designed with high strength and increased resistance to fatigue failure. These ligaments rely on their inherent mechanical properties to withstand forces over a prolonged period of time without any contribution from autogenous tissues or tissue ingrowth into the ligament.

The second type is a temporary prosthetic ligament used as a stent. It functions to augment the strength of an intraarticular biologic reconstruction. These devices increase the security of fixation of the tissue and increase the immediate strength of the composite graft. These ligaments are usually fixated at only one end of the graft to allow the transfer of stress to the underlying biologic tissue. Theoretically, as the tissue strength increases, the role of the ligament augmentation device becomes less important.

The third type of prosthetic ligament is the scaffold device, which allows ingrowth of tissue. These ligaments depend on autogenous tissue ingrowth. The collagen tissue may either grow into the existing graft, as in the Leeds-Keio ligament, or may actually replace the graft tissue as it is slowly degraded, as with the carbon ligaments. In these cases, the new collagen tissue matures into a replacement ligament that can theoretically last indefinitely without fatigue. Table 1 classifies the various prosthetic ligaments in this classification scheme.

FDA APPROVAL PROCESS

Currently there are only three prosthetic ligament devices approved by the FDA for use in ACL reconstruction. The FDA follows a systematic process before approving prosthetic devices for implantation (27) (Table

TABLE 1. *Classification of prosthetic ligaments*

Permanent prosthesis	Gore-Tex ligament
	Stryker Dacron ligament
	Richards polyflex ligament[a]
	ProCol xenograft bioprosthesis[a]
Stent	Kennedy ligament augmentation device
	Integraft stent[a]
Scaffold	Leeds-Keio ligament

[a] Ligament not currently available in the United States.

TABLE 2. *Steps in FDA approval of ligament prothesis*

Premarket notification to FDA (510 K)
↓
Laboratory and animal tests
↓
Clinical trials proposed
↓
Investigational device exemption status (IDE)
↓
Phase 1. Clinical trials (single investigator)
↓
Phase 2. Clinical trials (multiple investigators)
↓
Premarketing approval (PMA)
↓
Released for general use

2). Manufacturers are required to notify the FDA before marketing a new device. These premarket notification submissions are referred to as 510 K(S). During this 90-day period, the FDA determines whether the device is similar to a previously approved device. If the device is not substantially equivalent, it is required to undergo the approval process before marketing.

These devices must then be tested in laboratory and animal studies and found to be reasonably safe and effective. This first phase includes biomechanical studies performed in animal models. The animals are routinely examined for evidence of adverse reactions. Because prosthetic ligaments have no method to remodel once implanted, an important characteristic to measure is fatigue failure. This is usually measured as million of cycles (average cycles per year = 1.4 million) to failure. From these data an estimate of the life expectancy of the ligament in humans is calculated. Table 3 demonstrates the comparative biomechanical testing results for the normal ACL and those reviewed for six different prosthetic ligaments.

The next step for FDA approval involves submitting a proposed clinical trial with sufficient numbers and adequate follow-up to allow statistical determination of safety and efficacy. At this point, the device may be granted Investigation Device Exemption (IDE) status. Phase I clinical trials are confined to a single clinical investigator. In Phase II, multicenter trials are conducted using a common protocol. During phases I and II the device is not available for general use. After the data from the clinical trials have been evaluated, the FDA may grant premarketing approval (PMA) status. A PMA status means that a decision from the FDA is expected within 6 months. After analysis of the completed clinical trials and review by a panel of experts, the ligament may be approved and released for general use. At this point, the ligament is available to all orthopedic surgeons, but it may be marketed only for the indications specifically approved by the FDA. For example, the Gore-Tex and

Stryker ligaments are approved only for use in patients with previously failed intraarticular reconstructions and the ligament augmentation device as of September 1991 is approved for use with iliotibial tendon, semitendinosus tendon, and patellar tendon ACL reconstruction as a result of a multicenter phase II U.S. study. The individual surgeon may still use an approved ligament outside of the FDA guidelines, but must discuss with the patient the reasons and indications for the choice of a prosthetic ligament as opposed to an autogenous reconstruction.

THE GORE-TEX PROSTHETIC LIGAMENT

The Gore-Tex prosthesis (Fig. 3) is intended to serve as a permanent replacement for the ACL. The ligament is composed of expanded polytetafluorethylene (PTFE). The prosthesis is composed of a single strand of the material that is wound into multiple loops. The strands are then woven into a three-bundle multifilament with fixation eyelets incorporated at each end of the ligament. The eyelets allow fixation at each end of the prosthesis with cortical screws into the host bone. The screw fixation is intended to supply the initial fixation of the ligament, whereas permanent fixation is provided by tissue ingrowth into the strands of ligament contained in the bony tunnels. This ingrowth is estimated to take at least 6 months to occur. Bolton and Bruchman (10) performed static and cyclic creep tests measuring the *in vivo* loading stresses in the normal ACL. They found that ligament strength of approximately 4,400 N was necessary to prevent clinically significant elongation *in vivo*. The Gore-Tex prosthetic ligament can withstand a greater maximum load with approximately 8% to 10% elongation at failure (58).

Based on the encouraging preliminary biologic studies, clinical trials of the device were initiated in the United States in October 1982 under an IDE. As part of the study, 1,021 patients had a Gore-Tex ligament implanted for ACL insufficiency by 20 groups of investigators. The prospective study was performed with patients being evaluated at 3-month intervals for the first year and at 6 month intervals until 5 years postoperative follow-ups were obtained. The preliminary results of this study were satisfactory, and formal FDA approval was obtained in October 1986.

Results of Reconstruction

The Gore-Tex ligament has been implanted in over 18,000 patients worldwide. The W.L. Gore Company has reported the results of the Gore-Tex ligament reconstruction in the 186 patients included in the original study with at least 5 years of follow-up (39). The average age of the patients was 27.5 years. Seventy-six of these patients had prior surgical procedures on the involved knee. Objective examination preoperatively demonstrated that 84% of the patients had a Lachman >2+ and 83% of the patients had a positive pivot shift. After insertion of the Gore-Tex ligament, 30% of the patients had a Lachman >2+ and only 24% had residual positive pivot shift. The incidence of giving-way symptoms decreased from 89% before reconstruction to only 11% postoperatively.

Complications occurred in 14.3% of patients. Thirty-eight patients had the graft removed (3.8%), with 18 patients having actual failure of the graft (1.8%). An infection developed in 13 patients (1%), which required removal of the prosthesis in 10 patients. Recurrent instability developed in 8 patients (0.8%) without evidence of graft failure, with 5 of these 8 patients subsequently reconstructed successfully.

Recently, the original Gore-Tex investigators individually published the results of reconstruction in their patients. Ahfeld et al. (1) reported on 30 patients with an average follow-up of 2 years. They noted improvement of instability in 87% of patients and satisfactory results in 83%. Glousman et al. (37) evaluated 82 patients who underwent Gore-Tex ligament reconstruction with a

TABLE 3. *Comparison of ACL prosthetic ligaments*

	Normal ACL	Gore-Tex	LAD	Stryker	Leeds-Keio
Animal model	Human (16–26 yr)	Sheep	Goat	Dog	Pig
Fixation	Bone	Bone	Soft tissue	Bone	Bone
Type of prosthesis		Permanent	Stent	Stent	Ingrowth
Material		PTFE	Polypropylene braid	Dacron fabric	Dacron mesh
Ultimate tensile strength (N)	1,730	>4,448	1,730 (8 mm) 1,500 (6 mm)	3,110–3,631	2,000
Stiffness (N/mm)	182	322	56 N/mm (8 mm) 15 cm long 61 N/mm (6 mm) 15 cm long	39	>182
Ultimate strain (%)	60	9	22 (8 mm) 22 (6 mm)	18	35

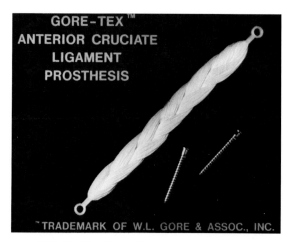

FIG. 3. The Gore-Tex ligament prosthesis.

mean follow-up of 18 months. The objective analysis, which included a Lachman test, anterior drawer test, and pivot shift test, demonstrated improvement at final follow-up in comparison with the patients' preoperative status. Complications noted in their study included four ligament ruptures, four chronic sterile effusions, two patients with partial attenuation of the ligament, one infection, and one loose body. Fourteen patients subsequently required additional surgery. Glousman et al. felt that the results were satisfactory, but cautioned that longer term follow-up was necessary. Of concern was a deterioration of the objective data when evaluated at 6-month intervals. The investigators speculated that the trend of graft loosening may be the result of some resorption of the bone tunnels adjacent to the graft due to interposed soft tissue, ligament creep, or possibly actual loosening of the graft. It is interesting that the subjective scores have not significantly changed in these patients. Johnson (48) reported on 59 patients who underwent a Gore-Tex ACL reconstruction with a minimum of 2 years' follow-up. Ninety-three percent of the patients were satisfied with the procedure. There were 12 objective failures, all of whom were asymptomatic. Only 5% of the patients were considered subjective failures. KT-1000 demonstrated a side-to-side difference of 2.0 mm at a 2-year follow-up, and 1.5 mm at a 3-year follow-up. Johnson suggested that this was evidence that the results did not deteriorate over time, but that there were only 13 patients in the 36-month follow-up group. Complications included 11% who had effusions and 5% who required secondary reconstruction after failure of the graft. Ferkel et al. (26) reported the results of an arthroscopic second look in 21 knees that had arthroscopically assisted implantation of the Gore-Tex prosthesis. Eight of the arthroscopies were performed for complaints of knee pain postreconstruction, whereas two were for giving-way symptoms, three for recurrent effusions, and eight for screw removal. The time interval from implantation to rearthroscopy was on average 11 months. The ligament was found to be intact in 11 knees, partially ruptured in 6, and completely ruptured in 4 patients. The majority of the patients had synovitis present at the time of the second-look arthroscopy, but this was similar in intensity to the synovitis present at the time of the original surgery and not thought to be due to a reaction to the graft. No PTFE particles were appreciated on histologic evaluation of the synovium when the Gore-Tex ligament was intact. Particular debris was found only when ruptured strands of the graft were present. However, there appeared to be no relation between the integrity of the graft and the presence of a synovial reaction. Ferkel et al. felt that the Gore-Tex ligament was inert and did not cause any significant synovial reaction or effusion when either intact or ruptured.

Despite the encouraging preliminary results of Gore-Tex ligament reconstruction, the results of 4- to 5-year follow-ups of many studies have demonstrated an apparent deterioration in both subjective and objective results. Karzel et al. (50) reported on 61 patients with a 4-year follow-up. A progressive increase in KT-1000 side-to-side differences was noted with longer follow-up, although 79% had good or excellent subjective results. There was a relatively high complication rate involving 49% of the patients, although most were minor. Seventeen percent of the patients subsequently required that the Gore-Tex ligament graft be removed. Of interest was that approximately one third of the patients who subjectively were scored as good to excellent had KT-1000 side-to-side differences of >5 mm. Karzel et al. noted that the subjective results did not always correlate well with the objective evaluation.

With doubts regarding the ultimate longevity of the Gore-Tex ligament, the apparent failure of the ligament after implantation with longer follow-up, and the recurrent and chronic effusions, a judicious approach to Gore-Tex prosthetic ligament implantation would appear to be justified. Currently, the ligament is approved by the FDA only for use in previously failed autogenous reconstructions.

New developments in the Gore-Tex ligament with the advent of the Gore-Tex II prosthesis may improve the results of reconstruction. The Gore-Tex II ligament (Fig. 4) addresses some of the biomechanical problems inherent in the original prosthesis. This prosthesis has been changed by compacting the diameter of the ligament with a tighter weave configuration, which may help pre-

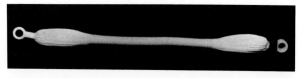

FIG. 4. The compact diameter Gore-Tex ligament (Gore-Tex II).

vent abrasion of the ligament on the bony edges in the intercondylar notch. Theoretically, this may increase the longevity of the implant and reduce PTFE shedding. *In vitro* testing has demonstrated that the prototype Gore-Tex II prosthesis has approximately twice the wear resistance and residual strength of the old Gore-Tex ligament. This ligament is currently being tested in Canada and is not commercially available in the United States.

THE STRYKER-DACRON LIGAMENT

The Stryker-Dacron ligament prosthesis is a composite of four Dacron tapes surrounded by a woven Dacron velour sleeve (Fig. 5). The components are combined to form a single prosthesis. The ends of the device are covered with plastic tips that facilitate passage of the graft within the knee. The development of the Stryker-Dacron ligament was preceded by the safety and efficacy of this material in vascular surgery. The implant was initially designed to be used as an augmentation device with the iliotibial band in ACL reconstructions, but the high strength of the ligament has led to its use as a permanent prosthesis. Animal studies in dogs had demonstrated significant bone and fibrous tissue ingrowth when used as an augmentation device (75). When used as a permanent type of prothesis, no synovial tissue ingrowth was noted intraarticularly (82). Mechanical testing has demonstrated the ultimate tensile strength (UTS) of the ligament to be 3,631 N (76). Fatigue testing showed the ability to withstand 134,000 fatigue cycles at 1,730 Newtons. This amount of force would presumably disrupt a normal ACL after a single cycle. The estimated *in vivo* life expectancy from the fatigue testing data is 8.5 years. The ligament can be used for combined intra-articular and extra-articular reconstruction, and is 8 mm in diameter with an overall length of 70 cm.

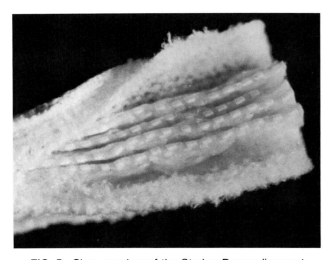

FIG. 5. Close-up view of the Stryker-Dacron ligament.

Results of Reconstruction

Lukianov et al. (61) reported results of ACL reconstructions for chronic instability using the Stryker-Dacron ligament in 513 patients from 19 investigational centers. Three hundred-thirty patients were available for at least 2 years of postoperative follow-up. Ninety-seven percent of these patients had a negative pivot shift at follow-up compared with 11% preoperatively. Complications included ligament rupture in 3.8% of the cases, infection in 2.3%, and synovitis in 1.5%. Lysholm scores improved from an average of 59 preoperatively to 93 at 2 years final follow-up.

Bartolozzi et al. (5) followed 53 patients with chronic ACL deficiency who had undergone Stryker-Dacron ligament reconstruction with a mean follow-up of 29 months. Subjectively, 83% of the patients had excellent/good results, 7.5% fair, and 9.5% poor. The percentage of poor subjective results tended to increase with longer follow-up. Objectively, only 35% of the patients had a <1+ Lachman test, and the jerk test was <1+ in 61.5% and 70.5% of all the patients who had a residual positive jerk test. These particular parameters were found not to deteriorate significantly with time. The KT-1000 data showed >3 mm side-to-side difference in approximately two thirds of the cases. Complications were present in 13% of the patients. There were no cases of persistent synovitis, but on radiographic evaluation after at least 1 year of ligament reconstruction 85% of the patients demonstrated periligamentous femoral osteolysis that was primarily located at the intraarticular portion of the distal femur tunnel. In this series, patients over 25 years of age tended to have worse overall results than younger patients.

Longer term follow-up studies have recently appeared in the literature and demonstrate further deterioration of results. Lopez-Vasquez et al. (60) observed 54 patients who had undergone Dacron prosthetic ligament implantation. Nineteen of these patients had had acute ACL injuries, whereas 36 had had chronic tears. Follow-up ranged from 2 to 5 years. Forty-eight percent of the patients had either detachment or elongation of the prosthesis. The majority of the failures occurred between the second and fourth postoperative years with no predilection for acute or chronic reconstructions. The Lysholm and Gillquist scores demonstrated deterioration with time. Vazquez et al. concluded that the prosthesis was not a durable substitute for ACL replacement or supplementation.

Tissue ingrowth into the ligament was evaluated in two cases where the Dacron ligament, used as a prosthesis, ruptured (82). The histologic and electron microscopic evaluation demonstrated fibroblastlike cells and elastic fibers in a lax connective tissue stroma immediately adjacent to the Dacron threads. The cells and collagen fibrils were located further from the Dacron threads.

This periprosthetic tissue did not demonstrate biomechanical properties or morphologic characteristics to resist tension stresses. Also noted were the infrequent occurrence of inflammatory cells in the synovium membrane, which indicated the relative inertness of the Dacron material.

The Stryker-Dacron ligament has been approved for general use in failed intraarticular ACL reconstructions by the FDA in January 1989. Recent studies demonstrate a significant failure rate at 5 years. Initially, the ligament was designed to act as a scaffold to allow soft tissue ingrowth, which would then ultimately provide its own tensile strength while simultaneously decreasing the role of the graft material. Subsequent investigations have demonstrated no significant differences of function and stability in the knees that underwent reconstruction with or without augmentation. This suggests that the Dacron ligament functions as a true prosthesis rather than as a scaffold type of implant. Because the graft material is biologically inert, there has been a lower reported incidence of synovitis than has been reported in the Gore-Tex ligament reconstructions. The results of this ligament reconstruction appear to be similar to those of the Gore-Tex, with continued deterioration and failure over time.

POLYESTER PROSTHESES

Outside the United States, several polyester prosthetic ACL implants have gained popularity equal to that of carbon fiber. One of the better known investigational polyester prostheses is the Leeds-Keio implant (Fig. 6). It has an open-weave configuration and functions as a scaffold-type prosthesis, allowing ingrowth of native tissue to build strength. Fixation is by means of femoral and tibial bone plugs and subsequent ingrowth. Its UTS is greater

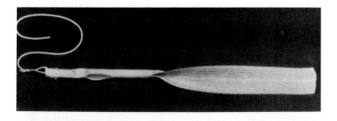

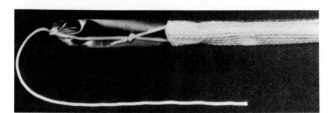

FIG. 6. The Leeds-Keio ligament (top). The implant is placed within a flexible polyethylene sheath to facilitate graft passage. (From ref. 84a, with permission.)

than 2,000 N with a stiffness of 195 N/mm, 262 N/mm, and 279 N/mm at 1%, 50%, and 100% strain rates, respectively. After 79 million cycles between 50 N and 500 N followed by 19 million cycles between 50 N and 700 N, its residual strength is 1,350 N (33).

After 9 months' postimplantation in pigs, the Leeds-Keio ligament and resultant fibrous ingrowth had a UTS of 950 N, compared with the contralateral, unoperated ACL value of 620 N. These values increased to 2,600 N and 1,450 N for the artificial and native ligaments, respectively (85), at 17 months. Implantation into a sheep model resulted in a 0% rupture rate at 1 year, but with evidence of implant wear in 50% of the animals (84). In addition, the polyester fibers did not appear to support collagenous ingrowth in this investigation.

However, histology from a failed Leeds-Keio clinical case demonstrated organized Type I collagen along the main tensile stress planes of the prosthesis, with adequate vascularization and an elastic component after 18 months (62). Fujikawa et al. (33) reported that of 450 Leeds-Keio prostheses implanted since 1982, 152 had at least a 4-year follow-up. At this time, 90% had a negative anterior drawer and Lachmans test. Range of motion was normal in 71.1% of the patients. One other study reported an 89% good or excellent subjective improvement over preoperative evaluation at an average of 27 months, with 88% having a 0 to 1+ Lachman test and 93% a negative pivot shift, and 71% of the patients resumed preoperative activity levels (44). Complications included a 4.6% loss of greater than 21 degrees in range of motion, and a 3.3% rupture rate, but no report of infection, effusion, or synovitis (33). Clinical trials for the Leeds-Keio prosthesis began in the United States in 1990.

The Leeds-Keio ligament has several potential advantages. The ligament is strong and relatively compact in size, allowing for an arthroscopically-assisted technique of insertion, without the need for a notchplasty. The ligament has the potential for soft tissue ingrowth, which would allow for potential long-term survival of the implant. Combining an intraarticular and extraarticular procedure at the time of reconstruction is also possible with this ligament. The method of fixation of the implant within the bony tunnels is innovative and appears to allow incorporation of the ligament into the bony tunnels for secure fixation. Backup staple fixation potentially leads to a more rapid rehabilitation by providing rigid fixation of the implant while the bony plug/ligament complex heals. The designers of the ligament emphasize the importance of placing the implant under tension so that the induced tissue can organize along the lines of stress and serve a load-bearing function. Also, current recommendations include attaching a piece of synovium to the ligament at the time of implantation to expedite tissue ingrowth.

Although the short-term results are encouraging,

longer term studies are necessary to determine the ultimate fate of soft tissue ingrowth. Of concern is the quality of soft tissue ingrowth into the ligament. The evidence of tissue ingrowth is primarily based on animal studies, with only a few recent reports in the literature performed after ligament implantation in humans. Unfortunately, these specific cases represent a small number of the ligaments implanted. Further long-term follow-up studies from groups other than the inventors are necessary to determine the general use efficacy of the Leeds-Keio ligament.

Another polyester ACL prosthesis is the Ligastic implant, studied mainly in France. The difference in this artificial ligament is its knitted structure, in which all the fibers are oriented longitudinally at their maximal length (54). There are several coated and uncoated sizes available, and they are denoted according to the number of polyester fibers incorporated. The UTS for the uncoated 60- and 72-fiber Ligastic implants are 3,500 N and 4,200 N, respectively. An approximate elongation at failure of 5% is noted.

In humans at 1 year the Ligastic prosthesis has been found to provide satisfactory results in 90% of the cases in returning patients to their preoperative level of activity (57). Laboureau and Cazenave (54,55) observed postoperatively 90% absent Lachmans, 94% absent anterior drawer, and 96% negative pivot shift. KT-1000 testing was normal or tighter than preoperative values in 90%. Complications included a 3% rupture rate, 1% reactive synovitis, and less than 1% infection rate (56).

New generation ultra high molecular weight polyester implants have improved on the biomechanical properties of this material, resulting in a UTS of up to 9,000 N and an estimated fatigue life of 840 billion cycles (29). Histology is unchanged with good fibrous encapsulation, but functional anterior stabilization decays over time in these investigational prostheses (2).

CONCEPT OF AUGMENTATION

In an effort to reduce the load on autografts and allografts, synthetic augmentation devices have been developed to share the load and prevent early graft weakness and failure (22,23,29,65,96). Although earlier *in vitro* studies showed that the ligament augmentation device (LAD) reduced loads in the graft, this initial advantage did not appear to be significant in *in vivo* studies, and graft vascularity was found to be reduced in the presence of the LAD. The role of extraarticular procedures in augmenting an intraarticular procedure has also been found to have no detectable effect on the outcome (73).

LAD

The LAD prosthesis is a permanent, nonabsorbable augmentation device made of woven polypropylene.

With fixation at one end only, its intended purpose is to provide structural integrity to an autogenous (or allograft) middle one third patellar tendon graft while the tissue undergoes the process of necrosis, revascularization, and remodeling. Other native tissues, such as the semitendinosus tendon and portions of the iliotibial band, have been implanted in conjunction with the LAD more recently (23). The load-sharing abilities of the LAD depend on the stiffness of the graft; as graft stiffness decreases (as it would during necrosis and revascularization), load on the LAD increases. Inversely, as graft stiffness increases (in remodeling), the load on the LAD decreases, theoretically allowing the forming ligament to assume more function. Implantation of the LAD with a patellar tendon graft at time zero results in the prosthesis bearing 28% of the tensile load, whereas implantation with a less stiff material, the semitendinosus tendon, requires the LAD to bear about 45% of the load (96).

In vitro testing demonstrates an initial UTS of 1,730 N, an elongation of 22% at failure, a stiffness of 200 N/mm, and cyclic elongation of 4% after 1 million cycles between 50 N and 500 N, resulting in a 9% strength loss (31,65,96). Bending fatigue parameters after 10 million cycles of 150 N to 300 N, with flexion between 15 and 40 degrees, yielded 4.5% cyclic elongation and 23% strength loss (96).

LAD augmentation of autogenous tissue in animal models has demonstrated a definite benefit. McPherson et al. (65) found that in the goat model at time zero, augmented grafts had a UTS of 364 N versus 260 N for nonaugmented grafts. At 2 years these values increased to 841 N and 520 N, respectively. Another canine study demonstrated at 6 months that LAD-augmented repairs exhibited 49.3% of native ACL strength, compared with 29.9% strength for nonaugmented groups (38). Initial fixation at one or both ends has been debated, and although double fixation provides a more rigid initial structure (30.8 N/mm of stiffness compared with 19.3 N/mm for one-ended repair), it does result in stress shielding of the graft (4). This is evidenced by the apparent dissolution and decreased cellularity in the double-fixed LAD augmentation. Animal rupture rates range from 12.5% at 1 year (18) to an alarming 100% complete or partial rupture at 10 months (67).

Clinical results with the LAD are encouraging (23,29,79,80). Telephone interviews of 94 patients at an average of 7.5 years postoperatively yielded 90% good or excellent results with respect to activity level, function, pain, swelling, and giving way (29). Ninety-six percent of the patients claimed that they would undergo the procedure again if necessary. Roth et al. (80) found that 32% of patients with nonaugmented ACL repairs had recurrent symptoms of instability at a mean follow-up of 64 months, whereas patients with LAD augmentation had only 11% incidence of recurrent giving way and greater anterior stability and functional testing at an average of 50 months' follow-up. In the largest series to date, Del

Pizzo (23) reported that LAD-augmented ACL reconstructions had a significant increase in range of motion compared with controls, and that they gained 130 degrees of motion at a mean of 6 months earlier than controls. Of the 721 patients, 269 had a minimum 2-year follow-up, and at this time 96% had a 0 to 1+ pivot shift, 79% had ≤3 mm of anterior laxity with KT-1000 testing at 20 pounds anterior force, and 95% had ≤5 degrees of extension restriction.

Complications from this series included a 1.4% infection rate and 3.9% sterile effusion, and 1.4% of the cases resulted in rupture of the prosthesis.

DESIGN CONSIDERATIONS

The ideal synthetic ligament should be tissue compatible and biomechanically competent. It should not incite any abnormal inflammatory response, and what reaction does occur should ideally be directed to the induction of fibrous tissue ingrowth and not scar. The material should be free of any systemic side effects and should be nonmutagenic. Design and technical factors should ensure a reliable and reproducible surgical technique.

The design of replacement materials used in the reconstruction of the ACL requires quantitative data on the normal function of the ligament. Given the multiplicity of roles that the ACL plays in normal knee kinematics, an overtly simplistic approach to the design of such materials may not be appropriate. In addition to contributing to the stability of the knee, particularly anterior translation (34,43,77), the ACL acts as a secondary restraint to tibial rotation and varus-valgus angulation, especially in full extension (64). The nonlinear behavior of the ligament is uniquely suited to providing support for maintaining normal knee kinematics. If the joint is subjected to excessively large forces, the nonlinear properties of the ligament (i.e., the increase in stiffness with load) limits excessive joint motion and protects the joint. Additionally, the unique twisting geometry of its two fiber bundles results in varying lengths and loads throughout knee range of motion (52,53,58,59,66,69,87, 91,95). This allows the ACL to stabilize the knee under different types of joint motion and to be functional at different flexion angles. Interestingly, an increase in length in a fiber bundle does not necessarily imply an increase in load in that bundle (91). It is unlikely that any synthetic substitute could replicate these changes in length and the corresponding load behavior.

The structural properties of the ACL have been intensively investigated despite the geometrically complex nature of the ligament and the difficulty of simulating the in vivo situation in the research setting (70,78,94,102). When considering a suitable replacement for the ACL, it is important that we concentrate not solely on the ultimate strength of the ACL, but also bear in mind the other parameters of the load-elongation behavior (101).

Along with the UTS, we should consider the linear stiffness and the energy absorbed to failure. There has been a considerable discrepancy in the values presented for UTS and linear stiffness in the literature. Factors responsible for this discrepancy include methods of testing, orientation of specimens, and whether the ligament was attached to bone when tested. Trent et al. (94) reported a linear stiffness of 141 N/mm and an average UTS of 633 N. Noyes et al. reported values of 182 ± 33 N/mm (mean ± SEM) and 1,725 ± 269 N for linear stiffness and ultimate load, respectively, for younger knees, and values of 129 ± 39 N/mm and 734 ± 660 N for older knees. Similarly, Woo et al. (102) have shown that the structural properties of the femur–ACL–tibia complex, as represented by the linear stiffness, ultimate load, and energy absorbed, were found to decrease significantly with the patient's age. In fact, the values for the younger specimens were roughly three times those of the older specimens. The values for linear stiffness and UTS for the younger group (242 ± 28N/mm and 2,160 ± 157 N) are higher than those previously recorded. With these values in mind, minimum requirements can be set for the design of prostheses for different age groups.

A replacement material might have the same or higher ultimate load as the ACL, but if its load-elongation curve is very different, it may not serve well as an ACL replacement. It is also important to remember that a graft with a failure strength several times larger than that of the ACL could be responsible for considerable damage to other knee structures when a large external load is applied to the knee that would fail the normal ACL.

Equally important properties are linear stiffness and the time-dependent viscoelastic properties that determine its response to cyclic stresses. During normal activity it is very unlikely that the graft would be exposed to loads that would cause it to fail. It has been suggested that when climbing stairs the native ACL is exposed to a cyclic load of about 70 N, around 200 N while level walking, and a load of 630 N when jogging (17). Early fatigue failure or excessive creep deformation could render an apparently adequate prosthetic material unacceptable. Unlike autogenous or allogenic grafts, which may have some ability to repair themselves, synthetic materials are unable to do so, meaning that the loss of prosthesis function over time is irreversible. Therefore, the most important mechanical, material properties to be determined are elastic modulus, yield point, creep, relaxation time, and fatigue characteristics (17).

Despite the extensive research on the biomechanics of the normal and the ACL-deficient knee, and the efforts to replicate these in the design of substitutes, both natural and synthetic, there is no proof that ACL reconstruction returns to normal the altered biomechanics of the ACL-deficient knee or that it has a protective effect on the knee with regards to future degenerative changes (28). Another limitation in the evaluation of these grafts is that there is no ideal laboratory device that totally evaluates flexion, rotation, and abrasion stresses that the ligament experiences in the knee. Consequently, ligaments that have been tested to 40 million cycles in the laboratory, rupture at 6 months in the human knee (31). Likewise, the desired combination of properties has not been adequately defined for ACL prostheses because there are a number of technical problems (e.g., finding mechanical grips to consistently secure the material being tested) in determining these values. Also, a standardized biomechanical testing protocol is needed to allow comparison between each of the synthetic ACL ligaments and the normal ACL. A uniform system of postoperative evaluation and rating is likewise lacking (58).

Whether the graft functions as a scaffold, an augmentation device, or a true prosthesis will also have some bearing on its required properties. If an ACL prosthesis acts as a scaffold or augmentation device, it is important that its mechanical properties are adequate to protect the knee during the early months of healing, while the scaffold is being replaced by fibrous tissue and the augmented allograft or autograft gains in strength. On the other hand, it is mandatory that a true (permanent) prosthesis replicates the function of the normal ACL as long as possible.

The other important parameters are the effects of graft placement and initial tension on knee function (13–15,42,103). Isometry is much discussed in relation to ACL replacement, but its true role, or even existence, has yet to be defined (32). True isometry implies that no elongation occurs in the ACL throughout the range of motion, and this appears not to be the case. Ideally, instead of discussing isometry, the minimum permissible change in length and tension should be addressed, because these are two of the most important factors that lead to failure of the reconstructive procedure. With the knee moving from 90 degrees of flexion to full extension, 3 mm is considered an acceptable change in length. Mueller (32) has suggested that instead of using the term isometric, we should use the term anatomometric. This implies that there are strict anatomic-biomechanic rules that should be adhered to in the placement of the ACL substitute.

Other factors that are thought to influence graft survival are the position of the graft fixation sites and the initial graft tension (14). Although the composite fibers of the ACL have no single isometric point, each individual fiber has an origin and an insertion. When the ACL is replaced by a synthetic graft of parallel fibers, the positioning of the graft is even more critical in order to avoid undue stresses during range of motions. If the graft lies too anteriorly, there is increased tension during flexion, and if the graft lies too posteriorly, there is increased tension during extension. Because the *in situ* load in the normal ACL is not known, it is difficult to prescribe an exact value for the *in situ* tension. However, if it is too low it will give insufficient joint stability, and if it is too

high it may lead to early graft failure. An initial graft tension of 20 N is advocated. Yoshiya et al. (103) found that when they applied loads of 1 N and 39 N, respectively, to autografts in dogs, there was no difference in the maximum load and linear stiffness 3 months postoperatively. However, the autografts tensioned to 39 N showed degeneration after 3 months, and both initial tensions demonstrated increased joint laxity. Increasing pretension in a synthetic graft of 10 to 40 N results in a significant increase in the amount of load in the graft at different flexion angles, in the presence or absence of a quadriceps force.

Abrasive resistance must be taken into account in the design of any prosthesis because the generation of wear particles gives rise to a number of adverse effects (74), and abrasion increases the risk of rupture. There are several technical considerations that can also alleviate this problem, such as correct surgical routing, smaller graft design, and various coverings for the graft. Increasing the hardness of the graft is not a desirable option because this induces increased stress on the adjacent bone (76). The emphasis should be on proper surgical technique and the removal of osteophytes, particularly from the intercondylar groove. Chamfering the edges of the bony tunnels is also thought to help.

The design features of the prosthesis should emphasize as small a graft as is compatible with normal function. Because of its multifascicular structure, Veltri (97) suggested that the best configuration for a synthetic graft is a two-bundle ligament that closely resembles the original ACL. The important technical considerations are that the graft should be amenable to open and arthroscopic placement. Correct tunnel placement and preparation of the edges, as with natural substitutes, are even more important with synthetic grafts.

CURRENT ADVANCES AND FUTURE DIRECTIONS

Prosthetic Coating

The current direction of prosthetic ACL replacements has been and continues to be guided by methods aimed at improving on the drawbacks of existing materials. Early fragmentation of carbon fiber implants noted in both animal and human trials has been partially amended by the application of a resorbable coat of either a copolymer (polylactic acid/polycapralactone or polyglycollic/polylactic acid) (6,35,99) or collagen (19,68). The end result has been an observable decrease in intrasynovial carbon fibers with continued good Type I and Type II collagen colonization (89). Similarly, to decrease abrasion of Dacron implants, a silicone coating was attempted. After a 70% failure rate of this prototype at 2 to 4 years, it was abandoned (41).

The variable results of tissue ingrowth into the scaffold-type prostheses has also been addressed. It has been shown that a suprapatellar synovial sheath sewn over a coated carbon fiber implant yielded a greater amount of fibrous tissue ingrowth and more fibroblasts, resulting in a neoligament twice the size of the native ACL (93).

Dacron covalently cross-linked with Type I collagen at a free amine site demonstrated improved cellular response to the implant and surrounding connective tissue *in vitro* and *in vivo* (90). Decreased inflammatory response (fewer polymorphonucleocytes and giant cells) and increased fibroblast response with new collagen production was noted.

In vitro seeding of Dacron grafts with autogenous cultured fibroblasts before *in vivo* implantation has also been attempted with a marked improvement in collagenous ingrowth (12).

Design Changes

Most notable in this category of synthetic ACL modifications is the restructuring of the Gore-Tex prosthesis into the prototypic compact design. The new model is composed of the same ePTFE, but has a decreased intra-articular cross-section of 28 mm², compared with the original dimension of 49 mm², with fibers arranged in parallel fashion. These two alterations are to reduce intercondylar abrasion and the resultant fragmentation/rupture that follows. It is easier to implant giving better visualization of the notch, which also apparently facilitates tensioning (49,86). In all nonwear parameters (cyclic elongation, bending fatigue, UTS) the compact design Gore-Tex matched or exceeded its predecessor, and lasted twice as long in abrasion testing.

In vivo testing could not demonstrate any new adverse biologic reaction, and resulted in a residual strength in goats at 6 months of 2,370 N (7) and at 1 year of 2,158 N (9). This corresponds to 1,180 N and 1,134 N for the original design at the same time intervals. The native goat ACL strength was measured at 1,810 N. Less impingement and less prosthetic abrasion was observed (7).

The compact design is currently being tested on a limited basis outside the United States, but it is reported that 15,000 have been implanted worldwide (8,11). In a series of 170 such patients with early follow-up at a mean of 17 months, there was a statistically significant subjective and objective improvement in stability over the original design at the same time interval. Overall complications decreased from 8.1% to 3.5%, with fewer effusions (none) and ruptures (1.2% versus 2.7%) (49,86).

New Materials

Few new promising synthetic materials have recently surfaced in the field of ACL prosthetics. One notable exception that could be considered a biologic replacement (such as the bovine xenograft) is reconstituted collagen. This implant consists of high-strength, biodegradable, composite Type I collagen prepared from purified bovine corium, and is cross-linked with either glutaraldehyde or by a dehydrothermal/carbodimide process (25,51). Fibers are 50 μm in diameter in each reconstituted ligament and are embedded in an un–cross-linked collagen matrix.

Further advancements in the field of prosthetic ACL technology are inevitable. The advantages of synthetic ACL reconstructions alone or in conjunction with tissue augmentation are evident: (a) elimination of the morbidity of autologous tissue harvest; (b) initial strength of the replacement; (c) technical ease of placement; and (d) reduction of rehabilitation to achieve preoperative levels of activity. Campbell et al. (17) polled orthopedic surgeons specializing in knee reconstruction and found the general consensus to be that the use of synthetics alone or with augmentation will increase from its present 5% of all ACL reconstruction to 33% within the next 10 years.

REFERENCES

1. Ahfeld SA, Larson RL, Collins HR. (1987): Anterior cruciate ligament reconstruction in the chronically unstable knee using an expanded polytetrafluoroethylene (PTFE) prosthetic ligament. *Am J Sports Med* 15:326–330.
2. Amis AA, Camburn M, Kempson SA, Radford WJP, Stead AC. (1992): ACL reconstruction with polyester fibers: long-term tissue results and joint stability in the sheep. In: 38th annual meeting of the Orthopaedic Research Society, Washington, DC.
3. Arnoczky SA, Warren RF, Ashlock MA. (1986): Replacement of the anterior cruciate ligament using a patellar tendon allograft. An experimental study. *J Bone Joint Surg* 68A:376–385.
4. Asahina S, Muneta T, Sakai H, Hokama R, Takakuda K. (1992): Biomechanical and histological study of ACL reconstruction augmented with LAD in rabbits. In: 38th annual meeting of the Orthopaedic Research Society, Washington, DC.
5. Bartolozzi P, Salvi M, Velluti C. (1990): Long-term follow-up of 53 cases of chronic lesions of the anterior cruciate ligament treated with an artificial Dacron Stryker ligament. *Ital J Orthop Trauma* 16:467–480.
6. Bercovy M, Goutallier D, Voisin MC, et al. (1985): Carbon-PGLA prostheses for ligament reconstruction. *Clin Orthop* 196:159–167.
7. Berman AB, Vireday C, Bain JR. (1989): The goat model for prosthetic anterior cruciate ligament reconstruction. In: 15th annual meeting of the Society of Biomaterials. Lake Buena Vista, FL.
8. Berman AB. (1990): The Gore-Tex compact diameter cruciate ligament prosthesis. In: 7th international symposium. Advances in cruciate ligament reconstruction of the knee: autogenous vs prosthetic, Palm Desert, CA.
9. Berman AB, Barnes T, Kovach L, Vireday C. (1990): In vitro and in vivo wear testing of ligament prostheses. In: 16th annual meeting of the Society for Biomaterials, Charleston, SC.
10. Bolton CW, Bruchman WC. (1985): The Gore-Tex expanded polytetrafluoroethylene prosthetic ligament. An in vitro and in vivo evaluation. *Clin Orthop* 196:202–213.
11. Bolton W. (1990): The Gore-Tex ligament: a historical review—1979–1990. In: 7th international symposium. Advances in cruciate ligament reconstruction of the knee: autogenous vs prosthetic, Palm Desert, CA.
12. Brody GA, Eisinger M, Arnoczky SP, Warren RF. (1988): In-vitro fibroblast seeding of prosthetic anterior cruciate ligaments. *Am J Sports Med* 16:203–208.

13. Burks RT, Daniel DM. (1984): Anterior cruciate graft preload and knee stability. *Orthop Trans* 8:52.

14. Butler DL, Martin ET, Kaiser AD, Grood ES, Chun KJ, Sodd AN. (1988): The effects of flexion and tibial rotation on the 3-D orientations and lengths of human anterior cruciate ligament bundles. In: Transactions of the Orthopaedic Research Society, Atlanta, GA.

15. Bylski-Austrow DI, Grood ES, Hefzy MS, Butler DL. (1990): Anterior cruciate ligament replacements: a mechanical study of femoral attachment location, flexion angle at tensioning and initial tension. *J Orthop Res* 8:522–531.

16. Campbell JD, Wills RP, Arnstone K, Feagin JA. Current trends in repair and rehabilitation of anterior cruciate ligament injuries, medial collateral ligament injuries, and meniscal injuries [*in press*].

17. Chen EH, Black J. (1980): Material design analysis of the prosthetic anterior cruciate ligament. *J Biomed Mater Res* 14:567–586.

18. Claes L, Durselen L. (1991): Results of ligament replacement in sheep using 8 different devices. In: 37th annual meeting of the Orthopaedic Research Society, Anaheim, CA.

19. Claes L, Neugebauer R. (1985): In vivo and in vitro investigation of the long-term behavior and fatigue strength of carbon fiber ligament replacement. *Clin Orthop* 196:99–111.

20. Cooper DE, Deng XH, Warren RF, Burstein AH. (1992): Strength of the central third patellar graft: a biomechanical study. In: Annual meeting of the American Academy of Orthopaedic Surgeons, Washington, DC.

21. Corner EM. (1914): Notes of a case illustrative of an artificial anterior cruciate ligament, demonstrating the action of that ligament. *Proc R Soc Med* 7:120–121.

22. Dahlstedt L, Dalen N, Jonnson U. (1990): Gortex prosthetic ligament vs. Kennedy ligament augmentation device in anterior cruciate ligament reconstruction. A prospective randomized 3 year follow-up of 41 cases. *Acta Orthop Scand* 61:217–227.

23. Del Pizzo W. (1990): US Kennedy LAD clinical experience. In: 7th international symposium. Advances in cruciate ligament reconstruction of the knee: autogenous vs prosthetic, Palm Desert, CA.

24. Denti M, Arosio A, Monteleone M, Peretti G. (1990): Preliminary assessment of anterior cruciate reconstruction with the Leeds-Keio artificial ligament. *Am J Knee Surg* 3:181–186.

25. Dunn MG, Kato YP, Tria AJ, Bechler JR, Zawadsky JP. (1991): ACL replacement using a composite collagenous material: preliminary implantation results. In: 37th annual meeting of the Orthopaedic Research Society, Anaheim, CA.

26. Ferkel RD, Fox JM, Wood D, Del Pizzo W, Friedman MJ, Snyder SJ. (1989): Arthroscopic "second look" at the Gore-Tex ligament. *Am J Sports Med* 17:147–153.

27. Ferl JG, Goldenthal KJ, Mishra NK. (1988): FDA regulation of prosthetic ligament devices. In: Friedman MJ, Ferkel RD, eds. *Prosthetic ligament reconstruction of the knee.* Philadelphia: WB Saunders, pp. 202–208.

28. Fischer SP, Ferkel RD. (1988): Biomechanics of the knee. In: Friedman MJ, Ferkel RD, eds. *Prosthetic reconstruction of the knee.* Philadelphia: WB Saunders.

29. Fowler PJ. (1990): Long-term follow up of intraarticular ACL reconstructions augmented with braided polypropylene (Kennedy LAD). In: 7th international symposium. Advances in cruciate ligament reconstruction of the knee: autogenous vs. prosthetic, Palm Desert, CA.

30. Fox J. (1977): Report on the clinical results of Polyflex ligament replacement. Presented to FDA Orthopedic Panel. April 15, 1977, Washington, D.C.

31. Friedman MJ. (1991): Prosthetic anterior cruciate ligaments. *Clin Sports Med* 10:499–513.

32. Fu FH, Daniel DM, Gillquist J, et al. (1990): Management of anterior cruciate ligament injuries. *Contemp Orthop* 21:393–424.

33. Fujikawa K. (1990): Clinical study on anterior cruciate reconstruction with the Leeds-Keio artificial ligament. In: 7th international symposium. Advances in cruciate ligament reconstruction of the knee: autogenous vs prosthetic, Palm Desert, CA.

34. Fukubayashi J, Torzilli PA, Sherman MF, Warren RF. (1982): An in vitro biomechanical evaluation of anterior-posterior mo-

tion of the knee. Tibial displacement, rotation and torque. *J Bone Joint Surg* 64A:258–264.

35. Funk FJ. (1987): Synthetic ligaments: current status. *Clin Orthop* 196:107–111.

36. Gaisser DM, Bauer TW, Shoda E, Moody JA, Reger SI. (1989): A polyethylene ACL prosthesis in sheep: mechanical and histologic evaluation after three months. In: 15th annual meeting of the Society for Biomaterials, Lake Buena Vista, FL.

37. Glousman R, Shields C, Kerlan R, Tibone J, Gambardella R. (1988): Gore-Tex prosthetic ligament in anterior cruciate deficient knees. *Am J Sports Med* 16:321–326.

38. Goertzen MJ, Mendenhall HV, Schulitz KP, Arnoczky SP. (1990): ACL reconstruction using anterior cruciate ligament allograft in dogs—results with and without ligament augmentation device (LAD). In: 36th annual meeting of the Orthopaedic Research Society, New Orleans, LA.

39. WL Gore and Associates. (1989). Gore-Tex cruciate ligament prosthesis: 5-year clinical results. Flagstaff, AZ.

40. Grood ES, Noyes FR. (1976): Cruciate ligament prostheses: strength, creep and fatigue properties. *J Bone Joint Surg* 58A:1083–1088.

41. Gupta BN, Brinker WO. (1969): An anterior cruciate ligament prosthesis in the dog. *J Am Vet Med Assoc* 154:1057–1061.

42. Hefzy MS, Grood ES. (1986): Sensitivity of insertion locations on length patterns of anterior cruciate ligament fibers. *J Biomech Eng* 108:73–82.

43. Heich HH, Walker PS. (1976): Stabilizing mechanisms of the loaded and unloaded knee joint. *J Bone Joint Surg* 58A:87–93.

44. Huylebrock J. (1990): Leeds-Keio ligament clinical results. In: 7th international symposium. Advances in cruciate ligament reconstruction of the knee: autogenous vs prosthetic, Palm Desert, CA.

45. Indelicato PA, Pascale MS, Huegel M. (1989): Early experience with the Gore-Tex polytetrafluoroethylene anterior cruciate ligament prosthesis. *Am J Sports Med* 17:55–62.

46. James SL, Woods GW, Homsy CA, Prewitt JM, Slocum DB. (1979): Cruciate ligament stents in reconstruction of the unstable knee: a preliminary report. *Clin Orthop* 143:90–96.

47. Jenkins DHR. (1978): The repair of cruciate ligaments with flexible carbon fibre. A longer term study of the induction of new ligaments and the fate of the implanted carbon. *J Bone Joint Surg* 60B:520–522.

48. Johnson DH. (1991): Arthroscopic reconstruction of the anterior cruciate ligament with Gore-Tex graft. *Am J Sports Med* 19:540.

49. Johnson DH. (1992): Arthroscopic reconstruction of the anterior cruciate ligament with the Goretex prosthetic ligament: a single centre clinical comparison of two expanded polytetrafluoroethylene (ePTFE) prosthetic ligament designs. In: 8th international symposium. Update 1992. New perspectives in arthroscopy and sports medicine, Palm Springs, CA.

50. Karzel RP, Diefendorf DR, Fox JM, et al. (1990): Four year experience with the Gore-Tex prosthetic ligament in anterior cruciate deficient knees. In: Annual meeting of the American Academy of Orthopaedic Surgeons, New Orleans, LA.

51. Kato YP, Dunn MG, Tria AJ, Zawadsky JP, Silver FH. (1990): Preliminary assessment of a collagen fiber ACL prosthesis. In: 16th annual meeting of the Society for Biomaterials, Charleston, SC.

52. Kennedy JC, Hawkins RJ, Willis RB. (1977): Strain gauge analysis of knee ligaments. *Clin Orthop* 129:225–229.

53. Kennedy JC, Hawkins RJ, Willis RB, Danylchuk KD. (1974): Tension studies of human knee ligaments. *J Bone Joint Surg* 56A:350–355.

54. Laboureau JP, Cazenave A. (1990): Presentation of the ligastic ligament. In: 7th international symposium. Advances in cruciate ligament reconstruction of the knee: autogenous vs prosthetic, Palm Desert, CA.

55. Laboureau JP, Cazenave A. (1990): A two bundle artificial plasty of the posterior cruciate ligament: surgical technique and results of an experience of eight years. In: 7th international symposium. Advances in cruciate ligament reconstruction of the knee: autogenous vs prosthetic, Palm Desert, CA.

56. Laboureau JP, Cazenave A, Abbink P. (1990): Fresh injuries of the anterior cruciate ligament. Future of a new reinforcement

ligament. Results after a five year experience. In: 7th international symposium. Advances in cruciate ligament reconstruction of the knee: autogenous vs prosthetic, Palm Desert, CA.

57. Laboureau JP, Dericks GH. (1992): 105 anterior cruciate ligament reconstruction cases using the ligament reconstruction system (ligastic) by arthroscopic technique. November 1989–December 1991. In: 8th international symposium. Update 1992. New perspectives in arthroscopy and sports medicine, Palm Springs, CA.

58. Larson RL. (1988): Prosthetic replacement of knee ligaments: overview. In: Feagin JA, ed. *The crucial ligaments.* New York: Churchill Livingstone, pp. 495–506.

59. Lewis JL, Lew WD, Engerbretsen E, Hunter RE, Kowalczky C. (1991): Factors affecting graft force in surgical reconstruction of the anterior cruciate ligament. *J Orthop Res* 8:514–521.

60. Lopez-Vasquez E, Juan JA, Vila E, Debon J. (1991): Reconstruction of the anterior cruciate ligament with a Dacron prosthesis. *J Bone Joint Surg* 73A:1294–1300.

61. Lukianov AV, Richard JC, Barret GR, Gilquist J. (1989): A multicenter study on the results of anterior cruciate ligament reconstruction using a Dacron ligament prosthesis in "salvage" cases. *Am J Sports Med* 17:380–385.

62. Marcacci M, Gubellini P, Busta R, et al. (1991): Histologic and ultrastructural findings of tissue ingrowth. The Leeds-Keio prosthetic anterior cruciate ligament. *Clin Orthop* 267:115–121.

63. Markolf KL, Pattee GA, Strum GM, Gallick GS, Sherman OH, Dorey FJ. (1989): Instrumented measurements of laxity in patients who have a Gore-Tex anterior cruciate ligament substitute. *J Bone Joint Surg* 71A:887–893.

64. Marloff KL, Mensch JS, Amstutz HC. (1976): Stiffness and laxity of the knee: the contribution of the supporting structures. A quantitative in-vitro study. *J Bone Joint Surg* 58A:583–594.

65. McPherson GK, Mendenhall HV, Gibbons DF. (1985): Experimental, mechanical and histological evaluation of the Kennedy ligament augmentation device. *Clin Orthop* 196:186–195.

66. Meglan D, Zueler W, Buck W, Berme N. (1986): The effects of quadriceps force upon strain in the anterior cruciate ligament. In: Transactions of the Orthopaedic Research Society, New Orleans, LA.

67. Mendenhall HV, Roth JH, Kennedy JC, Winter GD, Lumb WV. (1987): Evaluation of a polypropylene braid as a prosthetic anterior cruciate ligament in the dog. *Am J Sports Med* 15:543–546.

68. Mendes DG, Iusim M, Angel D, et al. (1985): Properties of the carbon fiber augmented ligament tendon: a laboratory and clinical study. *Clin Orthop* 196:51–60.

69. Monahan JJ, Grigg P, Pappas AM, et al. (1984): In-vivo strain patterns in the four major canine knee ligaments. *J Orthop Res* 2:408–418.

70. Noyes FR, Grood ES. (1976): The strength of the anterior cruciate ligament in humans and rhesus monkeys. Age-related and species related changes. *J Bone Joint Surg* 58A:1074–1082.

71. Noyes FR, Grood ES, Zernick RF, Hefzy MS. (1980): Biomechanical analysis of human ligament grafts in knee ligament repairs and reconstruction. *J Bone Joint Surg* 62A:687–695.

72. Noyes FR, Moar PA, Matthews DS, Butler DL. (1983): The symptomatic anterior cruciate deficient knee. *J Bone Joint Surg* 65A:1541–1562.

73. O'Brien SJ, Warren RF, Pavlov H, Panariello R, Wickewicz TL. (1991): Reconstruction of the chronically insufficient anterior cruciate ligament with the central third of the patellar ligament. *J Bone Joint Surg* 73A:278–286.

74. Olson EJ, Kang JD, Fu FH, Georgescu HI, Mason GC, Evans CH. (1988): The biochemical and histological effects of artificial ligament wear particles: in vitro and in vivo studies. *Am J Sports Med* 16:558–570.

75. Parke JP. (1991): Dacron ligament prosthesis for anterior cruciate ligament reconstruction. In: Scott WN, ed. *Ligament and extensor mechanism injuries of the knee.* St. Louis, MO: Mosby Yearbook, pp. 331–339.

76. Parke JP, Grana WA, Chitwood JS. (1985): A high-strength Dacron augmentation for cruciate ligament reconstruction. A two year canine study. *Clin Orthop* 196:175–185.

77. Piziali RL, Seering WC, Nagel DA, Schurman DJ. (1980): The function of the primary ligaments of the knee in anterior-posterior and medial-lateral motion. *J Biomech* 13:377–384.

78. Rauch G, Allzeit B, Gotzen L. (1988): Biomechanical studies of the tensile strength of the anterior cruciate ligament with special reference to age dependence. *Unfallchirurg* 91:437–443.

79. Roth JH. (1986): Polypropylene braid augmented and nonaugmented intraarticular anterior cruciate ligament reconstruction. In: 3rd annual symposium. Prosthetic ligament reconstruction of the knee, Scottsdale, AZ.

80. Roth JH, Kennedy JC, Lockstadt H, McCallum CL, Cunning LA. (1985): Polypropylene braid augmented and nonaugmented intraarticular anterior cruciate ligament reconstruction. *Am J Sports Med* 13:321–336.

80a. Rusch RM. (1988): Integraft anterior cruciate ligament reconstruction. In: Friedman MJ, Ferkel RD, eds. *Prosthetic ligament reconstruction of the knee.* Philadelphia: WB Saunders.

81. Rushton N, Dandy DJ, Naylor CPE. (1983): The clinical, arthroscopic and histological findings after replacement of the anterior cruciate ligament with carbon-fibre. *J Bone Joint Surg* 65B:308–309.

82. Salvi M, Velluti C, Misasi M, Bartolozzi P, Quacci D, Del Orbo C. (1991): Ultrastructure of periprosthetic Dacron knee ligament tissue. Two cases of ruptured anterior cruciate ligament reconstruction. *Acta Orthop Scand* 62:174–177.

83. Scharling M. (1981): Replacement of the anterior cruciate ligament with a polyethylene prosthetic ligament. *Acta Orthop Scand* 52:575–578.

84. Schindhelm K, Rogers GJ, Multhorpe BK, et al. (1991): Autograft and Leeds-Keio reconstructions of the bovine anterior cruciate ligament. *Clin Orthop* 267:278–293.

84a. Seedhom BB. (1988): The Leeds-Keio ligament: biomechanics. In: Friedman MJ, Ferkel RD, eds. *Prosthetic ligament reconstruction of the knee.* Philadelphia: WB Saunders.

85. Seedhom BB. (1990): The Leeds-Keio ligament concepts and mechanical aspects of the device. In: 7th international symposium. Advances in cruciate ligament reconstruction of the knee: autogenous vs prosthetic, Palm Desert, CA.

86. Settlage RA, Johnson DJ, Berman AB. (1992): Laboratory and clinical comparison of two Goretex ligaments. In: 8th international symposium. Update 1992. New perspectives in arthroscopy and sports medicine, Palm Springs, CA.

87. Sidles JA, Larson RV, Gabrini JL, Downey DJ, Matsen FA. (1988): Ligament length relationships in the moving knee. *J Orthop Res* 6:593–610.

88. Smith A. (1918): Diagnosis and treatment of injuries of the crucial ligaments. *Br J Surg* 6:176–189.

89. Strover AE, Firer P. (1985): The use of carbon fibre implants in anterior cruciate ligament surgery. *Clin Orthop* 196:88–98.

90. Suganama J, Pachence J, Alexander H, Ricci JL. (1991): In vitro and in vivo response to collagen-coated Dacron fibers. In: 17th annual meeting of the Society for Biomaterials, Scottsdale, AZ.

91. Takai S, Adams DJ, Livesay GA, Woo SL-Y. (1991): Estimation of loads in the ACL. In: Transactions of the Orthopaedic Research Society, Anaheim, CA.

92. Tietge RA, Rojas F. (1984): Anterior cruciate ligament reconstruction using a bovine xenograft prosthesis. In: American Orthopaedic Society of Sports Medicine, Atlanta, GA.

93. Townley CO, Fumich RM, Shall LM. (1985): The free synovial graft as a shield for collagen ingrowth in cruciate ligament repair. *Clin Orthop* 192:266–271.

94. Trent PS, Walker PS, Wolf P. (1976): Ligament length patterns, strength and rotational axes of the knee joint. *Clin Orthop* 117:263–270.

95. Vahey JW, Draganich LF. (1991): Tensions in the anterior and posterior cruciate ligaments of the knee during passive loading: predicting the ligament loads from in-situ measurements. *J Orthop Res* 9:529–538.

96. Van Kampen GL. (1990): Biomechanics of the 3M Kennedy LAD. In: 7th international symposium. Advances in cruciate ligament reconstruction of the knee: autogenous vs prosthetic, Palm Desert, CA.

97. Veltri D, Fulkerson J. (1989): Isometricity of Y-graft replacement in the anterior cruciate ligament. In: Transactions of the Orthopaedic Research Society, Las Vegas, NV.

98. Von Mironova SS. (1978): Spatresultate der rekonstruktion des bandapparates des uniegelenks mit lawson. *Zentralbl Chir* 103:432.

99. Weiss AB, Blazina ME, Goldstein AR, Alexander H. (1985): Ligament replacement with an absorbable copolymer carbon fiber scaffold: early clinical experience. *Clin Orthop* 196:77–85.

100. Whipple TL. (1988): Arthroscopic anterior cruciate ligament reconstruction with Procol xenograft bioprosthesis. In: Friedman MJ, Ferkel RD, eds. *Prosthetic ligament reconstruction of the knee.* Philadelphia: WB Saunders, pp. 112–117.

101. Woo SL-Y, Adams DJ, Takai S: Human anterior cruciate ligament and its replacement: biomechanical considerations. In: Niwa S, Perren SM, Hattori T, eds. *Biomechanics in Orthopedics.* Tokyo: Springer-Verlag, pp 13–30.

102. Woo SL-Y, Hollis JM, Adams DJ, Lyon RL, Takai S. (1991): Tensile properties of the human femur–anterior-cruciate ligament–tibia complex: the effect of specimen age and orientation. *Am J Sports Med* 19:217–225.

103. Yoshiya S, Andrish JT, Manley M, Bauer TW. (1987): Graft tension in anterior cruciate ligament reconstruction: an in-vivo study in dogs. *Am J Sports Med* 12:322–327.

The Anterior Cruciate Ligament: Current and Future Concepts, edited by D.W. Jackson, et al. Raven Press, Ltd., New York © 1993.

CHAPTER 31

Patellar Entrapment Following Anterior Cruciate Ligament Injury

Lonnie Paulos and Robert Meislin

When the orthopedic surgeon informs the patient of potential complications AFTER anterior cruciate ligament (ACL) surgery, postoperative stiffness as a generic possibility should headline the physician's informed consent. One only has to look at results from the various cruciate ligament articles to see how serious the problem of arthrofibrosis can be (4,6,12,13,15–23). In 1986 Paulos et al. presented patellar entrapment syndrome (PES) as a major cause of reduced range of motion after knee surgery (16). Unique to this group of patients was the combination of decreased knee extension and flexion associated with patella entrapment.

PES is defined as a loss of knee extension ≥10 degrees or loss of knee flexion ≥25 degrees of knee flexion with significantly reduced patellar mobility. Decreased patellar mobility is measured in extension and manifested by the loss of positive passive patellar tilt (Fig. 1), less than one quadrant of medial and lateral patellar glide (Fig. 2), and less than 5 mm of superior and inferior patellar glide (which may in reality be more a reflection of tilt than glide).

Traditionally, the extension contracture has been treated by suprapatellar, quadriceps, and peripatellar release, whereas the flexion contracture (in the past exclusive to pediatric and neuromuscular disorders) has been treated with posterior tendon lengthening and capsular release. Patients that meet the criteria of PES must be approached in a systematic and individualized manner.

BACKGROUND

Based on an initial review of 28 consecutive cases of PES, Paulos et al. described an entity that presented in two varieties: primary, an "exaggerated pathologic hyperplasia of the anterior soft tissues of the knee beyond that associated with normal healing," and secondary, a host of surgical factors that included postoperative immobility, quadriceps insufficiency, nonisometric liga-

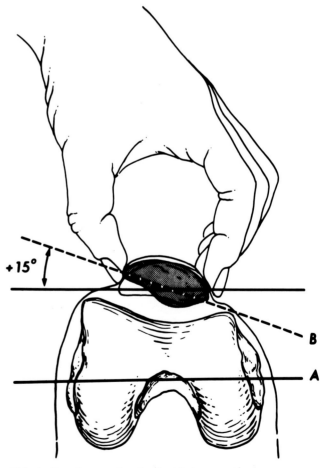

FIG. 1. Passive patellar tilt of +15 degrees is demonstrated. A tilt of 0 degrees or less indicates tight lateral restraints.

L. Paulos and R. Meislin: The Orthopedic Specialty Hospital, Salt Lake City, Utah 84107.

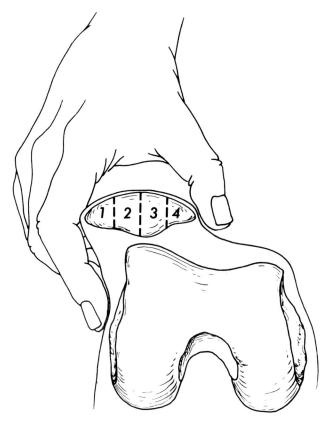

FIG. 2. Passive lateral glide test demonstrating a patella being subluxated laterally to its second quadrant. Decreased patellar mobility is manifested by less than one quadrant of medial and lateral glides.

ment surgery, graft impingement, excessive graft tension, infection, reflex sympathetic dystrophy, and an entrapped meniscus. In their experience, ACL surgery was the most common cause of patella entrapment and subsequent infrapatellar contracture syndrome (IPCS) (16).

In following these patients from acute presentation to patella infera, PES could be defined as a syndrome. It became clear that PES was a distinct clinical entity with a presentation, pathophysiology, and clinical course that was both diagnostic and, for the most part, predictable. Three stages of IPCS were identified: the prodromal stage (stage I), the active stage (stage II), and the residual or "burned out" stage (stage III) (16). For each stage there was a clinical presentation and period that was unique. We believe now that emphasis on staging should be based on clinical examination with the timing from surgery or injury used only as a general frame of reference.

PRODROMAL STAGE (STAGE 1)

This stage is characterized by diffuse edema present throughout the periarticular tissues, particularly in the area of the patellar tendon and fat pad. Physical examination demonstrates a painful active range of motion, tenderness along the patellar tendon, restricted patellar mobility, and a quadriceps lag. A quadriceps lag is defined as passive range of motion greater than active extension. Patients in this stage fail to progress during physical therapy, are unable to do full extension, and have associated pain and swelling. Toward the latter part of this stage, induration of the fat pad and retinacular tissues is noted. Although the prodromal stage was initially described to take effect within 2 to 8 weeks of the patient's surgery or injury, this initial stage may be seen to exist as late as 6 months.

ACTIVE STAGE (STAGE II)

At this stage, a quadriceps lag is no longer present. Rather, patients demonstrate restriction in both active and passive knee extension and flexion. As a result, significant quadriceps atrophy follows along with patellar crepitus. Decreased patellar mobility is noted with limitation of glides and tilts; superior glide is restricted the most. Extraarticular involvement is manifested by a "shelf sign" (Fig. 3). There is generally less swelling and warmth. This stage was initially recognized within 6 to 20 weeks of surgery or injury with the patients victims of vigorous, forceful physical therapy (including manipulations) that only aggravated their problem. Finally, the patients ambulate with a "short leg" gait due to their inability to actively gain full extension.

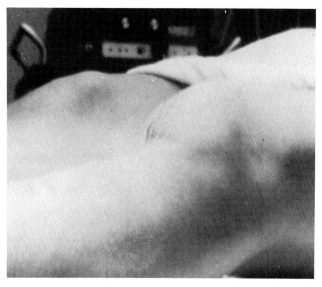

FIG. 3. Stage II (active stage): The presence of the "shelf sign" in the left knee is typical of this stage. Continued peripatellar swelling and induration with severely restricted patellar motion, particularly superior glide, is evident.

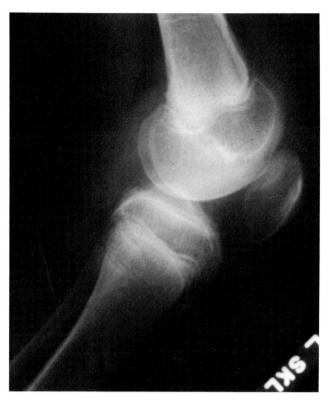

FIG. 4. Lateral radiograph illustrating marked patella infera secondary to infrapatellar contracture syndrome.

RESIDUAL STAGE (STAGE III)

Continued quadriceps atrophy is noted with restricted flexion and extension. Patellar mobility is decreased but is not as restricted as in stage II. This is attributed to diminished inflammation and induration about the peripatellar and retinacular tissues. Developmental patella infera may be the *sine qua non* of this stage (Fig. 4). Significant patellofemoral arthrosis is presented manifested by severe crepitus and decreased joint space in both lateral and merchant radiographs. If enough time has elapsed, residual infera and patellofemoral arthrosis may be the only symptoms.

PATELLA INFERA: DIAGNOSIS

There are currently several popular methods of identifying patella infera. The Blumensaat method is based on a 30-degree flexed knee lateral radiograph. The inferior pole of the patella should lie at the roof of the intercondylar notch (Blumensaat's line) (2). The Insall-Salvati method measures the length of the patellar tendon (LT) and the length of the patella (LP) measured at its greatest diagonal length. A ratio defined as LT:LP is determined and has an average of 1.02, with a standard deviation of 0.13 (8). Patella infera is considered present when the ratio is less than 0.8. Noyes et al. use a patellar vertical

height ratio, A:B, measuring the distance between the most ventral (anterosuperior) rim of the tibial plateau and the most inferior end of the patellar articular surface (A) to the maximum length of the patellar articular surface (B) and stress the importance of measuring the contralateral normal knee (13). If the difference between the two knees is greater than 11% to 15%, then "developmental patella infera" is suggested. The normal value is 1.04 (standard deviation 0.13) with infera present when the ratio is less than 0.75. Finally, the Blackburne-Peel method generates a ratio comparing the distance from the distal pole of the patellar articular cartilage with a perpendicular line drawn at the level of the tibial plateau (PA) and the length of the patellar articular surface (TA). A ratio defined as PA:TA is determined and ranges from 0.54 to 1.06. Patellar infera is considered present when the ratio is less than 0.54 (1). Because this method has the least amount of variability, we prefer this latter method for determining patella infera that occurs as a late presentation of PES.

PATHOLOGY

Insight into the pathophysiology was gained when Paulos et al. examined and correlated the cadaver sections of the anterior knee with the microscopic and macroscopic pathology from the treated patients (16).

In the active stage of the disease the patella becomes adherent to the fibrotic fat pad after fat pad inflammation. Histologically, the fatty tissue of the fat pad is replaced by a stroma of engulfing fibrous and inflammatory cells (Fig. 5). This fibrous tissue extends from the anterior fat pad, the medial and lateral gutters becoming involved with the anterior horns of the medial and lateral menisci, as well as the parapatellar plicae.

Patients in the residual stage may develop an invading fibrotic pannus that leads to anterior impingement and patellar tendon contraction. Like rheumatoid pannus, the fibrotic pannus of PES damages the articular cartilage by interfering with hyaline nutrition, and by causing mechanical injury to the knee joint by mass effect. Biopsy results demonstrate a loss of glycosaminoglycans. Flexion contracture and patella infera with resulting patellofemoral arthrosis is the end stage.

The potential for fibrotic formation with associated flexion contracture is understandable once the anatomy is reviewed. The patellar tendon is encompassed by fascial and fibrofascial planes. The fibrofatty pad is adherent to the inferior pole of the patella and the proximal patellar tendon. Anteriorly, bursal type tissues separate the tendon from the overlying deep fascia of the knee that contains organized collagenous tissue for the iliotibial band laterally and the medial patellofemoral ligaments. In addition, fibrous hyperplasia has its foundation in the patellomeniscal ligaments (Kaplan's liga-

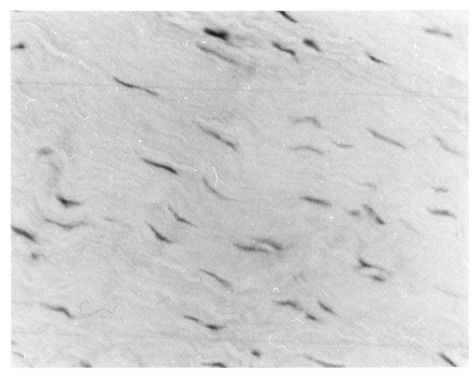

FIG. 5. Hematoxylin-eosin–stained capsular biopsy sample demonstrates diffuse fibrotic and inflammatory response with random collagen deposition.

ments) that arise from the inferior pole of the patella, as well as in the medial and lateral portions of the fat pad that attach to the anterior horns of both menisci (10). Decreased flexion has its basis in intraarticular adhesion bands in the suprapatellar pouch, as well as extraarticular patellofemoral bands that arise from the proximal pole of the patella and extend to the anterior surface of the femur (14). Sprague believes that these bands represent fibrotic fibers of the vastus intermedius muscle (22). These findings should all be differentiated from the "cyclops" lesion that Jackson described (9). The number of anatomical sites involved thus dictates the structures that must be addressed during surgical release and debridement.

TREATMENT

Critical to the management of PES is the orthopedic surgeon's ability to read the soft tissues about the knee. Initially, during the waiting period after surgery or injury when the patient shows no progress despite early range of motion and manual patellar mobilization, the physician should use corticosteroid dose packs, nonsteroidal antiinflammatory drugs (NSAIDs), and transcutaneous electrical nerve stimulation (TENS) units. Therapy should include a leg press program along with recommendations for swimming and cycling, because manual pushing on the knee should be avoided. During this period the patient must demonstrate a voluntary quadriceps

contraction, minimal swelling, pain, and warmth. This requires patience by the orthopedist as well as the patient, because it may require up to 4 months for the patient to gain an active quadriceps. A voluntary quadriceps contraction must exist with little or no lag before surgery.

The patient generally will not gain motion during stage I by a simple manipulation under anesthesia. Although Dodds et al. recently reported that manipulations were a safe and effective method for improving both flexion and extension in 86% of the knees that had restricted motion (less than 120 degrees of active flexion, less than 10 degrees of active extension within 6 months of surgery, and failure to gain motion more than 3 months after surgery), a closer examination is in order (5). In their report, Dodds et al. failed to report the patients' patellar mobility. This only accentuates the point that in patients that fail to progress after ACL surgery the patella must be examined for entrapment. If patellar entrapment is absent, then a 4- to 6-week course of aggressive physical therapy and drop-out casts are recommended. At that point, if no progress is achieved, arthroscopy followed by manipulation is our course of treatment. The 14% failure rate that Dodds et al. reported with manipulations performed at an average of 7 months after surgery was probably attributable to underlying PES (5).

Once stage II of PES sets in, the best treatment (because both flexion and extension is restricted) is to ap-

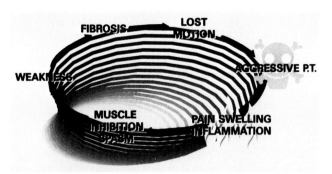

FIG. 6. Aggressive physical therapy only aggravates arthrofibrosis by causing constant pain, swelling, and inflammation.

proach extension first. Gaining extension is the priority. These patients require surgery and will only worsen with continued manual manipulation and forced passive motion (Fig. 6). If physical therapy is in place, it may be advisable to halt the therapy sessions. Open intraarticular and extraarticular debridement and release is recommended. Because of the associated flexion contracture secondary to infrapatellar and peripatellar contracture, arthroscopy will be near impossible. Open debridement includes lateral retinacular release, as well as anterior debridement of the fat pad attachments near the anterior horns of the medial and lateral menisci, and those near the intercondylar extensions to the notch. The patella and patellar tendon should be released medially, superiorly, and inferiorly, both intra- and extraarticularly, with particular attention to the retropatellar tendon bursae. A medial arthrotomy may be required to release the medial fat pad and medial patellomeniscal ligament. Often, however, incisions from the index surgery will be present and will dictate the surgical approach to the knee. Once the intra- and extra-articular regions of the knee are exposed, infrapatellar, peripatellar, and, if necessary, suprapatellar release and debridement can be performed. These incisions should be closed meticulously with staples for skin.

Because ACL surgery is such a leading factor for PES, evaluation for nonisometric placement, excessive graft tensioning, and notch impingement of the graft should be determined. Anteriorly placed tibial tunnels will helplessly result in graft impingement as the knee is extended. Howell et al. in a magnetic resonance imaging study demonstrated that eccentrically placed tibial tunnels (5 mm anteromedial to the center of ACL insertion) require 5 to 6 mm of bone removal from the intercondylar roof to prevent impingement (7). This compared with centrally placed tunnels requiring 2 to 3 mm of bone removal and minimal bone resection when the graft is placed within the bulk of the ACL fibers, 3 mm posterior to the center of the ACL insertion. A nonisometric and overtensioned graft may necessitate lengthening, if not excision. For the entrapped patella, patellar mobility must be returned to second quadrant glides and passive patellar tilt must exceed +15 degrees. If patella infera is present, a proximal tibial tubercle advancement may be performed (3,11).

Postoperatively, for both stages II and III continuous passive motion (CPM) and the use of a drop-out cast (especially at night) are necessary for a short period. Often an epidural anesthetic is helpful for the procedure so that the patient can observe the range of motion achieved at surgery and, with the epidural in place, effective painless CPM can proceed in the patient's room. These nighttime extension splints are encouraged until active extension is demonstrated by the patient. Extension is paramount; a flexion loss can always be obtained later with arthroscopy and manipulation.

Reflex sympathetic dystrophy (RSD) is differentiated from PES by the persistence and degree of pain (day and night) not normally seen in PES. In addition to a decreased range of motion, the patient with RSD will have hypersensitivity to touch with, a change in skin temperature from initial warmth to cold, to the point of becoming cyanotic with extreme exposure.

Patients with stage III PES will be refractory to vigor-

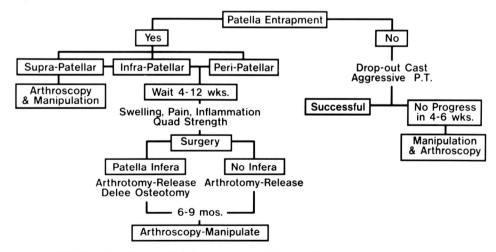

FIG. 7. Algorithm outlining our treatment for patellar entrapment syndrome.

ous physical therapy. Due to advanced arthrosis, debridement and retinacular release is of little value. Surgery should be reserved for salvage procedures such as patellectomy, Maquet osteotomy, proximal tibial tubercle advancement, and possibly total knee replacement.

An algorithm in Fig. 7 encapsulates our treatment protocol.

A CURRENT APPRAISAL

Paulos et al. recently conducted a retrospective study that outlined the long-term outcome of patients who developed PES (17). Forty-seven patients were evaluated at an average follow-up of 41 months after index procedure (range 24 to 72 months). The majority of patients had their initial surgery performed elsewhere. Primary PES predominated (66%) with most of the index cases ACL reconstructions (79%). The average number of secondary procedures for correction of entrapment was 2.6, with a range of 1 to 8. Average age for these patients was 29.9 years at the time of index surgery. Arthroscopic debridement was the most common secondary procedure.

Significant increases in range of motion and patellar mobility were noted. Extension gains averaged +11.7 degrees and flexion gains averaged +29.5 degrees. The final range of motion averaged −2.9 degrees of extension, from a preoperative range of −7 to −35 degrees (average 17), to 127.5 degrees of flexion, from a preoperative range of 60 to 139 degrees (average 98). Patellar mobility increased to an average passive patellar tilt of +5.7 degrees, superior and inferior glides of +6.5 mm, and medial and lateral glides of +1 quadrant. Lysholm scores (based on degree of pain, limp, squat, swelling, stairs, locking, instability, and need for support) averaged 72.2 of a possible total of 100. Scores for pain, limp, and squatting were low, whereas instability scores were high. KT-1000 measurements in 6 patients who required graft sacrifice for nonisometric placement confirmed this finding of continued stability. Average side-to-side differences for manual maximum was +3.08 (range +0.5 to +6). Eighty-three percent had decreased Tegner activity scores, an average reduction of 2.32 (preinjury versus follow-up).

Radiographic findings included patella osteopenia, decreased patellofemoral joint space with minor spurring, and patients with mild degenerative changes in the medial and lateral compartments. For patients who underwent proximal tibial tubercle advancement, the Blackburne-Peel patella height ratio increased from a preoperative value of 0.53 (contralateral normal knee 0.95) to a postoperative value of 0.8. Proximal advancement averaged 21.4 mm. Interestingly, patellar height indices demonstrated a tendency to recur to infera at long-term follow-up. Seventy-five percent of the patients were able to return to work, with the majority of those not working not disabled by knee symptoms. More than two thirds of the patients were athletically active at follow-up, and

75% reported that they would repeat their original decision regarding index surgery.

RISK FACTORS FOR PES

Various factors were examined that were felt to predict and affect outcome after PES presentation (17). These included patient characteristics, choice of graft, timing of index procedure, associated procedures at index surgery, and operative techniques for PES surgery.

Females who developed PES were found to predominate with good results. Those with poorer outcomes and patella infera requiring proximal advancement were predominately male and older. This was akin to the findings of Fu et al., who found male patients at a statistically significant higher risk for the development of a postoperative flexion contracture; older age only suggested a trend toward flexion contracture (6).

The timing of ACL surgery has become an increasingly popular topic as it relates to arthrofibrosis. Many investigators have reported statistically significant increases in arthrofibrosis on ACLs operated in the acute phase (defined as 3 to 6 weeks from injury) as compared with ACLs reconstructed in the subacute and chronic periods (6,12,19,20,23). Paulos et al. found an incidence of 71.4% among those acute patients requiring three or more secondary PES surgical procedures (17).

There are no data to decide whether patellar tendon autografts lead to a greater incidence of PES. Mohtadi et al. noted no difference based on the choice of autologous graft or type of reconstruction (open versus arthroscopically aided) (12). Fu et al. found a trend toward flexion contracture after autograft when compared with allograft placement (6). Paulos et al., in comparing patellar tendon autografts with other grafts (hamstring autografts, allografts), found both groups to do well (17). Patellar tendon autografts did have a greater reduction in Tegner activity score compared with other ACL reconstructive procedures. However, because most of the patellar tendon autografts were secondarily referred from other centers, with findings consisting of nonisometric placement and graft impingement (2-degree PES), firm conclusions could not be made.

Several investigators have found a relationship between associated ligamentous and meniscal injury with concomitant repair and decreased knee motion. Fu et al. found no correlation with associated meniscal repair and iliotibial band tenodesis, but did find an association with posterior oblique reefing and collateral ligament repair (6). Paulos et al. found a positive correlation between PES and associated extraarticular reconstruction and collateral ligament repair (17).

Other factors correlating with a good result with PES included patients with primary PES, and those requiring only one secondary procedure and whose secondary procedure was arthroscopic debridement. Poorer outcomes or more refractory forms of PES included secondary

PES, three or more secondary procedures, manipulation without debridement, and proximal tibial tubercle advancement.

If one believes the plethora of articles specific to the treatment of arthrofibrosis by arthroscopy, arthroscopic debridement has seemingly become a panacea for the management of arthrofibrosis. However, as our findings indicate, the good to excellent results reported from the various centers most likely reflect a less refractory form of arthrofibrosis. Sprague echoed our belief when he wrote ". . . although improvement in extension has been reported in some reviews following arthroscopic lysis of adhesion, the procedure does not reliably correct significant extension loss, and the primary indication for the procedure is to correct flexion limitation" (21).

PREVENTION

The key to prevent PES that we estimate occurs in 5% of all ACL knee reconstructions is to prevent all possible causes of secondary PES. Immobility is avoided by emphasizing immediate full knee extension, early weight-bearing, and a carefully outlined functional knee exercise program. Forceful manipulation is to be avoided at all times. Patellar mobilization as expressed by glides and tilts with neuromuscular stimulation will discourage PES. Precise ACL graft placement, adequate notchplasty, and attention to proper graft tensioning will lessen the chance of PES. The literature increasingly points to the proper timing of index surgery.

Once the first signs of PES present, the surgeon must be prudent and patient. The patient should be treated with an NSAID and/or a steroidal dose pack. A TENS unit may be added. Forceful range of motion is to be avoided with arthroscopic or open debridement individualized to the patient at the proper time. A manipulation under anesthesia without associated arthroscopic or open debridement is futile.

The best treatment we can hope for in PES is prevention. We believe that secondary PES is the most commonly seen presentation. The challenge for knee surgeons lies in technically performing the best ACL reconstruction possible with equally matched and individualized rehabilitation.

REFERENCES

1. Blackburne J, Peel T. (1977): A new method of measuring patellar height. *J Bone Joint Surg* 58B:241.
2. Blumensaat C. (1938) Die Lageabweichungen und verrenkungen der kneischeibe. *Ergen Chir Orthop* 31:149–223.
3. Cameron HU, Young-Bok J. (1988): Patella baja complicating total knee arthroplasty. A report of two cases. *J Arthrop* 3:188.
4. Caraffa A, Cerulli G, Buompadre, Proietti M. (1991): Loss of knee extension in cases of acute ACL tears following reconstructive arthroscopic and open surgery. Proceedings of the International Society of the Knee. Toronto, Canada, May 13 to 17, 1991. *Am J Sports Med* 19:559–560.
5. Dodds JA, Keene JS, Graf BK, Lange RH. (1991): Results of knee manipulations after anterior cruciate ligament reconstructions. *Am J Sports Med* 19:283–287.
6. Fu F, Paul JP, Harner C, et al. (1991): The development of flexion contractures following arthroscopic anterior cruciate ligament reconstruction. Proceedings of the International Society of the Knee. Toronto, Canada, May 13 to 17, 1991. *Am J Sports Med* 19:560.
7. Howell SM, Clark JA, Farley TE. (1991): A rationale for predicting anterior cruciate graft impingement by the intercondylar roof. A magnetic resonance imaging study. *Am J Sports Med* 19:276–281.
8. Insall J, Salvati E. (1971): Patella position in the normal knee joint. *Radiology* 101:101–104.
9. Jackson DW, Schaefer RK. (1990): Cyclops syndrome: loss of extension following intra-articular anterior cruciate ligament reconstruction. *Arthroscopy* 6:171–178.
10. Kaplan EB. (1957): Factors responsible for the stability of the knee joint. *Bull Hosp Joint Dis* 18:51–59.
11. Linclau L, Dokter G. (1984): Iatrogenic patella "baja." *Acta Orthop Belg* 50:75–80.
12. Mohtabi NG, Webster-Bogaert S, Fowler PJ. (1991): Limitation of motion following anterior cruciate ligament reconstruction. *Am J Sports Med* 19:620–625.
13. Noyes FR, Wojtys EM, Marshall MT. (1991): The early diagnosis and treatment of developmental patella infera syndrome. *Clin Orthop* 265:241–252.
14. O'Connor RL. (1977): *Arthroscopy*. Philadelphia: JB Lippincott.
15. Parisien JS. (1988): The role of arthroscopy in the treatment of postoperative fibroarthrosis of the knee joint. *Clin Orthop* 229:185–192.
16. Paulos LE, Rosenberg TD, Drawbert J, Manning J, Abbott P. (1987): Infrapatellar contracture syndrome: an unrecognized cause of knee stiffness with patella entrapment and patella infera. *Am J Sports Med* 15:331–341.
17. Paulos LE, Wnorowski DC, Rosenberg TD. Patellar entrapment syndrome: update. A clinical study with long-term follow up. (submitted for publication).
18. Richmond JC, Al Assal M. (1991): Arthroscopic management of arthrofibrosis of the knee, including infrapatellar contracture syndrome. *Arthroscopy* 7:144–147.
19. Sachs RA, Reznik A, Daniel DM, Stone ML. (1990): Complications of knee ligament surgery. In: Daniel DM, Akeson WH, O'Connor JJ, eds. *Knee ligaments: structure, function, injury, and repair*. New York: Raven Press, pp. 505–520.
20. Shelbourne KD, Wilckens JH, Mollabashy A, DeCarlo M. (1991): Arthrofibrosis in acute anterior cruciate ligament reconstruction: the effect of timing of reconstruction and rehabilitation. *J Sports Med* 19:332–336.
21. Sprague NF. (1991): Arthroscopic management of motion-limiting arthrofibrosis of the knee. In: McGinty JB, et al. *Operative arthroscopy*. New York: Raven Press, pp. 381–388.
22. Sprague NF, O'Connor RL, Fox JM. (1982): Arthroscopic treatment of postoperative knee fibroarthrosis. *Clin Orthop* 166:165–172.
23. Strum GM, Friedman MJ, Fox JM, et al. (1990): Acute anterior cruciate ligament reconstruction. Analysis of complications. *Clin Orthop* 253:184–189.

The Anterior Cruciate Ligament: Current and Future Concepts, edited by D.W. Jackson, et al. Raven Press, Ltd., New York © 1993.

CHAPTER 32

Cyclops Lesions

Scott K. Forman and Douglas W. Jackson

As anterior cruciate ligament (ACL) reconstructive surgical techniques have improved and postoperative results studied closer, arthrofibrosis has become recognized as one of the more significant complications following this procedure (3,11,13). Reestablishing full extension after ACL reconstruction has been the focus of physicians, physical therapists, and patients. Causes of failure to regain full extension after ACL reconstruction include graft impingement on the roof of the intercondylar notch, suprapatellar and/or intercondylar adhesions (4,5,8,15), fat pad fibrosis (13), patella entrapment, capsular contracture, patella infra syndrome, and joint capture by positioning or tensioning of the graft. Recently, a specific entity associated with loss of extension was described by Jackson et al. and was termed "cyclops" lesion (12). The cyclops is a form of intraarticular intercondylar notch fibrous proliferation. It results in a fibrous nodule anterior to and associated with the tibial graft insertion site in the intercondylar notch. The term cyclops was coined for the lesion's headlike appearance and characteristic focal bluish areas of coloration (Fig. 1). These pupil-like points arise from venous channels on the surface of the nodule that appear as bluish eyes at the time of arthroscopic visualization. The presence of a cyclops lesion may be subtle or large. It represents a spectrum of reactive tissue and usually is associated with a clunk on terminal extension. The more global involvement with capsular contracture may include an associated loss of flexion and extension of the postoperative knee. An audible, palpable clunk with terminal extension on physical examination is the most consistent finding in this diagnosis in those patients with less than 10 degrees of extension loss.

EPIDEMIOLOGY

Jackson et al. in 1990 originally described 13 cyclops lesions occurring in 230 consecutive patients undergoing primary patellar tendon autograft ACL reconstruction, for an incidence of 5% (12). Before Jackson's labeling of this lesion, other investigators had published detailed reports of a fibroproliferative response occurring within the intercondylar notch. Fullerton et al. in 1984 described a complication that demonstrated all the characteristics of a cyclops syndrome (6). His patient experienced a mechanical block to terminal extension at 10 weeks post–ACL reconstruction and discovered a hypertrophic mass measuring 1.5 cm in diameter on repeat arthroscopic inspection of the joint. The lesion was noted to contain surface blood vessels against a fibrous background. The mass abutted the intercondylar notch, blocking 15 degrees of terminal knee extension. Resection of the nodule resulted in an immediate 7-degree increase in range of motion. Full motion (0 to 135 degrees) was noted at 3 years' follow-up.

Since description of the cyclops syndrome, other reports have appeared in the world literature. Chassaing and Perraudin presented 19 cyclops syndromes out of 197 anterior ligament reconstructions (9.8% incidence) at the European Society of Knee Surgery and Arthroscopy meeting in March 1992 (1). Generous notchplasty and posterior placement of the tibial tunnel have been suggested as preventative measures to development of the cyclops lesion. Roof impingement on the distal graft may instigate and/or become a factor as the lesion develops (10). Gachter (7) published his retrospective review of 2,891 ACL reconstructions, noting 121 cases of extension lag (4.2% incidence). Thirty of the 121 cases were noted to have developed a "vascular fibrous tumor" located anterior to the tibial insertion. Impingement of the nodule against the femoral notch was felt to be the major cause of extension lag. Gachter theorized

S. K. Forman and D. W. Jackson: Southern California Center for Sports Medicine, Long Beach, California 90806.

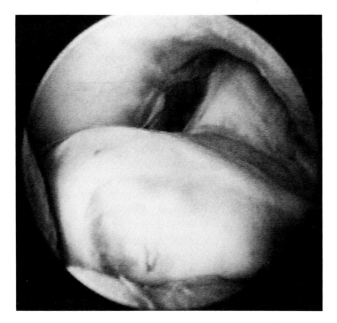

FIG. 1. Arthroscopic view, anterolateral portal. ACL reconstruction and femoral notch (background) and cyclops lesion (foreground). Note characteristic focal bluish areas of granulation tissue within the fibrous mass.

that malalignment of the transplanted graft at the time of ACL reconstruction was the primary etiologic factor in the development of these "tumors." All patients improved range of motion with resection of the mass with or without additional notchplasty. Our experience to date involves over 40 cases of this entity.

The incidence of cyclops that develops after ACL surgery is not clear at this time, but the range of these early investigations is 1 to 9.8%.

ETIOLOGY

The exact etiology of the fibroproliferative response seen with the cyclops lesions is not completely explained. We believe that the nidus of this lesion is stimulated by the debris raised from the drilling and preparation of the tibial tunnel. The angle and direction of the cannulated drill when it enters the knee joint may create an overhang of bone and/or cartilage anterior and lateral to the drill hole (Fig. 2). Some of the drilling debris of the subchondral bone and articular surface may remain attached to the overlying soft tissue and anterior horn of the lateral meniscus instead of being washed out with the irrigation fluid. Upon withdrawal of the drill from the tibial tunnel, irrigation fluid flows out, pulling tissue down into the tunnel and avoiding detection or debridement. If the graft is passed up through the tibial tunnel rather than the reverse, this tissue flap or debris is pushed up out of the tunnel and may present anterior to the graft on the tibial surface. This excess tissue may serve as a

nidus from which granulation and fibrous tissue proliferates to produce the cyclops lesion.

If the surgeon performs a generous enlargement of the anterior and lateral notch, or if the tibial tunnel is posteriorly displaced, reactive tissue, if it develops, may not create as much of a problem in regaining full extension. However, if the surgeon has anatomically created the tibial tunnel, which allows the graft to lie along the roof of the notch in full extension, very little clearance exists. Regardless of the instigating mechanism, the presence of a cyclops will then impinge with full extension.

It should be noted that treatment of the cyclops lesion may be successful without additional notchplasty if the tunnel is not too far anterior. This finding supports speculation that this lesion is not solely the result of impingement from inadequate debridement of the intercondylar notch.

Failure to establish and maintain extension as part of early motion enhances the intercondylar notch proliferation of fibrous tissue. Presence of associated capsular and intraarticular contracture syndrome makes localized excision of the cyclops less successful and more refractory. The most easily treated and responsive are those cases in which the intercondylar notch proliferation is the only factor accounting for the loss of extension.

Prior to the recognition of this entity, we were attempting to save as much of the stump of the ACL as

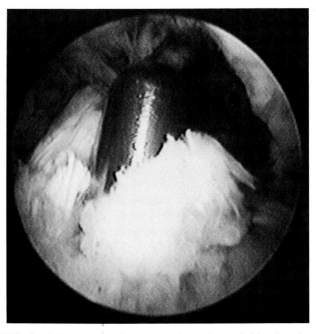

FIG. 2. Arthroscopic view, anterolateral portal. Metal probe inserted into the distal aspect of the tibial tunnel and exiting proximally through the intraarticular surface of the tibia. Note the flap of osteochondral tissue anterior and lateral to the probe. Failure to resect this overhang of tissue may act as a nidus for cyclops development.

possible for two reasons. First, it was hoped that native ACL fibroblasts would incorporate as part of the new composite grafts, and secondly, preservation of the remaining ACL neurosensory elements might be beneficial. Since the recognition of this entity, we have directed more attention to the tibial graft placement. Care is taken so that none of the graft or remaining ACL tissue extends beyond the previous confines of the ACL footprint. The graft is placed slightly more posterior, and meticulous attention is paid to removing overhanging cartilaginous margins and bony debris. Roof lateral notchplasty is more liberally performed if there is any concern that the graft may have roof impingement in its final position.

HISTOLOGY

Histologic sectioning of the cyclops lesion shows a dense, fibrous, well-circumscribed nodule of tissue. Centrally located granulation tissue comprised of vessels and immature hypercellular fibrous tissue account for the focal bluish areas of coloration seen on the surface of the nodule (Fig. 3). Centrifugal growth of the cyclops lesion is thought to occur from the progressive maturation and proliferation of fibrocytes located in the hypervascular epicenters. Histologically, mature fibrous tissue, characterized by parallel collagen fiber matrix, relative hypocellularity, and flattened, spindle-shaped fibrocytes, radiates from the centrally located granulation tissue (Fig. 4A,B). Several cyclops lesions have been found to contain bone. Pathogenesis of these bony fragments remains speculative. Histologic evaluation under polarized light show two types of bony deposits (Fig. 5A,B). Well-organized, mature bone, noted by its characteristic birefringent, laminated pattern of osteoid, was found to contain numerous "empty" lacunae. Immature, woven bone, demonstrated by irregular, disorganized appearance, was relatively hypercellular with prominent nuclei. These findings support the notion that the necrotic lamellar bone was incorporated into the lesion from the original osteocartilaginous tissue. Relative hypercellularity and an increased nuclear-to-cytoplasmic ratio of the woven or immature bone leads one to conclude that this bone is formed within the cyclops itself, nourished by the lesion's rich vascular supply. These observations are made solely on the basis of histologic sectioning. Further investigation, such as tetracycline labeling to determine intralesional new bone formation, would probably confirm such speculation.

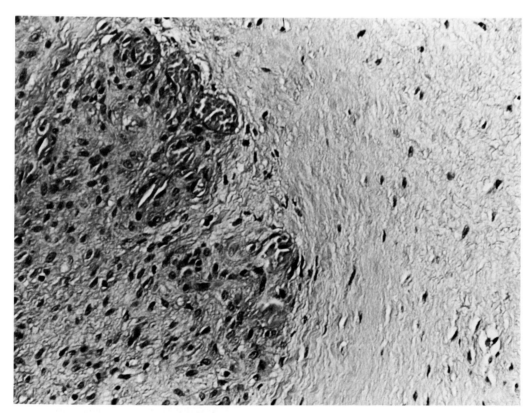

FIG. 3. Histologic section, cyclops lesion, hematoxylin and eosin stain, magnification ×10. Hypervascular granulation tissues surrounded by mature, well-organized fibrous capsule account for the lesion's pupil-like appearance on gross visualization.

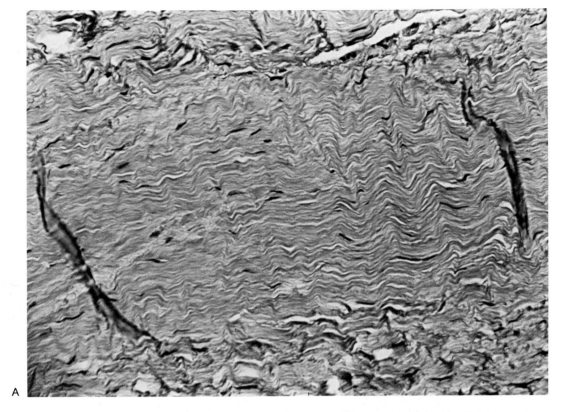

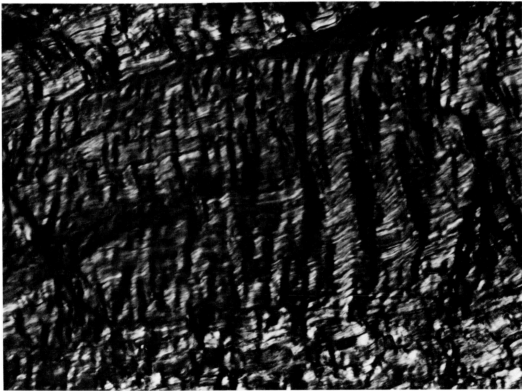

FIG. 4. Histologic section, cyclops lesion, hematoxylin and eosin stain, magnification ×50. **A:** Well-organized fibrous tissue found at periphery of lesion. Note parallel collagen fiber arrangement, relative hypocellularity, and flattened, spindle-shaped fibrocytes. **B:** Polarized light. Note crimp pattern of this mature fibrous tissue.

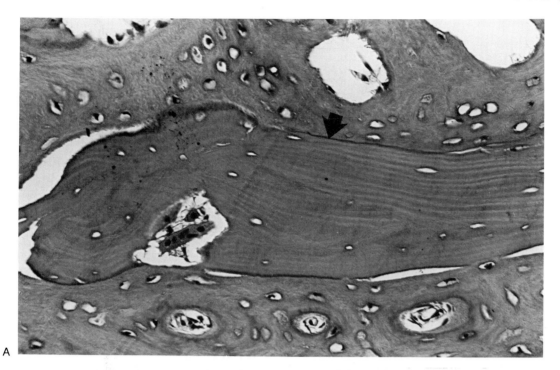

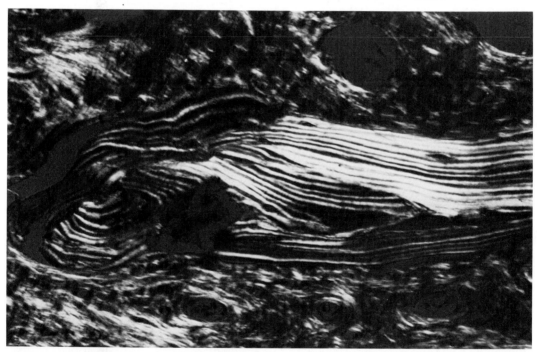

FIG. 5. Histologic section, cyclops lesion, hematoxylin and eosin stain, magnification ×10. **A:** Bony fragment within cyclops lesion containing two types of bone matrix. Large arrow points to well-organized bone characterized by birefringent laminated matrix with empty lacunae. It is surrounded by primary woven bone. Note relative hypercellularity, prominent nuclei, and disorganized matrix appearance. **B:** Histologic section, polarized light. Enhanced birefringent laminated pattern of central cortical bony fragment compared with random disorganized pattern of surrounding new bone.

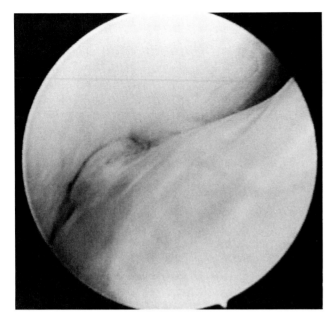

FIG. 6. Arthroscopic view, anterolateral portal of femoral cyclops lesion. Superior portion of intercondylar femoral notch (background) and ACL reconstruction (foreground). Note impingement of small 0.5 × 1 cm lesion with knee extension.

FEMORAL CYCLOPS

Recently, an analogous, less frequent kissing lesion has been identified occurring on the anteromedial corner of the femoral tunnel (Fig. 6). Gross and histological evaluation has confirmed similarity between this lesion and the tibial cyclops. It is speculated that a similar pathogenesis exists.

CLINICAL PRESENTATION

The most striking feature of this entity is the pathognomonic palpable and audible clunk that is heard upon terminal extension. Patients notice and experience a "popping" sensation or sound when they actively extend toward this endpoint. This sound may be associated with a block to extension and is generally not painful.

Four clinically distinct patterns have emerged. Patients may complain of a terminal extension clunk only (type 1) or terminal extension with a clunk, with an associated loss of extension that returns to full extension after a warm-up session (type 2). Another manifestation is a large lesion with or without bone associated with a fixed flexion contracture (type 3). The more difficult to treat lesions are associated with global fixed flexion and extension knee contracture (type 4). Consistent cyclops lesion types have been identified with each clinical presentation. Type 1 lesions are typically small (0.5 to 1.5 cm in diameter) and tend to be composed of "hard" tissue, such as bone or cartilage. Type 2 lesions are asso-

ciate with a small, "soft," immature fibrous proliferation. Type 3 lesions are large (2.0 to 4.5 cm in diameter), mature fibroproliferative tumors with or without associated bone or cartilage. These lesions tend to fill the entire intercondylar notch anterior to the ACL graft, thus preventing accommodation for the cyclops with terminal extension. Type 4 lesions are related to extensive fibrous proliferation in the intercondylar notch with associated global knee arthrofibrosis.

In Jackson's series of cyclops lesions, the average interval between ACL reconstruction and arthroscopic excision of the cyclops lesions was 16 weeks (range 8 to 36). In all patients, extension gain had plateaued. The average range of motion at the time of surgical intervention was 16 to 103 degrees. All knees had negative Lachman and anterior drawer tests. The range of extension loss was 6 degrees to a maximum of 25 degrees. After arthroscopic resection, average range of motion was improved to 6.0 degrees of extension and 130 degrees of flexion.

Any patient with a less than normal range of motion post–ACL reconstruction with the above findings should be considered suspect for this pathologic lesion. In addition to the diagnosis of cyclops lesion, other causes of postoperative contracture must be ruled out. The greater the loss of extension, the greater the chance for associated extraarticular contractures and associated roof impingement with the graft.

TREATMENT

A systematic approach is required in addressing these problems, because it is apparent that just removing the cyclops lesion in the more severe extension deficit is not

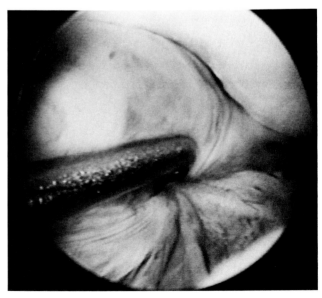

FIG. 7. Arthroscopic view, anterolateral portal. Probing of the cyclops mass between the lesion (foreground) and ACL reconstruction posteriorly.

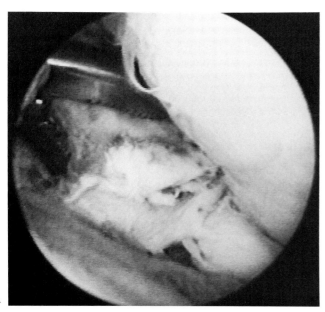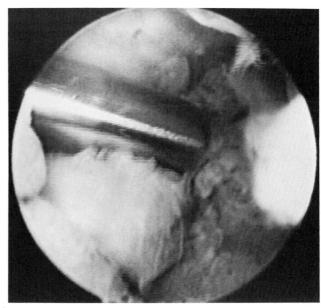

A   B

FIG. 8. Arthroscopic view, anterolateral portal. Debriding and resection of cyclops lesion.

enough (2,9,16–18). Several patients treated for symptomatic cyclops lesion and 10 degrees or greater loss of extension required more than one procedure (12). Repeat arthroscopy of these patients' knees varied on the recurrence of the cyclops lesion. Treatment should address all possible pathologies determined to cause knee contracture; suprapatellar and intercondylar adhesions must be identified and resected, graft impingement, if present, must be identified, patellar fat pad fibrosis may need to be released, and the cyclops lesion should be resected.

The junction between the cyclops and the reconstructed graft is defined by probing between the parallel fibers of the graft and the capsule of the lesion (Fig. 7). Resection of the cyclops can be performed by a combination of debriding instrumentation (Fig. 8A,B). Tourniquet pressure is released, and bleeding from the resected granulation tissue is controlled with the use of electrocautery (Fig. 9). After resection, a characteristic "fibrous fluff" appearance is noted overlying the remaining anterior cruciate graft (Fig. 10). The ACL grafts in our experience have been intact when this lesion is present. The

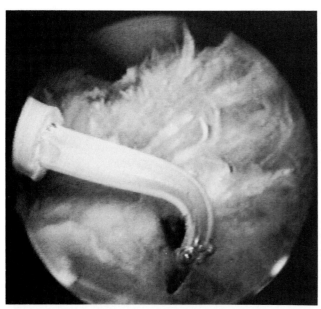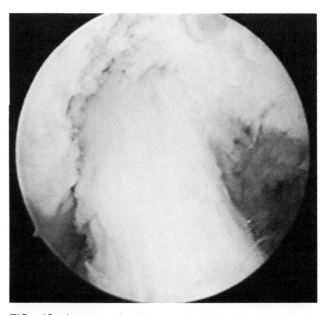

FIG. 9. Arthroscopic view, anterolateral portal. Electrocautery is used to stop bleeding after cyclops resection.

FIG. 10. Arthroscopic view, anterolateral portal. Post–cyclops resection. Note "fibrous fluff" appearance of ACL reconstruction after complete removal of the lesion.

patients notice almost immediate loss of terminal clunking and improved knee extension.

PREVENTION

Clinical experience indicates that tolerance to extension loss is extremely limited, and even minimal amounts of extension loss constitute an unacceptable result in the high-performance knee. Loss of as little as 5 degrees of symmetric knee extension is not well tolerated in the athletic population. A significant residual loss of extension can be more disabling than the preoperative instability.

Current ACL reconstruction techniques that are designed to avoid cyclops development include debriding the tissue anterior and lateral to the tibial tunnel after the tunnel is drilled, avoiding positioning the osseous tunnel too anteriorly, and performing a generous superior notchplasty to avoid impingement of the graft. Patients developing a plateau in regaining extension and/or an audible clunk should be considered for early surgical intervention, addressing all pathologies leading to the knee contracture. Arthroscopic debridement usually leads to near complete resolution of patient limitations in most cases if graft impingement is not a significant factor.

REFERENCES

1. Chassaing V, Perraudin JE. (1992): Cyclops Syndrome. Transactions from European Society of Knee Surgery and Arthroscopy meeting, Palma de Mallorca, Spain, May 25–29, 1992, S-98.
2. Conner AN. (1970): The treatment of flexion contractures of the knee in poliomyelitis. *J Bone Joint Surg* 52B:138–144.
3. DeHaven KE. (1988): Complications of knee ligament surgery. Meeting: Advanced concepts in arthroscopy of the lower extremity. American Academy of Orthopaedic Surgeons, San Diego, CA, December 1988.
4. DeLee JC. (1985): Complications of arthroscopy and arthroscopic surgery: results of a national survey. *Arthroscopy* 1:214–220.
5. Enneking WF, Horowitz M. (1972): The intra-articular effects of immobilization of the human knee. *J Bone Joint Surg* 54A:973–985.
6. Fullerton LR, Andrews JR. (1984): Mechanical block to extension following augmentation of the anterior cruciate ligament. *Am J Sports Med* 12:166–168.
7. Gachter A. (1990): Arthtoskopisches shaving nach kreuzbandersatzplastiken. *Orthopade* 19:103–106.
8. Graf B, Uhr F. (1988): Complications of intra-articular anterior cruciate reconstruction. *Clin Sports Med* 7:835–848.
9. Heydorian K, Akbarnia B, Jabalameli M, et al. (1984): Posterior capsulectomy for the treatment of severe flexion contractures of the knee. *J Pediatr Orthop* 4:700–704.
10. Howell SM, Clark JA, Farley TW. (1991): A rationale for predicting anterior cruciate graft impingement by the intercondylar roof. A magnetic resonance imaging study. *Am J Sports Med* 19:276–281.
11. Hughston JC. (1985): Complications of anterior cruciate ligament surgery. *Orthop Clin* 16:237–240.
12. Jackson DW, Schaefer RK. (1990): Cyclops syndrome: loss of extension following intra-articular ACL reconstruction. *Arthroscopy* 6:171–178.
13. O'Conner RL. (1977): *Arthroscopy.* Philadelphia: JB Lippincott, pp 14–16.
14. Paulos LE, Rosenberg TD, Drawbert J, Manning J, Abbott P. (1987): Infrapatellar contracture syndrome: an unrecognized cause of knee stiffness with patella entrapment and patella infera. *Am J Sports Med* 15:331–340.
15. Small NC. (1986): Complications in arthroscopy: the knee and other joints. *Arthroscopy* 2:253–258.
16. Sprague NF. (1987): Motion limiting arthrofibrosis of the knee: the role of arthroscopic management. *Clin Sports Med* 6:537–540.
17. Sprague NF, O'Conner RL, Fox JM. (1980): Arthroscopic treatment of postoperative knee fibroarthrosis. *Clin Orthop* 166:165–172.
18. Thompson TC. (1944): Quadricepsplasty to improve knee function. *J Bone Joint Surg* 26:366–379.

The Anterior Cruciate Ligament: Current and Future Concepts, edited by D.W. Jackson, et al.
Raven Press, Ltd., New York © 1993.

CHAPTER 33

Loss of Motion Following Anterior Cruciate Ligament Reconstruction

Freddie H. Fu, James J. Irrgang, and Christopher D. Harner

Loss of motion (LOM) after anterior cruciate ligament (ACL) reconstruction is a common and serious complication that has recently been recognized (3,9,12,13,16). LOM after ACL reconstruction can involve loss of both flexion and extension, but loss of extension is a potentially more significant problem. Patients with LOM fail to progress with physical therapy, and walk with a bent knee gait. They often require additional surgery and extended rehabilitation to regain their motion. Appropriate preoperative, intraoperative, and postoperative intervention is necessary in order to minimize the risk of developing LOM. If LOM develops, early recognition and appropriate management based on etiology of the LOM is necessary for a successful outcome.

INCIDENCE AND RISK FACTORS ASSOCIATED WITH LOM

Sachs et al. (13) reported loss of extension greater than 5 degrees in 24% of patients undergoing ACL reconstruction. Loss of extension was often associated with quadriceps weakness and patellofemoral pain. Mohtadi et al. (9) reported a 7% incidence of LOM defined as a flexion contracture ≥10 degrees and/or knee flexion less than 120 degrees at 3 months after ACL reconstruction. In their study, LOM was significantly associated with an acute reconstruction performed within 2 weeks of the index injury. No other risk factors were found to be statistically significant. Shelbourne et al. (16) retrospec-

tively determined that patients undergoing ACL reconstruction within the first 3 weeks after injury had a higher incidence of limited extension; however, their overall incidence of LOM was not reported.

Harner et al. (3) defined LOM as a knee flexion contracture ≥10 degrees and/or knee flexion ≤125 degrees at 2 months after ACL reconstruction. Two hundred forty-four patients undergoing ACL reconstruction between 1986 and 1989 were reviewed, and an 11.1% incidence of LOM was reported. All patients experienced loss of extension and two thirds also experienced loss of flexion. Factors that were statistically associated with LOM included gender (male), reconstruction within 4 weeks of injury to the knee, and concomitant ligament surgery. Age, type of graft, and postoperative physical therapy protocol also appeared to be associated with LOM but did not reach statistical significance. The incidence of LOM was higher in those who were older, those who received an autograft, and those who had limited extension imposed in the immediate postoperative period.

All of the above studies identified reconstruction soon after the index injury to be a significant risk factor for LOM. A similar observation was noted by DeHaven (1), who stated that LOM was heavily weighted toward acute versus chronic ligament surgery. Strum et al. (17) observed LOM in 35% of their acute (less than 3 weeks) reconstructions that required adhesiolysis and manipulation to restore range of motion (ROM). This was in contrast to the 12% incidence of LOM in their chronic reconstructions.

Several factors may explain the higher incidence of LOM after an acute ACL reconstruction. When ACL reconstruction is performed acutely, the knee still may be actively inflamed. Surgical insult during this period will further inflame the knee and accelerate the healing

F. H. Fu and C. D. Harner: Department of Orthopaedics, University of Pittsburgh School of Medicine, Pittsburgh, Pennsylvania 15261.

J. J. Irrgang: Sports Medicine Institute, University of Pittsburgh Medical Center, Pittsburgh, Pennsylvania 15261.

process, resulting in excessive fibrotic tissue formation. Other factors significantly associated with LOM included sex and concomitant ligament surgery (3). The higher incidence of LOM in males is unexplained. The risk associated with concomitant ligament surgery was primarily related to procedures involving the medial capsule (medial collateral ligament repair and POL reefing). Repair of the medial capsule may not precisely restore the normal tissue planes, which may interfere with restoration of motion. Surgery involving the medial capsule may accentuate the fibrotic response of the knee joint, resulting in greater scar tissue formation. Additionally, surgery of the capsule may result in more pain, which would inhibit restoration of motion.

Age, type of graft, and physical therapy protocol also appear to be associated with LOM (3). Patients who are older tend to experience more difficulty with LOM. This may be associated with age-related changes in connective tissue, which include increased stiffness and decreased elasticity.

Patients who receive an autograft as opposed to an allograft are more likely to experience LOM. Harvest of an autograft from the patellar tendon disrupts the extensor mechanism. This results in greater pain and inhibition of the quadriceps, both of which could contribute to increased incidence of LOM. Patients who had imposed limited extension in the immediate postoperative period experienced greater incidence of LOM (3). Similar findings were noted by Shelbourne and Nitz (15), who compared an accelerated rehabilitation program emphasizing early restoration of full extension with a rehabilitation program immobilizing the knee in flexion and restricting early extension of the knee. Early emphasis on obtaining full extension immediately after surgery resulted in a significant decrease in loss of extension. Placing the knee in full extension immediately after surgery engages the graft in the intercondylar notch. This may minimize hemorrhage formation and intercondylar notch scarring (ICNS), which is associated with LOM in approximately 50% of the cases.

ETIOLOGY OF LOM

The etiology of LOM after ACL reconstruction is multifactorial and may include ICNS, capsulitis, nonanatomic graft placement, concomitant ligament surgery, infection, and reflex sympathetic dystrophy.

ICNS is the result of scar formation in the intercondylar notch area that produces a physical block to extension. Patients presenting with ICNS usually have loss of extension only while flexion is full. The patient usually complains of stiffness in the morning upon awakening that improves with motion. The patient may also complain of a catching sensation as the knee is extended.

(Refer to section on cyclops lesion.) Swelling is usually minimal, and patellar mobility is normal.

The term capsulitis implies periarticular inflammation and swelling. Pain associated with this chronic inflammation results in quadriceps inhibition and weakness, and a quadriceps lag can develop. Loss of active knee extension allows a knee flexion contracture to develop. Capsulitis is characterized by complaints of constant pain and stiffness. The knee is actively inflamed and diffuse swelling is present. Usually both flexion and extension are limited, as is patellar mobility. If capsulitis is not recognized and treated, it may progress to patellar baja associated with the latter stages of patellar entrapment syndrome as described by Paulos et al. (12).

PREVENTION OF LOM

Prevention of LOM requires preoperative, intraoperative, and postoperative intervention. Preoperatively, unless the knee is severely unstable, reconstruction after acute injury is delayed until the symptoms of the initial insult have subsided and ROM has been restored. When the knee is severely unstable, surgery within the first 2 weeks is indicated as described by Palmer (10). Caution must be exercised when operating on a "locked" knee. A true locked knee from a torn meniscus is relatively rare. Often, limited extension immediately after injury is the result of pain and swelling. Immediately after injury, the patient is advised to use modalities to decrease pain and swelling. Cold and compression, such as that provided by the Cryocuff (Aircast Inc., Summit, NJ), has been an effective adjunct to treatment during this phase of recovery (Fig. 1). Additionally, during this period the patient is instructed to perform ROM exercises to recover motion and quadriceps and hamstring exercises to restore muscle function. Surgery is delayed until the acute symptoms of inflammation have resolved and the patient has recovered ROM and muscle function. Preoperatively, patients should be educated about the risk for developing LOM and warned that LOM may occur in 5% to 10% of cases.

Intraoperatively, prevention of LOM requires anatomic placement of the graft. Poor placement of the graft will "capture the knee" and will result in LOM and/or failure of the graft. A notchplasty is performed to provide adequate clearance for the graft in the intracondylar notch as the knee extends. If the graft impinges in the intracondylar notch when the knee is in the fully extended position, the notchplasty should be enlarged to allow full extension without impingement. Full extension and flexion should be achieved intraoperatively. Concomitant ligament surgery should be minimized in order to reduce the incidence of LOM and is only performed if the knee is severely unstable.

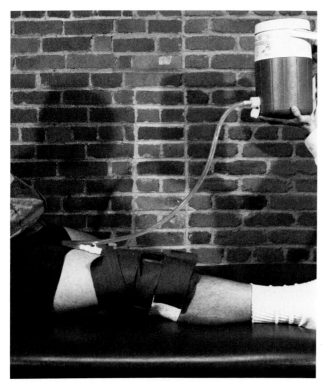

FIG. 1. Cold and compression as applied by the Cryocuff (Aircast Inc., Summit NJ) is effective in decreasing pain and swelling after acute injury and surgery.

Concomitant ligament surgery should anatomically repair or reconstruct the injured structures. Plications or advancements should be avoided to avoid overconstraining the knee. When concomitant ligament surgery is performed, prolonged immobilization should be avoided and early ROM with emphasis on extension should be initiated.

Postoperative management after ACL reconstruction to reduce the incidence of LOM should emphasize reduction of inflammation, early restoration of extension symmetrical to the uninvolved knee, early ROM and quadriceps exercises, and early resumption of normal gait. Cold and compression is used to minimize inflammation.

Postoperative management to minimize the risk of LOM must emphasize early restoration of extension. The goal is to attain full passive extension symmetrical to the noninvolved knee within 2 to 3 weeks after surgery. This is achieved by immobilizing the knee in full extension that engages the graft in the intercondylar notch to reduce hemorrhage and subsequent ICNS (Fig. 2). During the first week, the brace is unlocked several times per day to allow the patient to perform self-administered ROM exercises. The patient is encouraged to achieve full extension by lying prone with the lower leg unsupported or by sitting with the heel elevated and knee unsupported several times per day (Fig. 3).

Graded patellar mobilization is initiated several days after surgery to maintain patellar mobility. The patella is passively moved superiorly, inferiorly, medially, and laterally. Additionally, a patellar tilt lifting the lateral border of the patella is performed to maintain length of the lateral retinaculum. Patellar mobilization must be performed in a manner that does not increase pain or inflammation. Overly aggressive patellar mobilization can increase pain and inflammation, which may lead to capsulitis.

Early quadriceps activity is encouraged. Quad sets are performed with the knee in full extension to regain quadriceps control and maintain superior mobility of the patellofemoral joint. Quad sets produce minimal stress on the graft, because quadriceps contraction with the knee fully extended primarily produces compression of the tibiofemoral joint with little anterior translation of the tibia. Additionally, isometric quadriceps exercises in the range of 60 to 90 degrees of flexion are performed because they have been shown to produce little or no active quadriceps anterior drawer (14). Straight leg raises are

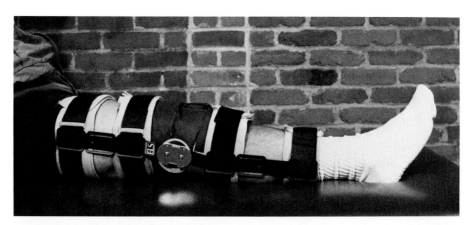

FIG. 2. Placing the knee in full extension engages the graft in the intracondylar notch and minimizes development of intracondylar notch scarring.

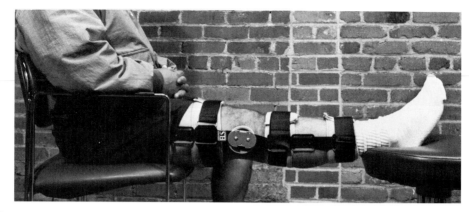

FIG. 3. The patient is encouraged to achieve full extension in the immediate postoperative phase. This is accomplished by sitting with the heel elevated and the knee unsupported.

performed if the patient can do so with less than a 10-degree knee extension lag. Closed-chain exercises for the lower extremity are initiated early in preparation for weight-bearing (Fig. 4). Closed-chain exercises improve functional strength while minimizing patellofemoral stress (5) and stress on the graft (2,7,11,18). Compression of the tibiofemoral joint during closed-chain exercises

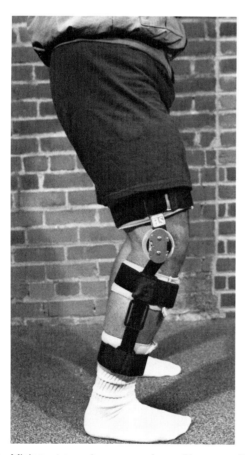

FIG. 4. Minisquat exercises are performed in preparation for weight-bearing. Closed-chain exercises are progressed as tolerated by the patient.

lends stability to the joint and minimizes tibial translation (2). Additionally, during closed-chain exercises the resistance is applied axially in relation to the tibia, which decreases the shear component at the tibiofemoral joint (11).

Initial ambulation after reconstruction is partial weight-bearing with the brace locked in full extension. After the first week the brace is unlocked during ambulation to allow a normal heel-to-toe gait. Weight-bearing is progressed as tolerated. Crutches are discontinued when the patient has full extension without a quadriceps lag and can demonstrate a normal gait pattern. Early return to normal ambulation presents low ACL strain during walking (4).

The current trend of aggressive postoperative physical therapy after ACL reconstruction to allow early restoration of motion, including full extension, early quadriceps activity, and immediate weight-bearing, must be done in a manner that minimizes inflammation and its associated symptoms of pain and swelling. Excessive inflammation during this period may lead to LOM. Complete disregard of sound rehabilitation principles in order to accelerate recovery must be avoided.

The effects of these measures to reduce the incidence of LOM was evaluated by a retrospective review of 231 consecutive patients undergoing endoscopic ACL reconstruction between 1990 and 1991. Only 4 patients (1.7%) experienced loss of extension greater than 10 degrees. Two patients required arthroscopic adhesiolysis and debridement to recover motion. The remaining two patients regained their motion with physical therapy only. Thirty two patients (13.9%) demonstrated less than 125 degrees of flexion 8 weeks postoperatively. Twenty-three of these patients (72%) regained full flexion with physical therapy by 6 months. Two patients required manipulation and arthroscopic adhesiolysis to regain their flexion (both patients also demonstrated loss of extension of 5 to 9 degrees). All patients regained full flexion and extension by 1 year.

RECOGNITION OF LOM

LOM is indicated by failure to achieve the expected range of motion. Full extension symmetrical to the uninvolved knee is expected within 2 to 3 weeks and full flexion is expected by 8 weeks. Failure to achieve this motion and/or lack of progression is cause for concern that the patient is developing a stiff knee. Once LOM is recognized, its etiology must be determined so that appropriate intervention can be planned. The etiology of LOM is ICNS in approximately 50% of cases and capsulitis in the remaining 50% of cases. Intercondylar notch scarring is indicated by complaints of stiffness in the morning that decrease with motion. The patient may also complain of a catching sensation as the knee is extended. Usually there is only loss of extension, whereas flexion is full. Additionally, with ICNS, swelling and inflammation is minimal and patellar mobility is normal.

Capsulitis is characterized by complaints of constant pain and stiffness. The knee is actively inflamed and diffuse swelling is present. Usually both flexion and extension are limited, as is patellar mobility. Primary capsulitis must be differentiated from secondary capsulitis. The latter is due to nonanatomic graft placement, infection, and/or reflex sympathetic dystrophy. Additionally, it must be kept in mind that capsulitis can overlap with ICNS.

MANAGEMENT OF LOM

Successful management of LOM is dependent on the etiology and length of time after surgery when it is recognized. When LOM appears to be due to ICNS and is recognized early (less than 2 months postoperatively), management consists of physical therapy to improve extension. Stretching to improve extension is performed using low-amplitude sustained forces to maximize creep and plastic deformation (8). This is performed by lying prone with the lower leg unsupported, with a light weight (2 to 3 pounds) placed around the ankle (Fig. 5). To maximize a permanent increase in length, heat should be applied simultaneously with the stretch, and the stretch should be maintained during the period of cooling (6). Neurophysiological stretching techniques, such as contract-relax and hold-relax, may be useful. A dropout cast is used overnight to provide a sustained stretch and prevent loss of extension while the patient sleeps (Fig. 6). Quadriceps exercises are performed to eliminate any quadriceps lag that may be present. If a quadriceps lag persists, it may facilitate development of a flexion contracture.

If extension fails to improve with physical therapy, or if ICNS is detected more than 3 months after surgery, then arthroscopic debridement of the intracondylar notch may be necessary to remove the physical block to extension. If full extension has not been restored after debridement of the notch, then a notchplasty to enlarge the notch may be required. After debridement and/or notchplasty, a drop-out cast is applied and physical therapy is initiated to recover the extension that was gained intraoperatively. The prognosis for improvement and recovery of normal motion and function when LOM is secondary to ICNS is excellent if recognized and managed appropriately. Surgical intervention should be considered if extension has not improved with physical therapy. Continuing aggressive physical therapy will not eliminate the physical block to extension and may lead to increased pain, graft failure, and/or frustration of the patient, physician, and physical therapist.

Capsulitis is characterized by loss of flexion and extension, with persistent pain and inflammation that is aggravated by aggressive activity. When recognized within the first 3 months during the acute inflammatory phase, the condition is usually reversible. Anti-inflammatory medications such as nonsteriodals or a Medrol dose pack are recommended to decrease inflammation. Addition-

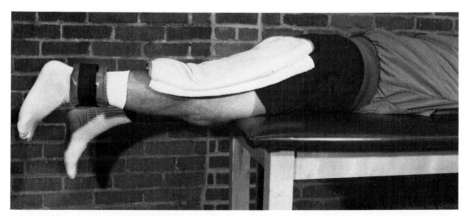

FIG. 5. Stretching to improve extension is performed by lying in the prone position with the lower leg unsupported and a light weight applied near the ankle. Heat is applied simultaneously to maximize lengthening.

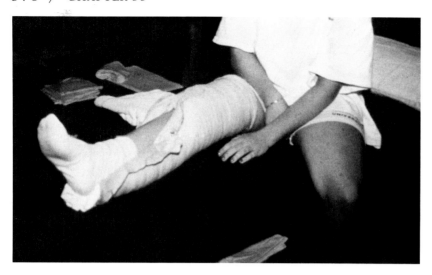

FIG. 6. A drop-out cast is used overnight to increase or maintain knee extension.

ally, anti-inflammatory physical agents, such as cold or mild forms of heat, may be used. Physical therapy during this period must not be overly aggressive. Aggressive physical therapy during this period will lead to further inflammation and delay restoration of motion. Stretching techniques should be gentle and should not exacerbate pain and swelling. Low-grade sustained stretch combined with mild heating is recommended. Efforts to increase motion should be directed toward gaining motion in one direction at a time. Because loss of extension is potentially more problematic, initial efforts should be directed at regaining extension. A drop-out cast can be used overnight to improve and/or maintain extension, but should only produce a low-grade stretch. Once extension has been recovered, emphasis should be placed on regaining flexion. Passive motion machines can be used to improve flexion, but have little value in improving extension.

Often, pain and swelling associated with capsulitis during the period of active inflammation inhibits muscle activity. Active and light resistive quadriceps and hamstring exercises should be performed to gain active control of the passive motion that has been developed through stretching. Emphasis should be on muscle reeducation rather than on strengthening. Use of biofeedback or electrical stimulation may be beneficial to facilitate muscle reeducation.

Gentle patellar mobilization can be used to increase patellar mobility. However, the patellar mobilization techniques must be graded appropriately for the stage of inflammation that the patient's knee demonstrates. Overly aggressive patellar mobilization will further inflame the peripatellar tissues and delay restoration of motion. Inferior excursion of the patella is necessary for flexion, and superior excursion is necessary for normal functioning of the extensor mechanism. Superior excursion of the patella can also be improved by performing quad sets in terminal extension.

During the acute inflammatory phase of capsulitis, manipulation and/or surgical debridement and adhesiolysis is of questionable value because it will only serve to further inflame the knee. During this time, patience on the part of the patient, physician, and physical therapist is crucial. The patient must be educated in the goals and philosophy of treatment in order to achieve optimum results. Likewise, the physical therapist must be educated to not be overly aggressive in stretching to recover motion. Discontinuing physical therapy for a period of time may be indicated if the patient's motion is not improving. This will allow the inflammatory process to subside and motion will subsequently improve.

When capsulitis is detected early and treated appropriately, good results can be achieved. When capsulitis is detected 3 to 6 months after surgery, it is in the fibrotic stage and less than optimal results can be expected. If the knee is still actively inflamed and swollen, nonoperative management as described above is recommended. Surgery at this time will further increase the inflammatory process and delay restoration of motion. If the knee is not actively inflamed, then surgical intervention to recover the lost motion is indicated. Surgery to recover lost motion during the fibrotic stage must be well planned to address the specific cause for the limited motion. An arthroscopic approach can be used, but occasionally an open arthrotomy must be performed to excise all of the scar tissue. Scar tissue should be excised from the anterior, medial, and lateral aspects of the knee. A lateral release may be necessary. For secondary capsulitis, a poorly placed graft may need to be removed. Postoperatively the patient should be admitted to the hospital for 2 to 5 days for an epidural block to eliminate pain. Cold and compression can be used to minimize inflammation.

Postoperative physical therapy should initially address regaining extension. A drop-out cast to increase and/or maintain extension can be used overnight. Quad sets and straight leg raises should be performed to gain control of the increased passive extension that has been gained. If active quad control is not regained, then passive extension will be lost and a flexion contracture will develop again. Work to increase flexion can begin once extension is under control. Occasionally a second manipulation is required in order to regain flexion.

End-stage capsulitis is characterized by patella baja. This condition is rare, but can lead to progressive degeneration of the patellofemoral joint and progressive disability. Surgical management for end-stage capsulitis with patella baja requires an open arthrotomy with a tibial tubercle slide to reestablish the normal position of the patella. The postoperative management is similar to that described above; however, loaded quadriceps exercises must be delayed for 6 weeks until the tibial tubercle has reunited.

RESULTS OF MANAGEMENT OF LOM

Harner et al. (3) reported on our initial results of management of 21 of 27 patients with LOM after ACL reconstruction who returned for a follow-up examination an average of 22.8 months after the index surgical procedure. These patients were compared with 24 patients who underwent ACL reconstruction but did not experience difficulty in regaining motion. Patients who had experienced LOM had persistent deficits in extension and flexion compared with the control group. At follow-up, 5 patients with LOM had a persistent knee flexion contracture ≥10 degrees and an additional 9 patients had a 5- to 9-degree flexion contracture. None of the normal knee motion patients had a knee flexion contracture ≥10 degrees and 2 had a 5- to 9-degree flexion contracture. Nine patients who experienced LOM had persistent limitation of flexion ≤125 degrees, whereas none of the normal motion patients had limited flexion.

Patients who experienced LOM had a higher incidence of decreased patellar mobility and use of a bent knee gait. There was no difference in anterior tibial displacement between patients who experienced LOM and those who had normal motion after ACL reconstruction. Additionally, both groups had similar functional strength as indicated by similar mean values and frequency distributions of hop and vertical jump scores.

A good to excellent subjective functional rating was obtained in 67% of the patients who experienced LOM compared with 80% in patients who had normal motion after ACL reconstruction. Five of the 21 (24%) patients with LOM had a poor subjective functional rating compared with only 1 of 24 (4%) patients who had normal knee motion. Of significance was the fact that all LOM motion patients with poor results had a significant knee flexion contracture. Of the 5 patients with a poor result, 2 had a knee flexion contracture greater than 10 degrees and 3 had a 5- to 9-degree knee flexion contracture. Four

of these patients were unable to perform the hop or vertical jump tests, and the remaining patient had hop and vertical jump indices of less than 80%. These data appear to indicate that poor functional results can be expected in patients who experience LOM and have a persistent knee flexion contracture ≥5 degrees and poor functional strength.

Our more recent experience appears to indicate that earlier recognition and appropriate management of LOM leads to more optimal results. All four of the patients who had a knee flexion contracture greater than 10 degrees between 1990 and 1991 regained full extension. Two required arthroscopic surgical intervention and the remaining two improved with physical therapy alone. Twenty-three of 32 (72%) with limited flexion regained full flexion with physical therapy by 6 months. Two patients with limited flexion required manipulation and arthroscopic debridement to recover their flexion (both also had knee flexion contractures of 5 to 9 degrees). All patients with limited flexion regained full flexion by 1 year after the index surgery.

SUMMARY

LOM after ACL reconstruction is a common and potentially devastating problem that occurs in 5% to 10% of patients undergoing ACL reconstruction. The incidence of LOM can be reduced by appropriate preoperative, intraoperative, and postoperative intervention. Management is dependent on the etiology of the LOM (ICNS versus capsulitis) and the inflammatory state of the knee. Aggressive physical therapy that results in increased pain and inflammation should be avoided. Often surgery is the most conservative form of treatment. Emphasis should initially be placed on regaining extension, because loss of extension is related to patellofemoral pain and functional disturbances. If LOM is recognized and appropriately managed, good results can still be achieved.

REFERENCES

1. DeHaven K. (1987): Letter. *Am J Sports Med* 15:340–341.
2. Drez D, Paine R, Neuschwander DC. (1991): In-vivo testing of closed versus open kinetic chain exercises in patients with documented tears of the anterior cruciate ligament. Presented at the annual conference of the American Orthopaedic Society for Sports Medicine, Orlando, FL, July 1991.
3. Harner CD, Irrgang JJ, Paul J, Dearwater S, Fu FH. (1992): Loss of motion following anterior cruciate ligament reconstruction. *Am J Sports Med,* 20:499–506.
4. Henning CE, Lynch MA, Glick KR. (1985): An in-vivo strain gauge study of elongation of the anterior cruciate ligament injury. *Am J Sports Med* 13:22–26.
5. Hungerford DX, Barry M. (1979): Biomechanics of the patellofemoral joint. *Clin Orthop* 144:9–15.
6. Lehmann JF, Masock AJ, Warren CG, Koblanski JN. (1970): Ef-

fect of therapeutic temperatures on tendon extensibility. *Arch Phys Med Rehabil* 51:481–487.

7. Lutz GE, Palmitier RA, An KN, Chao EYS. (1991): Comparison of tibiofemoral joint forces during open kinetic chain and closed kinetic chain exercises. Presented at the annual conference of the American Academy of Orthopaedic Surgeons, Anaheim, CA, February 1991.

8. Kisner C, Colby LA. (1977): *Therapeutic exercise. Foundations and techniques.* Philadelphia: FA Davis.

9. Mothadi NGH, Webster-Bogaert S, Fowler PJ. (1991): Limitation of motion following anterior cruciate ligament reconstruction: a case-control study. *Am J Sports Med* 19:620–625.

10. Palmer I. (1983): On the injuries to the ligaments of the knee joint: a clinical study. *Acta Chir Scand* 81(suppl 53).

11. Palmitier RA, An KN Scott SG, Chao EYS. (1991): Kinetic chain exercise in knee rehabilitation. *Sports Med* 11:402–413.

12. Paulos LE, Rosenberg TD, Drawbert J, Manning J, Abbott P. (1987): Infrapatellar contracture syndrome. *Am J Sports Med* 15:331–341.

13. Sachs RA, Daniel DL, Stone ML, Garfein RF. (1989): Patellofemoral problems after anterior cruciate ligament reconstruction. *Am J Sports Med* 17:760–765.

14. Sawhney R, Dearwater S, Irrgang JJ, Fu FH. (1990): Quadriceps exercises following ACL reconstruction without anterior cruciate ligament reconstruction without anterior tibial displacement. Presented at the annual conference of the American Physical Therapy Association, Anaheim, CA, June 1990.

15. Shelbourne KD, Nitz P. (1990): Accelerated rehabilitation after anterior cruciate ligament reconstruction. *Am J Sports Med* 18:292–299.

16. Shelbourne KD, Wilckens JH, Mollabashy A, Decarlo M, (1991): Arthrofibrosis in acute anterior cruciate ligament reconstruction: the effect of timing of reconstruction and rehabilitation. *Am J Sports Med* 19:332–336.

17. Strum GM, Friedman MJ, Fox JM, et al. (1990): Acute anterior cruciate ligament reconstruction: analysis of complications. *Clin Orthop* 253:184–189.

18. Voight M, Bell S, Rhoades D. (1991): Instrumented testing of anterior tibial translation in open versus closed chain activity. *Phys Ther* 71:S98.

The Anterior Cruciate Ligament: Current and
Future Concepts, edited by D.W. Jackson, et al.
Raven Press, Ltd., New York © 1993.

CHAPTER 34

Rehabilitation After Anterior Cruciate Ligament Surgery

Lonnie E. Paulos and Jeremy Stern

Successful outcome from an anterior cruciate ligament (ACL) surgery can be enhanced with a team approach. There is a chain of treatment decisions (Fig. 1) that involves the combined efforts of the surgeon, therapist, and patient, and is based on the skills and cooperation of these individuals. The chain begins with patient selection, moves to procedure selection and surgical techniques, and ends with rehabilitation. The rehabilitation link of this chain must take into consideration the balance between the effects of disuse on musculoskeletal tissues and the knowledge of the healing requirements related to the specific surgical procedure. There should be a progression in a logical fashion through the chronology of immobility, range of motion, progressive weight-bearing, and strengthening exercises. The strengthening phase can be subdivided into the separate phases of isometrics, isotonics, functional exercises, and isokinetics. The ultimate goal of the final phase is a safe return to full activity.

BASIC SCIENCE OF IMMOBILITY AND HEALING

To carefully plan a rehabilitative course, a balance must be achieved between too much activity, which has the potential to damage the repair, and not enough activity, which may not stress the graft and promote healing. The individual rehabilitation program should be based on the reaction of the musculoskeletal system to injury, disuse, and stress.

All tissues in the musculoskeletal system suffer from the atrophic effects of disuse and immobility. This is true

L.E. Paulos and J. Stern: The Orthopaedic Specialty Hospital, Salt Lake City, Utah 84107.

whether the immobility is from a brace, cast, or voluntary disuse by the patient. Disuse atrophy occurs after a short period of immobility (2,3,23–25,29,58). Eriksson and Haggmark showed 40% quadriceps atrophy after 5 weeks of immobilization, and noted a decrease in oxidative fast-twitch fibers and slow-twitch endurance fibers (22). In addition, immobilization in a shortened position (i.e., joint flexion) seemed to increase the rate of atrophy (21,22). Patients with joint effusions experience similar atrophic effects, although they are not immobilized. This stems from the neuromuscular inhibition to the quadriceps caused by the effusion.

Ligamentous attachments to bone are very sensitive to disuse and immobilization. The greatest reabsorption occurs at ligamentous insertion sites (39,57). Because collagen is laid down along lines of stress, the lack of stress allows collagen to deposit in a random fashion, leading to decreased compliance and tensile strength (1). After 8 weeks of immobility, Noyes saw a 40% decrease in strength and a 30% decrease in stiffness at the ligamentous insertion sites (43). This was reversible with the return of stress to the ligament, but took more than 1 year to return completely.

Hyaline cartilage is also sensitive to disuse and immobility. Motion and weight-bearing are critical to hyaline cartilage nutrition, because chondroblasts get nutrition through imhibition of synovial fluid via cyclic loading. Weight-bearing is also important to the maintenance of a strong subchondral bone plate. Buckwalter et al. showed that decreased stress is closely followed by changes in hyaline fluid dynamics (14). Rabbit studies showed histologic changes after 6 days, which included metachromasia, decreased water content, and increased metabolic activity (55). Although early motion seems to reverse these changes, they may become permanent after as little as 8 weeks (24,51). Ulceration can oc-

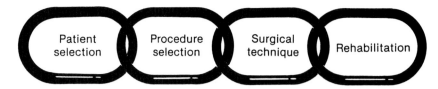

FIG. 1. Rehabilitaion is a critical link in the chain of treatment decisions regarding knees with anterior instability.

cur at points of cartilage abutment (23) and at areas of intraarticular adhesions that become avulsed during manipulation (47).

The effects of disuse and immobilization that effect ligaments and muscle also occur in the periarticular structures. As collagen deposition becomes random, ligamentous structure are remodeled in the position of immobilization. Articular adhesions form and the joint becomes stiff (2–4,6,23,29,48). Evans et al. have further shown that by 12 weeks a torque 12 times normal is required to move a joint through its normal arc of motion.

To avoid these disuse changes, immediate or early motion is required. Noyes et al. and Bassett et al. (13,42,43) advocate continuous passive motion (CPM) for early postoperative motion. It has been our experience that although CPM does provide early range of motion, it can be dangerous to the ACL reconstruction if the CPM unit is inappropriately placed on the patient or if limits for range of motion are inappropriately set. There is also the potential of damage to the graft through cycling fatigue, or sundial effect, at the notch margins (47). In view of these dangers, we do not recommend the use of CPM. Rosen et al. showed that there was no effect, positive or negative, with the use of CPM. We have found that it is beneficial to have patients involved in a more active manner with their early range of motion, so that they become part of the healing process. Our goal then is to initiate active and passive motion as early as possible, determined by patient type (i.e., hyperligamentous laxity or age) and surgical consideration (i.e., graft type, fixation type, or other associated procedures).

MUSCULOSKELETAL HEALING

The next phase to consider is that of musculoskeletal healing. There should be a balance between the stress needed to stimulate and align collagen production and the need to protect the weakened peri- and intraarticular tissue. Most surgeons would agree that the menisci are important structures of the knee. One of the goals of ACL reconstruction is to create an environment in which the menisci can survive if not damaged at the time of anterior cruciate injury, and heal if repair is needed. Healing in the peripheral vascular zone (red zone) occurs much like healing elsewhere in the body (10,16,32,36,

56). This occurs via migration of pleuripotential cells from the vascular channels outside the meniscal body. There cells differentiate into fibroblasts, which produce a collagen scar. This healing can occur only in a stable environment (47) without excess meniscal motion or shear stress.

More recently there has been an investigation into the ability of the meniscus to heal in the avascular or white zone (9,56). It is thought that this occurs by the action of meniscal fibroblasts that are nourished by synovial fluid, and possibly enhanced by fibrin clot through an intermediary such as platelet-derived growth factor (8,11).

Hyaline cartilage shows limited ability to heal insults to the cell matrix molecules, or proteoglycans. This is true regardless of the cause of injury (e.g., blunt trauma, surgical trauma, infection, or immobility). Defects superficial to the subchondral bone show healing potential that is limited to chondrocyte proliferation and matrix repair (14). Defects that penetrate into the subchondral bone heal with ingrowth of pleuripotential cells from the bony vascular bed, which differentiate to fibroblasts. These then change the initial fibrin clot to a fibrocartilage scar. This process, which takes 6 or more months to complete, ends with a scar cartilage that is inferior in quality and shows a greater wear over time than normal hyaline (26). For these defects to heal, whether traumatic or surgical, the knee must be protected. Large defects in high-stress, weight-bearing zones, those in the patellofemoral joint, or those in unstable knees do poorly, regardless of the mode of treatment.

There are several factors to consider related to the incorporation of the graft. The strength of the initial graft fixation, as well as healing at the fixation site and within the tunnels are factors affected by rehabilitation. Early loss of fixation occurs via creep, suture migration, tissue necrosis at the bony tunnels, and cyclical loading. Bone-to-bone healing has been shown to be more predictable and faster than soft tissue–to–bone healing (12,17,38). In addition, interference screw fixation of the bone plug to the tunnel has proven to be stronger than staple or screw fixation (20,37,38). Stronger initial fixation allows for earlier motion and weight-bearing, and thus decreases the surgical morbidity and the potential to develop arthrofibrosis (18). It is the superior fixation that has led to the acceptance of bone–patellar tendon–bone autografts as the standard for ACL reconstructions. The less commonly used hamstring graft (semitendinosus tendon with or without the gracilis tendon) raises concerns related to the weaker initial fixation and the rate of fixation that occurs within the bony tunnels. The modes of fixation using a screw and washer, or sutures through a button or around a post, allow for the potential adverse effects of soft tissue necrosis under the washer, necrosis secondary to suture techniques, or stress risers at the bony tunnel margins. Various investigators have noted that the healing of soft tissue grafts in bony tunnels is much like fracture healing or enchondral ossification (52,54). Many of the drawbacks of hamstring graft fixation and healing have been improved with newer washer design (33,34,44,49) but more documentation of techniques being developed for endoscopic placement of hamstring grafts will evolve.

The rate of incorporation of the intraarticular portion of the graft should effect any rehabilitation protocol. Cabaud et al. divided soft tissue healing into three phases (16). The acute or inflammatory phase lasts only the first 72 hours. The repair and regeneration phase lasts from 48 hours to 6 weeks. This phase is marked by fibroblast migration and proliferation, and in the production of Type III collagen. Phase III begins at 3 weeks and continues for an unknown period of time. During this phase, the Type II collagen is replaced by Type I collagen, and the collagen is oriented along the lines of stress. The ultimate graft strength attained is approximately 50% of the original graft strength by 3 to 12 months postsurgery in animal models (5,16,27,33,35,41). Allografts seem to undergo a similar progression of healing but over a different time frame. The period of healing is dependent, at least in part, on the allograft size, with larger allografts maturing more slowly and possibly never reaching full maturation in their central portions (unpublished data, Charles Beck).

Lastly, there are biologic variations in the healing process of different patients. Those patients who have generalized ligamentous laxity (i.e., hyperextension of the elbows, knees, and distal interphalangeal joints) may need to be protected longer. Those patients who tend to be "scar formers" or produce keloids are at greater risk for arthrofibrosis and would need a faster, more aggressive rehabilitation protocol (46).

BIOMECHANICS OF HEALING

There are biomechanical factors that must be considered during the rehabilitation phase of healing. As motion begins, the graft is subject to stresses in the form of cyclic loading, stretching past the graft elastic limit, or simple overloading. Cyclic stresses can cause fatigue failure at points of high stress concentration, such as at the bony tunnel margins. Cyclic stress can be decreased by accurate placement of the graft, and possibly by placing the bone block flush with the surface of the intercondylar

notch such that no tendon is in the femoral tunnel. Acute overload is of course possible, particularly if the patient is not compliant. This can occur in flexion or extension with sudden high loads. It is more likely to occur when the graft is weakest, during the early phases of healing, and if no brace is used. Less severe loads may cause stretching of the graft past its elastic limit, causing the graft to be permanently elongated (46). These grafts will be intact, but will lose function secondary to elongation. This can happen due to anterior drawer via quad contraction (7,28,45) or by walking down ramps, stairs, etc. (49). Even if the graft is isometric it is subject to strain with leg extension. This strain is greatest from 0 to 20 degrees and is increased with active leg extension against a distally applied force. In addition, the force generated by functional activities must be considered (19,41,45,49,53).

A last surgical consideration is the tensioning of the graft. It is necessary to tension the graft properly to avoid capturing the knee or leaving it unstable. More work in this area is needed, because no one has shown what is the proper graft tension for different ACL grafts. However, it seems that the proper tensioning will be tissue specific. Numerous investigators have shown that patellar tendon grafts are stiffer than hamstring or iliotibial band grafts. Thus, patellar tendon grafts require less tensioning than hamstring or iliotibial band grafts (15,41). In addition, the strength of the graft must be considered. As a rule, grafted tissue will lose up to 50% of its initial strength, so a graft must be selected that is twice as strong as needed. Noyes et al. in 1984 demonstrated clearly the relative strengths of various donor tissues (41).

GENERAL REHABILITATIVE PROGRAM

Our ACL rehabilitative program begins in the preoperative phase. Before surgery, all patients are instructed by a physical therapist in the exercises they will be required to perform in the acute postoperative period: straight leg raising, quad sets, patellar glides (Fig. 2), and ankle pumps. In addition, they are taught how to use a polar care unit, which is applied to all patients. We feel that the use of a cooling device decreases postoperative inflammation and pain, and is a valuable postoperative modality. Beginning on the first postoperative day, patients will be started on a protocol individualized for their injury and specific surgeries. In choosing this protocol, we again consider the possibility of ligamentous laxity or keloid formation. It is critical that as the patient proceeds through recovery, the physician and therapist maintain communication in regard to the patient's progress and signs of any potential problems. In addition, the surgeon should continue to assess the soft tissue healing of the patient and adjust the protocol as needed. Our protocols are printed so that both the therapist and the patient can

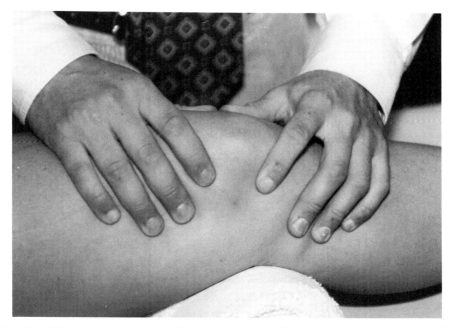

FIG. 2. Patellar glides maintain patellar motion and prevent patellar entrapment. It is important that these are not done too aggressively or they can cause patellar entrapment.

easily read and understand which exercises and what brace settings are to be used at any point postoperatively. We feel it is important to include patients as part of the rehabilitative team. They should be encouraged to be actively involved in their physical therapy.

BRACING, IMMOBILITY, AND RANGE OF MOTION

All patients are placed in a postoperative knee brace (Fig. 3) that is easy to apply, quickly changes flexion and extension stops, allows patellar mobilization, and facilitates wound inspection. In must also be able to accommodate the polar care pads and hoses now used. It is our goal to completely eliminate immobilization from almost all postoperative rehabilitation protocols. In general, our patients begin passive range of motion on the first postoperative day via wall slides (Fig. 4). If immobilization is felt to be necessary, it should not exceed 3 to 4 weeks. Bone–patella–bone allografts and autografts, and Achilles tendon allografts are allowed 0 to 90 degrees of passive motion and 40 to 90 degrees of active motion immediately postsurgery. Hamstring grafts are allowed

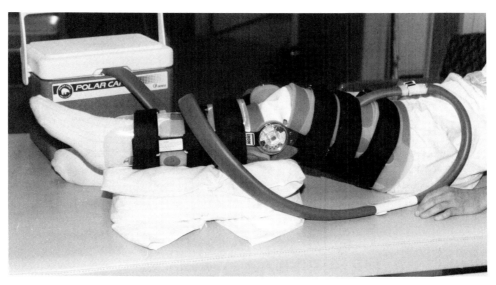

FIG. 3 Postoperative brace with polar care unit in place.

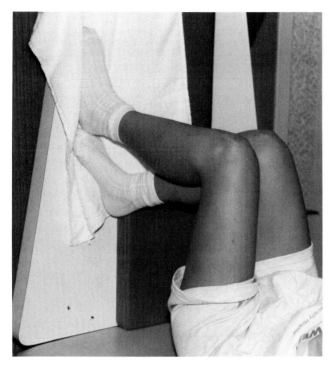

FIG. 4. Wall slides allow for good range of motion in a safe, effective manner, and keep the patients involved in their care.

10 to 70 degrees passively and 30 to 60 degrees actively due to their weaker initial fixation. We have not found a need to restrict range of motion in patients who have had meniscal repairs because this does not seem to affect the outcome. However, we do lock their braces between range of motion sessions. Again, we prefer patient involvement in active and passive range of motion via wall slides and collateral leg stretches, rather than CPM, which increases cost.

WEIGHT-BEARING

Even more than range of motion, weightbearing is procedure specific. Non–weight-bearing or partial weightbearing is needed to allow for healing of the graft within the tunnel for both bone-to-bone and tendon-to-bone healing. The onset of full weight-bearing is individualized. We prefer that the patient have no more than 5 degrees extension loss, no quadriceps lag, minimal swelling, and enough quadriceps strength to allow nearly normal gait. Meniscal repairs may alter weight-bearing status of the patient depending on the surgeon's preference. For full-thickness chondral defects that were treated with drilling or abrasion, we prefer that patients have 6 weeks of non–weight-bearing to allow metaplasia from fibrin clot to scar cartilage and to avoid damaging the neocartilage by shear stress or axial compression. For patients using a hamstring graft, our preference is to delay until the beginning of the sixth postoperative week. Fifty per-

cent weight-bearing is then allowed, progressing to full weight-bearing over 2 weeks.

ISOMETRIC EXERCISES

Isometric exercises are defined as those where muscular contraction occurs without change in length of the muscle or joint position. These are the first strengthening techniques that are allowed after ACL surgery. Quad setting and straight leg raising are the mainstays of this program. For these exercises, we prefer the brace be locked at 30 degrees, preventing inadvertent extension of the knee. The isometrics are performed on both legs to facilitate the cross-over effect (30,31), in which exercise of the nonsurgical leg leads to strengthening of the operated limb. For those patients who are not progressing as would be expected, electromyographic (EMG) biofeedback can be used to help retrain weakened quadriceps. EMG biofeedback has taken the place of neuromuscular stimulation, which we found ultimately to be of question-

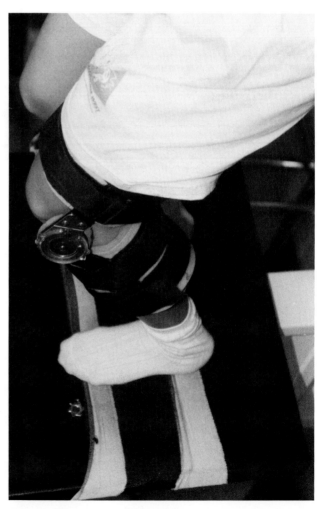

FIG. 5. Closed-chain PREs produce good strength safely, and can be started when weight-bearing is allowed.

able value. Using EMG biofeedback, the patient has a visual guide as to when the quadriceps muscle has been successfully contracted. For those patients who are having difficulty with their quadriceps strengthening, this can be a valuable tool, particularly in the early postoperative period.

ISOTONICS (PROGRESSIVE RESISTANCE EXERCISES)

Isotonic strengthening or progressive resistance exercises (PREs) are those in which muscle contraction produces constant tension over a given range of motion. These must be carefully instituted with strict attention paid to the arc of motion. The first PREs are those that isolate the agonist muscles, predominantly the hamstrings. These can be performed in a seated or prone position, and again should be performed on both surgical and nonsurgical limbs. PREs train both agonist and antagonist muscles in a cocontraction, such as leg press, and are followed lastly by antagonist muscle work. Our

preference is to use a brace during these exercises. The brace settings are determined according to the specific surgical procedures and reassessed depending on patient progress. As a starting point, 10% of the body weight is used for both quad and hamstring exercises with increases according to the patient progression. Recently, more emphasis has been placed on closed-chain progressive resistance exercises, which are more physiologic, probably safer, and more functional exercises (Fig. 5). Closed-chain exercises are those where the foot is fixed such that movement at any limb segment causes movement at all limb segments, as in squats or leg press. These can start at the time weight-bearing is allowed. The benefit of closed-chain activities is that while strengthening both agonist and antagonist muscle, the exercises also enhance coordination and proprioception. The patient will generally begin stretch cords (Fig. 6A) and minisquat (Fig. 6B) when they are allowed 50% weight-bearing. In our protocol this is at 3 weeks for bone–patellar–bone allograft and autograft, and Achilles tendon allograft in those patients who did not have meniscal

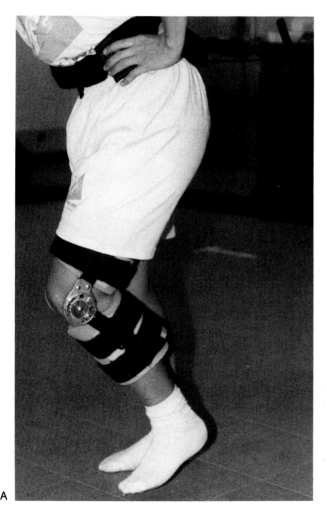

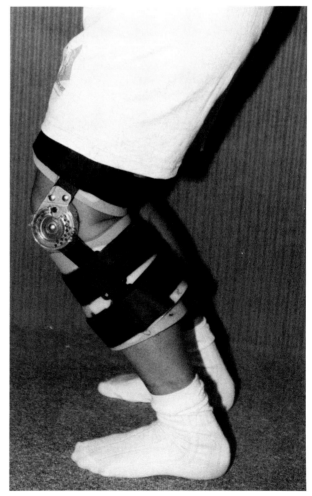

A   B

FIG. 6. Sports Cords (**A**) and minisquats (**B**) promote strength and balance, and can be started when weight-bearing is allowed.

repair, and at 6 weeks for meniscal repair patients and those patients with hamstring grafts. Swimming can be started when the wounds allow. Flutter kick only is allowed due to the marked ACL strain produced by a whip kick. Cycling can begin when range of motion is 105 degrees or greater. Hamstring grafts and those with meniscal repairs would again be delayed. Balance activities such as BAPS, KAT, sand dunes, balance board, and pogo ball should be delayed until 5 to 7 weeks, and then we prefer the patient be protected with bracing.

ISOKINETICS

Isokinetics are activities where the speed of motion is fixed and the resistance to motion accommodates to the amount of force input to the machine. These are the last strengthening exercises introduced after ACL reconstruction. These usually do not begin until 5 to 6 months postoperatively because they produce high joint-reactive forces. Initially, our patients use high-speed exercises because they produce lower joint forces than the slower speeds (Table 1). Our patients use a pyramid type workout starting from approximately 180 degrees per second, increasing at 30 degree per second intervals to 300 degrees per second, then working their way back down to the 180 degrees per second range. Again, the 60 to 180 degrees per second range exercises are avoided until very late in the rehabilitation schedule due to their increased joint-reactive forces. Also, because this is an open-chain exercise, it can lead to graft stresses. Patients with concomitant chondrosis, particularly in the patellofemoral joint, may not tolerate this type of work-out at all because it increases the patellofemoral joint-reactive forces dramatically. As closed-chain isokinetic devices are redeveloped, perhaps this form of exercise will become a more important part of our rehabilitation program for the reasons previously stated.

RETURN TO SPORTS

Return to sports is the usual goal after ACL reconstruction. For patellar tendon and Achilles tendon grafts, the patient is allowed to return to sports at 6 to 9 months if all of the following are achieved: no swelling, a completed jog/run program, isokinetic testing of the quads that shows 85% strength of the operative leg versus the nonoperative leg, isokinetic testing of the hamstrings that shows 90% strength of the operative leg versus the nonoperative leg, a single leg hop test that shows 85% of the distance on the operative leg as the nonoperative leg, and a full range of motion. Although the usefulness of braces in graft protection is questionable, we protect all of our ACL reconstructions during sporting activities for 1 year postoperatively. We use a functional ACL brace with a 20-degree extension stop because this allows us to limit the limb to 7 to 10 degrees of extension.

TABLE 1. *Protocol for isokinetic exercise*

Weeks post-op	Program	Criteria
3–4	Concentric Hamstring conditioning 30°/sec to 60°/sec speeds. Full spectrum conditioning for unaffected extremity (quads & hams)	Patient able to perform manual isokinetics with therapist. Delay 2 wks if patient has unstable meniscus.
5–7	Concentric hamstring conditioning 60°/sec to 120° sec speeds. Hamstring strength test @ 60°/sec. Goal of 50–60% of unaffected ext. (start fifth week)	Ability of patient to catch higher speeds. Painfree conditioning.
8–11	Concentric hamstring conditioning 60°/sec to 240°/sec speeds. Hamstring strength/endurance test @ 60°/sec and 240°/sec (start 8th week) Goal of 70–80% of unaffected ext. Endurance goal 50% Alternate concentric/eccentric conditioning if strength is 75% Full spectrum conditioning for unaffected extremity (quads & hams)	Ability of patient to catch higher speeds. Test endurance @ 180°/sec if patient is unable to exercise @ 240°/sec. 70% endurance is ideal. (20 reps, 20% comp.)
12–16	Limited range of quadriceps concentric conditioning (90° to 40° ROM) 60°/sec to 180°/sec (start 12th week) Continue hamstring conditioning Goal of 100% hamstring strength by 12th week Quadriceps strength test @ week 14 @ 60°/sec (90°–40° ROM) Goal of 50–60% of unaffected ext	Patient able to perform manual isokinetics with therapist. Normal, painfree PF mobility. Use of anti-sheer device for quad conditioning.
17–24	Full spectrum quad/ham concentric conditioning (100° to −20° ROM) Strength/endurance test @ 60°/sec and 240°/sec Goal of 80% of unaffected ext	Painfree conditioning. Release patient to independent conditioning program when quads are 75%.

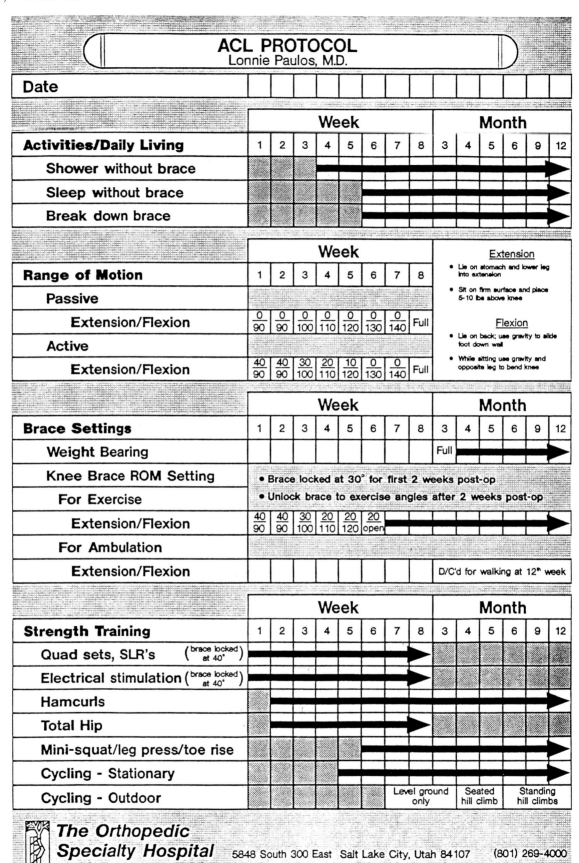

| ACL PROTOCOL | | | | | | | | | | | | | | | |
| Lonnie Paulos, M.D. | | | | | | | | | | | | | | | |

Date

| **Activities/Daily Living** | Week | | | | | | | | Month | | | | | |
	1	2	3	4	5	6	7	8	3	4	5	6	9	12
Shower without brace				→										→
Sleep without brace					→									→
Break down brace					→									→

| **Range of Motion** | Week | | | | | | | | Extension |
	1	2	3	4	5	6	7	8	• Lie on stomach and lower leg into extension
Passive									• Sit on firm surface and place 5-10 lbs above knee
Extension/Flexion	$\frac{0}{90}$	$\frac{0}{90}$	$\frac{0}{100}$	$\frac{0}{110}$	$\frac{0}{120}$	$\frac{0}{130}$	$\frac{0}{140}$	Full	Flexion
Active									• Lie on back; use gravity to slide foot down wall
Extension/Flexion	$\frac{40}{90}$	$\frac{40}{90}$	$\frac{30}{100}$	$\frac{20}{110}$	$\frac{10}{120}$	$\frac{0}{130}$	$\frac{0}{140}$	Full	• While sitting use gravity and opposite leg to bend knee

| **Brace Settings** | Week | | | | | | | | Month | | | | | |
	1	2	3	4	5	6	7	8	3	4	5	6	9	12
Weight Bearing									Full	→				
Knee Brace ROM Setting	• Brace locked at 30° for first 2 weeks post-op													
For Exercise	• Unlock brace to exercise angles after 2 weeks post-op													
Extension/Flexion	$\frac{40}{90}$	$\frac{40}{90}$	$\frac{30}{100}$	$\frac{20}{110}$	$\frac{20}{120}$	$\frac{20}{open}$	→							
For Ambulation														
Extension/Flexion									D/C'd for walking at 12ᵗʰ week					

| **Strength Training** | Week | | | | | | | | Month | | | | | |
	1	2	3	4	5	6	7	8	3	4	5	6	9	12
Quad sets, SLR's (brace locked at 40°)	→						→							
Electrical stimulation (brace locked at 40°)	→						→							
Hamcurls		→												→
Total Hip		→						→						
Mini-squat/leg press/toe rise			→											→
Cycling - Stationary														
Cycling - Outdoor								Level ground only	Seated hill climb		Standing hill climbs			

The Orthopedic Specialty Hospital 5848 South 300 East Salt Lake City, Utah 84107   (801) 269-4000

FIG. 7. Protocols for rehabilitation as specified by surgical procedure.

Date														

	Week								Month					
Balance/Coordination	1	2	3	4	5	6	7	8	3	4	5	6	9	12
Baps/KAT/Sandunes/ Rhomberg/Tape touch									→					
Profitter									→					
Sport cord lateral agility									→					

	Week								Month					
Conditioning	1	2	3	4	5	6	7	8	3	4	5	6	9	12
Cycle with well leg	→													
UBE (upper body conditioning)	→													
Swimming (refer to pool protocol)				20°	→									
Walking (100% weight)								10° →						
Stairmaster									20° →					
X-country ski machine									20° →					
Rowing									30°/90° →					
Run/jog (sports brace must be worn)													20° →	

	Week								Month					
Power Training	1	2	3	4	5	6	7	8	3	4	5	6	9	12
Low repetitions - leg press/Squats/Hamcurls									20°/90° →					
Isokinetics (refer to protocol)													→	

To Return to Sports:

- Minimum of 9 months post-operative
- No swelling
- Complete jog/run program
- Quadriceps strength 85% of opposite knee
- Hamstring strength 90% of opposite knee
- Hop distance 85% of opposite knee
- Range of motion 0° to 140°

FIG. 7. *Continued.*

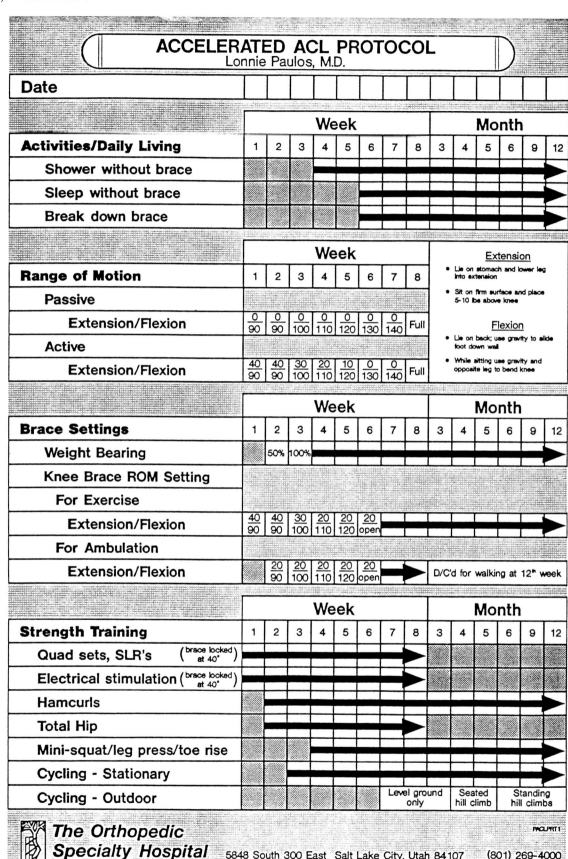

FIG. 7. *Continued.*

Date														

	Week								Month					
Balance/Coordination	1	2	3	4	5	6	7	8	3	4	5	6	9	12
Baps/KAT/Sandunes/Rhomberg/Tape touch						→→→→→→→→→→→→→→→→→→→→→→								
Profitter									→→→→→→→→→→→→→→					
Sport cord lateral agility									→→→→→→→→→→→→→→					

	Week								Month					
Conditioning	1	2	3	4	5	6	7	8	3	4	5	6	9	12
Cycle with well leg	→													
UBE (upper body conditioning)	→→													
Walking (100% weight)			10° →→→→→→→→→→→→→→→→→→→→→→→→→→→→→→→→→→→→											
Swimming (refer to pool protocol)				20° →→→→→→→→→→→→→→→→→→→→→→→→→→→→→→→→→→										
Stairmaster						20° →→→→→→→→→→→→→→→→→→→→→→→→→→→→→→→→								
X-country ski machine						20° →→→→→→→→→→→→→→→→→→→→→→→→→→→→→→→→								
Rowing							20° →→→→→→→→→→→→→→→→→→→→→→→→→→→→→→							
Run/jog (sports brace must be worn)												20° →→→→		

	Week								Month					
Power Training	1	2	3	4	5	6	7	8	3	4	5	6	9	12
Low repetitions: Leg press/Squats/Hamcurls									20°/90° →→→→→→→→→→→→→→					
Isokinetics (refer to protocol)											→→→→→→			

To Return to Sports:

- Minimum of 9 months post-operative
- No swelling
- Complete jog/run program
- Quadriceps strength 85% of opposite knee
- Hamstring strength 90% of opposite knee
- Hop distance 85% of opposite knee
- Range of motion 0° to 140°

PACLPRT2

FIG. 7. *Continued.*

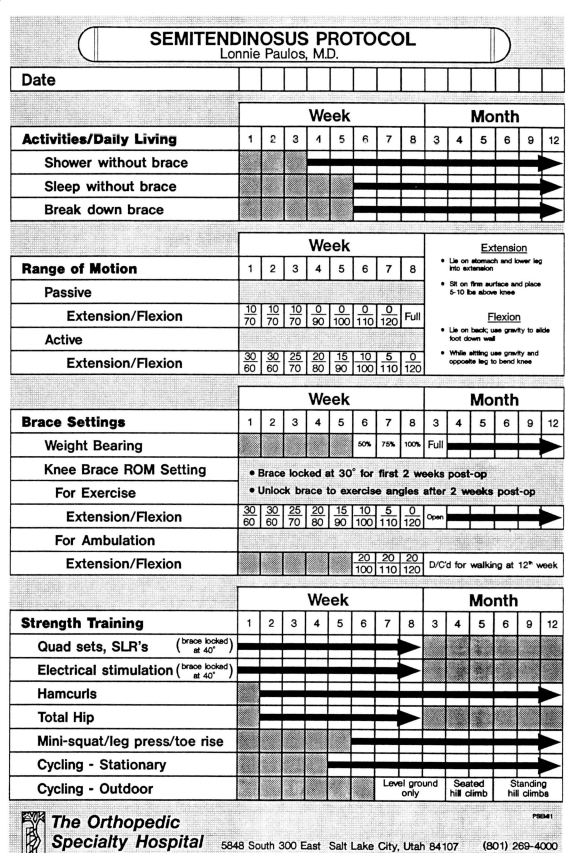

FIG. 7. Continued.

Date

	Week								Month					
Balance/Coordination	1	2	3	4	5	6	7	8	3	4	5	6	9	12
Baps/KAT/Sandunes/ Rhomberg/Tape touch								→→→→→→→→→→→→→→→→→						
Profitter									→→→→→→→→→→→→→					
Sport cord lateral agility									→→→→→→→→→→→→→					

	Week								Month					
Conditioning	1	2	3	4	5	6	7	8	3	4	5	6	9	12
Cycle with well leg	→→→→→→→													
UBE (upper body conditioning)	→→→													
Swimming (refer to pool protocol)					20° →→→→→→→→→→→→→→→→→→→→→→→→									
Walking (100% weight)								10° →→→→→→→→→→→→→→→→						
Stairmaster									20° →→→→→→→→→→→→→					
X-country ski machine									20° →→→→→→→→→→→→→					
Rowing									30°/90° →→→→→→→→					
Run/jog (sports brace must be worn)													20° →→	

	Week								Month					
Power Training	1	2	3	4	5	6	7	8	3	4	5	6	9	12
Low repetitions - leg press/Squats/Hamcurls									20°/90° →→→→→→→					
Isokinetics (refer to protocol)											→→→→			

To Return to Sports:

- Minimum of 9 months post-operative
- No swelling
- Complete jog/run program
- Quadriceps strength 85% of opposite knee
- Hamstring strength 90% of opposite knee
- Hop distance 85% of opposite knee
- Range of motion 0° to 140°

FIG. 7. Continued.

SPECIFIC PROTOCOLS

We use three ACL protocols (Fig. 7). Our standard protocol has weight-bearing and brace settings left blank. This allows us to individualize the protocol in accordance with the specific surgical procedure and patient situation. This protocol is used for patients with special requirements, or with another procedure in addition to the ACL reconstruction. For those patients with isolated ACL reconstructions, or with ACL reconstructions with partial meniscectomies only, an accelerated rehabilitation protocol allows earlier functional weight-bearing exercises. Lastly, our semitendinosus tendon protocol is slower to account for the weaker initial fixation, greater graft compliance, and slower soft tissue–to–bone healing.

For those grafts that allow bone-to-bone healing and interference screw fixation, immediate motion is started at 0 to 90 degrees. This, of course, may be changed depending on other surgeries. Generally, the patient is allowed an increase to 10 degrees per week after the third week. For meniscal repairs, the brace is locked at 30 degrees between range of motion sessions for 3 weeks, but the patient is still allowed 0 to 90 degrees immediately. Patients can shower without their brace after 3 weeks, sleep without the brace after 6 weeks, and walk without the brace after 12 weeks. After 12 weeks, the brace is used for exercises only. Functional braces are fit at 6 months or when the quadriceps mass is equal in both the operative and nonoperative legs.

One must remember the importance of patellar mobilization throughout the perioperative phase. It is important to stress to the patient that superior/inferior glides are the most important. We encourage the patient to perform patella glides and tilts at least five times a day to prevent a possible patellar entrapment syndrome. The patient and physical therapist should be counseled that these mobilization exercises should not cause the knee to become painful, swollen, or stiff, because this can actually increase the possibility of patellar entrapment.

Functional exercises, such as swimming and biking, are allowed early in the rehabilitative phase. Leg press from 20 to 90 degrees and mini squats are performed in place of leg extensions for quadriceps strengthening.

CONCLUSION

There is a chain of decisions that takes place after an ACL injury that links a patient to a successful return to sports. Care must be taken at each step not to use a cookbook technique, but to individualize the care of each patient, each surgery, each set of soft tissues, and each healing response. It is most important to make the patients feel part of the rehabilitation team and to encourage them to be active participants in their recovery.

REFERENCES

1. Akeson WH, Amiel D, Abel MF, et al. (1987): Effects of immobilization on joints. *Clin Orthop* 219:28–37.
2. Akeson WH, Amiel D, LaViolette D. (1967): The connective tissue response to immobility: a study of chondroitin-4 and -6 sulfate and dermatan sulfate changes in periarticular connective tissue of control and immobilized knees of dogs. *Clin Orthop* 51:183–197.
3. Akeson WH, Amiel D, Mechanic GL, et al. (1977): Collagen cross-linking alterations in joint contractions: changes in reducible crosslinks in periarticular connective tissue collagen after nine weeks of immobilization. *Connect Tissue Res* 5:15.
4. Akeson WH, Woo SL, Amiel D, et al. (1973): The connective tissue response to immobility: biomechanical changes in periarticular connective tissue of the immobilized rabbit knee. *Clin Orthop* 93:356–362.
5. Alm A, Ekstrom H, Gillquist J, et al (1974): The anterior cruciate ligament—a clinical and experimental study on tensile strength, morphology, and replacement by patellar ligament. *Acta Chir Scand (Suppl)* 445:15–24.
6. Andriacchi T, Sabiston P, Dehaven K, et al. (1987): Ligament injury and repair. In: Woo SL, Buckwalter JA, eds. *Injury and repair of musculoskeletal soft tissues.* Savannah, GA: American Academy of Orthopaedic Surgeons symposium.
7. Arms SW, Pope MH, Johnson RJ, et al. (1984): The biomechanics of anterior cruciate ligament rehabilitation and reconstruction. *Am J Sports Med* 12:8–18.
8. Arnoczky SP, McDevitt CA, Warren RF, et al. (1986): Meniscal repair using an exogenous fibrin clot—an experimental study in the dog. Presented at the 32nd annual meeting of the Orthopaedic Research Society, New Orleans, LA, February 1986.
9. Arnoczky SP, O'Brien SF, Dicarlo EF, et al. (1988): Cellular repopulation of deep-frozen meniscal autografts: an experimental study in the dog. Presented at the 34th annual meeting of the Orthopaedic Research Society, Atlanta, GA, February 1988.
10. Arnoczky SP, Warren RF. (1983): The microvasculature of the meniscus and its response to injury: an experimental study in the dog. *Am J Sports Med* 11:131–141.
11. Arnoczky SP, Warren RF, Kaplan N. (1985): Meniscal remodeling following partial meniscectomy—an experimental study in the dog. *J Arthrosc Rel Surg* 1:247–252.
12. Arnoczky SP, Warren RF, Kaplan N. (1986): Replacement of the anterior cruciate ligament using a patella tendon allograft—an experimental study. *J Bone Joint Surg* 68A:376–385.
13. Bassett FH II, Beck JL, Weiker G. (1980): A modified cast brace: its use in nonoperative and postoperative management of serious knee ligament injuries. *Am J Sports Med* 8:63–69.
14. Buckwalter J, Rosenberg L, Coutts R, et al. (1987): Articular cartilage: injury and repair. In: Woo SL, Buckwalter JA, eds. *Injury and repair of the musculoskeletal soft tissues.* Savannah, GA: American Academy of Orthopedic Surgeons symposium.
15. Burks RT, Leland R. (1988): Determination of graft tension before fixation in anterior cruciate ligament reconstruction. *J Arthrosc Rel Surg* 4:260–266.
16. Cabaud HE, Rodkey WG, Reagin JA. (1979): Experimental studies of acute anterior cruciate ligament injury and repair. *Am J Sports Med* 7:18–22.
17. Clancy WG Jr., Narechania RG, Rosenberg TD, et al. (1981): Anterior and posterior cruciate ligament reconstruction in rhesus monkeys: a histological, microangiographic, and biomechanical analysis. *J Bone Joint Surg* 63A:1270–1284.
18. Clancy WG Jr., Ray JM. (1987): Anterior cruciate ligament autografts. In: Jackson DW, Drez D Jr., eds. *The anterior cruciate deficient knee—new concepts in ligament repair.* St. Louis: CV Mosby.
19. Daniel DE, Akeson W, O'Conner J, eds. (1990): *Knee ligaments. Structure, function, injury, and repair.* New York: Raven Press.
20. Daniel DM, Robertson DB, Flood DL, Biden EN. (1987): Fixation of soft tissue. In: Jackson DW, Drez D Jr., eds. *The anterior cruciate deficient knee—new concepts in ligament repair.* St. Louis, MO: CV Mosby.
21. Dickinson A, Bennett KM. (1985): Therapeutic exercise. *Clinics Sports Med* 4:417–430.

22. Eriksson G, Haggmark T. (1979): Comparison of isometric muscle training and electrical stimulation supplementing isometric muscle training in the recovery after major knee ligament surgery. *Am J Sports Med* 7:169–171.

23. Evans EB, Eggers GWN, Butler JK, Blumel J. (1960): Experimental immobilization and remobilization of rat knee joints. *J Bone Joint Surg* 42A:737–758.

24. Finsterbush A, Friedman B. (1973): Early changes in immobilized rabbits knee joints: a light and electron microcopy study. *Clin Orthop* 92:305–319.

25. Finsterbush A, Friedman B. (1975): Reversibility of joint changes produced by immobilization in rabbits. *Clin Orthop* 111:290–298.

26. Furukawa T, Eyre DR, Koide S, Gilmcher MJ. (1980): Biomechanical studies on repair cartilage resurfacing, experimental defects in rabbit knee. *J Bone Joint Surg* 62A:79–89.

27. Gelberman RH, Menon J, Gonsalves M, et al. (1980): The effects of mobilization on the vascularization of healing flexor tendons in dogs. *Clin Orthop* 153:283–289.

28. Grood ES, Suntay WJ, Noyes FR, et al. (1984): Biomechanics of the knee-extension exercise. *J Bone Joint Surg* 66A:725–734.

29. Hall MC. (1963): Cartilage changes after experimental immobilization of the knee joint in the young rat. *J Bone Joint Surg* 42A:36–44.

30. Hallebrandt FA, Houtz SJ, Kirkorian AM. (1950): Influence of bimanual exercise on unilateral work capacity. *J Appl Physiol* 2:452–466.

31. Hallebrandt FA, Waterland JC. (1962): Indirect learning: the influence of uni-manual exercise on related muscle groups of the same and the opposite side. *Am J Physiol Med* 41:45–55.

32. Heatley FW. (1980): The meniscus—can it be repaired? An experimental investigation in rabbits. *J Bone Joint Surg* 62B:397–402.

33. Hirsch EF, Morgan RH. (1939): Casual significance to traumatic ossification in tendon insertions. *Arch Surg* 39:824–837.

34. Hurson DJ, Sheehan JM. (1981): The use of spike plastic washers in the repair of avulsed ligaments. *Acta Orthop Scand* 53:23–36.

35. Kennedy JC, Weinberg HW, Wilson AS. (1974): Anatomy of function of the anterior cruciate ligament. *J Bone Joint Surg* 56A:223–235.

36. King D. (1936): The healing of semilunar cartilages. *J Bone Joint Surg* 18:1069–1076.

37. Kurosaka M, Yoshiya S, Andrish JT. (1987): A biomechanical comparison of different surgical techniques of graft fixation in anterior cruciate ligament reconstruction. *Am J Sports Med* 15:225–229.

38. Lambert KL. (1983): Vascularized patella tendon graft with rigid internal fixation for anterior cruciate ligament insufficiency. *Clin Orthop Rel Res* 172:85–89.

39. Laros GS, Tipton CM, Cooper RR. (1971): Influence of physical activity on ligament insertions in the knees of dogs. *J Bone Joint Surg* 53A:275–286.

40. Deleted in proof.

41. Noyes FR, Butler DL, Grood ES, et al. (1984): Biomechanical analysis of human ligament grafts used in knee ligament repairs and reconstructions. *J Bone Joint Surg* 66A:344–352.

42. Noyes FR, Butler DL, Paulos LE, Grood EL. (1983): Intra-articular cruciate reconstruction I: perspectives on graft strength, vascularization and immediate motion after replacement. *Clin Orthop* 172:71–77.

43. Noyes FR, Mangine RE, Barber S. (1974): Biomechanics of ligament failure: analysis of immobilization, exercise, and reconditioning effects in primates. *J Bone Joint Surg* 56A:1406–1418.

44. O'Carroll P, Hurson VJ, Sheehan J, et al. (1983): A technique of medial ligament repair of the knee with cancellous screws and spiked washers. *Injury* 15:99–104.

45. Paulos LE, Noyes FR, Grood E, Butler DL. (1981): Knee rehabilitation after anterior cruciate ligament reconstruction and repair. *Am J Sports Med* 9:140–149.

46. Paulos LE, Payne FC, Rosenberg TD. (1987): Rehabilitation after anterior cruciate ligament surgery. In: Jackson DW, Drez D, eds. *The anterior cruciate ligament deficient knee.* St. Louis, MO: CV Mosby.

47. Paulos LE, Wnorowski DC, Beck CL. (1991): Rehabilitation following knee surgery. Recommendations. *Sports Med* 11:257–275.

48. Peacock EE Jr. (1963): Comparison of collagenous tissue surrounding normal and immobilized joints. *Surg Forum* 14:400.

49. Robertson DB, Daniel DM, Biden E. (1986): Soft tissue fixation to bone. *Am J Sports Med* 14:398–403.

50. Deleted in proof.

51. Salter RB, Simmonds DF, Malcolm BW, et al. (1980): The biological effect of continuous passive motion on the healing of full-thickness defects in anterior cartilage. *J Bone Joint Surg* 62A: 1232–1251.

52. Sisk TD, Stralka SW, Deering MB, Griffin JW. (1987): Effect of electrical stimulation on quadriceps strength after reconstructive surgery of the anterior cruciate ligament. *Am J Sports Med* 15:215–220.

53. Smidt G. (1973): Biomechanical analysis of knee flexion and extension. *J Biomech* 6:79–92.

54. Stratford P. (1981): Electromyography of the quadriceps femoris muscles in subjects with normal knees and acutely effused knees. *Phys Ther* 62:279–283.

55. Troyer H. (1975): The effect of short-term immobilization on the rabbit knee joint cartilage. *Clin Orthop* 107:249–257.

56. Webber RJ, Harris M, Hough AJ Jr. (1984): Intrinsic repair capabilities of rabbit meniscal fibrocartilage: a cell culture model. Presented at the 30th annual meeting of the Orthopaedic Research Society, Atlanta, GA, February 1984.

57. Woo SL-Y, Gomez MA, Seguchi Y, et al. (1983): Measurement of mechanical properties of ligament substance from a bone–ligament–bone preparation. *J Orthop Res* 1:22.

58. Woo SL-Y, Matthew JV, Akeson WH, et al. (1975): The connective tissue response to immobility: a correlative study of biomechanical and biochemical measurements of the normal and immobilized rabbit knee. *Arthritis Rheumatism* 18:257–264.

New Directions: Basic Science, Clinical Applications and Research

The previous sections in this text have presented and interpreted current information on the anterior cruciate ligament (ACL). This subsection expands the search for improved techniques and materials to be used for ACL reconstruction. These innovative and provocative concepts and approaches are still in their infancy and will require more investigation and evaluation to establish their usefulness.

Rapidly expanding advances in cellular and molecular biology are stimulating these new concepts for future treatment of ACL injuries and surgery. These have included increased insight into the role of growth factors, cytokines, integrins, and extracellular matrix, and the regulation of gene expression. This information must still be transferred to the clinical setting.

Coupled with new understanding of these biologic processes, advances in the field of biomaterials have restimulated the quest for an ACL prosthesis and augmentation device. New implantable synthetics can mimic natural tissues and offer the potential to physically stimulate or control the cellular responses. They may act as a substrate for cell growth and provide controlled release of chemical mediators and bioactive molecules. These new biomaterials may enhance attachment site formation for cells and increase localized cellular collagen synthesis. As information and understanding increases in the design and synthesis of biopolymers, these new materials will offer the potential to mimic the natural tissues they are intended to replace.

As we search for new approaches, the same questions arise. Is the treatment effective in the patient? What is the range of expected outcomes? Has the patient's quality of life improved? This quality of life assessment as an outcome in ACL reconstructive surgery continues to be an area that will impact the future treatment and health-care delivery systems.

Timothy M. Simon

The Anterior Cruciate Ligament: Current and Future Concepts, edited by D.W. Jackson, et al. Raven Press, Ltd., New York © 1993.

CHAPTER 35

Potential Clinical Applications of Growth Factors and Unique Cell Populations to Promote Anterior Cruciate Ligament Healing

David A. Hart, Cyril B. Frank, and Patricia G. Murphy

In many of the previous chapters of this monograph, specific aspects of the biochemistry, biomechanics, cell biology, and morphology of normal and healing ligaments have been discussed. From these discussions it is apparent that new understanding of the processes is evolving at a rapid rate and we are becoming poised to apply some of this information to foster anterior cruciate ligament (ACL) healing. Cell biology, growth modulators, inflammation, regulation of gene expression, and the role of the extracellular matrix (ECM) are all areas where some of the basic science information can now be molded to fit specific clinical applications. This chapter will identify some of these new directions, indicate the need for specific additional information, and speculate on how the information can be applied to the specific goal of augmenting ACL healing to achieve functional regeneration. Many of the principles underlying the rationale for the areas discussed have been addressed in Chapter 14. Therefore, they will not be reiterated here and the reader is referred to that chapter.

CLINICAL APPROACHES

Unique Cells and Biologic Matrix

There are likely many variables that could explain why the ACL heals less well than the medial collateral

D. A. Hart, and C. B. Frank: McCaig Centre for Joint Injury and Arthritis Research, Department of Microbiology and Infectious Diseases, University of Calgary Health Science Center, Calgary, Alberta, Canada T2N 4N1.

P. G. Murphy: Joint Injury and Arthritis Research Group, University of Calgary Health Science Center, Calgary, Alberta, Canada T2N 4N1.

ligament (MCL). One possibility is that total ACL transections might not have a scaffold upon which to heal. That is, the joint position and possible retraction of the ACL prevents it from having an attachment as well as a ground substance on which healing might occur. Therefore, providing the ACL with a synthetic matrix may enable this ligament to heal more effectively. There are several possibilities for the types of matrices that may be used for this purpose. One option is the use of fetal ligament tissue to replace the injured ACL. This option could be beneficial for several reasons, but may provoke ethical restraints. One beneficial effect could be related to the organization of the matrix, with oriented collagen fibrils. The cells used in other ligament healing may not be available to the ACL or may be in an unresponsive state (terminally differentiated). Thus, other factors may be required to activate the cells. Fetal tissue could provide a scaffold to the injured ACL, as well as providing the ACL with cells that are likely more pluripotent and undifferentiated. These cells may proliferate and form a more normal tissue. The fetal cells may proliferate in a scar matrix much more effectively than they would in a more "mature" matrix, because the matrix that is observed in scar more closely resembles immature or embryonic tissue (1,7,8,14,19,21,24,25,27). Some of the matrix components (collagen and fibronectin) detected in scar tissue are also observed in embryonic and fetal tissue (10,14). Interestingly, in other adult injury or wound-healing models, the cells in the wound appear to revert to an embryonic phenotype with regard to gene expression of molecules such as fibronectin (10) and collagen (14).

The reverse may occur as well. That is, the intrinsic cells within the ACL may also be more capable of participating in the healing response when exposed to a natural immature matrix. It is also conceivable to use only the cells from either fetal tissue or adult tissue and then introduce these cells into the joint or adhere them onto the scar in an attempt to repopulate the torn ACL. These cells may repopulate a matrix in which the ligament cells have been removed. This could prove to be technically more difficult, and the fetal cells may not be as successful in a mature matrix compared with a more immature one. Although using allogeneic tissue is a concern immunologically, this may not be as relevant in ligament tissue because of the relative avascularity. It is also possible to eliminate the potential immunological response by using autogeneic cells obtained from the patient, grown *in vitro*, and later reintroduced into the joint. The use of these types of cells may provide the ligament with the phenotypically correct type of cells in which a better healing response may occur.

Other possible explanations as to the mystery of ACL healing may relate to its vascularity. The ACL is thought to be less vascular than the MCL, and this may be critical during healing (3,4,11). As demonstrated in other wound healing, the formation of a blood clot at the site of injury is beneficial to wound repair (7,8). This has also been demonstrated using a fibrin clot in similar types of systems, including meniscal repair (18). The blood clot contains, among other components, platelets that upon activation release growth factors such as platelet-derived growth factor (PDGF) and transforming growth factor (TGF)-β. As mentioned previously, these growth factors recruit other cell types thought to be involved in the healing response (7,8). The application of a synthetic matrix, such as a fibrin clot or a composite fibrin-collagen gel, containing these factors or the introduction of a natural or augmented fibrin matrix around the torn ACL may provide the injury site with the factors necessary for healing.

In Vivo Augmentation with Growth Factors/Cytokines

It also may be possible to enhance healing of the ACL and ligaments in general by applying exogenous factors to the injured tissue. As previously indicated, fetal wound healing lacks an inflammatory response and is much more successful than adult wound healing (20,22,23,25,27). It also has been demonstrated that prolonged inflammation is deleterious to some wound healing. Therefore, improper regulation of inflammation may have a negative influence on repair of ligaments, although it has previously been shown that anti-inflammatory agents do inhibit ligament healing (9). However, it is possible that application of appropriate concentrations of anti-inflammatory drugs (such as aspirin, indomethacin, and corticosteroids) or natural anti-inflammatory molecules (such as the interleukin-1 antagonists), alone or in combination with other substances, could result in a less "hostile" environment (decreased proteinase secretion and cytokine expression) in which more effective healing/regeneration may occur.

Other agents that may enhance healing of ligaments *in vivo* are growth factors. Growth factors have been demonstrated to increase the proliferation of the scar of certain tissues *in vivo* (most notably skin). This also has been demonstrated in connective tissue such as bone, where there is an increase in bone formation (17). However, the bone formed in some of the reported studies is biomechanically weaker than control (5). This may be related to the experimental design of these studies. Whether the application of growth factors to wounds results in a more functional tissue is uncertain, but their potential is exciting. Although some of the growth factors tested thus far (fibroblast growth factor, IGF-1) did not result in a detectable response by ligament tissues and cells, other growth factors or combinations of growth factors may elicit an effective response, and studies with growth factors such as TGF-β are currently being evaluated. It should be noted that at the present time, such studies are somewhat empiric because the database regarding endogenous growth factors in normal and healing ligaments is deficient.

Alternate potential stimulators of ligaments *in vivo* would include possible biomechanical stimulation of ligaments with exogenous growth factors. Because immobilization and exercise may influence endogenous growth expression (and likely responsiveness to growth factors), appropriate biomechanical stimulation may be critical. Although the MCL produces a much better healing profile, the scar that forms is inferior to its uninjured predecessor (2,4,6,12,13). Its weaker nature may be related to a lack of appropriate biomechanical stimuli because it is thought that the biomechanical environment influences the cell biology of ligaments (26). Therefore, the application of a device that properly stimulates the ligament may lead to the healing or regeneration process. Obviously, it is also possible that the use of these modalities in combination with one another may enhance their effectiveness.

BASIC RESEARCH NEEDS

To improve on the chances for success with the clinical applications discussed above, more basic information on the processes involved is needed. Specific areas where new information would facilitate the clinical application of the approaches discussed include the following.

Phenotyping of Intrinsic Cells in Ligaments

There is a paucity of information regarding the heterogeneity of fibroblasts within a ligament or whether cells within specific ligaments are unique and different from those in other ligaments and/or tendons. Furthermore, more information on the plasticity of normal and scar cells will be necessary to assess the potential of growth factors or other modulatory agents to influence the healing/regeneration process.

Determination of the Growth Factor Milieu of Normal and Healing Ligaments

Information regarding the dependence of normal ligaments on autocrine, paracrine, and endocrine stimuli is just beginning to emerge. However, the question of whether growth factors unique to ligaments exist is still an unresolved issue. If paracrine regulation is operative, then the spatial arrangement of cell types and cells within the tissue becomes an important issue that is also not well understood. In the work of Hansson et al. (15,16), it was noted that exercise induced growth factor expression primarily in the peritenon cells rather than in the tendon cells. Do similar relationships hold true in ligaments?

Wound healing leads to a complex growth factor/cytokine milieu during the inflammatory phase that likely resolves during the remodeling process. Further information from animal models is needed to determine what is present at specific phases of the healing process, because the effectiveness of exogenous modulators will likely change as the wound proceeds from the inflammatory phase to a more mature tissue.

Better Understanding of the Mechanisms Involved in the Fetal Healing/Regeneration Process

As discussed above, and earlier in the Chapter 14, fetal wound healing appears to lead to regeneration rather than scar formation. The process in fetal tissues does not appear to involve an inflammatory response, resulting in an altered environment and growth factor milieu (7,20,25). Such observations lead to the question of whether fetal ligament healing also results in regeneration and, if so, can factors that contribute to this outcome be isolated and effectively applied to adult ligament healing? Considerable basic science research is ongoing in a number of fetal wound-healing models, but there is a paucity of information available in the ligament field. More information could enable investigators to determine the validity of extrapolating from other fields or determine whether ligaments have unique mechanistic features.

It is likely that inroads can be made into these questions over the next few years. Much of the technology (*in situ* hybridization, immunocytochemistry, etc.) is available but has not as yet been extensively applied to this field. Therefore, the merging of existing and evolving technology with a unique set of biological questions

should lead to the generation of a database that can then be used to develop rational clinical applications.

ACKNOWLEDGMENTS

We thank Judy Crawford for assistance in preparation of the manuscript, and the Canadian Arthritis Society, the Alberta Heritage Foundation for Medical Research (AHMFR), and the Medical Research Council of Canada for financial support of the studies leading to the generation of the ideas and concepts discussed. P.G.M. was supported by AHFMR and the Canadian Arthritis Society Studentships; C.B.F. and D.A.H. are AHFMR Scholars.

REFERENCES

1. Amiel D, Frank CB, Harwood FL, Akeson WH, Kleiner JB. (1987): Collagen alteration in medial collateral ligament healing in a rabbit model. *Connect Tissue Res* 16:357–366.
2. Andriacchi T, Sabiston P, DeHaven K, et al. (1988): Ligament: injury and repair. In: Woo SL-Y, Buckwalter JA, eds. *Injury and repair of the musculoskeletal soft tissues.* Illinois: American Academy of Orthopaedic Surgeons, Park Ridge, Ill. pp. 103–132.
3. Bray RC, Fisher AW, Frank CB. (1990): Fine vascular anatomy of adult rabbit knee ligaments. *J Anat* 172:69–79.
4. Bray RC, Frank CB, Miniaci A. (1991): Structure and function of diathrodial joints. In: McGinty JB, ed. *Operative arthroscopy.* New York: Raven Press, pp. 79–123.
5. Carpenter JE, Hipp JA, Gerhart TN, Rudman CG, Hayes WC, Trippel SB. 1992. Failure of growth hormone to alter the biomechanics of fracture healing in a rabbit model. *J Bone Joint Surg* 74A:359–366.
6. Chimich D, Frank C, Shrive N, Dougall H, Bray R. (1991): The effects of initial end contact on medial collateral ligament healing: a morphological and biomechanical study in a rabbit model. *J Orthop Res* 9:37–47.
7. Clark RAF, Henson PM. (1988): *The molecular and cellular biology of wound repair.* New York: Plenum Press.
8. Cohen IK, Diegelman RF, Linblad WJ. (1992): *Wound healing: biochemical and clinical aspects.* Philadelphia: WB Saunders.
9. Dahners LE, Gilbert JA, Lester GE, Taft TN, Payne LZ. (1988): The effect of a nonsteroidal antiinflammatory drug on the healing of ligaments. *Am J Sports Med* 16:641–646.
10. Dean DC. (1989): Expression of the fibronectin gene. *Am J Respir Cell Mol Biol* 1:5–10.
11. Eng K, Rangayyan RM, Bray RC, Frank CB, Anscomb L, Veale P. (1992): Quantitative analysis of fine vascular anatomy of articular ligaments. *IEEE Trans Biomed Eng* 39:296–306.
12. Frank CB, Amiel D, Woo SL-Y, Akeson WH. (1985): Normal ligament properties and ligament healing. *Clin Orthop Rel Res* 196:15–25.
13. Frank CB, Woo SL-Y, Amiel D, Gomez MA, Harwood FL, Akeson WH. (1983): Medial collateral ligament healing: a multidisciplinary assessment in rabbits. *Am J Sports Med* 11:379–389.
14. Hallock GG, Rice DC, Merkel JR, DiPaolo BR. (1988): Analysis of collagen content in the fetal wound. *Ann Plast Surg* 21:310–315.
15. Hansson HA, Dahlin LB, Lundborg G, Lowenadler B, Paleus S, Skottner A. (1988): Transiently increased insulin-like growth factor 1 immunoreactivity in tendons after vibration trauma. *Scand J Plast Reconstr Surg Hand Surg* 22:1–6.
16. Hansson H A, Engstrom AMC, Holm S, Rosenquist AL. (1988): Somatomedin C immunoreactivity in the Achilles tendon varies in a dynamic manner with the mechanical load. *Acta Physiol Scand* 134:119–208.
17. Harris WH, Heaney RP. (1969): Effect of growth hormone on skeletal mass in adult dogs. *Nature* 223:403–404.

18. Henning CE, Lynch MA, Yearout KM, Vequist SW, Stallbaumer RJ, Decker KA. (1990): Arthroscopic meniscal repair using an exogenous fibrin clot. *Clin Orthop* 260:64–72.
19. Huang YH, Ohsaki Y, Kurisu K. (1991): Distribution of type I and type III collagen in the developing periodontal ligament of mice. *Matrix* 11:25–35.
20. Krummel TM, Nelson JM, Diegelman RF, et al. (1987): Fetal response to injury in the rabbit. *J Pediatr Surg* 22:640–645.
21. McDonald JA. (1988): Fibronectin: a primitive matrix. In: Clark RAF, Henson PM, eds. *The molecular and cellular biology of wound repair.* Philadelphia: Plenum Press, pp 405–435.
22. Robinson BW, Goss AN. (1981): Intrauterine healing of fetal rat cheek wounds. *Cleft Palate* 18:251–255.
23. Rowsell AR. (1984): The intra-uterine healing of foetal muscle wounds: experimental study in the rat. *Br J Plast Surg* 37:635–642.
24. Sage H, Mecham R. (1987): Extracellular matrix-induced synthesis of a low molecular weight collagen by fetal calf ligament fibroblasts. *Connect Tissue Res* 16:41–56.
25. Siebert JW, Burd AR, McCarthy JG, Weinzweig J, Ehrlich HP. (1990): Fetal wound healing: a biochemical study of scarless healing. *Plast Reconstr Surg* 85:495–504.
26. Walsh S, Frank CB, Hart DA. (1992): Immobilization alters cell metabolism in an immature ligament. *Clin Orthop Rel Res* 277:277–288.
27. Whitby DJ, Ferguson MWJ. (1991): The extracellular matrix of lip wounds in fetal, neonatal, and adult mice. *Development* 112:651–668.

The Anterior Cruciate Ligament: Current and Future Concepts, edited by D.W. Jackson, et al. Raven Press, Ltd., New York © 1993.

CHAPTER 36

Mesenchymal Stem Cells and Tissue Repair

Arnold I. Caplan, David J. Fink, Tatsuhiko Goto, Anne E. Linton, Randell G. Young, Shigeyuki Wakitani, Victor M. Goldberg, and Stephen E. Haynesworth

Tissues do not live forever; indeed, the cells that fabricate and/or maintain specific tissues exist for definite time periods, then expire to be replaced by identical or similar units. The process of expiration of a cell and its replacement historically has been referred to as normal turnover. The normal turnover sequence is the basis by which tissues continuously rejuvenate themselves and, in the case of major injury, the rejuvenation dynamics are amplified to bring about major tissue repair. There appears to be a direct correlation between the observed turnover dynamics and the potential for tissue repair itself after injury. For example, adult articular cartilage has a very limited capacity to repair itself and an extremely slow turnover rate (20,44,45). In contrast, bone turns over relatively rapidly and has a high capacity for self-repair as seen in aspects of fracture healing (23). Therefore, it seems reasonable to assume that the initial formation of a tissue, its sequence of cellular turnover, and the cellular mechanisms governing repair all have common unifying control elements at both the cellular and molecular levels.

Many cell-mediated processes related to the production of skeletal tissue depend on the number of cells involved, both in the rate and magnitude of the effect. For example, in the *in vitro* production of connective tissue,

the rate of collagen gel contraction by fibroblasts embedded in the gel is dependent on the number of cells present in the culture (11). A similar gel-contracting activity has also been correlated with cell density–dependent secretion of a contraction-promoting factor by endothelial cells (34). In addition, the extent of fibroblast orientation in cultures grown on collagen gels is directly related to the initial cell density (40). This cell orientation effect has been correlated with the observation of "organizing centers" in the culture, the number of which has been suggested to be a direct indicator of morphogenetic capacity at the molecular and cellular levels (8).

In vitro culture of embryonic chick calvarial osteoblasts has been demonstrated to reproduce many of the stages of osteoid formation and mineralization observed *in vivo,* including the production of phosphoproteins involved in the mineralization process (28,29). In one culture system for calvarial-derived chick osteoblasts, cells in micromass culture on a dense collagen matrix began producing mineral within the matrix within 6 to 8 days when the collagen matrix was composed of organized (aligned) collagen fibrils (48). This biomineralization process is strongly dependent, both in the rate and extent of mineral formation, on the number of cells first introduced onto the collagen matrix; at low cell density, mineralization is never observed (O. Nakamura, D. J. Fink, and A. I. Caplan, unpublished data).

Cell density–dependent differentiation was clearly demonstrated in the culture of chick limb bud cells (22). When cultured at very low density (10^6 cells/35 mm dish), these cells do not exhibit chondrogenic or osteogenic properties. At intermediate cell culture densities (2×10^6 cells/35 mm dish), the cells exhibit the maximum frequency of osteogenesis, whereas at still higher density (5×10^6 cells) the maximum frequency of chondrocyte phenotypes is observed.

In each instance cited above, the number of cells initially present strongly influences the nature of cell-

A. I. Caplan, R. G. Young, and S. E. Haynesworth: Skeletal Research Center, Department of Biology, Case Western Reserve University, Cleveland, Ohio 44106.

D. J. Fink: CollaTek, Inc., Columbus, Ohio 43201.

T. Goto: Department of Orthopaedic Surgery, National Defense Medical College, Tokorozawa 354, Japan.

A. E. Linton: Department of Emergency Medicine, MetroHealth Medical Center, Cleveland, Ohio 44106.

S. Wakitani: Department of Environmental Medicine, Osaka University Hospital Medical School, Osaka 565, Japan.

V. M. Goldberg: Department of Orthopaedic Surgery, Case Western Reserve University School of Medicine, Cleveland, Ohio 44106.

mediated processes involved in skeletal tissue formation and the rate at which these developmental and physiological processes occur. If these observations are applied to the reparative processes of skeletal tissues, it seems clear that some minimum threshold of cell number may be required at the repair site before formation of normal neotissue can occur. We hypothesize that in many cases this minimum threshold may exceed the number of recruitable reparative cells, including less committed cells that can differentiate to repair-competent phenotypes; therefore, the extent to which the reparative process can occur may be limited by this single parameter.

Another example of such cell-mediated dynamics is available in the area of embryonic bone development. In this regard, we have previously suggested that the sequence of cellular events in embryological bone formation and adult bone repair involves a series of cellular transitions, a lineage, which originates from a primitive, undifferentiated stem cell and ultimately progresses to the unique phenotypic stages of secretory osteoblast or osteocyte (Fig. 1). The results of Bruder and Caplan's recent experiments (14–18) clearly indicate that unique cell surface antigens are formed that identify both the individual transitory stages in this osteogenic process as well as the unique end phenotypes, the osteoblast and osteocyte. Importantly, these same antigens have been observed to arise in sequential fashion when bone marrow cells are introduced into the closed space of a diffusion chamber, which is then incubated *in vivo* in the peritoneal cavity of an immunocompatible rodent (6–9,19). These experiments document that the same progenitor cell capable of forming the embryonic osteogenic sequence is present in bone marrow and is responsible for fabricating both bone and cartilage. Other studies from this laboratory further document that this same progenitor cell can be isolated from the periosteal tissues

of animals or humans (46,47). We have hypothesized that this progenitor cell can form a number of mesenchymal tissues and, thus, is a mesenchymal stem cell (Fig. 2). Inherent in this hypothesis is the suggestion that bone marrow– or periosteal–derived mesenchymal stem cells can develop into tendon or ligament fibroblasts that can form or repair these tissues.

These experiments form the basis for proposing that skeletal tissue reconstruction may be brought about by use of mesenchymal stem cells as a form of cell therapy. Cell therapy is perhaps more commonly associated with the use of isolated and expanded hematopoietic cells for systemic therapy (10,24). In the context of skeletal tissue repair, however, cell therapy is the local application of autologous (host-derived) cells to promote reconstruction of tissue defects caused by trauma, disease, or surgical procedures. This approach recognizes that all healing processes are cell mediated and regulated by specific cell phenotypes that coordinate the closure of the wound site and the eventual regeneration of reparative tissue.

It seems clear that the repair of complex skeletal structures is subject to the local availability of competent or undifferentiated cells, which are recruited to the site by a number of interacting molecular and cellular responses (endocrine, autocrine, and paracrine). Because the complexity of these local signals makes management of the healing process extremely difficult, the objective of the cell therapy approach is to deliver high densities of repair-competent cells (or cells that can become competent when influenced by the local environment) to the defect site in a format that optimizes both initial wound mechanics and eventual neotissue production.

The cell therapy approach is directed to the *in situ* cell-mediated generation of neotissue, which is intended to have properties similar to the missing (normal) tissue. Therefore, it is likely that the implant vehicle(s), used to (a) transport and constrain the autologous cells in the defect site and (b) provide initial mechanical stability to

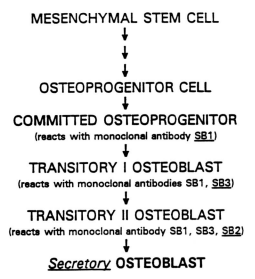

FIG. 1. Stages in the osteogenic lineage deduced from the studies of Bruder and Caplan (14–18).

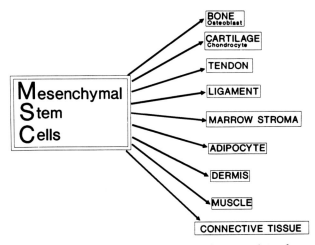

FIG. 2. Mesenchymal stem cells can produce a variety of mesenchymatous tissues.

the surgical site, will slowly biodegrade at a rate comparable with the production of and development of strength in the reparative tissue. The cell therapy approach contrasts significantly with more passive approaches to wound repair in which no attempt is made to deliver or recruit reparative cells to the defect site. For example, in the case of anterior cruciate ligament (ACL) repair with synthetic (presumably inert) polymer grafts, the healing process depends entirely on local cellular responses to initiate and control the incorporation of a permanent implant (13).

Recently, more active devices have been tested using matrix scaffolds designed to deliver and/or direct cellular processes. These have included tendon or ACL repair (25,31,37–39), meniscus repair (36,42,52,62), and articular cartilage repair (32,33,57,59). Alternatively, the use of locally delivered peptide factors, intended to stimulate recruitment of reparative cells and their attachment and/or differentiation, have also been investigated (43,54, 55,61).

In perhaps the best documented tendon repair experiments to date, Silver et al. described extensive investigations of the performance of collagen fiber prostheses for Achilles tendon (31,37,39) and ACL (25,38) repair in rabbits. They report that at 52 weeks postimplantation in the Achilles tendon defect, the reconstructed tendon (prosthesis and repair tissue) was about 66% as strong as the normal tissue for all implants tested, including an autologous tendon graft and glutaraldehyde- or carbodiimide-crosslinked collagen fiber composites (39). Both the autologous implants and the carbodiimide-crosslinked prostheses were observed to biodegrade rapidly, then regain strength rapidly as new tissue was produced. Glutaraldehyde cross-linked prostheses biodegraded much more slowly in the Achilles tendon model and became surrounded by a thick capsule that eventually stopped the degradation process. Although the neotendon developed in these studies was similar to normal, it was not identical. For example, the crimp angle of the neotendon collagen was similar to normal tendon in all implants, but the length of the neotendon crimp was less than 30% of normal for the collagen prosthetic devices. In addition, the moduli of the neotendons formed from the more rapidly degrading implants (autologous tendon and carbodiimide-crosslinked collagen fibers) were significantly lower than for normal tendon. Finally, the neotendon observed did not assemble with the fascicle microarchitecture of normal tendon. These researchers concluded that the rate of degradation of the prosthesis, and the consequent transfer of load to the new tissue, may be as important as the initial prosthesis tensile strength in determining the ultimate properties of the repair tissue (39). A similar generation of neoligament was observed in the ACL implants after 20 weeks, although the recovery of strength of the tissue may be somewhat slower in the avascular synovial environment (38).

Based on this evidence and from investigations with other implant materials (1,50,53,56), it is clear that at least in the healthy animal, repair-competent cells can be recruited from the tissues surrounding defects in tendons and ligaments, and that these cells will initiate the production of neotissue. It remains unclear from these investigations to what extent the recruited cells represented differentiated phenotypes (e.g., tendon fibroblasts), as opposed to undifferentiated stem cells, or whether increased numbers of such cells would enhance the rate of synthesis or the microarchitecture and mechanical properties of the neotissue produced.

Our studies have also shown that the number of mesenchymal stem cells in the bone marrow of humans decreases steadily with age—a population of 1 per 10,000 nucleated marrow cells in the newborn drops to less than 1 per 2,000,000 at age 80 years (S.E. Haynesworth and A.I. Caplan, unpublished data). Because our working hypothesis assumes that tissue repair is primarily initiated locally by mesenchymal stem cells responding to the molecular signals of the affected and adjacent tissues, the healing potential of these tissues should decrease with age. It also seems likely that other factors related to the health of the patient—diet, exercise, disease, pharmacological status, immunocompetence, etc.—may further decrease the population of mesenchymal stem cells in bone marrow, and therefore further compromise the ability of the patient to heal.

By providing an alternative pathway for enhancing the number of progenitor cells available to participate in the healing process, mesenchymal stem cell therapy should improve both the rate of new tissue formation and the control of the process, especially in older and/or diseased patients in which the number of reparative cells available for local recruitment is likely to be inadequate.

To illustrate the cell therapy approach, we review here our more advanced experimental efforts to use mesenchymal stem cells to repair bone and our recent exploratory approaches to cartilage, tendon, and ligament repair.

BONE REPAIR

Clinicians recognized long ago that bone marrow provided an enhancing capacity for repairing bone, either in simple or compound fractures, nonunions, or even for spinal fusions. Friedenstein et al. (26,27) and others (2–9,12,19) further refined these clinical observations by showing that a subset of cells within the marrow have osteogenic properties. These observations led to the isolation of marrow stromal cell lines that exhibit osteogenic properties or pluripotential cells from preparations of osteogenic cells (2–9,12,19,26,27). The reparative capacity of marrow in a large femoral gap model in the rat (Fig. 3) has been systematically studied using porous cal-

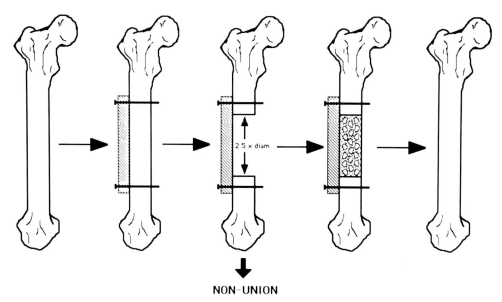

NON-UNION

FIG. 3. Sequence of construction of the rat femur gap model for massive, nonunion bone repair. A load-bearing polyethylene plate is anchored and supports the femur; a defect is created by removing a length of diaphyseal bone equal to more than 2.5 times the femur diameter. Unfilled defects or defects filled with ceramic only result in nonunions. Defects filled with marrow cell–loaded ceramic form unions.

cium phosphate ceramic to deliver such reparative cell preparations to *in vivo* sites (49). From this early experimentation, a standard assay for mesenchymal stem cells was established based on their capability to differentiate into osteoblasts and chondrocytes. This assay involves isolating cells from a tissue source, mitotically expanding the cell number in culture, and then loading such culture-expanded cells into 3-mm cubes of porous ceramic. When these cubes are implanted to subcutaneous sites, bone and/or cartilage forms on the walls or in the pores of the ceramic vehicle as illustrated in Fig. 4. Using this system, the conditions for optimally treating the ceramic and cells to maximize bone formation have been established, and the roles of both donor and host cells in these *in vivo* processes have been identified. These cul-

tured mesenchymal stem cells can be passaged many times [far exceeding their Hayflick (35) expiration number], while they still retain the capacity to form bone in the ceramic cube test system (30). For routine experiments, second- or third-passage cells are implanted back into *in vivo* circumstances, because it is presumed that such low-passage preparations may be used for human reconstructive surgery. Differentiation of mesenchymal stem cells from bone marrow or periosteum implanted in the standard ectopic rabbit assay is cell density dependent. At low loading cell density (less than 0.25×10^6 cells/ml), poor cellularity is observed after 1 to 2 months, and a scarlike connective tissue is found in the pores of the ceramic. At higher cell density (5×10^6 cell/ml), bone growth is initiated after about 2 to 3 weeks. At even higher cell loadings (10^7 cells/ml), only cartilage is observed within the ceramic pores, presumably because vascularization of the ceramic has been inhibited by the loaded cells and chondrogenesis is favored (J. E. Dennis, J. Goshima and A. I. Caplan, unpublished data). The implications of these studies that focus on bone are that

1. mesenchymal stem cells reside in both marrow and periosteum
2. these cells can be isolated, purified, culture expanded, and reintroduced back into *in vivo* locations where they fabricate *de novo*, live bone
3. these cultured cells are not transformed (no tumor has been observed in thousands of such implants)
4. these cells can respond to local molecular signals or cues (i.e., vascularized pores coated with mesenchymal stem cells yield bone, whereas nonvascular aggregates yield cartilage)

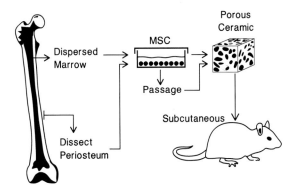

FIG. 4. A representation of our standard subcutaneous implant assay for cartilage and bone formation controlled by implanted mesenchymal stem cells in a porous ceramic (cube) vehicle.

5. such development can take place at either heterotopic or orthotopic sites
6. mesenchymal stem cells from marrow can be isolated and expanded from chicken, rodent, dog, goat, rabbit, and, most importantly, from human bone marrow. All such preparations make bone in ceramic cubes when implanted into syngeneic or immuno-unreactive hosts by the standard mesenchymal stem cell assay.

CARTILAGE REPAIR

A number of bioactive factors (proteins) have been isolated that can induce progenitor cells to become chondrocytes when tested in both *in vitro* and *in vivo* systems. These factors include the BMPs, transforming growth factor (TGF)-β2, chondrogenic stimulating activity (CSA), chondrogenic inducing factor (CIF), and so forth (43,54,55,61). More important than the identification of these bioactive proteins is the fact that responding cells reside at or can be drawn to specific *in vivo* locations. We believe that the primary skeletal cells responding to these cues are mesenchymal stem cells.

When the capability to isolate mesenchymal stem cells was established, we originally proposed to expose these cells to one or a combination of bioactive factors in culture to induce their chondrogenic differentiation; such chondrocytes would then be autologously transplanted into cartilage defects to affect the repair of a lesion. We abandoned this approach when we discovered that implanted mesenchymal stem cells alone would rapidly develop into chondrocytes when introduced appropriately into full-thickness lesions.

In order to establish a useful model for articular cartilage repair, we studied the self-repair of small and large full-thickness lesions, which extended into the subchondral bone of the distal medial femoral condyle of adult (3 kg) New Zealand white rabbits (21,51,59). The rabbits were all given full cage motion immediately after surgery. Of importance is the observation that small defects (i.e., less than 2 mm) have a substantial capacity for complete repair of both the subchondral bone and articular cartilage; only a small percentage of larger defects can repair themselves to some extent. The repair of both small and large defects was observed to involve fibrous accumulation of fibroblastic cells in the defect and, in some cases, full bony repair topped with hyalinelike cartilage. The long-term durability of this cartilage was not tested.

We speculate that the observed repair of both small and large defects involves the migration and infiltration of mesenchymal stem cells from the marrow subjacent to the defect. With the invading vascular front, these infiltrating cells differentiate into bone except at the bone-cartilage junction where, presumably, synovial factors inhibit vascular ingrowth. Thus, an avascular distal zone is created where the mesenchymal stem cells differentiate into chondrocytes and then fabricate a cartilaginous tissue. This thesis is based on the assumption that all reparative tissue must emanate from undifferentiated progenitor cells.

Based on these studies, a larger defect measuring 6 × 3 × 3 mm (length × width × depth) was created by curetting out the bridging tissue between two touching 3-mm drill holes on the medial aspects of the distal femoral condyle of adult rabbits (58). These defects cover 40% to 60% of the weight-bearing surface of the condyle. Implants included a Type I collagen gel containing either no cells, autologous culture-expanded mesenchymal stem cells from marrow or periosteum, or allogenic-cultured articular chondrocytes (Fig. 5) into the 6 × 3 × 3 mm defects; the rabbits were returned immediately postoperatively to cages for 1, 2, 4, 12, or 24 weeks. Preliminary results and a more detailed report of our experimental finding will appear elsewhere.

The observations important to this treatise are that the mesenchymal stem cells in the defect very rapidly differentiated uniformly throughout the full defect into fully functional, highly synthetic chondrocytes. Likewise, the allogenic chondrocytes rapidly fabricated cartilaginous matrix throughout the defect (60). The empty collagen delivery vehicle was inhibitory to fibroblast infiltration into the empty defect; without added cells, a fibrous plug formed and, eventually, reparative bone was observed.

At 1 month postoperatively, the mesenchymal stem cell plug had progressed from a full cartilage plug to one where host subchondral bone had endochondrally replaced almost all of the donor cell–produced cartilage, whereas the cartilage above this tide line was maintained (58). In distinct contrast, after 1 month, the allogenic chondrocyte plug remained almost completely intact and showed no signs of endochondral bony replacement (60). In a number of specimens of mesenchymal stem cell origin at 6 months, remodeling of the new subchondral bone was observed to a similar thickness and density comparable with the surrounding host bone, whereas the new cartilage appeared to be functionally intact. In sev-

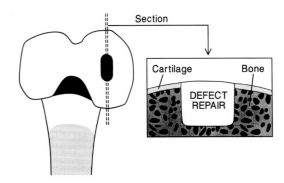

FIG. 5. Schematic diagram of the rabbit femoral condyle model for cartilage repair.

eral animals, aliquots of the same preparations of mesenchymal stem cells, which were incorporated into the collagen delivery vehicles, were introduced into 3-mm porous ceramic test cubes and then implanted into subcutaneous sites near the operative knee lesion of the donor-host rabbit. In these implants, the input cells fabricated bone onto the walls of the pores of the ceramic, again fulfilling the standard *in vivo* test for mesenchymal stem cells.

We speculate that the rapid conversion of the implanted mesenchymal stem cells to chondrocytes in the defect is due to the relatively massive influx of bioactive factors (such as TGF-β or BMP) from the surrounding bone walls of the defect (Fig. 6). Clearly, mesenchymal stem cells are very sensitive to such peptide signals, and they enter the chondrogenic lineage and rapidly fabricate a cartilaginous matrix. Those chondrocytes at the base of the defect continue to lineage progress rapidly to become hypertrophic chondrocytes; these hypertrophic chondrocytes attract host vasculature and, together with host mesenchymal stem cells and resorptive cells, replace the cartilage and subsequently fabricate bone. More distal cartilage in the defect is inhibited from such a progression and replacement sequence, presumably by the influence of synovial factors, whose diffusion into the newly fabricated cartilaginous tissue is sufficient to reestablish the tide line and limit subchondral bone replacement of the articular cartilage (Fig. 7). Various aspects of this speculation are amenable to experimental verification and are now being elaborated in our laboratory. Suffice to say that mesenchymal stem cells are highly sensitive to

local cuing and, because they are immature progenitor cells, are capable of lineage progression to a variety of phenotypes; on the other hand, already differentiated and expressive cells, such as the allogenic articular chondrocytes, have reached terminal phenotypes and cannot lineage progress further.

Conclusions from these investigations with cartilage are pertinent to cell therapy for tendon/ligament repair:

1. Mesenchymal stem cells are highly sensitive to local molecular cuing. Because they are immature progenitor cells, they are capable of differential lineage progression that depends on the local environment. In the cartilage defect model, it appears that the entire population of implanted mesenchymal stem cells initially progresses to the chondrocyte phenotype. At this stage, molecular cues, presumably arising from the bone surrounding the defect, appear to stimulate cells in the subchondral zone to differentiate further into hypertrophic chondrocytes; however, chondrocytes in the articular zone must be inhibited, presumably by other cues arising from the synovium, and are locked into the chondrocyte phenotype. Subchondral hypertrophic chondrocytes then appear to stimulate vascular invasion, followed by the tissue resorption process, and the eventual development of bone, presumably from locally recruited progenitor cells. This sequence is identical in all respects to the sequence of bone development observed (a) at the growth plate, (b) at sites of heterotopic implantation of demineralized bone chips, or (c) at sites of BMP release. Thus, by their differential responses to local cues, the

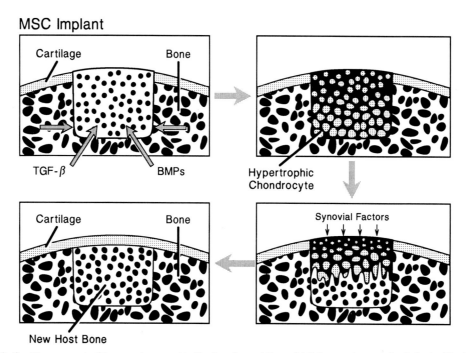

FIG. 6. Cartilage repair. Stages observed in the healing of the rabbit femoral condyle defects filled with a collagen gel containing mesenchymal stem cells.

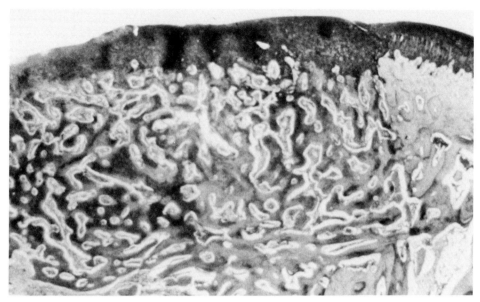

FIG. 7. Photomicrograph of a sagittal section of mesenchymal stem cell–filled femoral condyle defect 1 month after surgery (58).

same initial population of mesenchymal stem cells develops into, or leads to the formation of, two distinctly different, adjacent, and joined tissues, articular cartilage and bone. The implication for ligament repair is that direct fixation of implants to bone may be accelerated by the mesenchymal stem cell therapy approach, if the cells can be appropriately delivered to the bone-implant interface.

2. Articular neocartilage formed in this cartilage defect model appears to be fully integrated with the subjacent bone. In these experiments, however, integration of neocartilage to the surrounding articular cartilage was not always complete. In many cases, clear histological evidence for a distinction between old and new cartilage was observed, which is presumed to indicate a weakened reconstruction of the surgical site. Although investigations are underway to improve the integration of new cartilage to adjacent existing cartilage, cell-mediated attachment/stabilization of implants may be easier through bone than through soft tissue junctions.

3. Histological evaluation of cartilage defects 24 weeks after implantation of mesenchymal stem cells also indicates that the cartilage layer is thinner than in earlier stages of repair. This thinning, which also correlates with mechanical (indentation) testing of normal and repair tissue, may be related to the postsurgical rehabilitation/exercise regimen. In this experimental series, rabbits were returned to full cage activity immediately after surgery; a more gradual return to weight-bearing, which may be indicated to prevent subsequent thinning of the repair tissue, is currently being investigated in this cartilage defect model.

TENDON/LIGAMENT REPAIR

We have recently begun to investigate the cell therapy approach in a tendon repair model in the Achilles tendon of the rabbit. As illustrated in Fig. 8, there are three components to this model: the defect, the cells, and the vehicle to deliver the cells to the defect site. The delivery vehicle in this model must restrain the cells at the defect site, stabilize the tissue mechanics, then slowly biodegrade as new tissue is produced.

The defect is created by excising a 1-cm section from the middle of the three-tendon bundle of the Achilles

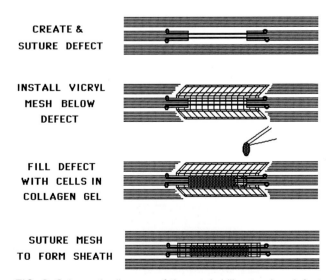

CREATE &
SUTURE DEFECT

INSTALL VICRYL
MESH BELOW
DEFECT

FILL DEFECT
WITH CELLS IN
COLLAGEN GEL

SUTURE MESH
TO FORM SHEATH

FIG. 8. Schematic diagram of the rat Achilles tendon defect model.

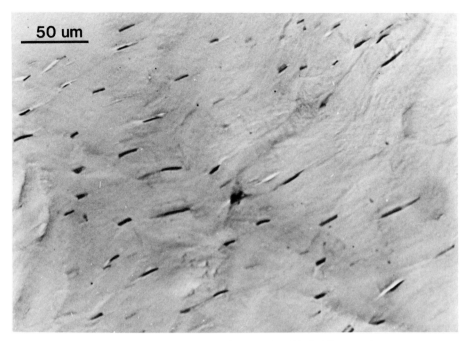

FIG. 9. Longitudinal section of normal rabbit Achilles tendon.

tendon. The length of the defect is secured by two passes of either a resorbable suture (Dexon-"S" 4-0, polyglycolic acid, code nos. 7114-31 or 7609-31, Davis and Geck, Inc., Danbury, CT) or a reconstituted collagen fiber (primarily Type I collagen; approximately 500 μm diameter wet; glutaraldehyde cross linked; prepared by a proprietary process by CollaTek, Inc., Columbus, OH).

Autologous mesenchymal stem cells and autologous tendon fibroblasts are isolated by the following procedure. A 1-cm piece of the Achilles tendon is first excised from the left Achilles tendon, and processed to provide autologous tendon fibroblasts. Alternatively, tibial bone marrow aspirate is drawn from the animal, then processed to provide mesenchymal stem cells using published procedures (30). Two to four weeks later, both culture-expanded cell types (i.e., autologous mesenchy-

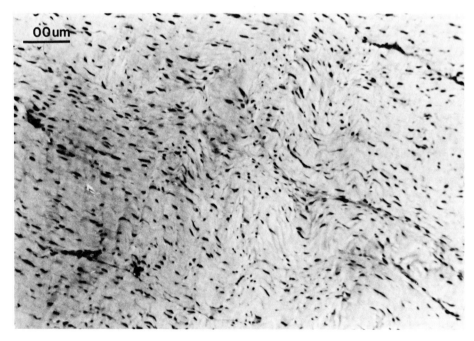

FIG. 10. Longitudinal sections of control (Vicryl sheath only) rabbit Achilles tendon defect after 12 weeks. Regions of relatively high cell density can be observed; the general organization of the neotissue is judged to be poor.

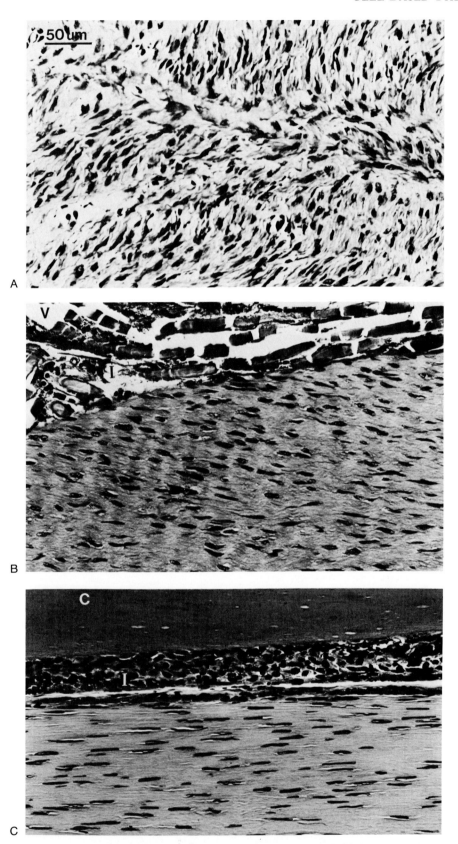

FIG. 11. Longitudinal sections of autologous mesenchymal stem cell implants in the rabbit Achilles tendon model: **(A)** 3 weeks postsurgery; **(B)** 6 weeks postsurgery; **(C)** 12 weeks postsurgery. Of note are the inflammatory responses (I) to Vicryl mesh [V in **(B)**] and collagen fiber suture [C in **(C)**].

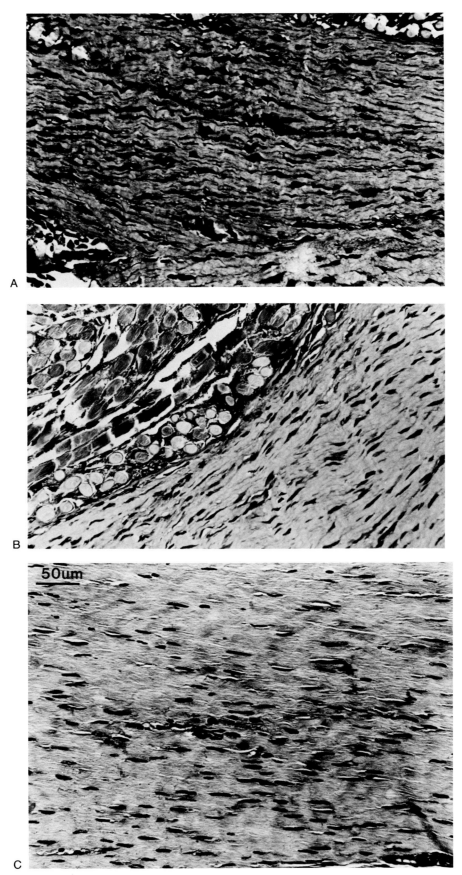

FIG. 12. Longitudinal sections of autologous tendon fibroblast implants in the rabbit Achilles tendon model: **(A)** 5 weeks postsurgery; **(B)** 7 weeks postsurgery; **(C)** 12 weeks postsurgery.

mal stem cells or tendon fibroblasts) are available for implantation into fresh right Achilles tendon defects.

Initial experiments have used a cylindrical sheath of Vicryl knitted mesh (Polyglactin 910, code no. VKM-L, Ethicon Inc., Somerville, NJ), which is sutured around the defect to create a cavity to contain the cells. Autologous cells (4 to 5×10^6 cells/ml), suspended in a loose collagen gel (approximately 1.5 ml collagen/ml in F-12 medium) are then transferred into this cavity and the Vicryl cylinder is sutured closed to contain the gel.

Control surgeries were performed with no delivery vehicle (suture only, no Vicryl sheath or cells) and delivery vehicle with no cells (collagen gel only in the Vicryl sheath). Animals were sacrificed at 3, 6, and 12 weeks, and the defects were examined histologically. Observations to date indicate the following:

1. Control surgeries (no cells; suture only or Vicryl sheath only) resulted in reparative tissue that was similar to normal tendon (Fig. 9) based on its histological morphology. These observations are consistent with those of Silver et al. (31,39), who found that in healthy animals, ingrowth of host cells was rapid. After 6 or 12 weeks (Fig. 10), however, the control tissues were more cellular than normal tendon, displayed a variety of cellular morphologies, and generally showed low cellular alignment.

2. Bone marrow–derived mesenchymal stem cells implanted in this model differentiated into fibroblastic phenotypes in 6 to 12 weeks (Fig. 11).

A. After 3 weeks, nearly all of the implanted cells retained a rounded morphology with an indication that the cells were beginning to assume an elongated shape, and with only local alignment of cell axes (Fig. 11a). Based on the high cell density compared with control implants, it seems clear that the majority of cells present in the 3-week implants must have been derived from the implanted mesenchymal stem cells.

B. After 6 to 7 weeks (Fig. 11b), the cell density had decreased in most of the implant, and they displayed a more extended morphology, although a mixture of cell shapes was observed, and more axial alignment was present.

C. After 12 weeks (Fig. 11c), cellular orientation was very high and nearly all of the cells were extended into the typical tendon fibroblastic shape. The cell density had decreased still further from the 6 to 7 weeks date, but remained slightly higher than in the normal tendon.

3. Autologous tendon fibroblast implants (Fig. 12) appeared very similar to mesenchymal stem cell implants (Fig. 11).

4. The resorbable suture (Dexon), Vicryl sheath, and collagen fibers remained intact at both the 6- and 12-week points. All of these structures stimulated a low-grade, local inflammatory response after 6 weeks (Fig. 11a), which persisted after 12 weeks, especially in the collagen-fiber implants where inflammatory cell density

appeared to increase from 6 to 12 weeks (Fig. 11b). The inflammatory response did not interfere with the development of neotendon tissue.

Based on these preliminary implants, in which both differentiated tendon fibroblasts and mesenchymal stem cells produced tendonlike neotissue within 12 weeks, we are encouraged that autologous cell therapy can facilitate the regeneration of tendon (and probably ligament) tissue. The long-term durability and mechanical properties of the repair tissue remain to be evaluated. Experiments are underway using goat and rabbit ligament models to extend these primitive beginning experiments into new cell therapy treatment protocols for ligament or tendon repair.

SUMMARY AND PROSPECTUS

This laboratory is now exploring several experimental model systems that use autologous mesenchymal stem cells as a source of reparative cells for defects not currently amenable to reconstructive repair logic. This approach is based on the relative ease of obtaining starting cell preparations containing mesenchymal stem cells from marrow, their isolation into culture, their mitotic expansion, and their eventual delivery into repair sites. We have shown that mesenchymal stem cells so delivered are influenced by local bioactive factors or cytokines, and that these progenitor cells differentiate and integrate into reparative tissues. We predict that an era of cell therapy will evolve from these efforts, which will give rise to new technologies to repair skeletal tissues previously not capable of self-repair because of their relatively low turnover dynamics.

ACKNOWLEDGMENTS

This work was supported in part by grants from the National Institutes of Health and the Ohio Edison Bio-Technology Center.

REFERENCES

1. Aragona J, Parsons JR, Alexander H, Weiss AB. (1981): Soft tissue attachment of a filamentous carbon-absorbable polymer tendon and ligament replacement. *Clin Orthop* 160:268–278.
2. Ashton B, Allen T, Howlett C, Eaglesom C, Hattori A, Owen M. (1980): Formation of bone and cartilage by marrow stromal cells in diffusion chambers in vivo. *Clin Orthop* 151:294–307.
3. Ashton B, Cave F, Williamson M, Sykes B, Couch M, Poser J. (1985): Characterization of cells with high alkaline phosphatase activity derived from human bone and marrow: preliminary assessment of their osteogenicity. *Bone* 6:313–319.
4. Ashton B, Eaglesom C, Bab I, Owen M. (1984): Distribution of fibroblastic colony-forming cells in rabbit bone marrow and assay of their osteogenic potential by an *in vivo* diffusion chamber method. *Calcif Tissue Int* 36:83–86.
5. Ashurst D, Ashton B, Owen M. (1988): Bone marrow stromal cells

raised in diffusion chambers produce typical bone and cartilage matrices. *Calcif Tissue Int* 42(suppl):2.

6. Bab I, Ashton B, Gazit D, Marx G, Williamson M, Owen M. (1986): Kinetics and differentiation of marrow stromal cells in diffusion chambers *in vivo. J Cell Sci* 84:139–151.

7. Bab I, Ashton B, Syftestad G, Owen M. (1984): Assessment of an *in vivo* diffusion chamber method as a quantitative assay for osteogenesis. *Calcif Tissue Int* 36:77–82.

8. Bab I, Howlett C, Ashton B, Owen M. (1984). Ultrastructure of bone and cartilage formed *in vivo* in diffusion chambers. *Clin Orthop* 187:243–254.

9. Bab I, Passi-Even L, Gazit D, et al. (1988): Osteogenesis in *in vivo* diffusion chamber cultures of human marrow cells. *Bone Mineral* 4:373–386.

10. Barr E, Leiden JM. (1991): Systemic delivery of recombinant proteins by genetically modified myoblasts. *Science* 254;1507–1512.

11. Bell E, Ivarsson B, Merrill C. (1979): Production of a tissue-like structure by contraction of collagen lattices by human fibroblasts of different proliferative potential *in vitro. Proc Natl Acad Sci USA* 76:1274–1278.

12. Beresford J. (1989): Osteogenic stem cells and the stromal system of bone and marrow. *Clin Orthop* 240:270–280.

13. Bonnarens FO, Drez D Jr. (1987): Biomechanics of artificial ligaments and associated problems. In: Jackson DW, Drez D Jr., eds. *The anterior cruciate deficient knee: new concepts in ligament repair.* St. Louis: CV Mosby, pp. 226–238.

14. Bruder SP, Caplan AI. (1989): Discrete stages within the osteogenic lineage are revealed by alterations in the cell surface architecture of embryonic bone cells. In: Glimcher MJ, Lian JB, eds. *Third international conference on the chemistry and biology of mineralized tissue.* New York: Gordon & Breach, pp. 65–71.

15. Bruder SP, Caplan AI. (1989): First bone formation and the dissection of the osteogenic lineage in the embryonic chick tibia is revealed by monoclonal antibodies against osteoblasts. *Bone* 11:359–375.

16. Bruder SP, Caplan AI. (1990): A monoclonal antibody against the surface of osteoblasts recognizes alkaline phosphatase in bone, liver, kidney and intestine. *Bone* 11:133–139.

17. Bruder SP, Caplan AI. (1990): Osteogenic cell lineage analysis is facilitated by organ cultures of embryonic chick periosteum. *Dev Biol* 141:319–329.

18. Bruder SP, Caplan AI. (1990): Terminal differentiation of osteogenic cells in the embryonic chick tibia is revealed by a monoclonal antibody against osteocytes. *Bone* 11:189–198.

19. Bruder SP, Gazit D, Passi-Even L, Bab I, Caplan AI. (1990): Osteochondral differentiation of avian bone marrow cells in diffusion chambers *in vivo. Bone Mineral* 11:141–151.

20. Buckwalter JA, Rosenberg LC, Hunziker E. (1990): Articular cartilage: composition, structure, response to injury, and methods of facilitating repair. In: Ewing JW, ed. *Articular cartilage and knee joint function: basic science and arthroscopy.* New York: Raven Press, pp. 19–56.

21. Buckwalter J, Rosenberg L, Coutts R, Hunziker E, Reddi AH, Mow V. (1987): Articular cartilage: injury and repair. In: *Injury and repair of the musculoskeletal soft tissue.* Park Ridge, IL: American Academy of Orthopaedic Surgeons, pp. 456–482.

22. Caplan AI. (1970): Effects of the nicotinamide-sensitive teratogen 3-acetylpyridine on chick limb cells in culture. *Exp Cell Res* 62:341–355.

23. Caplan AI. (1989): Cell delivery and tissue regeneration. *J Contr Release* 11:157–165.

24. Crombleholme TM, Langer JC, Harrison MR, Zanjani EO. (1991): Transplantation of fetal cells. *Am J Obstet Gynecol* 164:218–229.

25. Dunn MG, Kato YP, Tria AJ, Bechler JR, Zawadsky JP, Silver FH. (1989): ACL replacement using a composite collagenous material: preliminary implantation results. Proceedings of the 37th annual meeting of the Orthopaedic Research Society, Abstract 597, Anaheim, CA.

26. Friedenstein AJ. (1976): Precursor cells of mechanocytes. *Int Rev Cytol* 47:327–359.

27. Friedenstein AJ, Chailakhyan RK, Gerasimov U. (1987), (1968): Bone marrow osteogenic stem cells: *in vitro* cultivation and transplantation in diffusion chambers. *Cell Tissue Kinet* 263–272. *Transplant* 6:230–247.

28. Gerstenfeld LC, Chipman SD, Glowacki J, Lian JB. (1987): Expression of differentiated function by mineralizing cultures of chicken osteoblasts. *Dev Biol* 122:49–60.

29. Gerstenfeld LC, Lian JB, Gotoh Y, et al. (1989): Use of cultured embryonic chicken osteoblasts as a model of cellular differentiation and bone mineralization. *Conn Tiss Res* 21:215–225.

30. Goshima J, Goldberg VM, Caplan AI. (1991): The osteogenic potential of culture-expanded rat marrow mesenchymal cells assayed *in vivo* in calcium phosphate ceramic blocks. *Clin Orthop* 242:262–298.

31. Goldstein JD, Tria AJ, Zawadshy JP, Kato YP, Christiansen D, Silver FH. (1989): Development of a reconstituted collagen tendon prosthesis: a preliminary study. *J Bone Joint Surg* 71A:1183–1191.

32. Grande DA. (July 11, 1989): Technique for healing lesions in cartilage. U.S. patent number 4,846,835.

33. Grande DA, Pitman MI, Peterson L, Menche O, Klein M. (1989): The repair of experimentally produced defects in rabbit articular cartilage by autologous chondrocyte transplantation. *J Orthop Res* 7:208–218.

34. Guidry C, Hohn S, Hook M. (1990): Endothelial cells secrete a factor that promotes fibroblast contraction of hydrated collagen gels. *J Cell Biol* 110:519–528.

35. Hayflick L. (1977): The cellular basis for biological aging. In: Finch CE, Hayflick L, eds. *Handbook of the biology of aging.* Reinhold, NY; Van Nostrand, pp. 159–179.

36. Henning CE, Lynch MA, Yearout KM, Vequist SW, Stallbaumer RJ, Decker KA. (1990): Arthroscopic meniscal repair using an exogenous fibrin clot. *Clin Orthop* 252:64–72.

37. Hsu SYC, Cheng JCY, Chong YW, Leung PC. (1989): Glutaraldehyde-treated bioprosthetic substitute for rabbit Achilles tendon. *Biomaterials* 10:258–264.

38. Kato YP, Dunn MG, Tria AJ, Zawadsky JP, Silver FH. (1991): Preliminary assessment of a collagen fiber ACL prosthesis. Proceedings of the 17th annual meeting of the Society for Biomaterials, Abstract 265, Scottsdale, AZ.

39. Kato YP, Dunn MG, Zawadsky JP, Tria AJ, Silver FH. (1991): Regeneration of Achilles tendon with a collagen tendon prosthesis: results of a one-year implantation study. *J Bone Joint Surg* 73A:561–574.

40. Klebe RJ, Caldwell H, Milam S. (1989): Cells transmit spatial information by orienting collagen fibers. *Matrix* 9:451–458.

41. Klebe RJ, Overfelt TM, Magnuson VL, Steffensen B, Chen D, Zardeneta G. (1991): Quantitative assay for morphogenesis indicates the role of extracellular matrix components and proteins. *Proc Natl Acad Sci USA* 88:9588–9592.

42. Klompmaker J, Jansen HWB, Veth RPH, de Groot JH, Nijenhuis AJ, Pennings AJ. (1991): Porous polymer implant for repair of meniscal lesions: a preliminary study in dogs. *Biomaterials* 12:810–816.

43. Lucas PA, Syftestad GT, Caplan AI. (1988): A water-soluble fraction from adult bone stimulates the differentiation of cartilage in explants of embryonic muscle. *Differentiation* 37:47–52.

44. Mankin HJ. (1974): The reaction of articular cartilage to injury and osteoarthritis: Parts I and II. *N Engl J Med* 291:1285–1292; 1335–1340.

45. Mankin HJ. (1982): Current concepts review: the response of articular cartilage to mechanic injury. *J Bone Joint Surg* 64A:460–466.

46. Nakahara H, Bruder SP, Haynesworth SE, et al. (1990): Bone and cartilage formation in diffusion chambers by subcultured cells derived from the periosteum. *Bone* 11:181–188.

47. Nakahara H, Goldberg VM, Caplan AI. (1991): Culture-expanded human periosteal-derived cells exhibit osteochondral potential *in vivo. J Orthop Res* 9:465–476.

48. Nakamura O, Fink DJ, Caplan AI. (1991): Oriented collagen matrices: the control of biomineralization in bone. In: Alper M, Calvert P, Frankel R, Rieke P, Tirrell D, eds. *Materials synthesis based on biological processes.* Vol. 218. Pittsburgh, PA: Materials Research Society, pp. 275–280.

49. Ohgushi H, Goldberg VM, Caplan AI. (1989): Repair of segmental long bone defect by composite graft of marrow cells and porous calcium phosphate ceramic. *Acta Scand Orthop* 60:334–339.

50. Ozaki J, Fujiki J, Sugimoto K, Tamai S, Masuhara K. (1989): Reconstruction of neglected Achilles tendon rupture with marlex mesh. *Clin Orthop* 238:204–208.

51. Pineda SJ, Pollack A, Stevenson S, Goldberg VM, Caplan AI.

(1992): A semiquantitative scale for grading articular cartilage repair. *Acta Anat* 143:335–340.

52. Stone KR, Rodkey WG, Webber RJ, McKinney L, Steadman JR. (1990): Collagen based prostheses for meniscal regeneration. *Clin Orthop* 252:129–135.

53. Suganuma J, Pachence J, Alexander H, Ricci JL. (1991): *In vitro* and *in vivo* response to collagen-coated dacron fibers. In: Proceedings of the 17th annual meetinq of the Society for Biomaterials, Abstract 265, Scottsdale, AZ.

54. Syftestad GT, Lucas PA, Caplan AI. (1985): The *in vitro* chondrogenic response of limb bud mesenchyme to a water-soluble fraction prepared from demineralized bone matrix. *Differentiation* 29:230–237.

55. Syftestad GT, Lucas PA, Ohgushi H, Caplan AI. (1987): Chondrogenesis as an *in vitro* response to bioactive factors extracted from adult bone and nonskeletal tissues. In: Thornhill T, Senna, eds. *Development and diseases of cartilage and bone matrix.* UCLA Symposium Volume. New York: Alan Liss, pp. 187–199.

56. Tauro JC, Parsons JR, Ricci J, Alexander H. (1991): Comparison of bovine collagen xenografts to autografts in the rabbit. *Clin Orthop* 266:271–284.

57. von Schroeder HP, Kwan M, Amiel D, Coutts RD. (1991): The use of polylactic acid matrix and periosteal grafts for the reconstruction of rabbit knee articular defects. *J Biomed Mater Res* 25:329–339.

58. Wakitani S, Goto T, Pineda SJ, et al. (1993): Mesenchymal cell-based repair of large full-thickness defects of articular cartilage and underlying bone. *J Bone Joint Surg* [*in press*].

59. Wakitani S, Kimura T, Hirooka A, et al. (1989): Repair of rabbit articular surfaces with allograft chondrocytes embedded in collagen gel. *J Bone Joint Surg* 71B:74–80.

60. Wakitani S, Goto T, Young RG, et al. (1993): A comparison of the repair of large full-thickness defects in weight-bearing and partial weight-bearing articular surface with allograft articular chondrocytes embedded in collagen gel. (submitted for publication).

61. Wang EA, Rosen V, D'Alessandro JS, et al. (1990): Recombinant human bone morphogenetic protein induces bone formation. *Biochem* 87:220–224.

62. Wood DJ, Minns RJ, Strover A. (1990): Replacement of the rabbit medial meniscus with a polyester-carbon fibre bioprosthesis. *Biomaterials* 11:13–16.

The Anterior Cruciate Ligament: Current and Future Concepts, edited by D.W. Jackson, et al. Raven Press, Ltd., New York © 1993.

CHAPTER 37

Gene Therapy for Ligament Healing

Christopher H. Evans, Geethani Bandara, Paul D. Robbins, Gunhild M. Mueller, Helga I. Georgescu, and Joseph C. Glorioso

Damage to the anterior cruciate ligament (ACL) is one of the most frequent soft tissue injuries (17). Because a spontaneous healing process is lacking, various surgical strategies for the repair or replacement of the ACL have been developed (1,2,13,20). Although surgical approaches to treating the injured ACL have received considerable attention, biological approaches have not. There are good grounds for suspecting that the ability of the ACL to repair would be greatly improved if its biological environment were appropriately modified. In particular, there is the likelihood that the provision of suitable growth factors will trigger spontaneous healing. Gene transfer techniques offer a system for delivering these factors to the ACL that we feel has great promise.

CONNECTIVE TISSUE HEALING

Studies of wound healing in skin have provided the most detailed information on how connective tissues repair (7,9,12). Hemorrhage at the time of injury is quickly followed by an inflammatory response that sees the influx of neutrophils, and then macrophages, into the wounded area. The cellularity of the wound subsequently increases through division of the resident mesenchymal cells, as well as through immigration of undifferentiated stem cells. These cells first synthesize a new extracellular matrix that then undergoes a slow process of maturation. Neovascularization, which progressively occurs as the tissue heals, is essential for successful repair.

Much less information is available on the healing of ligaments. Although the ACL does not heal spontaneously, the medial collateral ligament (MCL) has considerable reparative capacity. Several stages of MCL healing have been identified in a rabbit model (10); these resemble those found in skin. The first response is hemorrhage, followed by inflammation and the subsequent influx of fibroblastic cells of unknown origin. Cellular recruitment and cell division lead to a hypercellular tissue that becomes progressively hypervascular as neovascularization continues. This scar tissue is more hydrated than normal, has less collagen, and is biomechanically weak. It is progressively remodeled into a tissue in which vascularity and cellularity return to normal, and the extracellular matrix is better organized. Histologically this tissue resembles normal MCL, but it remains mechanically weaker than normal. Repair of the MCL is hindered by immobilization, but there is little other information on how environmental factors affect healing.

Despite the absence of a natural repair process, it is nevertheless possible to gain some information on ACL healing by studying the natural history of allografts (1,2). Cells resident within the allograft are lost within a few days of implantation. However, host cells that repopulate the graft proceed to synthesize and remodel a new collagenous matrix. Revascularization occurs, with new blood vessels entering from the fat pad and synovium.

CYTOKINES AND WOUND HEALING

From experiments with skin, it is clear that cellular factors provide the key signals for successful healing (8,11,12,29). Collectively, these factors regulate chemotaxis, angiogenesis, and mitogenesis, while promoting cellular differentiation, matrix synthesis, and matrix re-

C. H. Evans, G. Bandara, and H. I. Georgescu: Ferguson Laboratory, Department of Orthopaedic Surgery, University of Pittsburgh School of Medicine, Pittsburgh, Pennsylvania 15261.

P. D. Robbins, G. M. Mueller, and J. C. Glorioso: Department of Molecular Genetics and Biochemistry, University of Pittsburgh School of Medicine, Pittsburgh, Pennsylvania 15213.

modeling. At various phases during wound healing, these factors are derived from platelets, neutrophils, macrophages, and tissue mesenchymal cells.

Within seconds of injury, platelets degranulate, releasing (among other things) platelet-derived growth factor (PDGF), prostaglandins, leukotrienes, platelet factor 4, transforming growth factors α and β (TGF-α, TGF-β), epidermal growth factor (EGF), and β-thromboglobulin (8). The neutrophils and macrophages that follow produce additional factors, such as interleukin-1 (IL-1) and basic fibroblast growth factor (bFGF) (22); many of these cytokines are also synthesized by skin cells. The potential of such cytokines to regulate wound healing has been indicated by numerous *in vitro* and *ex vivo* studies using cell and organ cultures. Their ability to do so has been confirmed in several animal studies that have identified PDGF, TGF-α, TGF-β, bFGF, and EGF as particularly promising vulnerary agents (4,18,21,28). Animal studies also have provided the important result that skin which heals under the influence of exogenously applied cytokines is indistinguishable from native tissue.

As noted in clinical studies, the degranulation products of platelets strongly improve the healing of human skin (14). Purified PDGF, bFGF, EGF, and TGF-β also have entered phase II or phase III clinical trials. The data from these continuing trials appear to be confirming the utility of PDGF and EGF, whereas the results with FGF and TGF-β are disappointing. The insulinlike growth factors are also of potential clinical use in wound healing, and there is interest in the application of specific binding proteins that increase their stability *in vivo*. Cytokine interactions with ligament cells have been poorly studied. Most information has been obtained with fibroblasts derived from the peridontal ligament. These cells produce prostaglandin E_2 in response to IL-1, tumor necrosis factor-α (TNF-α) and Γ-interferon (25,26). IL-1 also induces collagenase (23). Autoradiography using 125I-labeled ligands provides results consistent with the presence of receptors for EGF (6), but not nerve growth factor (5). Endothelial cell growth factor and bFGF are of interest because they enhance the adhesion, migration, and proliferation of peridontal ligament fibroblasts (27). PDGF and certain components of the extracellular matrix are chemotactic for these cells (15).

Cell culture conditions for the growth of ACL cells have only recently been developed (19,24). Nothing to date has been published about the responses of these cells to cytokines. Studies are underway in our laboratory to identify those cytokines that show the most promise in promoting ligament repair (Blomstrom and Evans, unpublished data). Of particular interest is evidence that peridontal ligament cells produce an autocine growth factor that is distinct from other known cytokines (E. Dick, personal communication). Such a factor would be of great utility in the present context, because it would provide a specificity lacking in existing factors.

GENE THERAPY FOR THE ACL

Targeting molecules to joints is exceedingly difficult. Traditional methods of drug delivery rely on vascular perfusion of the synovium to carry the agent to the joint. Transfer of the drug to the intraarticular compartment then follows by passive diffusion. This inefficient, nonspecific system is particularly difficult for large molecules such as proteins. Cytokines present an even bigger problem because they are quickly cleared from the circulation.

As an intraarticular ligament, the ACL is subject to the same pharmacologic inaccessibility as other tissues within the joint. Direct intraarticular injection of cytokines would be ineffective because of the rapidity with which they are cleared from the joint. Surgically implanted delivery systems, such as infusion pumps or slow-release devices, are invasive and cumbersome. Cost is another factor, because cytokines remain extremely expensive despite the ability of genetically engineered bacteria to produce them recombinantly in copious amounts.

Because of difficulties such as these, we are developing methods with which to transfer genes to the joint. The products of these genes will accumulate intraarticularly where they are needed. This approach obviates problems such as targeting, minimizes concerns about side effects, and permits a sustained synthesis of the gene product. In addition, because a single gene can be copied many millions of times into its gene product, the cost of a gene is inherently much less than the cost of the protein for which it codes.

As reviewed recently by Bandara et al. (3) we are developing two general approaches for introducing genes into joints (Fig. 1). In one approach, the gene(s) of interest are incorporated into a vector that can be injected directly into the joint. In an alternative approach, cells are removed, genetically modified *in vitro,* and transplanted back into the joint. In each case the genetically modified cells secrete the products of their foreign genes intraarticularly.

Because this idea was originally developed in the context of treating arthritis, until now we have been targeting genes to the synovium. Ligament healing factors produced by genetically modified synoviocytes presumably can diffuse to the ACL and thus promote repair. However, the appropriate genes could also be introduced into cultures of ligament cells or mesenchymal stem cells (see Chapter 36) before their transplantation to joints for ligament regeneration. An advantage of this approach would be to reduce exposure of intraarticular tissues other than the regenerating ACL.

These gene transfer techniques not only provide an efficient way to deliver cytokines to the ACL, but also offer considerable potential for fine regulation. For example, it is unlikely that a single cytokine will suffice to

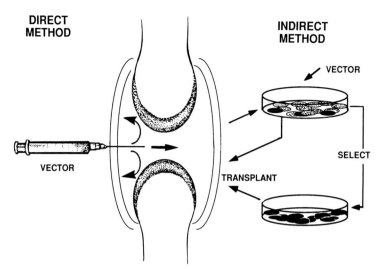

FIG. 1. Two strategies for transferring genes into the synovial lining cells. (From ref. 3, with permission.)

regenerate a normal ACL. Rather, it is much more likely that different combinations of cytokines will be needed at different stages of repair. By the judicious selection of promoters, it should be possible to provide the necessary sequential, transient expression of cytokine genes. Furthermore, this approach will allow cytokine genes to be switched off after healing has finished, thus avoiding complications such as arthrofibrosis. The repression of these genes could be accomplished by the manipulation of negative, regulatory genetic elements. Alternatively, we might take advantage of transient expression vectors that deliver genes episomally. In this case, the foreign DNA is intrinsically unstable, thus permitting temporary expression of the cytokines for which it codes.

We are presently investigating the use of several types of vectors, including retroviruses, adeno-associated virus, herpes virus, and liposomes. The first two of these integrate their genetic material, and that of their passenger genes, into the genome of the host cell. Thus, expression and repression of selected genes will be best achieved through manipulation of their genetic controlling elements. Herpes virus and liposomes, in contrast, deliver genes episomally. They are thus good candidates for delivering genes whose expression is required to be transient; ligament healing provides a good context for such a requirement.

SUMMARY AND CONCLUSIONS

Although the ACL does not normally heal, it may do so when provided with the appropriate growth factors. These factors remain to be identified, but the wider literature on wound healing suggests TGF, FGF, and especially PDGF and EGF as good candidates. Data from clinical trials confirm that topical application of the appropriate cytokines not only accelerates wound healing, but promotes the healing of wounds which otherwise would not heal at all.

The gene delivery systems potentially hold promise as an economical, efficient way of exposing the healing or reconstructed ACL to high concentrations of whatever cytokines are found to be necessary. Moreover, gene expression can potentially be regulated in such a way as to provide a timed sequence of different cytokines, as healing requires. Depending on the experimental results, this type of gene therapy could be used to improve the performance of ligament reconstructions. However, if cytokines prove able to initiate and sustain biological repair by the ACL itself, surgical intervention for acute ruptures may be limited to securing the severed ends of the ligament.

The gene therapeutic approach to connective tissue healing need not be limited to the ACL, or indeed, to ligaments. These general approaches can be used to modify the local biochemical environment in ways that enhance the repair or regeneration of many, if not most, tissues in the body.

ACKNOWLEDGMENTS

We thank Drs. David Steed and Gail Blomstrom for critical review of an earlier draft of this article, and Lou Duerring for typing the manuscript.

REFERENCES

1. Arnoczky SP, Tarvin GB, Marshall JL. (1982): Anterior cruciate ligament replacement using patellar tendon. *J Bone Joint Surg* 64A:217–224.
2. Arnoczky SP, Warren RF, Ashlock MA. (1986): Replacement of the anterior cruciate ligament using a patellar tendon allograft. An experimental study. *J Bone Joint Surg* 68A:376–385.
3. Bandara G, Robbins PD, Georgescu HI, Mueller GM, Glorioso JC, Evans CH. (1992): Gene transfer to synoviocytes: prospects for gene treatment for arthritis. *DNA Cell Biol* 11:227–231.
4. Buckley A, Davidson JM, Kameroth CD, Wolt TB, Woodward SC. (1985): Sustained release of epidermal growth factor accelerates wound healing. *Proc Natl Acad Sci USA* 82:7340–7344.

5. Byers MR. (1990): Segregation of NGF receptor in sensory receptors, nerves and local cells of teeth and periodontium demonstrated by EM immunocytochemistry. *J Neurocytol* 19:765–775.

6. Cho MI, Lee YL, Garant PR. (1988): Radioautographic demonstration of receptors for epidermal growth factor in various cells of the oral cavity. *Anat Rec* 222:191–200.

7. Clark RA. (1989): Wound repair. *Curr Opinion Cell Biol* 1:1000–1008.

8. Duel TF, Kawahara RS, Mustoe TA, Pierce GF. (1991): Growth factors and wound healing: platelet-derived growth factor as a model cytokine. *Ann Rev Med* 42:567–584.

9. Eckersley JR, Dudley HA. (1988): Wounds and wound healing. *Br Med Bull* 44:423–436.

10. Frank C, Woo SL-Y, Amiel D, Harwood F, Gomez M, Akeson W. (1983): Medial collateral ligament healing: a multidisciplinary assessment in rabbits. *Am J Sports Med* 11:379–389.

11. Grotendorst GR. (1988): Growth factors as regulators of wound repair. *Int J Tissue React* 10:337–344.

12. Hudson-Goodman P, Girard N, Jones MB. (1990): Wound repair and the potential use of growth factors. *Heart Lung* 19:379–384.

13. Jenkins DHR, McKibbin B. (1980): The role of flexible carbon fibre implants as tendon and ligament substitutes in clinical practice. *J Bone Joint Surg* 62B:497–499.

14. Knighton CR, Fiegel VD, Austin LL, Ciresi KF, Butler EL. (1986): Classification and treatment of chronic nonhealing wounds. Successful treatment with autologous platelet-derived wound healing factors (PDWHF). *Ann Surg* 204:322–329.

15. Kubota M. (1989): Biochemical study on the TGF-β like growth factor derived from bovine periodontal ligament. *Kanagawa Shigaku* 24:157–168 (in Japanese Medline AN 91237757.91000).

16. Leibovich SJ, Wiseman DM. (1988): Macrophages, wound repair and angiogenesis. *Prog Clin Biol Res* 266:131–145.

17. Miyasaka KC, Daniel DM, Stone ML, Hirshman P. (1991): The incidence of knee ligament injuries in the general population. *Am J Knee Surg* 4:3–8.

18. Mustoe TA, Pierce GF, Morishima C, Deuel TF. (1991): Growth factor-induced acceleration of tissue repair through direct and inductive activities in a rabbit dermal ulcer model. *J Clin Invest* 87:694–703.

19. Nagineni CN, Amiel D, Green MH, Beruchuck M, Akeson WH. (1992): Characterization of the intrinsic properties of the anterior cruciate and medial collateral ligament cells: an in vitro cell culture study. *J Orthop Res* 10:465–475.

20. Park JP, Grana WA, Clintwood JS (1985): A high strength Dacron augmentation for cruciate ligament reconstruction. A two year canine study. *Clin Orthop Rel Res* 196:175–185.

21. Pierce GF, Mustoe TA, Senior RM, et al. (1988): In vivo incisional wound healing augmented by platelet-derived growth factor and recombinant c-sis gene homodimeric proteins. *J Exp Med* 167:974–987.

22. Rappolee DA, Werb Z. (1988): Secretory products of phagocytes. *Curr Opinion Immunol* 1:47–55.

23. Richards D, Rutherford RB. (1990): Interleukin-1 regulation of procollagenase mRNA and protein in peridontal fibroblasts in vitro. *J Peridont Res* 25:222–229.

24. Ross SM, Joshi R, Frank CB. (1990): Establishment and comparison of fibroblast cell lines from the medial collateral and anterior cruciate ligaments of the rabbit. *In Vitro* 26:579–584.

25. Saito S, Ngan P, Saito M, et al. (1990): Effects of cytokines on prostaglandin E and cAMP levels in human peridontal ligament fibroblasts in vitro. *Arch Oral Biol* 35:387–395.

26. Saito S, Saito M, Ngan P, Lanese R, Shanfeld J, Davidovitch Z. (1990): Effects of parathyroid hormone and cytokines on prostaglandin E synthesis and bone resorption by human peridontal ligament fibroblasts. *Arch Oral Biol* 35:845–855.

27. Senior RM, Huang SS, Griffin GL, Huang JS. (1986): Brain-derived growth factor is a chemoattractant for fibroblasts and astroglial cells. *Biochem Biophys Res Commun* 141:67–72.

28. Tsuboi R, Rifkin DB. (1990): Recombinant basic fibroblast growth factor stimulates wound healing in healing-impaired db/db mice. *J Exp Med* 172:245–251.

29. Wahl SM, Wong H, McCartney-Francis N. (1989): Role of growth factors in inflammation and repair. *J Cell Biochem* 40:193–199.

The Anterior Cruciate Ligament: Current and Future Concepts, edited by D.W. Jackson, et al. Raven Press, Ltd., New York © 1993.

CHAPTER 38

The Role of Integrin Adhesion Receptors in Anterior Cruciate Ligament Physiology

Paul J. Schreck, David Amiel, Virgil L. Woods, Jr., and Wayne H. Akeson

The extracellular matrix (ECM) of the anterior cruciate ligament (ACL) contains collagen, proteoglycans, and a variety of glycoproteins, including fibronectin (3). Fibronectin is thought to play a key role in events occurring during wound healing, especially cell migration, and elaboration and maintenance of ECM. Through its multiple specific adhesive domains, fibronectin attaches simultaneously to collagen or fibrin and its cell surface receptors to permit fibroblastic migration through connective tissue or blood clots (47). The cell surface linkage depends on the action of specific types of adhesion receptors termed the integrins (66).

The integrins are a recently identified family of cell surface proteins that serve as the principal mechanical links between the ECM surrounding the cell and the actin-containing cytoskeleton inside the cell. In a wide variety of tissues, these receptors mediate many essential cellular functions, including adhesion, migration, proliferation, and regulation of the ECM composition (2,67). It is likely that they serve similar functions in the physiology of the ACL.

The term integrin reflects the ability of these integral transmembrane proteins to link the extracellular environment of the cell with the cell cytoskeleton (82). Various forms of integrin receptors are present on the cells of virtually every tissue of the body studied thus far (53), including the ACL (35). Most integrins identified are involved in cell-ECM interaction, whereas others mediate cell-cell adhesion (53). The importance of the integrins can scarcely be overemphasized. They have been shown to mediate a wide variety of events critical to embryogenesis, tissue morphogenesis, hemostasis, and tumor metastasis (2). To add to the fundamental understanding of the mechanical-physiological interplay within the ACL, this section will focus on the ECM–integrin–cytoskeleton complex.

INTEGRIN STRUCTURE

Each integrin molecule is composed of two noncovalently associated, integral membrane glycoproteins (Fig. 1). One chain is termed α and one is termed β, and the associated pair is referred to as a heterodimer (48,69). At least eight highly related but structurally distinct β subunits and at least 13 unique α subunits have been identified to date (9,19,30,38,43,45,48,53). These subunits are very well characterized and the DNA sequences of most have been described (43,44,57,64,73,81). There is approximately 40% to 48% amino acid sequence homology between β subunits (95 to 130 kD), including a highly conserved region of cysteine residues residing in four repeating units (2,43). The amino terminus of the β subunit is folded into a loop due to an intrachain disulfide bond between cysteine residues (7). The α subunits (142 to 180 kD) possess more sequence heterogeneity than the β subunits, and certain α subunit isotypes contain a heavy and a light chain interconnected by a disulfide bond (2). The pairwise associations of the various subunits produce a wide variety of heterodimers, each with distinct structural and functional properties. The large extracytoplasmic regions of the integrin heterodimers have specific subregions capable of binding an array of ECM ligands, whereas the intracellular portion of integrins contain regions that can specifically associate with

P. J. Schreck, D. Amiel, and W. H. Akeson: Department of Orthopaedics, University of California San Diego, La Jolla, California 92093.

V. L. Woods, Jr.: School of Medicine, University of California San Diego, La Jolla, California 92093.

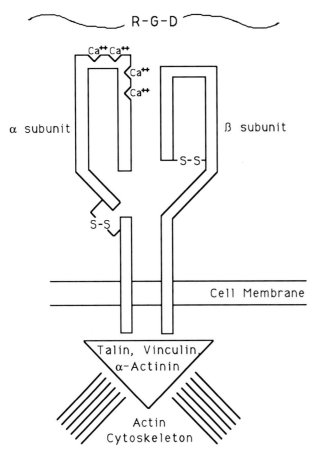

R-G-D

α subunit

β subunit

Cell Membrane

Talin, Vinculin,
α-Actinin

Actin
Cytoskeleton

FIG. 1. Integrin structure. This schematic representation of a typical integrin demonstrates the large globular extracellular region, the single short membrane–spanning domain, and the short carboxy terminal cytoplasmic domain of each subunit. The ligand binding site structure is occupied by an RGD peptide, and the intracellular linkage via talin, vinculin, and α-actinin to the actin cytoskeleton is shown. Due to intrachain disulfide bonds between cysteine residues, the amino terminus of the β subunit is folded into a loop. The extracellular domain of the α subunit contains the calcium-binding regions.

THE SUBFAMILY ORGANIZATION OF INTEGRINS

β1 Subfamily

This subfamily contains the largest number of distinct heterodimers, which were initially characterized by their appearance on lymphocytes days to weeks after cellular activation by a variety of stimuli, and thus are termed the very late activation antigens (VLA). All members of this family possess the same β1 chain. Eight α-chain forms have been identified in this subfamily, and each heterodimer has distinct ligand specificities (9,19,53). Each integrin has the ability to bind to a specific set of ligands, with some integrins being capable of binding solely to one ligand. For example, the classic fibronectin receptor α5β1 binds exclusively to fibronectin. Other integrins can bind to multiple alternative ligands, such as α3β1 to collagen, fibronectin, or laminin. The ligand specificity of the β1-β3 subfamilies is shown in Fig. 2.

β2 Subfamily

The β2 subfamily, also termed the Leu-CAMs (LFA-1, Mac-l, pl50,95), are leukocyte adhesion receptors and are restricted to white blood cells (2,80). Members of this subfamily subserve important roles in cell-cell interactions critical to the functioning of polymorphonuclear leukocytes, monocytes, and the immune system.

β chain	α chain	Ligand
β1	α1	laminin, collagen
	α2	laminin, collagen, fibronectin
	α3	laminin, collagen, fibronectin
	α4	fibronectin (CSI-1), VCAM
	α5	fibronectin (RGD)
	α6	laminin
	α7	laminin
β2	αL	ICAM
	αM	C3bi, fibrinogen
	αX	C3bi ?
β3	αIIb	vitronectin, vWF, fibrinogen, TSP, fibronectin, laminin
	αv	vitronectin, fibrinogen, vWF, fibronectin, TSP, OP, laminin

FIG. 2. Integrin heterodimers and their ligands. Each integrin is composed of two noncovalently associated subunits, one α and one β, which together form a functional heterodimer with distinct ligand binding specificities. VCAM, vascular cell adhesion molecule; ICAM, intercellular adhesion molecule; C3bi, complement breakdown product; vWF, von Willebrand factor; TSP, thrombospondin; OP, osteopontin.

elements of the cytoskeleton (61). Evidence indicates that the presence of both the α and β subunits is required for the connection of the heterodimer with the cytoskeleton as well as with the ECM (2,41,76,78,85). Certain integrins are unique to the cell type on which they are expressed. For example, αIIbβ3 [also known as glycoprotein (GP)IIb/IIIa] is exclusively expressed by platelets and their precursors, and the β2 integrins [the leukocyte cell adhesion molecules (Leu-CAMs)] are only expressed by leukocytes (37,79,80).

Initially, three β-chain forms were identified and all α subunits known at that time appeared to associate solely with a single β chain. For this reason, integrin heterodimers were grouped into three separate subfamilies based on the particular β subunit present (48).

β3 Subfamily

The β3 subfamily is also termed the cytoadhesin group. This subfamily includes the platelet GPIIb/IIIa complex (αIIbβ3) and the vitronectin receptor (αvβ3). GPIIb/IIIa was the first integrin to be identified, and its characterization has served as the basis for understanding the subunit composition, morphology, and receptor function of many members of the integrin family (62). It is the most abundant platelet cell surface protein and thus has been readily available for study (2). Unlike GPIIb/IIIa, which is restricted to platelets and their precursors, the vitronectin receptor (αvβ3) has a much wider distribution. Our current studies have demonstrated its presence in the ACL. The β3 integrins are the most broad in their ligand binding capabilities. They have the ability to bind to multiple ligands, including vitronectin, fibrinogen, von Willebrand factor, thrombospondin, osteopontin, fibronectin, and laminin (17, 18,21,52,54,65). These ligands all contain the amino acid sequence arginine-glycine aspartic acid (RGD). With the subsequent identification and characterization of additional β chains (β4-β6, βp, βs, and additional α chains), this initial categorization has broken down. Furthermore, it is now known that particular α chains can associate and form heterodimers with more than one β chain. For example, the αv subunit has been found to be associated with each of the β1, β3, β5, and β6 subunits (8,20,57,63,64,73,77,85). The ligand binding specificities of heterodimers containing a particular α chain varies with the associated β chain, indicating that it is the combined structure of the α and β chains together that forms the precise ligand binding site (55,85).

EXTRACELLULAR LIGAND BINDING AND THE IMPORTANCE OF THE RGD SEQUENCE

The extracellular ligand binding domain of a particular integrin is created by an association of the amino-terminal domains of both the α and β chains (8,26,59,75,76,85). The ligand binding region of the integrin α subunit contains a divalent cation binding domain that is homologous in amino acid sequence with the cation binding sites of calmodulin. Removing calcium from this region reduces or eliminates the ligand binding capacity and thus receptor function (26,48,55, 62,75,76). Other evidence suggests that additional factors may modulate ligand binding, including a recently described 50-kD integrin-associated protein that seems to modulate integrin αvβ3 function (11). Moreover, cellular regulation may determine the ligand binding specificities of the integrins expressed on the cell surface. In platelets, for example, the α2β1 integrin is a collagen receptor, whereas in certain other cells it binds to la·

minin and fibronectin as well (51). Ligand recognition by these binding pockets uses specific amino acid sequences within the ligand peptide. The best described is the tripeptide amino acid sequence arginine-glycine-aspartic acid (RGD). The RGD sequence is involved in binding a variety of ligands including fibronectin, fibrinogen, thrombospondin, vitronectin, laminin, and Type I collagen (66,69). It appears that the protein conformation surrounding the RGD region maintains the specificity of the receptor-ligand interaction and determines which particular integrin an RGD protein will bind (69). With their broad binding capabilities, the β3 integrin subfamily likely recognizes the RGD sequence in multiple conformations, possibly using accessory binding sites to ultimately regulate which ligand binds to a particular receptor (19,62). Experimentally, it is possible to inhibit the binding of these ligands by adding short synthetic RGD-containing peptides to block the integrin-binding pocket. These RGD-containing peptides have been shown to block various cellular functions known to involve integrins, such as the formation of platelet thrombi (15).

RGD is not the only known integrin recognition sequence. Alternative binding sequences on certain ECM ligands have been discovered. The α4β1 heterodimer recognizes a specific peptide sequence of fibronectin within its CS-1 region that does not contain an RGD sequence (31,40,86). Thus, adhesion by a given cell to a particular ligand such as fibronectin may occur through multiple receptors and multiple ligand domains. If these peptides were one day used therapeutically, there is a potential for side effects due to lack of specificity because a significant number of integrins bind the RGD sequence (62). Therefore, using alternative binding sequences gives promise to the possibility of developing high-affinity, specific inhibitors or activators of integrins (70).

In response to binding of a specific ligand by its integrin, cell surface conformational changes occur that have been observed as a focal aggregation of receptors within the plane of the membrane. These focal domains seem to be associated with a corresponding condensation of cytoskeletal elements (13,62,74,87). Interestingly, the integrins seem to remain diffusely distributed in motile cells (1,28). Thus, ligand binding by integrin isoforms may potentiate changes in receptor distribution and cell shape that may enable cellular adherence, or alternatively, locomotion (19).

THE INTRACELLULAR LINKAGE

Attachment to the cytoskeleton seems to require the cytoplasmic domain of the β subunit and possibly of the α subunit (41,78). The integrin cytoplasmic domains are physically linked to the actin-containing cytoskeleton, probably through intermediary cytoplasmic proteins, including talin, vinculin, and α-actinin (14,33,46,60,61). This linkage has been demonstrated in focal contacts formed at the end of actin filaments (14,16,24,25,74,87). The physical linkage between the extracellular ligand and the cell cytoskeleton is better understood than the biochemical pathway of signal transmission. However, a tyrosine residue in the β subunit cytoplasmic domain has been implicated as a potential phosphorylation site for tyrosine kinases (82).

FUNCTIONAL ROLES OF INTEGRINS

Cellular Adhesion and Migration

Integrins were first characterized as the principal mediators of cellular attachment to ECM, a function clearly necessary for tissue integrity (12). Under suitable conditions, a given integrin can bind to elements outside of the cell and at the same time bind to cytoskeletal components inside the cell, and thereby form a mechanical link. Further, the importance of integrins in cellular locomotion is well recognized, and is clinically important in the genetic deficiency of the $\beta2$ integrin subunit, which makes leukocytes of the affected individuals incapable of migrating to sites of tissue inflammation (80). In general, cell adhesion and motility on particular ligand substrates are mediated by the integrin or integrins that recognize that ligand. This specific receptor-ECM interaction can be altered or eliminated by the addition of short peptides that contain the arginine-glycine-aspartic acid (RGD) sequence (32,43).

Particularly implicated for its crucial role in cell motility is the classic fibronectin receptor $\alpha5\beta1$, which specifically binds the RGD-containing sequence in the cell-binding domain of fibronectin and is widely expressed on several cell types (53,66). The $\alpha5\beta1$ receptor seems to be required for cell migration even on a ligand substratum, for which other integrins mediate cellular adhesion (6). Studies using cells deficient in the fibronectin receptor demonstrated that motility on a fibronectin substrate was nearly abolished. Further, even motility on a vitronectin substrate was eliminated despite an unperturbed amount of vitronectin receptor and a continued ability to adhere to vitronectin (71). After transfection of fibronectin receptor–deficient cells with human $\alpha5$ subunit cDNA, motility on fibronectin and vitronectin was restored (36). Thus, a coordinated role between the fibronectin and vitronectin receptors in regard to cell adhesion and migration is implicated (74). Further, overexpression of the $\alpha5\beta1$ integrin in a tumorigenic Chinese hamster ovary cell model suppressed cell migration and even made the cells nontumorigenic (36,72). A balance certainly must exist between adhesion and migration in the physiologically active cell. Strong adhesion immobilizes cells, as does no adhesion, analogous to trying to run on a frictionless surface. Moderate or "appropriate" adhesion permits and promotes cell motility (68). Not all ECM components induce adhesion and migration. Particular proteins, including tenascin and other not fully characterized inhibitory glycoproteins, may contain cell substrate antiadhesive domains that act via cell surface receptors. These proteins may in fact provide directionality to cellular migration by producing regulatory signals that direct cells away from them (50).

Transmission of Mechanical Force Across the Cellular Membrane

It has been suggested that the actin–integrin–fibronectin complex is crucial in tissue remodeling by providing for the transduction of biomechanical signals to the cellular machinery to modulate the phenotypes of fibroblasts (84). Conversely, integrins allow the cytoskeleton of the cell to exert mechanical force on the surrounding ECM. In a skin wound model, as migrating fibroblasts move into the wound to form granulation tissue, they are devoid of the $\alpha5\beta1$ integrin. Shortly before wound contraction occurs, approximately 1 week after the injury, large amounts of $\alpha5\beta1$ are expressed on the granulation tissue fibroblasts (23). Actin, a prominent contractile protein in the cytoskeleton of fibroblasts, appears to have a coordinated role in this process. Intracellular actin bundles have also been shown to increase in cellular focal adhesions in the course of tissue repair (88).

ECM Construction

Integrins also appear to play a central role in the construction of ECM. In tissue culture, fibroblasts first produce the soluble building blocks of the ECM, including procollagens and fibronectin dimers, and then assemble these soluble precursors into an insoluble three-dimensional structure. Monoclonal antibodies specific for the fibroblast fibronectin receptor $\alpha5\beta1$ have been found to block this second assembly step, most likely by inhibiting the cell surface retention of fibronectin (1,29). Apparently, fibroblast-secreted fibronectin dimers bind to the fibroblast $\alpha5\beta1$ integrin receptors and are then incorporated into the insoluble matrix. Based on these observations, it has been proposed that integrins may serve as "molecular knitting needles" on the fibroblast surface, weaving the monomeric units of their ligands into newly formed ECM. Other studies have postulated a causative relationship between a cytokine-mediated increase in the $\alpha2\beta1$ heterodimer and an increase in fibroblast collagen matrix deposition (22).

Transmembrane Signal Transduction

Although poorly understood, cells likely derive signals that direct their physiologic response from the adhesive ligand receptor interactions involving integrins (48). For example, under certain conditions, the engagement either of the fibronectin receptor $\alpha5\beta1$, the classic vitronectin receptor $\alpha v\beta3$, or the platelet integrin aIIb$\beta3$ (GPIIb/IIIa) may lead to intracellular events that result in the increased production and release of proteases functionally capable of enhancing invasion in a tumor model (4,89). An *in vivo* study demonstrated that melanoma cells grown on a laminin substrate disseminated more than the same cells grown on a fibronectin substrate after the cells were injected intravenously (83). Further, other recent work demonstrated that ligand binding by an unstimulated platelet integrin (GPIIb/IIIa) may stimulate platelets, activate the integrin receptor, and therefore induce platelet aggregate formation. RGD peptide binding to GPIIb/IIIa thus may serve as a trigger to effect high-affinity fibrinogen-binding function (activation) and subsequent platelet aggregation (27). Moreover, it seems likely that the differential response of two cell types to particular environmental cues in part reflects the differential complement of or regulation of cell surface integrin receptors.

INTEGRINS IN THE ACL

Recent study has established that a restricted set of $\beta1$ integrins is present in the ACL. Using immunohistochemical techniques and monoclonal antibodies specific for the various $\beta1$ integrin isoforms, the ACL fibroblasts were found to express the $\alpha1\beta1$ and $\alpha5\beta1$ heterodimers. The integrins $\alpha2\beta1$, $\alpha3\beta1$, $\alpha4\beta1$, and $\alpha6\beta1$ were absent. Monoclonal antibodies specific for the $\beta1$ subunit pro-

duced very strong staining of the ACL fibroblasts, whereas monoclonals specific for the $\alpha1\beta1$ and $\alpha5\beta1$ heterodimers stained the fibroblasts about equally but less intensely than the $\beta1$ subunit. The strong relative $\beta1$ subunit staining likely represents the cumulative amount of $\beta1$ subunits present in $\alpha1\beta1$ and $\alpha5\beta1$ heterodimers (35). These findings are represented in the photomicrographs in Fig. 3. More recent work has demonstrated the presence of the αv subunit and the $\alpha v\beta3$ heterodimer in human ACL.

ROLE OF INTEGRINS IN ACL REPAIR

The ACL generally does not heal after injury. The complex healing process is affected not only by environmental factors such as nutrient delivery, but also intrinsic cellular factors such as the capacity to synthesize particular ECM components. When ligament injury or altered biomechanics occurs, it is likely that the external force experienced by integrins changes, which triggers a signal transmission event to alter the resting cell physiology. The fibroblastic cell is the principal ACL cell type, and fibroblastic function is essential in the healing process. This has been examined in some detail in other tissues. After tissue injury, inflammatory cells become established in the wound, and tissue fibrocytes are activated into fibroblasts and stimulated to migrate. Fibronectin, collagen fragments, and various growth factors are some of the many substances involved in this activation process, which presumably occurs via integrins and other cell membrane receptors. Next, there is a proliferation of fibroblastic cells that likely represents the combined effects of migration and division. Wound closure and contraction of granulation tissue follows. This process is considered a cellular rather than an extracellular event. The fibroblast generates the contractile force via

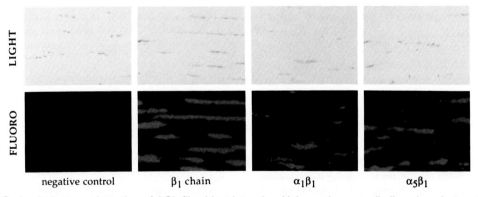

FIG. 3. *In situ* immunodetection of ACL fibroblast integrins. Using an immunoalkaline phosphatase/Fast Red detection system, human ACL sections were stained with monoclonal antibodies specific for $\beta1$ integrin heterodimers. A monoclonal specific for the platelet integrin αIIb$\beta3$ (GPIIb/IIIa) was used as a negative control. Representative fields were photographed using bright field and fluorescent techniques. A bright red precipitate that is highly fluorescent localizes monoclonal binding.

its cell surface receptors, which link the actin cytoskeleton with the maturing ECM. It has been proposed that the migratory fibroblast propulses forward on the scaffold of collagen and glycoproteins, exerting a shearing force on the substratum and thus effecting wound contraction. Finally, the fibroblast primarily synthesizes collagens, but also produces glycoproteins (fibronectin), glycosaminoglycans, and other matrix elements (39). In light of the foregoing discussion on the role of integrins in cellular function, it is apparent that integrins are essential to the fibroblastic recognition of tissue injury and the response to it.

Recent work supports the idea of physiologic differences between the ACL and the medial collateral ligament (MCL) at the cellular level, which may affect their relative healing capabilities. Ultrastructurally, fibroblasts from ACL demonstrate significant phenotypic differences from those of other ligament types that likely reflect subcellular differences (56). Functionally, fibroblasts from MCL tissue explant cultures have been shown to exhibit a more rapid cellular outgrowth than those from the ACL. Further, MCL fibroblasts demonstrated more rapid regeneration of cell-free zones in an *in vitro* wound model than did ACL fibroblasts (58). This may represent a combination of more rapid cellular migration and faster cellular proliferation. Another recently presented study demonstrated that the migration rate of cells from MCL explants is faster than that of cells from ACL explants onto plastic culture dishes and glass slides (34). In other cell types, monoclonal antibody to the alpha subunit of $\alpha5\beta1$ was shown to considerably stimulate the migratory rates of fibroblasts (1), whereas overexpression of the $\alpha5\beta1$ fibronectin receptor was associated with decreased migratory ability in an *in vitro* model (36). Thus, a higher level of functional expression of $\alpha5\beta1$ seems to be inversely related to cellular migration. These studies lend support to the hypothesis that a difference exists between the cellular physiology of the ACL and the MCL, specifically the amount of or regulation of or regulation of the complement of integrin receptors, particularly $\alpha5\beta1$, present on the cell surface. Given the role of the fibroblast in wound healing, such differences at the level of fibroblastic integrin receptors would affect the native healing capacity of the ACL.

In light of the complexity of cellular physiology, it is possible but unlikely that the understanding of a single receptor could explain differential cellular migration. In particular, the $\alpha v\beta3$ integrin heterodimer, which is also present on the ACL has been shown to closely cooperate with the $\alpha5\beta1$ receptor in adhesion and migration (6,17,74). Other studies have emphasized the ability of the vitronectin ligand (serum-spreading factor) to promote directed migration of certain cell lines (5) or to modulate keratinocyte motility on collagen (10). Thus, expression and regulation of the $\alpha v\beta3$ heterodimer could

prove crucial in understanding ACL fibroblast migration and function.

SUMMARY AND FUTURE APPLICATIONS

The biological effects that the integrins mediate are complex, and manipulation of the integrin activity can be used to either enhance or suppress certain cellular activities, such as migration and elaboration of ECM. Certainly, further study is needed before synthetic peptides or other integrin-targeting agents such as monoclonal antibodies could be used as an adjunct to facilitate ACL repair. Another area of interest surrounds growth factors such as transforming growth factor-β, which have been shown to modulate integrin expression *in vitro* (42,49). This could provide a further approach to the regulation of the adhesive and migratory properties of fibroblasts via integrin receptors.

ACKNOWLEDGMENT

This work was supported by National Institutes of Health Grants AR14918, AR34264, and AR07484.

REFERENCES

1. Akiyama SK, Yamada SS, Chen W-T, Yamada KM. (1989): Analysis of fibronectin receptor function with monoclonal antibodies: roles in cell adhesion, migration, matrix assembly, and cytoskeletal organization. *J Cell Biol* 109:863–875.
2. Albelda SM. Buck CA. (1990): Integrins and other cell adhesion molecules. *FASEB J* 4:2868–2880.
3. Amiel D, Billings E, Akeson WH. (1990): Ligament structure, chemistry, and physiology. Chapter 5. In: Daniel DM, Akeson WH, O'Connor JJ, eds. *Knee ligaments: structure, function, injury, and repair.* New York: Raven Press, pp. 77–91.
4. Banga HS, Simons ER, Brass LF, Rittenhouse SE. (1986): Activation of phospholipases A and C in human platelets exposed to epinephrine: role of glycoproteins IIb/IIIa and dual role of epinephrine. *Proc Natl Acad Sci USA* 83:9197–9201.
5. Basara ML, McCarthy JB, Barnes DW, Furcht LT. (1985): Stimulation of haptotaxis and migration of tumor cells by serum spreading factor. *Cancer Res* 45:2487–2494.
6. Bauer JS, Schreiner CL, Giancotti FG, Ruoslahti E, Juliano RL. (1992): Motility of fibronectin receptor-deficient cells on fibronectin and vitronectin: collaborative interactions among integrins. *J Cell Biol* 116:477–487.
7. Beer J, Coller BS. (1989): Evidence that platelet glycoprotein IIIa has a large disulfide-bonded loop that is susceptible to proteolytic cleavage. *J Biol Chem* 264:17564–17573.
8. Bodary SC, McLean JW. (1990): The integrin $\beta1$ subunit associates with the vitronectin receptor αv subunit to form a novel vitronectin receptor in a human embryonic kidney cell line. *J Biol Chem* 265:5938–5941.
9. Bossy B, Bossy-Wetzel E, Reichardt LF. (1991): Characterization of the integrin $\alpha8$ subunit: a new integrin $\beta1$ associated subunit, which is prominently expressed on axons and on cells in contact with basal laminae in chick embryos. *EMBO J* 10:2375–2385.
10. Brown C, Stenn KS, Falk RJ, Woodley DT, O'Keefe EJ. (1991): Vitronectin: effects on keratinocyte motility and inhibition of collagen-induced motility. *J Invest Dermatol* 96:724–728.

11. Brown E, Hooper L, Ho T, Gresham H. (1990): Integrin associated protein: a 50-kD plasma membrane antigen physically and functionally associated with integrins. *J Cell Biol* 111:2785–2794.

12. Buck CA, Horwitz AF. (1987): Cell surface receptors for extracellular matrix molecules. *Annu Rev Cell Biol* 3:179–205.

13. Burridge K, Fath K. (1989): Focal contacts: transmembrane links between the extracellular matrix and the cytoskeleton. *Bioessays* 10:104–108.

14. Burridge K, Fath K, Kelly T, Nuckolls G, Turner C. (1988): Focal adhesions: transmembrane junctions between the extracellular matrix and the cytoskeleton. *Annu Rev Cell Biol* 4:487–525.

15. Cadroy Y, Houghten RA, Hanson SR. (1989): RGDV peptide selectively inhibits platelet-dependent thrombus formation in vivo: studies using a baboon model. *J Clin Invest* 84:939–944.

16. Carter WG, Wayner EA, Bouchard TS, Kaur P. (1990): The role of integrins α2β1 and α3β1 in cell-cell and cell-substrate adhesion of human epidermal cells. *J Cell Biol* 110:1387–1404.

17. Charo IF, Nannizzi L, Smith JW, Cheresh DA. (1990): The vitronectin receptor αvβ3 binds fibronectin and acts in concert with α5β1 in promoting cellular attachment and spreading on fibronectin. *J Cell Biol* 111:2795–2800.

18. Cheresh DA. (1987): Human endothelial cells synthesize and express an Arg-Gly-Asp-directed adhesion receptor involved in attachment to fibrinogen and von Willebrand factor. *Proc Natl Acad Sci USA* 84:6471–6475.

19. Cheresh DA. (1991): Structure, function and biological proper ties of integrin αvβ3 on human melanoma cells. *Cancer Metastasis Rev* 10:3–10.

20. Cheresh DA, Smith JW, Cooper HM, Quaranta V. (1989): A novel vitronectin receptor integrin (αvβx) is responsible for distinct adhesive properties of carcinoma cells. *Cell* 57:59–69.

21. Cheresh DA, Spiro RC. (1987): Biosynthetic and functional properties of an Arg-Gly-Asp-directed receptor involved in human melanoma cell attachment to vitronectin, fibrinogen and von Willebrand factor. *J Biol Chem* 262:17703–17711.

22. Clark JG, Dedon TF, Wayner EA, Carter WG. (1989): Effects of interferon-Γ on expression of cell surface receptors for collagen and deposition of newly synthesized collagen by cultured human lung fibroblasts. *J Clin Invest* 83:1505–1511.

23. Clark RAF. (1990): Fibronectin matrix deposition and fibronectin receptor expression in healing and normal skin. *J Invest Dermatol* 94:128S–134S.

24. Damsky CH, Knudsen KA, Bradley D, Buck CA, Horwitz AF. (1985): Distribution of the cell substratum attachment (CSAT) antigen on myogenic and fibroblastic cells in culture. *J Cell Biol* 100:1528–1539.

25. Dejanna E, Colella S, Conforti G, Abbadini M, Gaboli M, Marchisio PC. (1988): Fibronectin and vitronectin regulate the organization of their respective Arg-Gly-Asp adhesion receptors in cultured human endothelial cells. *J Cell Biol* 107:1215–1223.

26. D'Souza SE, Ginsberg MH, Burke TA, Lam SC-T, Plow EF. (1988): Chemical cross-linking of arginyl-glycyl-aspartic acid peptides to adhesion receptors on platelets. *Science* 242:91–93.

27. Du X, Plow EF, Frelinger AL, O'Toole TE, Loftus JC, Ginsberg MH. (1991): Ligands "activate" integrin αIIbβ3 (platelet GPIIb-IIIa). *Cell* 65:409–416.

28. Duband J-L, Nuckolls GH, Ishihara A, et al. (1988): Fibronectin receptor exhibits high lateral mobility in embryonic locomoting cells but is immobile in focal contacts and fibrillar streaks in stationary cells. *J Cell Biol* 107:1385–1396.

29. Fogerty FJ, Akiyama SK, Yamada KM, Mosher DF. (1990): Inhibition of binding of fibronectin to matrix assembly sites by anti-integrin (α5β1) antibodies. *J Cell Biol* 111:699–708.

30. Freed E, Gailit J, van der Geer P, Ruoslahti E, Hunter T. (1989): A novel integrin β subunit is associated with the vitronectin receptor α subunit (αv) in a human osteosarcoma cell line and is a substrate for protein kinase C. *EMBO J* 8:2955–2965.

31. Garcia-Pardo A, Wayner EA, Carter WG, Ferreira OC. (1990): Human B lymphocytes define an alternative mechanism of adhesion to fibronectin: the interaction of the α4β1 integrin with the LHGPEILDVPST sequence of the type III connecting segment is sufficient to promote cell attachment. *J Immunol* 144:3361–3366.

32. Gehlsen KR, Argraves WS, Pierschbacher MD, Ruoslahti E. (1988): Inhibition of in vitro tumor cell invasion by Arg-Gly Asp-containing synthetic peptides. *J Cell Biol* 106:925–930.

33. Geiger B. (1979): A 130 K protein from chicken gizzard: its localization at the termini of microfilament bundles in cultured chicken cells. *Cell* 18:193–205.

34. Geiger MH, Amiel D, Green MH, Most D, Berchuck M, Akeson WH. (1992): Rates of migration of ACL and MCL derived fibroblasts. *Orthop Trans* 16(2):409.

35. Gesink DS, Pacheco HO, Kuiper SD, et al. (1992): Immunohistochemical localization of β1-integrins in anterior cruciate and medial collateral ligaments of human and rabbit. *J Orthop Res* 10(4):596–599.

36. Giancotti FG, Ruoslahti E. (1990): Elevated levels of the α5β1 fibronectin receptor suppress the transformed phenotype of Chinese hamster ovary cells. *Cell* 60:849–859.

37. Ginsberg MH, Loftus JC, Plow EF. (1988): Cytoadhesins, integrins, and platelets. *Thromb Haemost* 59:1–6.

38. Gresham HD, Goodwin JL, Allen PM. Anderson DC, Brown EJ. (1989): A novel member of the integrin receptor family mediates Arg-Gly-Asp-stimulated neutrophil phagocytosis. *J Cell Biol* 108:1935–1943.

39. Grierson I, Joseph J, Miller M, Day JE. (1988): Wound repair: the fibroblast and the inhibition of scar formation. *Eye* 2:135–148.

40. Guan J-L, Hynes RO. (1990): Lymphoid cells recognize an alternatively spliced segment of fibronectin via the integrin receptor α4β1. *Cell* 60:53–61.

41. Hayashi Y, Haimovich B, Reszka A, Boettiger D, Horwitz A. (1990): Expression and function of chicken integrin β1 subunit and its cytoplasmic domain mutants in mouse NIH 3T3 cells. *J Cell Biol* 110:175–184.

42. Heino J, Ignotz RA, Hemler ME, Crouse C, Massaque J. (1989): Regulation of cell adhesion receptors by transforming growth factor-β: concomitant regulation of integrins that share a common β1 subunit. *J Biol Chem* 264:380–388.

43. Hemler ME. (1990): VLA proteins in the integrin family: structures, functions, and their role on leukocytes. *Annu Rev Immunol* 8:365–400.

44. Hogervorst F, Kuikman I, von dem Borne AE, Sonnenberg A. (1990): Cloning and sequence analysis of beta-4 cDNA: an integrin subunit that contains a unique 118 kd cytoplasmic domain. *EMBO J* 9:765–770.

45. Holzmann B, McIntyre BW, Weissman IL. (1989): Identification of a murine peyer's patch-specific lymphocyte homing receptor as an integrin molecule with an α chain homologous to human VLA-4α. *Cell* 56:37–46.

46. Horwitz A, Duggan K, Buck C, Beckerle MC, Burridge K. (1986): Interaction of plasma membrane fibronectin receptor with talin—a transmembrane linkage. *Nature* 320:531–533.

47. Humphries MJ, Obara M, Olden K, Yamada KM. (1989): Role of fibronectin in adhesion, migration, and metastasis. *Cancer Invest* 7:373–393.

48. Hynes RO. (1987): Integrins: a family of cell surface receptors. *Cell* 48:549–554.

49. Ignotz RA, Heino J, Massague J. (1989): Regulation of cell adhesion receptors by transforming growth factor-β: regulation of vitronectin receptor and LFA-l. *J Biol Chem* 264:389–392.

50. Keynes R, Cook G. (1990): Cell-cell repulsion: clues from the growth cone? *Cell* 62:609–610.

51. Kirchhofer D, Languino LR, Ruoslahti E, Pierschbacher MD. (1990): α2β1 integrins from different cell types show different binding specificities. *J Biol Chem* 265:615–618.

52. Kramer RH, Cheng,Y-F, Clyman R. (1990): Human microvascular endothelial cells use β1 and β3 integrin receptor complexes to attach to laminin. *J Cell Biol* 111:1233–1243.

53. Kramer RH, Vu M, Cheng Y-F, Ramos DM. (1991): Integrin expression in malignant melanoma. *Cancer Metastasis Rev* 10:49–59.

54. Lawler J, Weinstein R, Hynes RO. (1988): Cell attachment to thrombospondin: the role of Arg-Gly-Asp, calcium, and integrin receptors. *J Cell Biol* 107:2351–2361.

55. Loftus JC, O'Toole TE, Plow EF, Glass A, Frelinger AL, Ginsberg MH. (1990): A β3 integrin mutation abolishes ligand binding and alters divalent cation-dependent conformation. *Science* 249:915–918.

56. Lyon RM, Akeson WH, Amiel D, Kitabayashi LR, Woo SL-Y. (1991): Ultrastructural differences between the cells of the medial collateral and the anterior cruciate ligaments. *Clin Orthop* 272:279–286.

57. McLean JW, Vestal DJ, Cheresh DA, Bodary SC. (1990): cDNA sequence of the human integrin β5 subunit. *J Biol Chem* 265:17126–17131.

58. Nagineni CN, Amiel D, Green MH, Berchuck M, Akeson WH. (1992): Characterization of the intrinsic properties of the anterior cruciate and medial collateral ligament cells: an in vitro cell culture study. *J Orthop Res* 465–475.

59. Nermut MV, Green NM, Eason P, Yamada SS, Yamada KM. (1988): Electron microscopy and structural model of human fibronectin receptor. *EMBO J* 7:4093–4099.

60. Nuckolls GH, Turner CE, Burridge K. (1990): Functional studies of the domains of talin. *J Cell Biol* 110:1635–1644.

61. Otey CA, Pavalko FM, Burridge K. (1990): An interaction between α-actinin and the β1 integrin subunit in vitro. *J Cell Biol* 111:721–729.

62. Phillips DR, Charo IF, Scarborough RM. (1991): GPIIb IIIa: the responsive integrin. *Cell* 65:359–362.

63. Pytela R, Pierschbacher MD, Ruoslahti E. (1985): Identification and isolation of a 140 kd cell surface glycoprotein with properties expected of a fibronectin receptor. *Cell* 40:191–198.

64. Ramaswamy H, Hemler ME. (1990): Cloning, primary structure and properties of a novel human integrin β subunit. *EMBO J* 9:1561–1568.

65. Reinholt FP, Hultenby K, Oldberg A, Heinegard D. (1990): Osteopontin—a possible anchor of osteoclasts to bone. *Proc Natl Acad Sci USA* 87:4473–4475.

66. Ruoslahti E. (1988): Fibronectin and its receptor. *Annu Rev Biochem* 57:375–413.

67. Ruoslahti E. (1991): Integrins. *J Clin Invest* 87:1–5.

68. Ruoslahti E, Giancotti FG. (1989): Integrins and tumor cell dissemination. *Cancer Cells* 1:119–126.

69. Ruoslahti E, Pierschbacher MD. (1987): New perspectives in cell adhesion: RGD and integrins. *Science* 238:491–497.

70. Scarborough RM, Rose JW, Hsu MA, et al. (1991): Barbourin: a GPIIb-IIIa-specific integrin antagonist from the venom of Sistrurus m. barbouri. *J Biol Chem* 266:9359–9362.

71. Schreiner CL, Bauer JS, Danilov YN, Hussein S, Sczekan MM, Juliano RL. (1989): Isolation and characterization of Chinese hamster ovary cell variants deficient in the expression of fibronectin receptor. *J Cell Biol* 109:3157–3167.

72. Schreiner CL, Fisher M, Hussein S, Juliano RL. (1991): Increased tumorigenicity of fibronectin receptor deficient Chinese hamster ovary cell variants. *Cancer Res* 51:1738–1740.

73. Sheppard D, Rozzo C, Starr L, Quaranta V, Erle DJ, Pytela R. (1990): Complete amino acid sequence of a novel integrin β subunit (B6) identified in epithelial cells using the polymerase chain reaction. *J Biol Chem* 265:11502–11507.

74. Singer II, Scott S, Kawka DW, Kazazis DM, Gailit J, Ruoslahti E. (1988): Cell surface distribution of fibronectin and vitronectin receptors depends on substrate composition and extracellular matrix accumulation. *J Cell Biol* 106:2171–2182.

75. Smith JW, Cheresh DA. (1988): The Arg-Gly-Asp binding domain of the vitronectin receptor: photoaffinity cross-linking implicates amino acid residues 61-203 of the βsubunit. *J Biol Chem* 1988;263:18726–18731.

76. Smith JW, Cheresh DA. (1990): Integrin ($\alpha v \beta$3)-ligand interaction: identification of a heterodimeric RGD binding site on the vitronectin receptor. *J Biol Chem* 265:2168–2172.

77. Smith JW, Vestal DJ, Irwin SV, Burke TA, Cheresh DA. (1990): Purification and functional characterization of integrin $\alpha v \beta$5: an adhesion receptor for vitronectin. *J Biol Chem* 265:11008–11013.

78. Solowska J, Guan J-L, Marcantonio EE, Trevithick JE, Buck CA, Hynes RO. (1989): Expression of normal and mutant avian integrin subunits in rodent cells. *J Cell Biol* 109:853–861.

79. Springer TA. (1990): Adhesion receptors of the immune system. *Nature* 346:425–434.

80. Springer TA, Dustin ML, Kishimoto TK, Marlin SD. (1987): The lymphocyte function-associated LFA-1, CD2, and LFA-3 molecules: cell adhesion receptors of the immune system. *Annu Rev Immunol* 5:223–252.

81. Suzuki S, Naitoh Y. (1990): Amino acid sequence of a novel integrin β4 subunit and primary expression of the mRNA in epithelial cells. *EMBO J* 9:757–763.

82. Tamkun JW, DeSimone DW, Fonda D, et al. (1986): Structure of integrin, a glycoprotein involved in the transmembrane linkage between fibronectin and actin. *Cell* 46:271–282.

83. Terranova VP, Williams JE, Liotta LA, Martin GR. (1984): Modulation of the metastatic activity of melanoma cells by laminin and fibronectin. *Science* 226:982–985.

84. Unemori EN, Werb Z. (1986): Reorganization of polymerized actin: a possible trigger for induction of procollagenase in fibroblasts cultured in and on collagen gels. *J Cell Biol* 103:1021–1031.

85. Vogel BE, Tarone G, Giancotti FG, Gailit J, Ruoslahti E. (1990): A novel fibronectin receptor with an unexpected subunit composition ($\alpha v \beta$1). *J Biol Chem* 265:5934–5937.

86. Wayner EA, Garcia-Pardo A, Humphries MJ, McDonald JA, Carter WG. (1989): Identification and characterization of the T lymphocyte adhesion receptor for an alternative cell attachment domain (CS-1) in plasma fibronectin. *J Cell Biol* 109:1321–1330.

87. Wayner EA, Orlando RA, Cheresh DA. (1991): Integrins $\alpha v \beta$3 and $\alpha v \beta$5 contribute to cell attachment to vitronectin but differentially distribute on the cell surface. *J Cell Biol* 113:919–929.

88. Welch MP, Odland GF, Clark RAF. (1990): Temporal relationship of F-actin bundle formation, collagen and fibronectin matrix assembly, and fibronectin receptor expression to wound contraction. *J Cell Biol* 110:133–145.

89. Werb Z, Tremble PM, Behrendtsen O, Crowley E, Damsky CH. (1989): Signal transduction through the fibronectin receptor induces collagenase and stromelysin gene expression. *J Cell Biol* 109:877–889.

The Anterior Cruciate Ligament: Current and Future Concepts, edited by D.W. Jackson, et al. Raven Press, Ltd., New York © 1993.

CHAPTER 39

Synthesized Biologics as Potential Anterior Cruciate Ligament Substitutes

Timothy M. Simon and Douglas W. Jackson

Reconstruction of the anterior cruciate ligament (ACL) currently is accomplished using either biologic grafts (autografts or allografts) or synthetic materials. The complex structural and material properties of the ACL have not been duplicated with tendons or current synthetics. Material engineers and clinicians continue to search for improved substitutes for the ACL (30). The ideal ACL substitute (a) would not be harvested from the patient; (b) would be available in a variety of sizes; (c) would be easily usable in surgery without much pretreatment; (d) would not be toxic, immunogenic, mutagenic, or carcinogenic; (e) would be free from the possibility of disease transmission; (f) would duplicate the mechanical and structural properties of the ACL; (g) would be compatible with adequate fixation; (h) would resist fraying, breakage, and producing particulate debris; (i) would provide a suitable substrate for cell ingrowth and allow for gradual stress transfer to biologic tissue; and (j) would be easily revisable in the small percentage that fail.

One area of potentially improved ACL substitutes may develop as a polymer. These polymers are formed through a chemical reaction (polymerization) in which two or more small molecules combine to form a larger molecule with repeating structural units of the original molecules. In synthetic polymers, the repeating small molecules (monomers) are of man-made origin. Biopolymers are formed in biologic systems from natural or biologically synthesized molecules.

To date, the ACL substitutes made from synthetic polymers have been used as either a prosthesis or augmentation device. A true ligament prosthesis provides joint stability without depending on future tissue ingrowth to provide strength. The augmentation devices are intended to protect and provide strength to a biologic graft during the early healing phase when the associated remodeling results in a reduction of the graft's strength. A common problem associated with the currently available synthetic ACL replacements has been the consequence of fatigue and wear within the substitute, resulting in an increasing incidence of graft failure with time.

The ACL is a complex, nonhomogeneous structure that owes its properties to the interaction of natural biopolymers synthesized by cells. The homogeneous synthetic polymers that are currently available do not duplicate the mechanical and surface properties of complex tissues. The ability to produce such materials with the inherent characteristics of the ACL has been a difficult goal to achieve. Material engineers have been further challenged to offer techniques and processes that can duplicate the properties of the naturally occurring numerous biopolymers synthesized in the human body. The challenge remains to duplicate the structure and the methods of formation of such structural composites as dentin, cartilage, and bone from readily available material at physiologic temperature and in aqueous conditions. Some material engineers, as an alternative to synthesis of new materials, have attempted to used synthesis techniques that simulate the natural process of producing biopolymers. This approach has been termed biomimics. The rapidly developing field of polymer chemistry, with both numerous natural and synthetic polymers, should offer new approaches for tissue repair and reconstruction.

HYDROGELS

Hydrogels can be described as water-swollen polymer networks of either natural or synthetic origin. A hydrogel is classically defined as a gel that has water as its dispersion medium.

T. M. Simon and D. W. Jackson: Southern California Center for Sports Medicine, Long Beach, California 90806.

Hydrogels can be formed from naturally occurring substances, such as collagen and alginate, and from numerous synthetic polymers, such as phosphazene, methyacrylate, hydroxyethylmethacrylate (HEMA), and polyvinylalcohol (2,6,7,15). An example of how unsaturated monomers (with a functional side group that is interactive with water) begins polymerization to form a homogeneous hydrogel polymer is shown in Fig. 1.

The appeal of hydrogels is their versatility for potential biomedical applications. There is an extensive list of hydrophilic monomers that are available to form hydrogels. The type of monomers used can control the amount of water binding within the matrix. The biomedical applications of hydrogels have grown dramatically. They are being used in soft contact lenses, intraocular lenses, drug delivery systems with graded release, synthetic articular cartilage, reproductive system implants, potential artificial pancreas, and wound dressings (18,19,35).

The role of these water-loving hydrogels in biomaterial applications is best demonstrated by comparing properties of existing non–hydrogel-forming polymers with natural tissues. Polymer compounds such polyethylene and polypropylene are hydrophobic. The interaction of water on the surface of these polymers is significantly influenced by their hydrophobic nature. The more hydrophobic the polymer, the less water can penetrate or wets its surface. This has led to their success in nonbiologic applications. Biologic systems are dependent on water interaction at nearly all biologic interfaces for transport of molecules. The water interaction at the cell surface in the biologic environment is affected by more hydrophilic groups. Similarly, the way water interacts with the variety of soft tissue interfaces in the body also contrasts with the hydrophobic polymers.

The advantages of hydrogels rest in their unique properties (3,17,26–29,36,40). Hydrogels allow cell attachment and growth, and can be cross-linked to change various properties (strength, solubility, etc.). Growth factors can be incorporated into hydrogels for modulated release. Hydrogels are water soluble, are usually biocompatible, can be bioerodible with nontoxic breakdown products, provide a means for controlled release of substances linked to the hydrogel matrix, and have permeable membranes. Hydrogels appear to be stable in an environment where pH, temperature, and tonicity may vary.

The water content within the polymer substrate is the key component that imparts the gel its characteristic properties. The amount of water that a gel can absorb is defined as its equilibrium water content (EWC) and is expressed in the following equation:

$$EWC = \frac{\text{Weight of water in the gel}}{\text{Total weight of hydrated gel}} \times 100\%$$

The mechanical properties, permeability, surface properties, and interaction in the biological environment of hydrogels are affected by this relationship. The hydrostatic swelling pressure in hydrogels can be significant. Other factors affecting the water content include density of cross-linking within the polymer, pH of the hydrating solution, temperature, and tonicity. Further, there is evidence that the water can exist in a "bound" or nonfreezing water state that is closely associated with the polymer network, or as "free" or freezing water that is not affected by the polymer network and as such has a much greater mobility. In actuality, there is probably a continuum in the states of water within the gel between the two

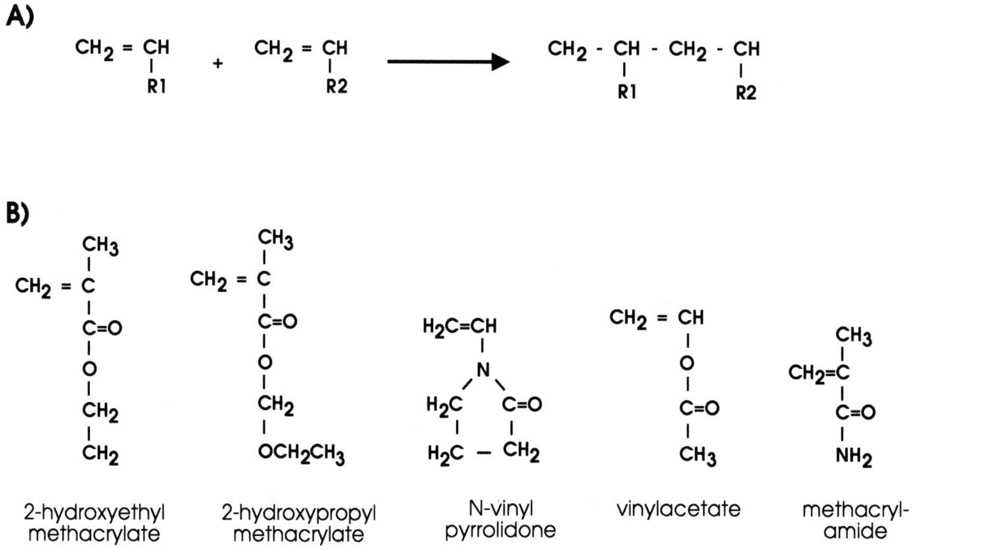

FIG. 1. A: Scheme demonstrating the polymerization of a monomer with a water-interacting side chain to form a hydrogel polymer. **B:** Structures of a few representative monomers used in the synthesis of hydrogels.

states. Hence, the mechanical and surface properties of the gel are greatly affected by both the water content and the ratio of freezing to nonfreezing water (6).

Temperature is an important consideration in the water content of the hydrogel. In general, the gel will increase its water content and therefore dimension with increased temperature. The size of the hydrogel at room temperature may vary when exposed to body temperature.

Another desirable characteristic of hydrogels is the permeability of oxygen, which potentially makes it available to adjacent or underlying tissues. This has been an important factor in contact lens development (24). This may have implications in the knee, where oxygen tension may be low.

The mechanical properties of hydrogels are difficult to measure because the test methods result in deformation and redistribution of the water within the gel. Despite this drawback, the microindentation technique has provided the most useful information to date on the hydrogels (33,37). In general, fully hydrated hydrogels are mechanically weak. This can be overcome through integrating a strong synthetic fiber or weave within the hydrogel. Such composites have been formed with Dacron for use as synthetic tendons (14,23). Increased strength characteristics may also be achieved with crosslinking and formation of composites (1,2).

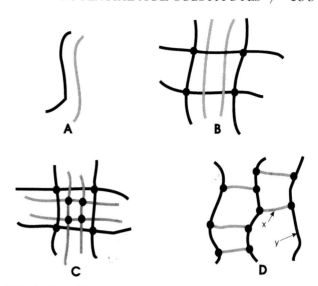

FIG. 2. Possible combinations of simple polymers. A: Polymer blend. B: Semi-interpenetrating polymer network. C: Full interpenetrating network. D: XY cross-linked polymer.

include chain stiffness, water structuring properties, molecular weights, and reactivity of attached "pendant" groups. Interpenetrating networks produce stronger and stiffer but less elastic gels than the homogeneous hydrogel copolymers of equal water content.

INTERPENETRATING POLYMER NETWORKS

Research in blending of two or more polymers has resulted in new materials having superior mechanical properties over the constituent polymers (10,16,31,32, 34). A polymer blend material refers to a mixture of components that are inseparable and indistinguishable. This differs from a polymer composite material in which each component remains identifiable. Using blends and composites techniques, the development of numerous synthetic polymer materials is possible. Little work has been devoted to hydrogel blends. However, this is expected to increase as there is a demand for more sophisticated biocompatible and biomimic materials.

Hydrogels formed into interpenetrating networks may also develop unique properties. Interpenetrating networks are defined as a combination of two polymers in network formed with at least one constituent being synthesized and/or cross-linked in the presence of the other (6). A possible interpenetrating network formation scheme is shown in Fig. 2. Interpenetrating networks may enable the development of hydrogels that mimic biologic composites such as ligaments and cartilage (the latter being a natural hydrogel). The use of interpenetrating networks offers an approach to alter the hydrogels, especially in the area of mechanical strength and water binding. Factors influencing interpenetrating networks

BIOCOMPATIBILITY

There has been considerable research into what makes a material biocompatible after it is positioned in the body (4,5,11,21). A material may be compatible in one application but not in another depending on its required function and location in the body. For example, a synthetic ACL could allow for cell ingrowth and deposition of matrix into the implant, whereas cell ingrowth and deposition of matrix would not be desired in a synthetic vascular graft composed of the same material. Perhaps a more appropriate definition of biocompatibility is the "ability of a material to perform with an appropriate host response in a specific application" (41).

Tissue culture methods have been used in an attempt to demonstrate *in vivo* biocompatibility. Tissue culture studies with hydrogels often demonstrate luxuriant cell growth that may be similar to cell growth observed on *in vivo* hydrogels (9,38). However, these findings should not be mistaken as an indicator of biocompatibility. Protein coatings of *in vitro* cell growth surfaces is similar to the protein interface that quickly forms on implants placed *in vivo*. Although the cell growth characteristics observed *in vitro* and *in vivo* may appear similar, they do not directly correlate to biocompatibility testing, and caution is suggested in interpreting such results. The tissue culture technique is a carefully controlled isolated *in vitro* environment that can support cell growth. This has been invaluable for studying the biology of these cells. The biologic environment is a much more dynamic and complex system, where cells can continually interact with implant materials. These interactions may lead to cellular changes in metabolism, mutations, or stimulation of the body's defense system, or may induce changes within the materials, leading to their degradation and release of potential toxic breakdown products.

A number of reports have focused on *in vivo* biocompatibility of HEMA gels, which are now considered to be less than ideal hydrogels for implantation (12). There are still limited reports published on the biocompatibility of other hydrogels, and much work needs to be done in this area. Despite the paucity of these studies, the potential to design new hydrogels with improved compatibility for different biologic environments is encouraging.

EFFECTS OF HYDROGELS ON CELLULAR FUNCTIONS

The properties of the hydrogel influence how forces are distributed throughout the hydrogel. The distortion stress, shear stress, strain energy, and hydraulic stress/strain can influence the surrounding tissues and cells on the surface or within the hydrogel. In this way, the physical forces the hydrogel encounters can be transmitted to the cells and affect their response. Physical forces that push and pull cells and the extracellular matrix can create structural patterns and alter cellular metabolism. At the cellular level, physical forces can affect cell shape, intracellular pressure, matrix interaction, and electric potential. At the molecular level, these forces could af-

fect the cytoskeleton, as well as activate ion transport channels and surface receptors on the cell. Two common forces that influence cells are hydrostatic stress and shear stress. Hydrostatic stress can affect the cells without changing their shape (Fig. 3a), whereas shear stress can alter the cells' shape (Fig. 3b). Such forces are naturally encountered within the tissues and cells of the body, and are responsible for directing and shaping the structure and function of these tissues.

DRUG DELIVERY FROM BIOERODIBLE HYDROGELS

An interesting aspect of hydrogels is their potential for controlled bioerosion and the utilization of this as a means for drug delivery. It may be possible to introduce and control the release of growth factors by using a hydrogel intended to erode over time. There are several potential release mechanisms that could be used, including the hydrolysis of a cross-linked hydrogel polymer releasing such molecules locked within the polymer matrix, and the aqueous solubilization of insoluble polymers by reactions such as ionization, hydrolysis, or protonation of side chains (6).

HYDROGEL-FORMING COMPOUNDS

Polyphosphazenes

The monomers in this group of hydrogels have water-soluble molecules that can be cross-linked with gamma irradiation to form hydrophilic water swelling membranes and hydrogels (Fig. 4). The amount of cross-linking in polyphosphazenes is related to the gamma irradiation dose. This in turn alters how water hydrates the gel and enables the properties of the hydrogel to be modified (1,2). Hydrogels in this group have been used to immobilize bioactive agents for controlled release (20,22).

Collagen Alginate Hydrogels

Collagen hydrogels exhibit good cell attachment and adhesion *in vitro,* often stimulating increased metabolic activity of these cells. Such gels can be coated to improve cell growth potential. Alginate-coated collagen gel fibers can be formed into stands or a mesh. These materials consist of a collagen gel matrix for cell attachment with an outer gel to capture and retain the implanted cells. The outer gel also provides some degree of mechanical stability to the complex.

A simple device consisting of two concentric small-diameter tubes can be used to prepare such a combination gel. Collagen and cells are expressed from the cen-

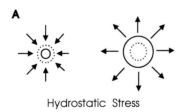

A

Hydrostatic Stress

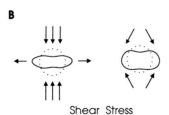

B

Shear Stress

FIG. 3. Effects of forces that the cell may encounter within or on the surface of a hydrogel. Dotted lines represent the original shape of the cell before application of the force. **A:** Hydrostatic force can change the size but not the shape of the cell. **B:** Shear stress can affect the cell shape. Both forces can have effects on the function of the cell.

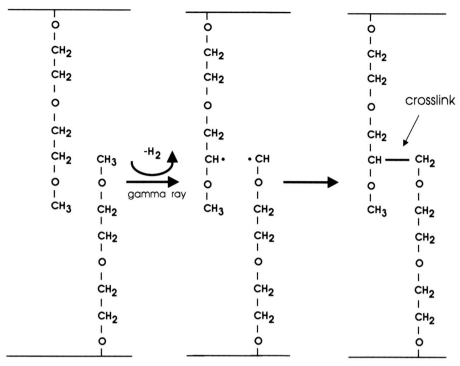

FIG. 4. Possible cross-linking reactions induced by gamma irradiation in the methoxyethoxyethoxy portion of the phosphazene molecule.

tral inner tube, and the alginate is extruded from the outer tube into a warm $CaCl_2$ solution. The inner collagen solution is gelled by warming, and the outer alginate is gelled instantly on contact with $CaCl_2$ (8).

Alginates

Alginates are polysaccharides with gel-forming properties. They are composed primarily of 1,4-linked beta-D-mannuronic acid (M) and alpha-L guluronic acid (G) in alternating M-G blocks. Varying the MG ratio has specific effects on stimulating certain cytokines [interleukin-1 (IL-1) and tumor necrosis factor (TNF)-alpha], and it has been determined that the mannuronic acid residues are the active cytokine inducer in alginates (25). IL-1 and TNF-alpha are inflammatory cytokines with strong fibroblast growth activity. Because it is considered important to not create an inflammatory response to the implant material, selecting an alginate high in G blocks and low in M blocks would be desired. Alginate hydrogels also have been shown to support good growth of tissue-cultured cells (15).

The studies of Edelman demonstrated that a controlled release of fibroblast growth factor (FGF) could be achieved using alginate gels (7). Fibroblast growth factor is usually degraded rapidly if injected or ingested. If FGF is mixed with conventional polymers, nearly 99% of the FGF activity is lost. However, binding the FGF to a heparin sepharose bead, and then encapsulating the bead

with alginate, results in 77% efficiency and 87.5% retention of the biologically active form of FGF.

NATURAL BIOPOLYMERS

Collagen

Solubilized collagen can be polymerized as fine strands with improvements in biological properties achieved using various cross-linking agents. Increased crosslinking is usually achieved by adding proteoglycans, or by chemical treatment with cyanamide or glutaraldehyde. Glutaraldehyde has fallen into disfavor as a treating agent due to apparent immunogenic and toxic properties. The reconstituted collagen is biocompatible and erodes with time. Cellular attachment and ingrowth into collagen *in vitro* and *in vivo* is excellent. Through control of the tanning process, it is possible to alter the reabsorption properties of the collagen so it is gradually absorbed, providing for gradual stress transfer. The collagen fibers can be formed into meshes or weaves for specific application similar to other synthetic fibers. Making fine collagen fibrils can be laborious, but should be easier in the future as new production techniques become available.

Collagen Graft Preparation

The methodology for preparing collagen for use as an implant device has been described in the literature (13).

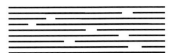

Extended Chain Fiber

- Very high molecular weight
- Minimum chain folding
- Very high degree of orientation

Conventional Fiber

- Moderate orientation
- Relatively low molecular weight
- Crystalline regions chain folded

FIG. 5. Comparison of the very high strength extended-chain polyethylene with conventional polyethylene. The highly oriented fibers are produced by a process in which the polymer is dissolved so that the polymer can become disentangled after gel spinning. This results in a product with a high modulus and high tensile strength.

This method uses insoluble collagen from bovine corium. This material can be washed with distilled water and isopropanol, and lyophilized and stored until needed.

A 1% (w/v) collagen dispersion is made by blending the lyophilized collagen with an HCl solution (pH 2.0). The collagen dispersion is degassed in a vacuum and stored in syringes at 4°C. The collagen dispersion is expressed through polyethylene tubing (inner diameter 0.58 mm) into a 37°C bath of fiber formation buffer (pH 7.5). After 45 minutes, fibers are transferred to an isopropanol bath (4 hours), then washed for 20 minutes in distilled water, and air-dried under tension overnight.

Dehydrothermal/cyanamide cross-linking is performed in a vacuum oven followed by cyanamide vapor cross-linking in a sealed desiccator (39).

The cross-linked collagen fibers (mean fiber diameter 60 μm), are assembled into a composite graft and then coated with a 1% (w/v) collagen dispersion in pH 2.0 HCl. The composite is air dried, then extensively washed in distilled water. For implantation, the composite is sterilized (60 minutes) in a glutaraldehyde-free cold sterilant, and washed (60 minutes) in sterile saline.

INNOVATIVE APPROACHES FOR MANUFACTURE OF HIGH-STRENGTH POLYMERS

The gel-spinning process has been successfully used in the manufacture of extremely strong fibers of extended-chain polyethylene. These molecules have molecular weights of 1 to 5 million, with a very high degree of orientation and a minimum amount of chain folding (Fig. 5). This is in contrast to conventional polyethylene fibers, which have a relatively low molecular weight (approximately 50,000), moderate orientation, and crystalline chain-fold areas. Typically, these extended-chain fibers have high abrasion resistance and high strength, are fairly supple, and have a low specific gravity. Because of the fibers' high tensile strength, their first applications have been for ballistic-proof vests. Combining the fibers' strength with a bias weave pattern results in a fabric that, when placed in several layers, can effectively prevent a bullet's penetration. These types of materials may have potential application for use as synthetic ligaments and tendons.

Synthetic polymers are usually simple homogenous materials such as polyethylene or polypropylene. Scientists are attempting to better understand how these polymers react in the biologic environment in order to improve the design of future polymers. New manufacturing techniques should improve the properties of these materials through molecular structuring and selecting specific pendant side chains to control the microstructure of the polymer.

CONCLUSIONS

Hydrogels appear to be a versatile group of materials that have not yet reached their full potential in biomedical applications. The development of new preparative techniques are enabling new properties to be applied to established polymers. The demand is on to provide a precise combination of physical, biologic, and chemical properties to simulate natural tissues. As information and understanding accumulates, it should be possible to design biopolymers for a specific application rather than finding a successful material by chance. These new materials offer the potential to mimic the natural tissues they will replace.

REFERENCES

1. Allcock HR, Gebura M, Kwon S, Neenan TX. (1988): Amphiphilic polyphosphazenes as membrane materials: influence of side group on radiation cross-linking. *Biomaterials* 9:500–508.
2. Allcock HR, Kwon S, Riding GH, Fitzpatrick RJ, Bennett JL. (1988). Hydrophilic polyphosphazenes as hydrogels: radiation cross-linking and hydrogel characteristics of poly[bis(methoxyethoxyethoxy)phosphazene]. *Biomaterials* 9:509–513.
3. Andrade JD, ed. (1976): *Hydrogels for medical and related applications.* ACS Symposium Series, No. 31. Washington, DC: ACS.
4. Baier RE, Dutton RC, Gott VL. (1970): Surface chemical features of blood vessels walls and of synthetic materials exhibiting thromboresistance. *Adv Exp Med* 7:235.
5. Cooper SL, Peppas NA, eds. (1989): *Biomaterials: interfacial phenomena and applications.* ACS Symposium Series, No. 199. Washington, DC: ACS.
6. Corkhill PH, Hamilton CJ, Tighe BJ. (1990): The design of hydrogels for medical applications. In: Peppas NA, ed. *Hydrogels in medicine and pharmacy. Vol. III. Properties and application.* Boca Raton, FL: CRC Press, pp. 363–436.
7. Edelman ER, Mathiowitz E, Langer R, Klagsbrun M. (1991): Controlled and modulated release of basic fibroblast growth factor. *Biomaterials* 12:619–626.

8. Enami J, Arai O, Saito N, Yamaoka S, (1990): Growth of nerve cells cultured in alginate-coated collagen gel fibers. *Jpn J Physiol* 40(suppl):S20.

9. Franzblau C, Faris BS, Civerchia-Perez L. (1986): Hydrogels capable of supporting cell growth. *Official Gazette US Patent Trademark Office* 10b2:1132.

10. Frisch HL, Frisch KC, Klempner D. (1981): Advances in interpenetrating polymer networks, *Pure Appl Chem* 53:1557.

11. Horbett TA. (1986): Protein adsorption to hydrogels. In: Peppas NA, ed. *Hydrogels in medicine and pharmacy.* Vol. I. Boca Raton, FL: CRC Press, p. 127.

12. Imai Y, Masuhara E. (1982): Long-term *in vivo* studies of poly (2-hydroxyethyl methacrylate). *J Biomed Mater Res* 16:609.

13. Kato YP, Christiansen DL, Hahn RA, Shieh S-J, Goldstein JD, Silver FH. (1989): Mechanical properties of collagen fibers: a comparison of reconstituted and rat tail tendon fibres. *Biomaterials* 10:38–42.

14. Kilarik J, Migliaresi C, Nicolais L. (1981): Mechanical properties of model synthetic tendons. *J Biomed Mater Res* 15:147.

15. King GA, Daugulis AJ, Goosen MFA. (1989): Alginate concentration: a key factor in growth of temperature sensitive baculovirus infected insect cells in microcapsules. *Biotechnol Bioeng* 34:1085–1091.

16. Klempner D, Berkowski L. (1987): Interpenetrating polymer networks. In: Kroschwitz JI, ed. *Encyclopedia of polymer science and engineering.* Vol. 8. New York: Wiley-Interscience, p. 279.

17. Kudula V. (1987): Hydrogels. In: Kroschwitz JI, ed. *Encyclopedia of polymer science and engineering.* Vol 7. New York: Wiley-Interscience, p. 783.

18. Larke JR, Pedley DG, Tighe BJ. (1977): National Research Development Corporation. British Patent 1,478,455.

19. Larke JR, Tighe BJ. (1975): National Research Development Corporation. British Patent 1,395,501.

20. Laurencin CT, Koh HJ, Neenan TX, Allcock HR. (1987): Controlled release using a new bioerodible polyphosphazene matrix system. *J Biomed Mater Res* 21:1231–1246.

21. Leonard EF, Toritto VT, Vroman L, eds. (1987): Blood in contact with natural and artificial surfaces. *Ann NY Acad Sci* 516:1–688.

22. Lora S, Carenza M, Palma G, Pezzin G, Caliceti P, Battaglia P, Lora A. (1990): Biocompatible polyphosphazenes by radiation induced graft copolymerization and heparinization. *Biomaterials* 12:275–280.

23. Migliaresi C, Nicolais L. (1980): Composite material for biomedical applications. *Int J Artif Organs* 3:114.

24. Ng CO, Pedley DG, Tighe BJ. (1976): Polymers in contact lens applications. VII. Oxygen permeability and surface hydrophobicity of poly (4-methyl pent-1-ene) and related polymers. *Br Polym J* 8:124.

25. Otterlei M, Ostgaard K, Skjak-Braek G, Smidsrod O, Soon-Shiong P, Espevik T. (1991): Induction of cytokine production from human monocytes stimulated with alginate. *J Immunother* 10:286–291.

26. Pedley DG, Skelly PJ, Tighe BJ. (1980): Hydrogels in biomedical applications. *Br Polym J* 12:99.

27. Ratner BD. (1981): Biomedical applications of hydrogels. A review and clinical appraisal. In: Williams DF, ed. *Biocompatibility of clinical implant materials.* Vol 2. Boca Raton, FL: CRC Press, p. 145.

28. Ratner BD, Hoffman AS. (1976): Synthetic hydrogels for biomedical applications. In: Andrade JD, ed. *Hydrogels for medical and related applications.* ACS Symposium Series No. 31. Washington, DC: ACS, p. 1.

29. Roorda WE, Bodde HE, de Boer AG, Junginger HE. (1986): Synthetic hydrogels as drug delivery systems. *Pharm Weekbl (Sci)* 8:165.

30. Silver FH, Tria AJ, Sawadsky JP, Dunn MG. (1991): Anterior cruciate ligament replacement: a review. *J Long-Term Effects Med Implants* 1:135–154.

31. Sperling LH. (1981): *Interpenetrating polymer networks and related materials.* New York: Plenum Press.

32. Sperling LH. (1985): Pure and applied research on interpenetrating polymer networks and related materials. In: Walsh DJ, Higgins JS, Maconnachie A, eds. *Polymer blends and mixtures.* NATO ASI Series, Series E, Vol. 89. Dordrecht, The Netherlands: Martinus Nijhoff, p. 267.

33. Taylor DJ, Kragh AM. (1970): Determination of the rigidity modulus of thin soft coatings by indentation measurements. *J Phys Part D: Appl Physics* 3:29.

34. Thomas DA, Sperling LH. (1978): Interpenetrating polymer networks. In: Paul DR, Neuman S, eds. *Polymer blends.* Vol 2. New York: Academic Press, p. 1.

35. Tighe BJ (1989): Contact lens materials. In: Phillips AJ, Stone J, eds. *Contact lenses.* 3rd ed. London: Butterworths, p. 72.

36. Tighe BJ. (1989): Hydrogel materials: the patents and the products (parts I and 11). *Optician* 17:197.

37. Timoshenko S, Goodier JN. (1951): *Theory of elasticity.* 2nd ed. New York: McGraw-Hill.

38. Toselli P, Mogayzel PJ Jr., Faris B, Ferrera R, Franzblau C. (1984): Mammalian cell growth on collagen hydrogels. *Scan Electron Microsc* 3:1301–1312.

39. Weadock K, Olson RM, Silver FH. (1984): Evaluation of collagen crosslinking techniques. *Biomat Med Dev Artif Organs* 11:293–318.

40. Wichterle O. (1971): Hydrogels. In: Mark H, Gaylord N, eds. *Encyclopedia of polymer science and technology.* Vol. 15. New York: Interscience, p. 273.

41. Williams DF. (1989): A model for biocompatibility and its evaluation. *J Biomed Eng* 11:185.

The Anterior Cruciate Ligament: Current and
Future Concepts, edited by D.W. Jackson, et al.
Raven Press, Ltd., New York © 1993.

CHAPTER 40

Quality of Life Assessment as an Outcome in Anterior Cruciate Ligament Reconstructive Surgery

Nicholas G. H. Mohtadi

An often quoted statement is "assessment and account-ability, the third revolution of the medical care of patients" (42). Although the stimulus for this revolution is the spiralling cost of health care the assessment of outcome is foremost in this process (53). Without clear knowledge of the effectiveness of treatment, specifically that of anterior cruciate ligament (ACL) reconstruction, accounting for the costs is an exercise in futility. Accountability can also be interpreted in another light, that of being accountable to our patients. Here again, the determination of the outcomes of reconstructive surgery are an absolute requirement in this process (9,16).

WHAT IS MEANT BY OUTCOME ASSESSMENT?

The assessment of outcome after surgical treatment can take on many different formats. To determine whether any surgical or nonsurgical treatment has benefitted the patient, the outcome of that treatment must be assessed in an appropriate way (51).

When planning a surgical reconstruction for a patient with an ACL-deficient knee, the orthopedic surgeon must weigh the potential benefits of the procedure against the risks or complications. The decision of whether to operate is further compounded, because it is likely that only a minority of patients require reconstructive surgery. The surgeon is faced with two dilemmas. The first is patient selection. This involves the process of discriminating between patients to determine who

should and who should not have the reconstructive procedure. The second dilemma is how to determine the effectiveness of the procedure. Effectiveness refers to the efficacy of the procedure as performed in actual practice. It can also be called the appropriateness of the procedure. An understanding of the outcome of surgery is a necessary step in addressing these dilemmas (51). Outcome with respect to the ACL in the past has involved looking at symptoms, objective measures such as the KT arthrometer (6), functional assessment (1), and acknowledgment of the emotional impact of the injury (32,33,36). An ideal outcome assessment would be all inclusive and comprehensive, and deemed to be a reliable, responsive, and valid measure of ACL outcome.

At the present time there is no such ideal outcome measure. Historically outcomes have been based on the history and physical examination. The surgeon examined a patient preoperatively, and determined that the knee was unstable and that the patient was having symptoms sufficiently severe to warrant a surgical solution (41). During follow-up, the history and physical were repeated, and if symptoms had decreased in frequency and severity and if the knee was more stable, then the surgery was considered a success. From this logical beginning the outcome assessment process developed into the formation of various scales (5,28,32), questionnaires, and scoring systems (49) to further elucidate the results of reconstructive surgery (7,23,24,27,33). These indices incorporated functional considerations (50), as well as those more classically part of the history and physical examination (17,45). This process was started by O'Donoghue in 1955 (39) and has blossomed into a whole system of knee evaluation as described and advo-

---

N. G. H. Mohtadi: University of Calgary, Sport Medicine Center, Calgary, Alberta, Canada 22N 1N4.

cated by Noyes (37,38). More recently the indices and evaluators have looked at other issues such as the emotional response to injury (40,46) and proprioception (2). One of the main problems is the inability to compare one index with another (4). The future of outcome research and assessment is in the area of quality of life assessment (9,14). This is not to say that the current measures (11,48) are no longer important, but they do not include all of the relevant outcomes necessary to evaluate patients completely. The more traditional measures complement the quality of life assessment.

QUALITY OF LIFE ASSESSMENT: WHAT DOES IT MEAN?

The concept of quality of life has a variety of different meanings and interpretations (47). It can refer to economic issues such as the standard of living, employment, and housing. It can refer to individual satisfaction or community and neighborhood issues (3). From a healthcare perspective, it is an evolving area with several definitions. Nevertheless, quality of life is similar to the World Health Organization definition of health, which is a state of complete physical, mental, and social well being, and not merely the absence of disease or infirmity (47,52).

The assessment of quality of life is the current trend in many areas of medicine (18). This has resulted because of the changing pattern of disease in the 20th century. No longer is mortality an appropriate outcome measure (47). The chronic nature of afflictions such as heart disease and cancer (8) demand that quality of life issues be assessed to determine how a patient is really doing. This is independent of the number of coronary arteries present or whether or not pulmonary metastases are detected. The same can be said of chronic ACL deficiency. It is not sufficient to comment on the amount of anterior translation compared with the opposite knee or whether a pivot shift phenomenon is present to determine a patient's outcome. There are many other issues that are equally or possibly more important, and the assessment of quality of life should be considered an important and complementary outcome measure. Quality of life assessment is patient based (13). It considers the subjective or softer scientific measures of outcome. The following definitions of quality of life are being used in the context of chronic ACL deficiency (43,44):

1. The functional definition is that of the "patients' perception of performance in four areas: physical and occupational function, psychological state, social interaction and somatic sensation."
2. "A concept encompassing a broad range of physical and psychological characteristics and limitations which describe an individual's ability to function and derive satisfaction from doing so."

The key is that this is based on the individual (19) and not what a surgeon thinks is important. It is good to have a consensus of experts decide on the evaluation scheme in a clinical trial of cruciate surgery, but is this what is important to the patients?

Quality of life assessment can be looked at from two perspectives. One way is to consider that quality of life is a global concept that can be applied across all disciplines (10). This implies that a generic instrument could be used to assess outcome in patients with ACL deficiency as well as in patients with coronary artery disease. The generic approach has considerable appeal, especially for health-care planners and administrators (52). It would allow for direct comparisons between how we treat different patients and diseases. Allocation of funding would be based on treatment that improves quality of life. Many of these measures have been validated, but not in any conditions similar to ACL deficiency. The validated generic quality of life measure is useful when validation of a new measure is sought.

The second approach is to consider disease-specific quality of life outcome measures. Although this suggests that every disease should have a fully evaluated and valid separate measure, not every disease is suitable. An acute disease with a well-defined natural history and treatment effect is not really going to impact on a patient's quality of life. Anterior cruciate deficiency is clearly not a disease of this kind.

Because the generic approach has been used primarily in those populations with chronic diseases such as heart disease, arthritis (30,31), and pulmonary disease, as well as in the aging population, it appears that the population of ACL-deficient patients has decidedly different concerns. The logical approach is a disease-specific outcome measure.

DEVELOPING A QUALITY OF LIFE OUTCOME MEASURE FOR CHRONIC ACL DEFICIENCY

There are different potential applications of a quality of life measure (21). It can be considered predictive, discriminative, or evaluative (29). A predictive index is a way of classifying individuals based on a standard. Because the standard test is not available for the outcome of ACL reconstructive surgery, this is currently not an appropriate application. A discriminative index can distinguish between patients to classify them into groups with respect to quality of life. This would then allow an intervention to take place to improve the situation. There are currently many separate issues that are taken into account when considering who should be operated upon, including patient demographics, amount of instability, level of sporting activity, type of job, and other considerations. However, these variables have not been considered under the label of quality of life. Nevertheless, the main concern is how to evaluate patients. The focus of this evaluation is a clinical trial (18). The evaluative index of quality of life is by definition an outcome measure. The basic property of any outcome measurement is that it should evaluate patients at a particular point in time or over a period of time. In ACL reconstruction it would be necessary to have a way of using the outcome measure at intervals after surgery and with at least 2 years' follow-up. An important property of the measure is that it could reflect clinically important changes (13,25) over time if they occur. This is known as responsiveness (20). A responsive index of quality of life will detect changes if they occur. This must be addressed in any situation where a new instrument is being devised. From a development standpoint, the other considerations are selecting appropriate items to be evaluated, scaling the items, and reducing the items into a manageable number. This ensures that the information is a reliable and valid measure of quality of life (19) as it pertains to patients with anterior cruciate deficiency.

A quality of life measure has been developed with these principles in mind (35). Initially an item pool was created by reviewing the literature specifically about the outcome measures in ACL surgery. The literature relating to quality of life assessment was also reviewed (34). The main issue in this stage of instrument development was that the items generated should be comprehensive. Nothing could be left out. Following this, surveys were given to knee surgeons, sport medicine physicians, and therapists experienced in the management of ACL deficiency. The final step was to administer a survey to patients with cruciate problems. The surveys asked for each health-care professional and patient to list items of concern with respect to ACL deficiency. The items were generated within five separate domains that satisfied the above definitions of quality of life. These included symptoms and physical complaints, sport/recreational concerns, work-related concerns, life-style, and social/emotional concerns. An additional domain related to the treatment of ACL was also included. This involved questions on surgical or nonsurgical treatment and was included because of its obvious clinical relevance. Methodologically, however, the use of treatment concerns in an evaluative outcome measure is flawed. An outcome measure is by definition a dependent variable with respect to the analysis of results. Treatment is an independent variable. To evaluate patients relative to different treatment methods mitigates against using treatment concerns in the quality of life instrument. The information gathered from this domain has relevance to a discriminative instrument, and hence the usefulness of collecting this information for future purposes. To determine whether the surveying process was comprehensive, it was repeated over and over on a subset of individuals until no new items had been identified. This resulted in a list of 167 items, an unmanageable number for the purposes of a practical outcome measure.

The next stage was to reduce the number of items. Again the focus had to be the patient. This list of items was formulated into a questionnaire. Patients were asked to fill in the questionnaire and rate every item with respect to how important the item was to them. Items were retained based on the frequency with which they were endorsed and the importance of the item based on a 6-point scale. The scale ranged from 0, which meant that the item was not experienced by the patient, to a 5, which indicated that the item in question was experienced and extremely important. Another consideration was the responsiveness of the item. This is a subjective appreciation of whether the item can reflect a change during the disease. Responsiveness is also important in the determination of the necessary sample size when setting up a clinical trial. The sample size is based on the power of the instrument to detect a clinically important change. The more an instrument can detect a change, the lower the sample size requirements.

The item reduction questionnaire was distributed to more than 100 patients with chronic ACL deficiency. A response rate of 75% was achieved. The forms were analyzed based on frequency, importance, and responsiveness. Thirty-four items were decided upon within the original six domains. The three items in the treatment domain were modified and incorporated into other domains to satisfy the concern outlined above regarding the dependent nature of an outcome measurement.

The next step for the quality of life measure was to develop another questionnaire with only the 34 items. Again, several issues had to be addressed. It was felt that a self-administered questionnaire was much more practical than one that would require an interviewer. The response options could be a scale with verbal descriptions or a visual analogue scale (15,26). A 7-point verbal descriptor scale was used. The questionnaire was then pretested on another group of chronic ACL-deficient patients. This pretesting stage is again a critical step. It helps to ensure that the questionnaire is understandable and appropriate to the patients. The other purpose of this stage of development is to evaluate whether the response options are being used. If any of the questions are always answered with the same option, then this question is not responsive and should be eliminated from the questionnaire. The questionnaire has now undergone modification and will be used in the future to establish the other properties of responsiveness, and validity.

The following domains are represented in this instrument of quality of life assessment for chronic ACL deficiency of the knee:

1. Symptoms and physical complaints (i.e., somatic sensation)
2. Work-related concerns (i.e., occupational function)
3. Recreational activities, sport participation or competition (i.e., physical function)
4. Life-style (i.e., social interaction, life function, and satisfaction)
5. Emotional aspects (i.e., psychological state)

It is important to recognize that unless these domains (as defined by the definitions above) are included, then this cannot represent a true quality of life measure.

Within the domain related to symptoms, this question is an example of the format used:

With respect to your overall knee function, how much are you troubled by stiffness?

1. *Severely troubled*
2. *A great deal of trouble*
3. *A good deal of trouble*
4. *Moderate trouble*
5. *Some trouble*
6. *Only a little trouble*
7. *Not troubled at all*

Within the work-related domain, the following example:

How much of a concern is it for you to lose time from school or work because of the treatment of your ACL-deficient knee?

1. *An extremely significant concern*
2. *A very great concern*
3. *A good deal of concern*
4. *A moderate concern*
5. *A little concern*
6. *Hardly a concern*
7. *No concern at all*

Within the recreational and sport-related domain, the following example:

With respect to the activities or sports that you currently desire to be involved with, how much have your overall expectations changed because of the status of your knee?

1. *Expectations totally lowered*
2. *Expectations extremely lowered*
3. *Expectations very much lowered*
4. *Expectations moderately lowered*
5. *Expectations a little lowered*
6. *Expectations hardly lowered at all*
7. *Expectations not lowered at all*

Within the life-style domain, the following example:

How much has your enjoyment of life been limited by your knee problem?

1. *Totally limited*
2. *Extremely limited*
3. *Very limited*
4. *Moderately limited*
5. *Somewhat limited*
6. *A little limited*
7. *Not limited at all*

Within the emotional domain, the following example:

How fearful are you of reinjuring your knee?

1. *Extremely fearful*
2. *A great deal of fear*
3. *A good bit of fear*
4. *Some fear*
5. *A little fear*
6. *Hardly any fear*
7. *Not fearful at all*

From these examples it can be seen that the better the quality of life, the higher one's score. In some of the questions there is a response option that scores a 0, and in others an option that scores an 8. These responses are included to reflect situations where the patient cannot endorse any of the options from 1 to 7. Two examples of this are as follows:

Are you worried about having to change your current occupation because of the problems in your knee?

1. *Have already changed occupation because of knee*
2. *Extremely worried*
3. *Terribly worried*
4. *Very worried*
5. *Moderately worried*
6. *Somewhat worried*
7. *A little worried*
8. *Not worried at all*

How much of the time does it bother you that your competitive needs are no longer being met because of your knee?

1. *All of the time*
2. *Most of the time*
3. *A good bit of the time*
4. *Some of the time*
5. *A little of the time*
6. *Hardly any of the time*
7. *None of the time*
8. *My competitive needs are being met*

There are many issues to be addressed. With respect to scoring this instrument: should an overall quality of life score be reported or separate scores for each of the domains or subscales? An overall score is more clinically attractive, but when analyses are made they by necessity are combining dissimilar items of information. It is important to realize that quality of life scores are to be recorded at different points in time in a repetitive fashion. When comparing one form of treatment with another in a clinical trial, it is the magnitude of change within each treatment group that forms the comparison. In this way each patient is his or her own control and the obvious individual variation is taken into account. This concept is critical when dealing with subjective information.

THE FUTURE IN QUALITY OF LIFE ASSESSMENT OF CHRONIC ACL DEFICIENCY

The nature of subjective information is that we are always skeptical about whether we are going to rely on its usefulness. Methodological principles must be adhered to in order to satisfy the skeptics. The quality of life measure as it stands will require further testing to show that it is a reliable, responsive, and valid measure of patients with chronic ACL deficiency.

Reliability can be assessed through repeated administrations of the instrument to the same patients under stable circumstances where no change in clinical status has occurred. Responsiveness is the ability to measure a clinically important change if this has occurred. This can be determined by seeing that the instrument reflects change in situations where it is clear that a change has occurred (18,22) If a group of ACL-deficient patients is followed for a period of time without surgical intervention, and deterioration in their clinical situation occurs, then a clinically relevant change has occurred. This should be reflected in a change in their quality of life as measured by the instrument. The same should apply in situations where obvious improvement has occurred. Finally, the instrument should prove to be valid. There are many ways to assess validity (12), and all will be demonstrated.

This instrument is considered to have face validity if it is measuring ACL deficiency from the observer's point of view. During the process of instrument development, all patients were asked to add any items to the original pool. They were asked if the questions represented relevant problems associated with ACL deficiency, and only those items that were considered to be important were included. It is concluded that face validity is not in question.

The next type of validity is content validity. This refers to the comprehensiveness of the instrument. Does it cover all the important areas of quality of life. Content validity can be determined by giving the instrument to a group of experts. The experts can be asked to answer the following questions:

Do the questions address quality of life issues related to chronic ACL deficiency?
Does each item represent an area of concern that is amenable to treatment with nonoperative and operative means?
Is the instrument comprehensive in addressing all areas of quality of life?
Are the response options appropriate?

Content validity reflects a consensus of opinion. If there were more than 20% of these experts doubting the validity of the instrument, then it would have to be modified.

The last type of validity is that of construct validity. A construct is a hypothesis, prediction, or theory. Overall, one would suggest or hypothesize that if this instrument were valid then it would reflect a patient's quality of life in a new and better way compared with other methods of assessment. It should be more sensitive than a generic quality of life measure. It should correlate highly with a global assessment of function as rated by the patient, because it purports to measure similar functional characteristics. The correlation should be higher than that reported by the surgeon or therapist involved in the patient's care. It should also correlate with other outcomes such as objective ligament laxity testing, strength testing, and occupational and sport performance. The irony of this process is that these other outcomes, although well accepted in the literature, are in themselves not proven reliable and valid instruments of assessing outcome of ACL deficiency.

In conclusion, improvement in the quality of life of our patients should be our primary goal with respect to the management of ACL deficiency. To ensure that we are administering the right treatment, we can assess this treatment with quality of life in mind. This demands that we use a reliable, responsive, and valid instrument of quality of life assessment. The current trend in orthopedic clinical research is to recognize the importance of outcome assessment and accountability to our patients. Orthopedic sport medicine practitioners have spent a generation looking at the ACL. We have to continue with today's trend and continue to evaluate our results critically in the future.

REFERENCES

1. Barber SD, Noyes FR, Mangine RE, McCloskey JW, Hartman W. (1990): Quantitative assessment of functional limitations in normal and anterior cruciate deficient ligament knees. *Clin Orthop* 225:204–214.
2. Barrett DS. (1991): Proprioception and function after anterior cruciate reconstruction. *J Bone Joint Surg* 73B:833–837.
3. Bergner M. (1989): Quality of life, health status, and clinical research. *Med Care* 27(suppl):S148–S156.
4. Bollen S, Seedhom BB. (1991): A comparison of the Lysholm and Cincinnati knee scoring questionnaires. *Am J Sports Med* 19:189–190.
5. Charlson ME, Johanson NA, Williarns PG. (1991): Scaling, scoring and staging. In: Troidl HEA, ed. *Principles and practice of research: strategies for surgical investigators.* New York: Springer-Verlag, pp. 192–200.
6. Daniel DM, Malcolm LL, Lossee G, Stone ML, Sachs R, Burks R. (1985): Instrumented measurement of anterior laxity of the knee. *J Bone Joint Surg* 67:720–725.
7. Daniel DM, Stone ML, Riehl B. (1990): Ligament surgery: the evaluation of results. In: Daniel DM, Akeson WH, O'Connor JJ, eds. *Knee ligaments structure, function, injury and repair.* New York: Raven Press, pp. 521–534.

8. Donovan K, Sanson-Fisher RW, Redman S. (1989): Measuring quality of life in cancer patients. *J Clin Oncol* 7:959–968.
9. Ellwood PM. (1988): Shattuck lecture—outcomes management. *N Engl J Med* 318:1549–1556.
10. EuroQol Group. (1990): EuroQol—a new facility for the measurement of health-related quality of life. *Health Policy* 16:199–208.
11. Feagin JA, Blake WP. (1983): Postoperative evaluation and result recording in the anterior cruciate ligament reconstructed knee. *Clin Orthop* 172:143 147.
12. Feinstein AR. (1987): *Clinimetrics.* New Haven, CT: Yale University Press.
13. Feinstein AR, Josephy BR, Wells CK. (1986): Scientific and clinical problems in indexes of functional disability. *Ann Intern Med* 105:413–420.
14. Flanagan JC. (1982): Measurement of quality of life: current state of the art. *Arch Phys Med Rehabil* 63:56–59.
15. Flandry F, Hunt JP, Terry GC, Hughston JC. (1991): Analysis of subjective knee complaints using visual analogue scales. *Am J Sports Med* 19:112–118.
16. Gartland JJ. (1988): Orthopaedic clinical research: deficiencies in experimental design and determinations of outcome. *J Bone Joint Surg* 70A.
17. Geens S, Clayton ML, Leidholt JD, Smyth CJ, Bartholomew, BA. (1969): Synovectomy and debridement of the knee in rheumatoid arthritis. *J Bone Joint Surg* 51A:626–641.
18. Guyatt GH. (1987): Measuring quality of life: a review of means of measurement in clinical trials of new medicines. *Pharmaceut Med* 2:49–60.
19. Guyatt GH, Bombardier C, Tugwell PX. (1986): Measuring disease-specific quality of life in clinical trials. *Can Med Assoc J* 134:889–895.
20. Guyatt GH, Deyo RA, Charlson M, Levine MN, Mitchell A. (1989): Responsiveness and validity in health status measurement: a clarification. *J Clin Epidemiol* 42:403–408.
21. Guyatt GH, Veldhuyzen Van Zanten SJO, Feeny DH, Patrick DL. (1989): Measuring quality of life in clinical trials: a taxonomy and review. *Can Med Assoc J* 140:1441–1447.
22. Guyatt GH, Walter S, Norman G. (1987): Measuring change over time: assessing the usefulness of evaluative instruments. *J Chronic Dis* 40:171–178.
23. Harter RA, Osternig LR, Singer KM, James SL, Larson RL, Jones DC. (1988): Long-term evaluation of knee stability and function following surgical reconstruction for anterior cruciate ligament insufficiency. *Am J Sports Med* 16:434–443.
24. Hughston JC, Barrett GR. (1983): Acute anteromedial rotatory instability. *J Bone Joint Surg* 65A:145–153.
25. Jaeschke R, Singer J, Guyatt GH. (1989): Measurement of health status: ascertaining the minimally clinically important difference. *Cont Clin Trials* 10:407–415.
26. Jaeschke R, Singer J, Guyatt GH. (1990): A comparison of seven point and visual analogue scales. *Cont Clin Trials* 11:43–51.
27. Jensen JE, Slocum DB, Larson RL, James SL, Singer KM. (1983): Reconstruction procedures for anterior cruciate ligament insufficiency: a computer analysis of clinical results. *Am J Sports Med* 11:240–248.
28. Kettlekamp DB, Thompson MS. (1975): Development of a knee scoring scale. *Clin Orthop* 107:93–99.
29. Kirschner B, Guyatt GH. (1985): A methodological framework for assessing health indices. *J Chronic Dis* 38:27–36.
30. Liang MH, Fossel AH, Larson MG. (1990): Comparisons of five health status instruments for orthopaedic evaluation. *Med Care* 28:632–642.
31. Liang MH, Katz JN, Ginsburg KS. (1990): Chronic rheumatic disease. In: Spilker, ed. *Quality of life assessments in clinical trials.* New York: Raven Press, pp. 441–458.
32. Lysholm J, Gillquist J. (1982): Evaluation of knee ligament surgery results with a special emphasis on use os a scoring scale. *Am J Sports Med* 10:150–154.
33. Marshall JL, Fetto JF, Botero MB. (1977): Knee ligament injuries: a standardized evaluation. *Clin Orthop* 123:115–129.
34. McDowell I, Newell C. (1987): *Measuring health.* New York: Oxford University Press.
35. Mohtadi NGH. (1990): *Development of a disease specific quality of life measure for chronic anterior cruciate ligament deficiency* (Masters Thesis). Hamilton, Ontario, Canada: McMaster University.
36. Muller W, Biedert R, Hefti F, Jakob RP, Munzinger U, Staubli HU. (1988): OAK knee evaluation: a new way to assess knee ligament injuries. *Clin Orthop* 232:37–50.
37. Noyes FR, Barber SD, Mooar LA. (1989): A rationale for assessing sports activity levels and limitations in knee disorders. *Clin Orthop* 264:238–249.
38. Noyes FR, Mooar LA, Barber SD. (1991): The assessment of work-related activities and limitations in knee disorders. *Am J Sports Med* 19:178–188.
39. O'Donoghue DH. (1955): An analysis of end results of surgical treatment of major injuries to the ligaments of the knee. *J Bone Joint Surg* 37A:1–13.
40. Ogilvie BC. (1988): Counselling patients with career-ending injuries. In: Feagin JA, ed. *The crucial ligaments.* New York: Churchill Livingstone, pp. 357–368.
41. Paulos L, Noyes FR, Malek M. (1980): A practical guide to the initial evaluation and treatment of knee ligament injuries. *J Trauma* 20:498–506.
42. Relman AS. (1988): Assessment and accountability: The third revolution in medical care. *N Engl J Med* 319:1220–1222.
43. Schipper H. (1990): Quality of life: principles of the clinical paradigm. *J Psychosocial Oncol* 8:171–184.
44. Schipper H, Clinch J, Powell V. (1990): Definitions and conceptual issues. In: Spilker B, ed. *Quality of life assessments in clinical trials.* New York: Raven Press, pp. 11–24.
45. Smillie IS. (1974): *Diseases of the knee joint.* Edinburgh, Scotland: Churchill Livingstone.
46. Smith AM, Scott SG, O'Fallon WM, Young ML. (1990): Emotional responses for athletes to injury. *Mayo Clin Proc* 65:38–50.
47. Spitzer WO. (1987): State of science 1986: quality of life and functional status as target variables for research. *J Chronic Dis* 40:465–471.
48. Straub T, Hunter RE. (1988): Acute anterior cruciate ligament repair. *Clin Orthop* 227:238–250.
49. Tegner Y, Lysholm J. (1985): Rating systems in the evaluation of knee ligament injuries. *Clin Orthop* 198:43–49.
50. Tibone JE, Antich TJ, Fanton GS, Moynes DR, Perry J. (1986): Functional analysis of anterior cruciate ligament instability. *Am J Sports Med* 14:276–284.
51. Troidl H, Kusche J, Vestweber K-H. Eypasch E, Koeppen L, Bouillon B. (1987): Quality of life: an important endpoint both in surgical practice and research. *J Chronic Dis* 40:523–528.
52. Ware JE. (1991): Conceptualizing and measuring health outcomes. *Cancer* 67 (suppl):774–779.
53. Wennberg JE. (1990): Outcomes research, cost containment, and the fear of health care rationing. *N Engl J Med* 323:1202–1204.

Section VI

Future Directions

For this final section, the contributors were asked to share their views on the future directions in their respective fields of expertise. Though the scope of the responses was broad and varied, they were distilled into five areas in basic research and five areas in clinical research. These concepts provide us with a perspective comparing past accomplishments with the sizable amount of important and exciting research remaining to be done. Greater integration of the clinical and basic science related to the anterior cruciate ligament has been recommended. Lastly, a caution is provided with respect to clinical application of promising areas of basic research, e.g., growth factors, that still requires extensive basic investigation to increase understanding.

Cyril B. Frank

The Anterior Cruciate Ligament: Current and Future Concepts, edited by D.W. Jackson, et al.
Raven Press, Ltd., New York © 1993.

CHAPTER 41

Future Directions of Anterior Cruciate Ligament Research

Cyril B. Frank

Although significant progress has been made in our experimental and clinical understanding of the anterior cruciate ligament (ACL), as reflected in the preceding sections of this book, all of the contributors to this book agree that a great deal of exciting and important work remains to be done. At the conclusion of the meeting at which this book was written, the authors were polled to submit their concepts of important future directions for work in each of their respective areas. These concepts were then discussed and refined into certain themes. This chapter represents a brief synthesis of that survey and discussion, purposely presented in no intended order of priority to reflect the theme that only through a multidisciplinary assessment of the ACL will its true structure and functions become apparent and its healing or replacement optimized. Clinical and basic science needs have been separated in this chapter, only to facilitate a clearer understanding of each, not to imply their discordance. In fact, a clearly stated deficiency at the time of this review was the lack of clinical and basic science integration. The reader is therefore encouraged to attempt to appreciate both clinical and basic needs in order to make contributions to as many areas as possible, so that problems with ACL deficiency identified in this book can be solved in our lifetimes.

BASIC RESEARCH

The first basic science topic that clearly requires further attention is the better definition of ACL structure at all levels, particularly its microstructure. Although some insights into the gross and microscopic arrangement of the major components of the ACL are already in place, very little is known about the "minor components"

(minor in a quantitative, not a functional sense), or about the interactions between components in its substance or its insertions. Distributions of components is likely to vary within the ACL and a thorough mapping of component distributions at all levels of organization is required in order to even begin to speculate on their functional significance. Fiber mapping, including measurements of axial twisting of fibers, fiber dimensions (both longitudinally and transversely), and fiber interactions will be important. In pericellular and intercellular areas, the roles of the adhesion proteins described in the previous section will likely be very important, both in normal ACLs and in ACL grafts.

A second fundamental area that is still deficient is the better definition of ACL mechanical functions, both *in vitro* and *in vivo,* and the relationships of these functions to ACL structures. Three-dimensional models of the knee are required and account taken of the articular surfaces and menisci. Associated anatomical studies are needed to provide more accurate information concerning model parameters: insertion locations in a three-dimensional sense, tension reference positions of different fiber groups, and variations in mechanical properties between different fiber groups. Three-dimensional models of the joints and entire locomotor apparatus of the leg should be used to define the circumstances leading to injury, the role of the menisci in stabilizing the cruciate-deficient joint, and the definition of optimal methods of rehabilitation. Explanations for viscoelastic behaviors and their significance; understanding actual load, stress, and strain conditions during functionally relevant activities; and improved assessments of functional interfaces (e.g., ligament to bone, ligament to ligament, cell to matrix, etc.) are required as precursors to understanding potential deficiencies of grafts or of scar tissue. Effects of applied stresses to tissue properties must be defined both in normal tissue and healing tissue. The mechanical definition of partial ACL injuries is required, along with

C. B. Frank: McCaig Centre for Joint Injury and Arthritis Research, Department of Surgery, University of Calgary, Calgary, Alberta, Canada T2N 4N1.

measures of potential recovery after such an injury. Better tools for assessing these behaviors are also needed, including better approaches for noninvasive, or at least less invasive, assessments of ACL functions. Relationships between graft loads and joint function (joint kinematics) must be defined.

A third area relating to definition of ACL structure that requires further thought is the mapping of ACL neurovascular structures. The possibility still exists that there are important neurological or vascular elements that have thus far been either missed or perhaps defined incompletely by current methods of staining and identification. Development of alternative methods of examining tissues, therefore, will also be of interest.

A fourth critical area, which is generally perceived to be a major deficiency at the present time, is the need for a clearer understanding of ACL cell biology. Cells need to be characterized phenotypically in various ways—morphologically, biochemically, metabolically, and genetically—in order to understand their potential roles and interactions, both normally and in grafts. This is an essential precursor to defining sources of cells and their potential deficiencies in ACL healing or grafting, and further, is a precursor to attempting to manipulate cell populations to improve healing. Reactions of cells, both *in vitro* and *in vivo*, to exogenous factors can then be defined quantitatively rather than empirically. Factors that may promote cellular ingrowth, specific matrix production, matrix modification, or matrix remodeling, in particular, should be emphasized. Again, interfaces between biology and biomechanics must be understood so that combined forms of treatment have some hope of being optimized. Effects of loading on quantities and qualities of new tissue formation must be understood in the milieu of the joint and the graft matrix. In fact, the mechanisms by which load interfaces with any cell behaviors are of enormous biological importance.

A fifth area relates more specifically to issues of ACL replacement itself. Allograft technology needs to be optimized, as does the technology of prosthetic replacements. The concept of optimized augmentations or replacements holds great excitement, particularly the prospects of biosynthetic (or biodegradable) grafts made of exogenous or "expanded endogenous" (e.g., cultured host tissues) materials that may promote healing, ingrowth, or actual ligament tissue regeneration. Networks for the use of allografts must be established, and such grafts must be better screened for disease (human immunodeficiency virus, hepatitis, etc.) and proven to be sterilized, stored, and handled optimally.

CLINICAL RESEARCH

There are still many fruitful areas of clinical research that should be pursued. Many of these are being pursued, but as far as the authors are aware, some are not.

One area identified was that of neuromuscular con-

trol. Neuromuscular control of knee function and alterations with ACL deficiency can still be defined better. The amount of disability due to neurosensory loss must be defined, and it must be determined whether neurosensory loss ever constitutes the major source of disability. Distinguishing neurosensory from structural loss remains a challenge, and the potential for restoration of neurosensory deficits (if present) must be established. Mechanisms of restoration then need to be optimized in ways that must be defined. Such restoration then needs to be related to therapeutic regimes (e.g., physiotherapy) and studied prospectively in some fashion.

Secondly, it was felt that we are still in need of better ACL outcome assessments. These tools (disease-specific quality of life measures) need to be assessed for reproducibility, reliability, and validity, and used to study populations in various centers.

Third, it was clear that there is relatively little investigation in ACL injury prevention. Although there is some work on modification of sport-specific equipment, these studies need to be extended to many other aspects of injury (surfaces, rules, coaching, training, etc.). There is still a need for further work in prophylactic bracing and its effects, the effects of hamstring quadriceps ratios on prevention, the possible influence of preinjury laxity, and the true implications of relevant anatomical abnormalities (e.g., notch sizes, joint shapes, predisposing laxities, etc.) on ACL injury.

Fourth, it is clear that the factors that lead to osteoarthritis in the ACL-deficient knee require definition. The possibility of iatrogenic osteoarthritis (secondary to inappropriate tensioning of grafts or unnecessary meniscectomies, for example) must be considered. A very important connection may be found in the further definition of the natural history of "bone bruises." Surgical approaches to the prevention of all of these causes of arthritis then will be needed.

Finally, there are still many potential improvements in surgical equipment and surgical approaches that may further refine anatomical and appropriate biological replacement of the ACL. In this area there should be strong input from basic science investigations into factors that may influence ACL healing or graft recoveries over time.

As a final note, there was a consensus that, as advocated by many investigators in other publications, there is a need for more consistency of surgical and rehabilitative techniques, improvements in the standardization of reporting of results (using agreed-upon measurement tools and scales), and less "individual experimentation" with only short-term follow-up. Only through such standardization across centers with long-term follow-up will the true effectiveness of any treatment program be validated for external (i.e., general) use. A particular caution should be extended toward the experimental clinical use of powerful biological tools (e.g., growth factors, etc.) until their safety is proven and there is some indication of their efficacy in basic science studies.

Index

Page numbers in italics refer to figures.